Nelson Yuan-sheng Kiang

Springer
Berlin
Heidelberg
New York
Barcelona
Hong Kong
London
Milan
Paris
Singapore
Tokyo

D. H. W. Grönemeyer
R. B. Lufkin (Eds.)

Open Field Magnetic Resonance Imaging

Equipment, Diagnosis and Interventional Procedures

With a Foreword by A. R. Margulis

With 233 Figures in 399 Separate Parts

Springer

Dr. D. H. W. GRÖNEMEYER
Professor and Chairman
Department of Radiology and Microtherapy
Universitätsstr. 142
D-44799 Bochum
Germany

Professor Robert B. LUFKIN, M. D.
University of California
Department of Radiological Sciences
UCLA School of Medicine
10833 Le Conte Avenue
Los Angeles, California 90095-1721
USA

ISBN 3-540-63781-8 Springer-Verlag Berlin Heidelberg New York Tokyo

Library of Congress Cataloging-in-Publication Data
Open field MRI/[edited by] D. Grönemeyer, R. Lufkin. p. cm. Includes bibliographical references and index. Cover title: Open field magnetic resonance imaging. ISBN 3-540-63781-8 (hardcover: alk. paper). 1. Magnetic resonance imaging. I. Grönemeyer, Dietrich H. W. II. Lufkin, Robert B. III. Title: Open field magnetic resonance imaging. [DNLM: 1. Magnetic Resonance Imaging – methods. 2. Diagnostic Imaging. WN 185 061 1999]. RC78.7.N83064 1999 616.07′548–dc21 DNLM/DLC for Library of Congress 99-25519

Cover-Design: de'blik, 10435 Berlin
Typesetting: K+V Fotosatz GmbH, 64743 Beerfelden
Printing and binding: Universitätsdruckerei H. Stürtz AG, 97017 Würzburg

SPIN 10544543 21/3135-5 4 3 2 1 0 – Printed on acid-free paper

To our families
and
Brian, Francisco, Graham, Larry, Matt, Michael

Foreword

Until the advent of the Access open magnet, introduced by Diasonics in 1988, claustrophobia and the loud hammering noise were considered part of the price patients had to pay for the benefits of this superb imaging approach. The fact that it was possible to obtain images of acceptable diagnostic quality while the patient was resting comfortably in pleasant airy surroundings reminiscent of a four-poster bed was certainly a great advantage.

It became obvious, however, that the open magnet also offered the opportunity for the interventional radiologist or surgeon to perform procedures, as access to the patient was immediate and can be continuous during the scanning. It was also necessary to develop methods for real-time imaging and also vary the spatial resolution, obtaining the best when speed was not essential.

After this instrument showed the potential of revolutionizing both the approach to imaging as well as interventional radiology by eliminating the exposure to ionizing radiation, allowing more complicated interventions to be image guided, several other companies embraced the idea of open magnets. These instruments have started to proliferate and now occupy a significant portion of the market.

This book edited by two leaders in the use of MR in interventional radiology covers the basic physics and engineering principles involved in open magnet imaging, the use of contrast media and the demands on ancillary instrument design with regard to safety, patient monitoring, MR compatibility and avoidance of image distortion. These chapters are written by teams of experts with long experience in the field, some of them among the original initiators.

The chapters on diagnostic studies of the brain, extremities and pediatric applications are similarly authored by leaders in the field.

The most valuable chapters of this book at this particular time, when MR is beginning to be used in image-guided minimally invasive surgery and radiology, are those on interventional procedures covering the entire anatomic spectrum. These chapters too are authored by experts, most of whom have been in the field since it began and have richly contributed to it.

I am convinced that this book will be a worthy precursor to a large body of literature on the subject, as it is becoming obvious that the performance of long, complicated, high-resolution image-guided procedures is coming to involve prohibitively high ionizing radiation doses to them and a less hostile environment is essential. Open magnets provide the solution to many problems presently plaguing image-guided interventions, and the present technical disadvantages and limitations of this technology will be successfully addressed. Software problems presently limiting the acquisition of high-resolution images in real time, in the proper planes and with the right contrast resolution will be solved, as many similar difficulties were overcome in the past. Interest and need are superb motivators.

ALEXANDER R. MARGULIS

Preface

Disease desperate grown
By desperate appliance are relieved
Or not at all.

Hamlet

The most significant and exciting development in recent development in magnetic resonance imaging has been the availability of open design instruments. This is evidenced by the fact that open design MR scanners now outsell closed systems worldwide and represent the fastest growing segment of the MRI industry.

Open field MR design offers significant advantages for both diagnostic as well as interventional applications of MRI. In the diagnostic area, open field systems allow greater patient comfort, lower scan failure rates due to claustrophobia, the capability to perform studies on larger patients, as well as the possibility to perform studies requiring additional space for the patient (i.e. kinematic studies). In the area of interventional studies, open systems allow unprecedented access to the patient for "hands on" interventional and more involved procedures requiring close monitoring and patient support not possible with current closed MR systems.

While it is possible to perform interventional MR studies in closed systems (and many are) there are significant advantages to performing such cases in open systems. Similarly, diagnostic studies may be and will continue to be performed in closed systems, however, there are a number of advantages in having them performed in an open system. But there is one important limitation in open-field MRI! Because of reduced local tissue discrimination, routine spinal diagnosis must be realized in systems with field strengths higher than 0.5 Tesla. This is why a chapter about spinal diagnosis is missing in this book. We are sure that in the future industry will market open designed high-field systems to solve this problem.

This book is unique in that it addresses both aspects (diagnostic and interventional) of this exciting new world of open MRI. It contains the latest on diagnostic studies in open systems as well as the state of the art in interventional MRI written by an international panel of leading experts in the field.

D.H.W. Grönemeyer
R.B. Lufkin

Contents

List of Contributors

Elliot Abemayor, MD
Department of Head and Neck Surgery, University of California, School of Medicine, 10833 Le Conte Avenue, Los Angeles, CA 90095, USA

S. Anderson, MD
Department of Radiology, University of California, San Francisco, 400 Grandview Drive, South San Francisco, CA 94080, USA

Yoshimi Anzai, MD
Radiology Services, Department of Radiology, University of Michigan Hospital, Ann Arbor, MI 48109, USA

Mitsuaki Arakawa, B.S.
Radiologic Imaging Laboratory, University of California, San Francisco, 400 Grandview Drive, South San Francisco, CA 94080, USA

Keith L. Black, MD
Cedars-Sinai Medical Center, 8635 West 3rd Street, no. 490, West Tower, Los Angeles, CA 90048, USA

Keith Blackwell, MD
Department of Head and Neck Surgery, School of Medicine, University of California, 10833 Le Conte Avenue, Los Angeles, CA 90095, USA

Ines Boechat, MD
Department of Radiological Sciences, School of Medicine, University of California, Los Angeles, 10833 Le Conte Avenue, Los Angeles CA 90095-1721, USA

Axel Bornstedt, MD
Deutsches Herzzentrum Berlin, Augustenburger Platz 1, 13353 Berlin, Germany

Alexandra Borges, MD
Department of Radiological Sciences, University of California, Los Angeles, 10833 Le Conte Avenue, Los Angeles, CA 90095-1721, USA

Bruce Breneman, MD
Applied Superconetics, Inc., 8980 Crestmar Pt., San Diego, CA 92121, USA

Martin Busch, PhD
Department of Radiology and Microtherapy, University Witten/Herdecke, Universitätsstr. 142, 44799 Bochum, Germany

Joseph Carlson, MD
Radiologic Imaging Lab, 400 Grandview Drive, South San Francisco, CA 94080, USA

Dan Castro, MD
Department of Head and Neck Surgery, School of Medicine, University of California, Los Angeles, 10833 Le Conte Avenue, Los Angeles, CA 90095-1721, USA

Lawrence E. Crooks, PhD
5439 Sacramento Avenue, Richmond, CA 94804, USA

John Curran, MD
Department of Radiological Sciences, University of California, Los Angeles, 10833 Le Conte Avenue, Los Angeles, CA 90095-1721, USA

Martin Deli, Dipl. Ing.
Department of Radiology and Microtherapy, University Witten/Herdecke, Institute of Microtherapy, Universitätsstr. 142, 44799 Bochum, Germany

Antonio DeSalles, PhD
Department of Neurosurgery, School of Medicine, University of California, Los Angeles, 10833 Le Conte Ave., Los Angeles, CA 90095-1721, USA

Elisabeth Dion, MD
Department of Radiology M-392, University of California, San Francisco, 505 Parnassus Avenue, San Francisco, CA 94143-0628, USA

Jay S. Dworkin, MD
Fonar Corporation, 110 Marcus Drive, Melville, NY 11747-4292, USA

Thomas Frenzel, MD
Schering AG, Forschung Kontrastmittel für Kernspintomographie, Müllerstr. 178, 13342 Berlin, Germany

Harry K. Genant, MD
Department of Radiology, University of California, San Francisco, 521 Parnassus Avenue, Box 0628, San Francisco, CA 94143, USA

Arthour Gevargez, MD
Department of Radiology and Microtherapy,
University Witten/Herdecke, Institute of Microtherapy,
Universitätsstr. 142, 44799 Bochum, Germany

Jonathan Goldin, MD
Department of Radiological Sciences, School of Medicine,
University of California, Los Angeles, 10833 Le Conte Avenue,
Los Angeles, CA 90095-1721, USA

D.H.W. Grönemeyer, MD
Department of Radiology and Microtherapy,
Institute of Microtherapy, University Witten/Herdecke and
Research and Development Center of Microtherapy Bochum,
Universitätsstr. 142, 44799 Bochum, Germany

Theodore Hall, MD
Department of Radiological Sciences, School of Medicine,
University of California, Los Angeles, 10833 Le Conte Avenue,
Los Angeles, CA 90095-1721, USA

Margaret A. Hall-Craggs, MD
Middlesex Hospital, UCL Hospital Trust, Mortimer Street,
London, W1N 8AA, UK

Yen-Hwa Hsu, MD
Applied Superconetics, Inc., 8980 Crestmar Pt, San Diego,
CA 92121, USA,

Nola M. Hylton, MD,
University of California, San Francisco, San Francisco, CA
94143, USA

Ferenc Jolesz, MD
Department of Radiology, Harvard Medical School,
Division of MRI and Image Guided Therapy,
Brigham and Women's Hospital, 75 Francis Street,
Boston, MA 02115, USA

Leon Kaufmann, PhD
University of California, San Francisco, Radiologic Imaging
Laboratory, 400 Grandview Drive,
South San Francisco, CA 94080, USA

Ron Kikinis, MD
Surgical Planning Laboratory, Department of Radiology,
Brigham and Women's Hospital, 75 Francis Street, Boston,
MA 02115, USA

Susanne Kossler, MD
Heiligendammer Str. 36, 14199 Berlin, Germany

David M. Kramer, PhD
P.O. Box 6864, San Rafael, CA 94903-0864, USA

Andrew Li, MD
Toshiba America, MRI, South San Francisco, CA, USA

R. B. Lufkin, MD
Department of Radiological Sciences, School of Medicine,
University of California, Los Angeles, 10833 Le Conte Avenue,
Los Angeles, CA 90095-1721, USA

David S.K. Lu, MD
Department of Radiological Sciences, School of Medicine,
University of California, Los Angeles, 10833 Le Conte Avenue,
Los Angeles, CA 90095-1721, USA

M. Mack, MD
Zentrum für Radiologie, Universitätsklinikum Frankfurt,
Theodor-Stern-Kai 7, 60590, Frankfurt, Germany

K. Matsutani, MD
Applied Superconetics, Inc., 8980 Crestmar Pt.,
San Diego, CA 92121, USA

A. Melzer, MD
Department of Radiology and Microtherapy,
Mülheim Radiology Institute, University of Witten/Herdecke,
Schulstrasse 10, 45468 Mülheim/Ruhr, Germany

H. Mumtaz, MD
Middlesex Hospital, UCL Hospital Trust, Mortimer Street,
London W1N 8AA, UK

William W. Orrison, Jr., MD
Department of Radiology, School of Medicine,
1A71 Medical Center, Salt Lake City, UT 84132, USA

Thomas Oshiro, PhD
Department of Radiological Sciences, University of California,
Los Angeles, 10833 Le Conte Avenue, Los Angeles,
CA 90095-1721, USA

C.G. Peterfy, MD
Department of Radiology, M-392, 505 Parnassus Avenue,
San Francisco, CA 94143-0628, USA

Johannes Platzek, MD
Grottkauer Str. 55, 12621 Berlin, Germany

Bernd Radüchel, MD
Gollanczstr. 132, 13465 Berlin, Germany

Gregory Rubino, MD
Department of Neurosurgery, University of California,
Los Angeles, 10833 Le Conte Avenue, Los Angeles,
CA 90095, USA

Joel Sercarz, MD
Department of Head and Neck Surgery, School of Medicine,
University of California, Los Angeles, 10833 Le Conte Avenue,
Los Angeles, CA 90095, USA

Rainer Seibel, MD
Department of Radiology and Microtherapy,
Mülheim Radiology Institute, University of Witten/Herdecke,
Alfred-Herrhausen-Str. 50, 58448 Witten, Germany

F.G. Shellock, PhD
7511 McConnell Avenue, Los Angeles, CA 90045-1037, USA

Stuart G. Silverman, MD
Division of MRI and Image Guided Therapy,
Brigham and Women's Hospital, 75 Francis Street, Boston,
MA 02115, USA

Shantanu Sinha, PhD
Department of Radiological Sciences, University of California,
Los Angeles, 10833 Le Conte Avenue,
Los Angeles, CA 90095-1721, USA

Usha Sinha, PhD
Department of Radiological Sciences, University of California,
Los Angeles, 10833 Le Conte Avenue, Los Angeles,
CA 90095-1721, USA

V. Tronnier, MD
Bleichwiesenweg 4, 69245 Bammental, Germany

Pablo Villablanca, MD
Department of Radiological Sciences, University of California,
Los Angeles, 10833 Le Conte Avenue,
Los Angeles, CA 90095-1721, USA

Thomas Vogl, MD
Zentrum für Radiologie, Universitätsklinikum Frankfurt,
Theodor-Stern-Kai 7, 60590 Frankfurt, Germany

Hans-Joachim Weinmann, MD
Schering AG, Forschung Kontrastmittel für
Kernspintomographie, Müllerstr. 178, 13342 Berlin, Germany

Michael Wendt, PhD
Case Western Reserve University, Department of Radiology,
Bolwell B124, 11100 Euclid Avenue, Cleveland, OH 44106, USA

Sjirk Westra, MD
Department of Radiological Sciences, University of California,
Los Angeles, 10833 Le Conte Avenue, Los Angeles, CA 90095-
1721, USA

M.L. Williams, PhD
Radionics Corp., 22 Terry Avenue, Burlington, MA 01803, USA

Leping Zha, MD
Toshiba America MRI, 400 Grandview Drive, South San
Francisco, CA 94080, USA

Basic Principles A

Basic Physics

1

L. Crooks · L. Kaufman · N. Hylton

■ Introduction

In MRI the intensity assigned to each pixel in the image is a measurement of the amount of signal generated from a small voxel (volume element) in the body. (Strictly, for the imaging methods usually used, it is impossible to generate images that do not contain information from neighboring pixels [4].) The magnitude of the signal is determined by properties of the tissue contained within the voxel, namely the number of nuclei in the element of interest (usually hydrogen), the T1 and T2 relaxation parameters that characterize how the nuclei respond to magnetic fields, chemical shift, diffusion, and motion. For flowing blood the phase of the signal is also important. Phase measures the direction of the voxel's nuclei. This depends mainly on field gradients and velocity.

Nuclear magnetic resonance is the phenomenon that generates the signal for imaging [1, 7]. It is caused by the interactions between the nuclei of the atoms within the tissue and an external magnetic field. Two properties of the nucleus contribute to the effect: the fact that its subparticles, protons and neutrons, contain charge, and that they have a spinning motion. (Although neutrons have a net charge of zero, they consist of charged matter that is distributed unevenly along the radial direction.) A charged particle in motion produces a magnetic field. The spinning and internal orbital motions of the nuclear particles cause them to generate a magnetic field. For the simplest cases (the spin of the proton in the hydrogen nucleus, for instance) this field is referred to as a *magnetic dipole*, and the particles are said to possess a magnetic dipole moment, μ. When a nucleus is

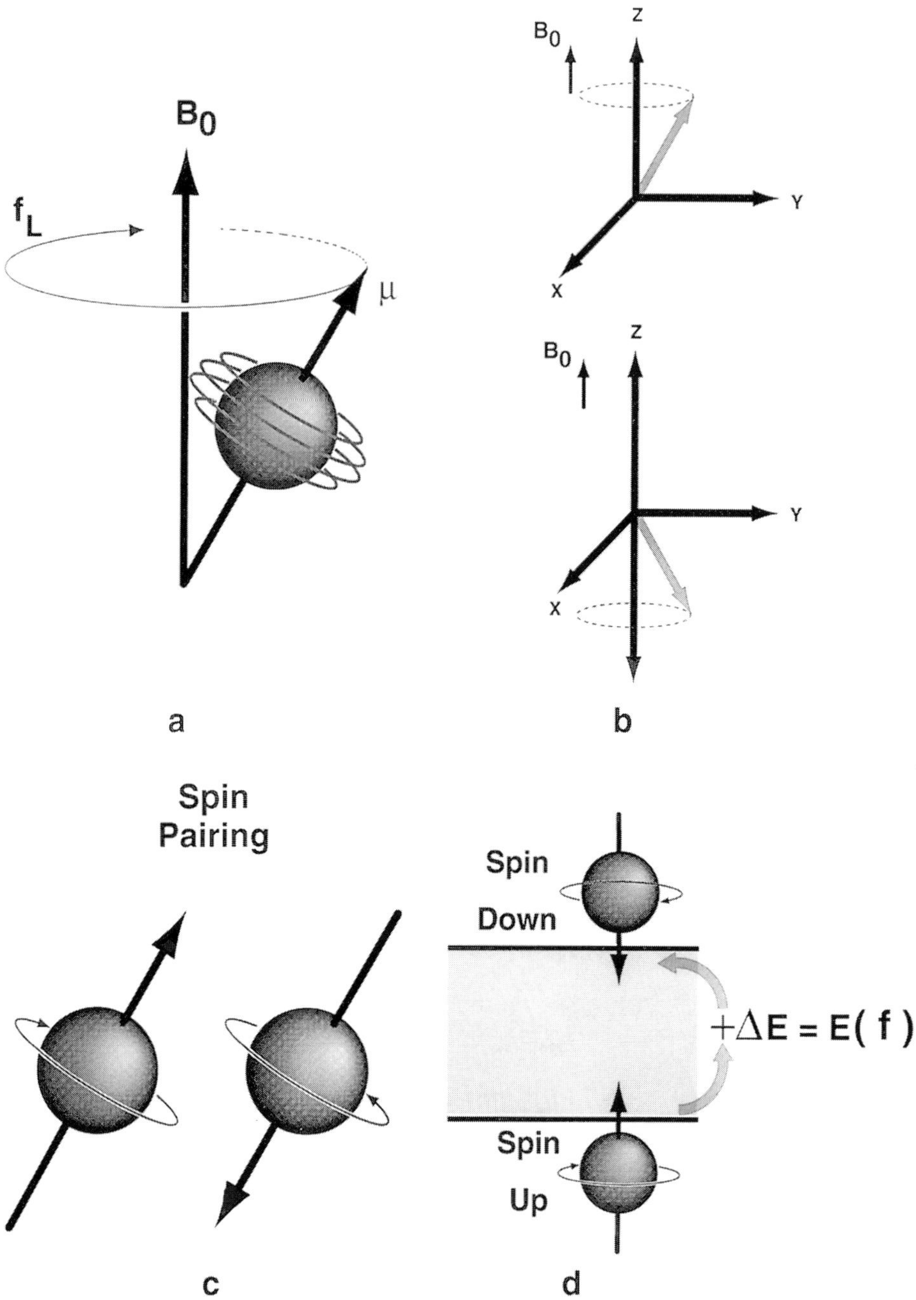

Fig. 1. a A magnetic dipole, μ, in magnetic field, B_0, precesses about the direction of B_0 at the Larmor frequency, f_L. **b** The two allowed orientations for a spin in a magnetic field. When the spin is aligned along the direction of B_0, it is in the lower energy, spin-up state. When aligned opposite the direction of B_0, it is in the higher energy or spin-down state. **c** Each pair of spins orient themselves in opposite directions, an energy-lowering process known as pairing. **d** A transition from the spin-up to the spin-down state requires the addition of an amount of energy exactly equal to the difference between the two energy states. This energy difference depends on the precession frequency of the spins, f_L. Electromagnetic energy must be at frequency f_L of the system to provide photons of this amount

placed in a magnetic field, B_0, the magnetic dipoles behave similarly to a bar magnet in the earth's magnetic field by tending to align with the field. Unlike the bar magnet which points in the direction of the field, because the charges are spinning, the magnetic dipole precesses as a top about the direction of B_0 (Fig. 1a). Every different nuclear specie precess with a unique frequency, called the Larmor frequency. The *Larmor frequency* depends on the strength of the field B_0

and a constant for the nuclei called the magnetogyric ratio, γ. The relationship between Larmor frequency, f_L, and magnetic field strength, B_0, is given by Eq. 1:

$$f_L = \gamma\, B_0 \quad (1)$$

The angular momentum of a particle can be positive or negative depending on the two directions of rotation called spin up (aligned with B_0) and spin down (aligned opposite B_0; Fig. 1b). Each proton and neutron contributes its angular momentum to the total angular momentum of the nucleus. Systems of particles orient themselves so as to lower the overall energy state of the system. In the nucleus this is done by pairing, in which every pair of like particles occupy opposing spin directions thus canceling each other's angular momentum and magnetic dipole contributions (Fig. 1c). It follows that if the nucleus has an even number of protons and an even number of neutrons, the net angular momentum and net magnetic dipole moment of the nucleus is zero. Only nuclei with a nonzero angular momentum and dipole moment can undergo nuclear magnetic resonance. The magnetic dipole of the nucleus is not free to assume any orientation with respect to the direction of the field B_0. It is restricted to occupy orientations that have certain exact energy levels. This implies that to change from one orientation to another energy must be absorbed or released in an amount exactly equal to the difference between the two energy states (Fig. 1d). The magnetic component of an oscillating electromagnetic field can be used to transfer energy to the magnetic dipole. To be exactly equal to the difference between the two energy states the electromagnetic field must be oscillating at the Larmor frequency of the nucleus. This is the phenomenon of *nuclear magnetic resonance*. If energy is added at a frequency other than the Larmor frequency, transitions, and resonance, do not occur.

A group of nuclei in a field B_0 at a given temperature form a natural distribution among their allowed orientations defined by the Boltzmann equation:

$$N_+/N_- = e^{(-E/kT)} \quad (2)$$

where N_+ and N_- are the relative numbers of spins in two allowed orientations, E is the energy difference between the two states, T is the absolute temperature, and k is Boltzmann's constant. If energy is added at the Larmor frequency using an oscillating field B_1, transitions to the higher energy states are made, and the distribution of energy states of the spins is shifted away from equilibrium. When B_1 is removed, nuclei return to the lower state by releasing energy, and equilibrium is reestablished. The released energy is transferred to the molecular lattice structure in which the nuclei are embedded and detected as a current oscillating at the Larmor frequency induced in a surrounding receiver coil.

The simplest nucleus is that of the hydrogen atom. Hydrogen is the most commonly used nucleus for MRI because of its great abundance in water-containing soft tissue. It also generates the largest amount of nuclear magnetic resonance signal of all the stable elements. The hydrogen nucleus consists of a single proton, and therefore the nucleus has a net angular momentum equal to that of the proton. The two spin states of the nucleus generate two allowable energy states in the magnetic field, one aligned with the field, the lower energy or parallel state, and one against the field, the higher energy or antiparallel state. Energy must be added at the Larmor frequency for hydrogen in order for resonance to occur. For a fixed field strength of 1 T, for example, and hydrogen's magnetogyric ratio of 4.258×10^7 Hz/T the Larmor frequency is 42.58 MHz. When a body in a magnetic field of 1 T is irradiated with a B_1 field of 42.58 MHz, only the hydrogen nuclei experience resonance. Because of their different magnetogyric ratios all other nuclei have Larmor frequencies different than 42.58 MHz and are therefore unaffected by the B_1 field.

The B_1 field is generated using an oscillating electromagnetic field at the frequency f_L. The B_1 field must be directed perpendicular to the B_0 field and is turned on to create resonance and turned off to allow the system to return to equilibrium. Because we usually pulse the B_1 field, and since f_L is in the frequency range of radiowaves for typical whole-body imaging, the use of the B_1 field is generally referred to as the radiofrequency *RF pulse* [10, 11]. A common term with MRI is a pulse of 90° (or any angle) to describe RF excitation sufficient in amplitude and duration to cause the net magnetic moment to rotate 90° away from the direction of B_0. A transmitter coil is usually placed in close proximity to the region being imaged and is designed to generate a B_1 field in the direction orthogonal to the main magnetic field.

The receiver coil is oriented along one axis in the plane transverse to the B_1 field. It samples one magnetic component of the spinning nuclei. A second coil can be placed orthogonal to this first coil to sample the complementary component of the nuclei. Phase shifting the second signal by 90° and adding it to the first improves the signal-to-noise ratio (S/N) by $\sqrt{2}$. This is known as quadrature reception.

■ Magnetization Vector in a Rotating Frame of Reference

To facilitate our understanding of what happens in a magnetic resonance experiment it is convenient to use the net magnetic moment vector **M** to represent the vector sum of all of the spins in a single voxel. Consider vector **M** in the frame of reference shown in Fig. 2a. The magnetic field B_0 is directed along the z-axis, also called the longitudinal direction. The plane formed by the x and y axes is called the transverse plane. As we mentioned above, the magnetic moments of individual nuclei precess about the direction of the magnetic field B_0. Because of the random nature of the precession, the sum of all of the magnetic moment vectors in the voxel has no net transverse magnetic moment, only a longitudinal component **M** (Fig. 2a). If energy is added at the Larmor frequency using an oscillating magnetic field B_1 directed in the transverse plane, individual spins absorb energy and make transitions to the upper energy state. The effect on the vector sum **M** is for it to begin to move away

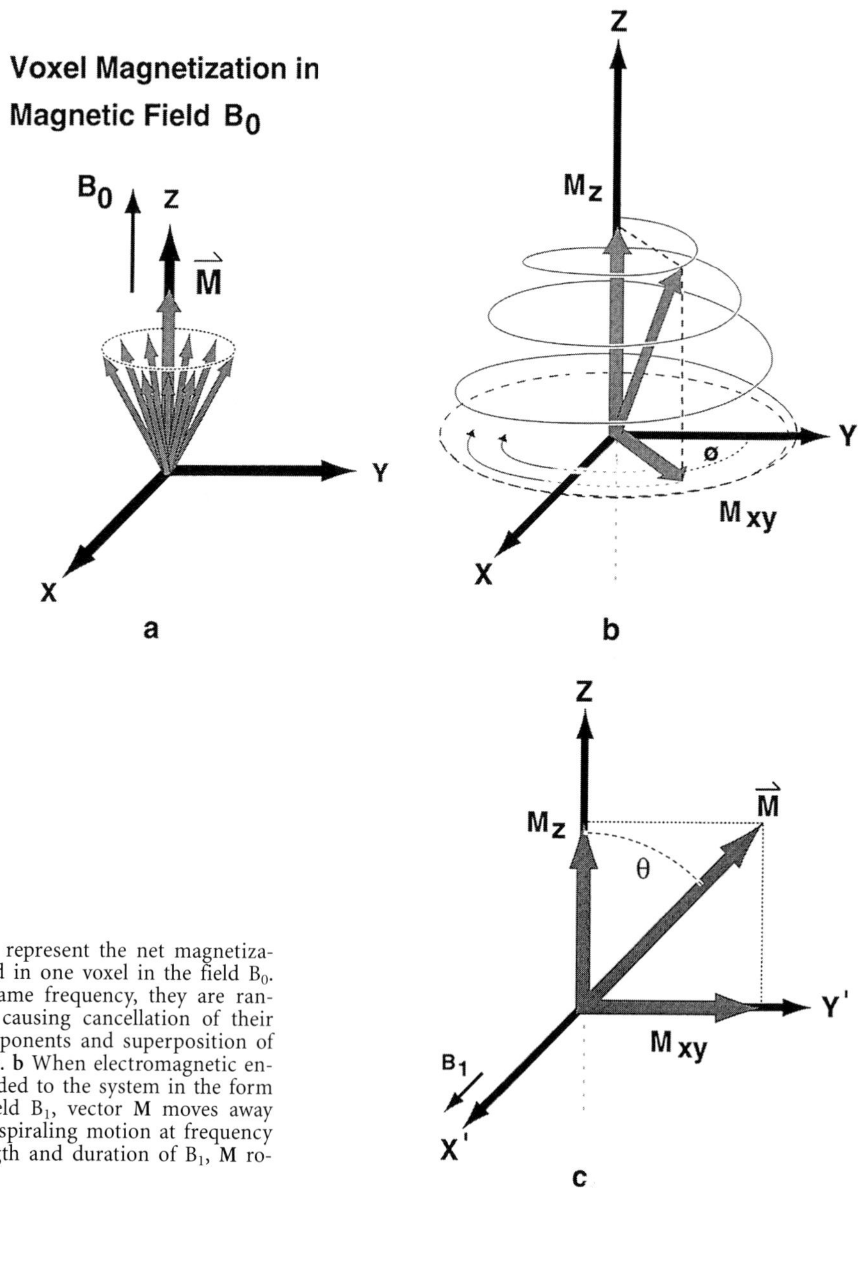

Fig. 2. a Vector **M** is used to represent the net magnetization of all the spins contained in one voxel in the field B_0. While all precessing at the same frequency, they are randomly distributed about B_0, causing cancellation of their transverse magnetization components and superposition of their longitudinal components. **b** When electromagnetic energy at the frequency f_L is added to the system in the form of an oscillating magnetic field B_1, vector **M** moves away from the direction of B_0 in a spiraling motion at frequency f_L. **c** Depending on the strength and duration of B_1, **M** rotates through an angle of $\theta°$

from the z-axis towards the transverse plane while precessing about z. This spiraling motion (shown in Fig. 2b) continues as long as B_1 remains on. As **M** begins to move away from the z-axis, a component in the transverse plane appears. **M** can be represented by its two components M_z and M_{xy} as shown. We refer to the M_z component as the longitudinal magnetization and M_{xy} as the transverse magnetization. Because of the precessing motion of M, the transverse component M_{xy} rotates in the xy plane. The angle that M_{xy} makes with the y-axis (or any arbitrary fixed direction in the plane) changes with time and is called the *phase angle* θ. While the size of the vector M_{xy} ultimately determines the intensity of the pixel, the direction described by the phase angle is also important. The phase angle is shown in Fig. 2b.

Depending on the strength and duration of the B_1 pulse, **M** rotates through an angle θ away from the z axis known as the *flip angle* shown in Fig. 2c. After the pulse, spin lattice relaxation allows the system to return to its equilibrium state (**M** aligned along positive z). While this happens, magnetic oscillations due to spin rotation at f_L induce current in the receiver coil generating the MR signal. The receiver coil is sensitive only to the transverse component of vector **M**. As the system relaxes and **M** realigns with the z direction, the transverse component decreases in size and eventually dies out. The signal is known as the *free induction decay* (FID), and it decays over time.

■ Relaxation Parameters

The processes by which the signal decays and longitudinal magnetization is restored after RF excitation are characterized by two relaxation parameters. Both are exponential in nature. The high intrinsic contrast obtained with MRI arises mostly from its sensitivity to these relaxation parameters, T1 and T2 [6, 23]. Differences in T1 and T2 between neighboring tissues give rise to signal differences and may provide discrimination when some diseases are present [6, 8].

T1 Relaxation

Spin-lattice, or T1 relaxation, is the process by which equilibrium is reestablished after the absorption of RF energy. Following absorption, energy can be released to the surrounding molecular structure or lattice. In the same way that RF energy is absorbed by a spin if the frequency matches its Larmor frequency, energy can be transferred from the spin to a neighboring process that is also oscillating at the Larmor frequency. As this happens, the excited spin system returns to its equilibrium distribution at a rate characterized by the relaxation constant T1. The molecular makeup of different tissues give them characteristic values of T1. T1 also depends on the frequency of the applied external field and is known to increase with frequency (i.e., magnetic field), typical T1 values ranging from 100 to 1500 ms [21].

T2 Relaxation

A second process called *spin-spin*, or T2 *relaxation*, reduces the measurable transverse magnetization. To discuss T2 and the idea of dephasing in general we need to remember that the magnetization **M** is really the vector total of the magnetic moments of many individual nuclei. In a perfectly homogeneous magnetic field all of the nuclei precess at exactly the same frequency. They remain coherent, or in phase, meaning that as they rotate they always have the same phase angle. If, however, slight variations exist in the strength of the field from location to location, there also exist slight variations in the frequencies at which individual nuclei are precessing. If this happens, faster precessing nuclei begin to get ahead of slower nuclei, causing phase differences to appear (Fig. 3a). As the phase dispersion increases, cancellation of individual spin magnetic moment vectors causes a decrease in the net value M_{xy}, decreasing the signal detected by the receiver coil. When the nuclei are uniformly dispersed over 360°, no signal is measurable.

There are several sources of this loss of phase coherence. The first is the intrinsic, irreversible process of T2 relaxation. Individual spins, being magnetic entities, themselves make small contributions to the total magnetic field. Each spin experiences the main static magnetic field plus small contributions from each of the spins around it. Since the configuration is slightly different from the vantage of each spin, the total magnetic field felt by a spin is slightly different from that of its neighbor. This creates a variation in field values over the voxel causing the value of **M** to decay over time at a rate described by the exponential constant T2. For hydrogen in tissues the rate of T2 decay is much faster than the rate at which longitudinal magnetization recovers as characterized by T1. In other words, after RF excitation and the rotation of the net magnetization **M** into the transverse plane, signal in the receiver coil dies out as transverse magnetization dephases. However, although no longer measurable, trans-

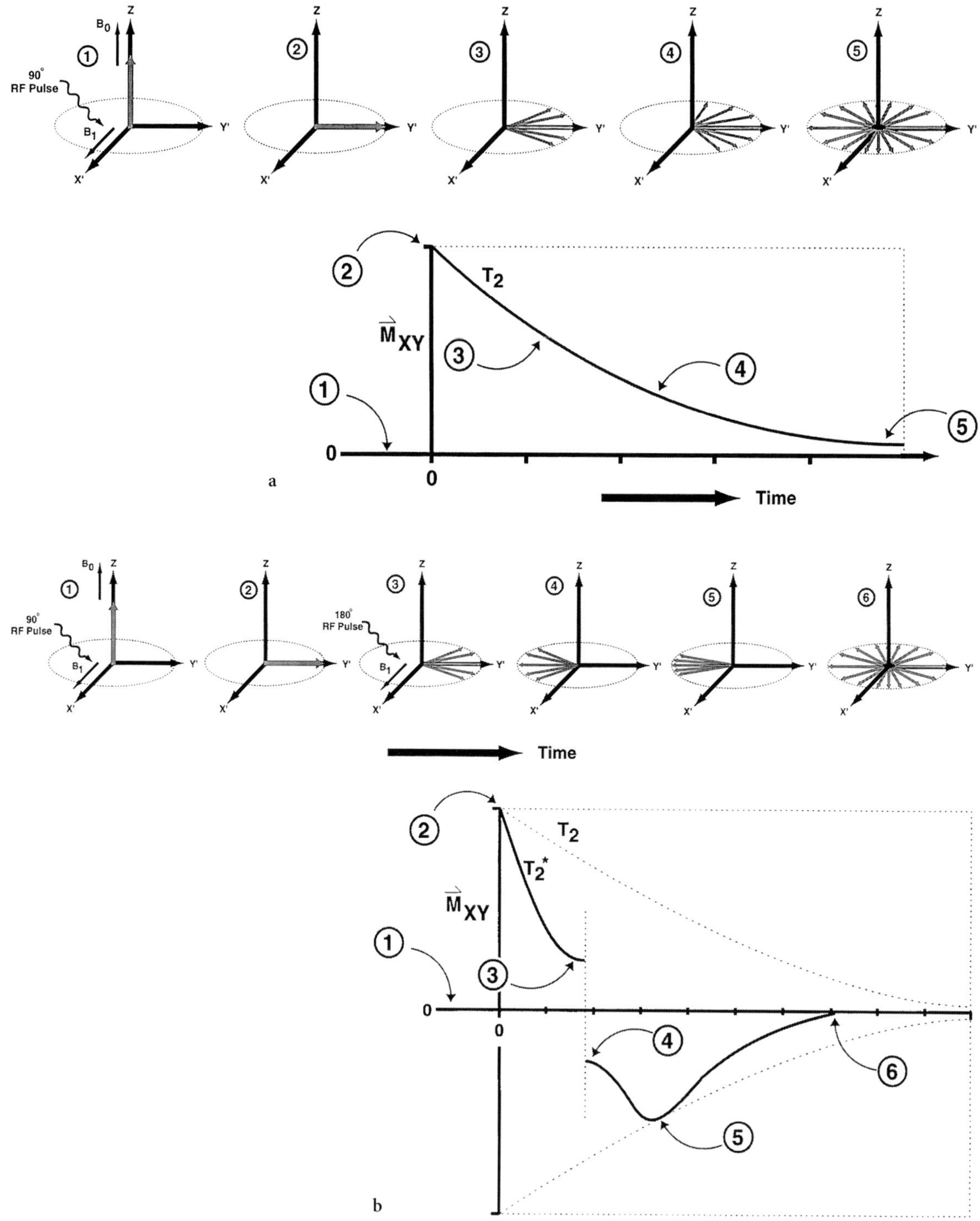

Fig. 3. a After B_1 excitation the free induction decay signal is measured in the receiver coil. The signal decays according to the relaxation constant T2 as spin dephasing occurs. **b** Field inhomogeneity causes additional dephasing and results in signal decay at a faster rate given by T2*. The effect of inhomogeneity can be overcome using a 180° refocusing pulse to reverse the spin system and refocus the spins. This is known as a spin-echo technique

verse magnetization still exists. The T1 relaxation process by which energy is transferred away from the spin system to the lattice and longitudinal magnetization is restored is still occurring.

Typical T2 values for soft tissue in the human body range from 20 to 100 ms and decrease with increasing field strength [5]. Differences in the T1 and T2 values among body tissues is largely responsible for the contrast in MR images [16].

Other phenomena that can cause dephasing and signal loss are field inhomogeneity and magnetic field gradients. These are reversible to some extent and can be corrected. Added to spin-spin relaxation, these effects cause the FID to decay at a rate faster than that given by T2. The constant T2* is often used to describe the rate of decay due to the collective dephasing effects.

Inhomogeneities in the main magnetic field contribute frequency variations within a voxel in the same manner as described above. A spin located in a slightly higher field develops a phase lead over a slower moving spin, as described in Fig. 3b. By using a 180° RF pulse about the x-axis, the system of spins can be reflected about that axis as shown. The precession direction is still the same, but the faster moving spin is now situated behind the slower moving spin. In a time equal to that required to develop the phase lead, the faster spin catches up with the slower spin. A regrowth of the signal occurs as the spins rephase, creating a signal echo. This is known as a *spin-echo* technique [15]. Because of the dynamic nature of the T2 dephasing process it is not reversible as is the dephasing caused by field inhomogeneity. The peak of the echo created by the refocusing pulse still reflects T2 decay.

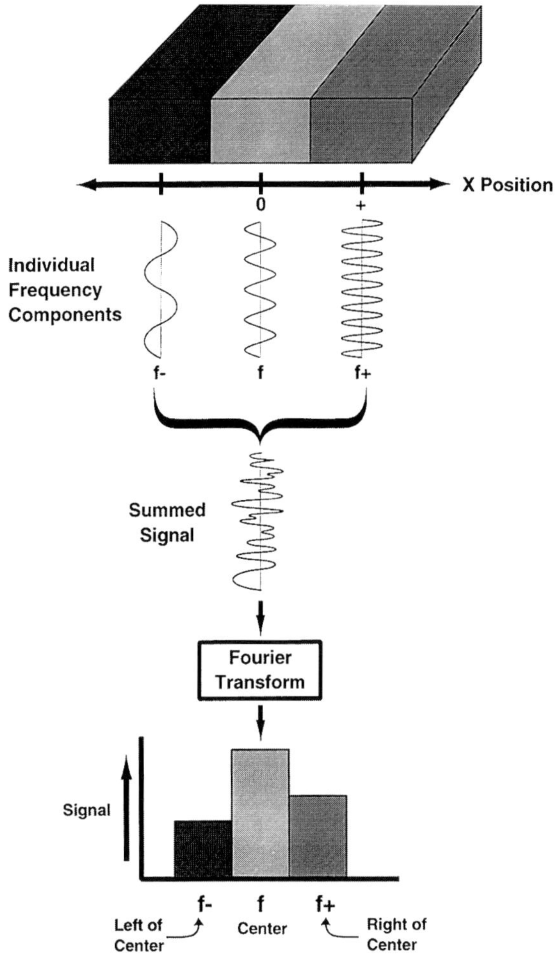

Fig. 4. In Fourier imaging the collective FID from spins with different Larmor frequencies is measured and processed by a Fourier transform to regain the individual frequency components of the input signal. By using magnetic field gradients to spatially vary the main field frequency can be interpreted to give the location of the signal

■ Fourier Transform and Data Collection

The basic magnetic resonance experiment consists of placing a sample in a magnetic field. A transmitting coil excites the spin system with an RF pulse causing the net magnetization vector to rotate into the transverse plane. When the pulse ceases, the spin system begins to return to equilibrium. The receiver coil is turned on and measures the FID. One way to create an image would be to repeat this process at every location within the object. This is impractical for many reasons, particularly because of the excessive amount of time it would take to complete an image with for example, 256×256 elements. The process is expedited by taking advantage of a mathematical tool known as the *Fourier transform* [2]. The principle behind the Fourier transform is that any signal can be represented as a sum of sine and cosine waves of many frequencies and can be decomposed into its individual frequency components.

In the case of MRI, if several voxels were placed in different field strengths and excited simultaneously, they would each generate an FID at a different Larmor frequency (Fig. 4). The signal measured by the receiver coil is the sum of these signals. This signal is processed by Fourier transform and yields the distribution and content of the frequencies from each of the contributing voxels. Furthermore, once we have the frequencies we can deduce the value of the field at each voxel due to the one-to-one relationship between frequency and field strength given in Eq. 1. If the spatial pattern of the field is known, the location of the voxel is known to within the precision that the Fourier transform permits [4]. In this way the signal values can be assigned to the appropriate location in the digital image.

The MR signal is complex valued. This means that we can think of it as having two components that are orthogonal to each other, called the real and imaginary parts of the signal (not much significance should be placed on this nomenclature). Ordinarily it is the display of the magnitude of the signal that shows the soft tissue anatomy. Alternatively, the phase of the signal or the real or imaginary components of the signal can be displayed. Under ideal conditions for tissues with the same magnetic susceptibility values, the phase angle at every position in the image is the same and displaying phase values is uninformative. However, field inhomogeneity, an improperly tuned imaging sequence or disturbances such as flow can result in variations in the phase. Another cause of phase disturbance are differences in the magnetic susceptibilities of different tissue. This is seen particularly at boundaries between air and tissue or between tissue and blood. The phase image is frequently used to detect these occurrences. Phase can also be made to depend on velocity. Alternatively, phase may be measured as a way to quantitate velocity. With the appropriate sequences, phase images can be used to provide chemical shift images, a use demonstrated in the imaging of breast implants, where protons in water, fat, and silicon can be differentiated [9].

In standard MRI data acquisition Fourier transform is an essential step in digital image processing before a recognizable image is obtained. Additional levels of digital signal processing are often used such as smoothing and edge enhancement to improve the appearance of the image. The image data can be manipulated to present a different form of the data, for example, an image composed of the T1 or T2 values at every pixel. There are an inexhaustible number of ways in which the data can be processed to provide different forms for display [18, 25].

■ Spatial Localization

Throughout the development of MRI techniques there have been many methods used for data acquisition and image reconstruction, including the sensitive point and line methods and a number of variants of Fourier imaging. A number of texts provide details about the development and historical significance of each of these [19, 26]. We describe here the two-dimensional Fourier transform method that has become the standard for the majority of commercial systems today. In this method the signal measured by the receiver has spatial information encoded into its frequency and phase. The "raw data" as collected (the FIDs or spin echoes) do not make a recognizable image until it is decoded by two-dimensional Fourier transform. In a typical data acquisition the position along the x direction is encoded into the frequency and position along the y direction into the phase.

Three steps are used to localize points spatially along the three axes in space. In a two-dimensional data acquisition the first of these is the slice selection. Consider the following example of a transaxial slice acquisition. Slice selection is performed by turning on a magnetic field gradient in the slice direction, shown along the z axis in Fig. 5. A linear gradient G_z is used such that with the z gradient on every position along z has a different field value. The RF pulse used for excitation is tailored to contain frequencies corresponding only to the Larmor frequency of spins contained within the slice **z**. Only these spins are affected and experience rotation of their magnetization vectors. This is called *selective excitation*. These spins now have a transverse component to their magnetization and can generate signal.

Once a slice has been selected, phase encoding is used to provide differentiation along the y direction. It is convenient to first skip to the third axis of spatial localization and discuss frequency encoding. This is performed along the readout direction, shown as x in Fig. 6. The readout gradient remains on while the FID is being sampled. Spins at different positions along x generate signals at different frequencies. The combined FID is decomposed by Fourier transformation to give the individual frequency components. These correspond to x position.

Between the time of the RF excitation with slice selection and the time of the signal readout the phase-encoding gradient along the y axis is turned on. This phase encoding gradient is turned on for a short period of time and then removed. Slice excitation and signal readout is repeated for N_{pe} different values of the phase-encoding gradient. During the time that the phase-encoding gradient is on, spins in different rows along the y direction precess at different frequencies. When the phase encoding gradient is turned off, the spins are again in the same field B_0 and all return to the same precession frequency f_L. However, they will have gained or lost a phase angle as a function of the y direction. In subsequent phase encoding cycles this is repeated but at increasing strengths of the phase-encoding gradi-

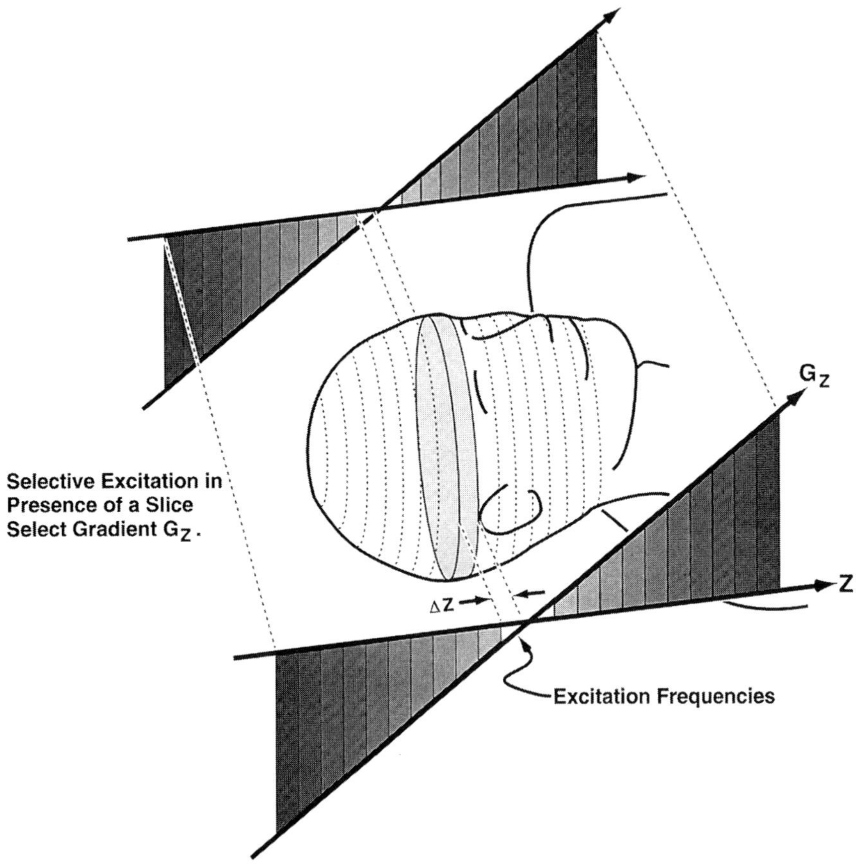

Fig. 5. In this example of a transaxial image acquisition a selected plane of tissue is excited by using RF excitation that contains a narrow bandwidth of frequencies corresponding to a section z along the z direction in the presence of the gradient G_z

ent. Looking along each column, the combined FID is increasingly distorted with each phase-encoding step. The effect on the FID of a changing gradient over N_{pe} steps is the same as the effect of sampling the FID continuously in the presence of a constant gradient, as in the readout direction. Figure 6 demonstrates the effect of three increasing values of the phase-encoding gradient on the FID signal. Fourier transform along the y direction gives the frequency components along y and thus position. The two dimensions of Fourier transform performed in x and y are identical.

The acquired data is in the form of rows of sampled FIDs with increasing phase-encoding gradient values. Because of the unique relationship between position and precession frequency, established by the use of the magnetic field gradients, the acquired data represent the spatial frequency contributions of the image and are therefore often referred to as k space data, where k is the wave number or value of the spatial frequency. In the majority of images encountered when imaging humans and animals with MRI, the largest contributions to the image are made by the low spatial frequencies with decreasing contributions at higher k values. The highest k values contribute details such as edges and features of small dimension.

The three gradients of the magnet can be used interchangeably to perform slice selection, phase encoding or signal readout. This allows images of any orientation (transaxial, sagittal, coronal or oblique) to be defined.

An alternative to collecting slice images is three-dimensional data acquisition. A thick slab is excited rather than individual slices, and an additional dimension of phase encoding is used to spatially localize planes within the slab. There is an increase in imaging time proportional to the number of phase encoding steps used in the slice dimension with a concurrent improvement in S/N, which depends on the square root of the number of slices. To compensate for the increased imaging time, very short TR values are usually used in three-dimensional acquisitions. This in turn lowers S/N, so that whether this parameter is improved de-

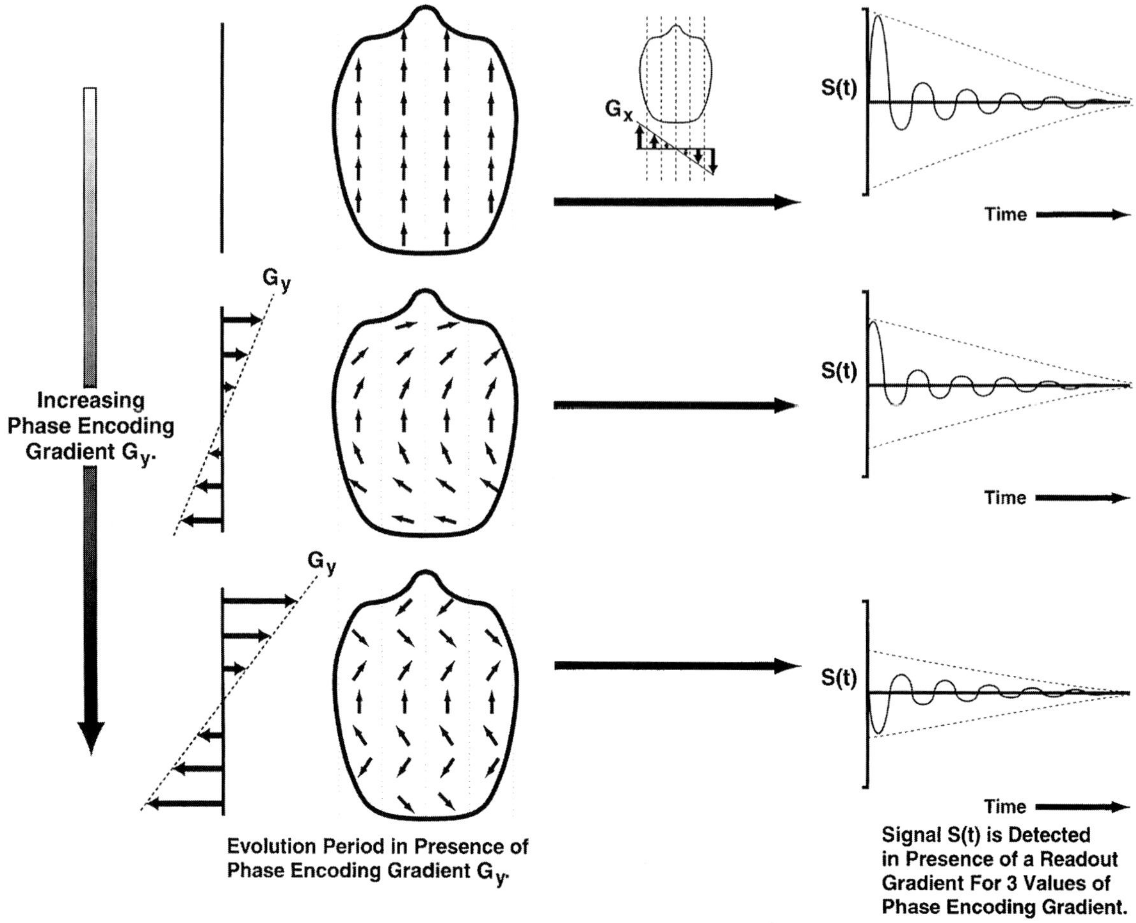

Fig. 6. Increasing values of the phase-encoding gradient cause increasing distortions of the signal that is read out in the presence of an x gradient

pends on the tissues being imaged and the particulars of the imaging sequence [22].

■ Imaging Parameters

Relaxation Time Dependences

There are many adjustable parameters of an MRI procedure that can have an effect on image appearance. Three important parameters are the *pulse repetition interval* (TR), the *echo delay time* (TE), and the *flip angle* (θ). TR is the time between successive RF excitations of a given slice. The intrinsic T1 value of the tissue determines the rate at which longitudinal magnetization recovers. By choosing TR appropriately one can control whether a portion or all of that magnetization is allowed to recover. A long TR means a higher signal level but also lengthens the total imaging time. Since in most cases a heterogeneous group of tissues with a range of T1 values are imaged simultaneously, TR must be chosen judiciously to best portray all the tissues of interest, and paying attention to operating field strength [25].

TE is the time delay between the RF excitation and the measurement of the signal. Transverse magnetization created by the RF pulse begins to dephase immediately after the pulse due to T2 and other effects such as field inhomogeneity. A 180° refocusing pulse at time TE/2 creates a spin echo at time TE that is corrected for field inhomogeneity effects. If no spin echo is performed, the rate of signal decay is faster, as characterized by T2*. A short TE measures maximal signal early in the decay while a long TE measures less signal later in the decay.

The flip angle is the angle through which the magnetization vector **M** is rotated away from the longitudinal direction by the RF pulse. A 90° pulse maximizes the transverse component but also requires a long recovery time before the next excitation to fully restore longitudinal magnetization. Since the recovery rate varies for different tissues depending on T1, a single choice of flip angle has a different effect on each tissue. Choice of TR, TE, and flip angle determines image contrast and S/N as well as the total imaging time and the ability to obtain multiple sections in a single experiment.

Image Contrast

Changing the above parameters gives MRI a powerful control over image contrast. Contrast is defined by the expression:

$$C=(I_A-I_B)/I_B \qquad (3)$$

where I_A is the feature signal, and I_B is the background signal. The MR image intensity depends not only on the hydrogen density distribution but on the relaxation characteristics of the nuclei. The intensity dependence in a spin-echo experiment is approximated by the following expression:

$$I=N(H)[1-e^{(-TR/T1)}]e^{(-TE/T2)}\sin\theta/[1-\cos\theta\, e^{(-TR/T1)}] \qquad (4)$$

Since water content in human soft tissue varies by only about 20%, hydrogen density N(H) accounts for only part of the contrast seen with MRI. Certain pathological conditions, such as edema or fluid-containing cysts, have a more marked increase in water content and may be detectable on this basis alone. The contrast is generated by an interplay of N(H), T1 and T2 differences among tissues. The T1 value of a tissue determines the rate at which its longitudinal magnetization M_z recovers after RF excitation, the longer the T1 the slower the recovery. The rate of the signal decay is characterized by the T2 value of the tissue, the longer the T2 the slower the decay. In a conventional spin echo sequence ($\theta=90^\circ$) for equal T1 and T2 the tissue with the highest N(H) has the larger signal. For the same T1 and N(H), the tissue with the longer T2 has the larger signal. For the same T2 and N(H), the tissue with the longest T1 will have the smaller signal.

Typically, when pathology is present N(H), T1 and T2 are all elevated. Then, in this kind of sequence, N(H) and T2 work to raise signal and T1 reduces signal in the pathological tissue. To make it hyperintense it is important to reduce T1 effects by allowing for a sufficiently long TR (TR>2T1), so that N(H) and T2 provided the desired contrast. Such an image is misnamed "T2-weighted"; it is in fact non-T1-weighted. The pathology can be made hypointense by shortening TR so that T1 effects prevail. To maximize hypointensity TE must be shortened as much as possible, but N(H) effects cannot be avoided. Such images, called T1-weighted are in fact closer to non-T2-weighted.

In addition to adjusting TR, the flip angle θ can be used to affect T1-related contrast. In *partial-flip* sequences, by rotating the longitudinal magnetization vector only partway into the transverse plane, less time is required for it to recover. This allows TR to be reduced substantially and lowers the total imaging time. Many sequences combine these features, most notably the FLASH [14] or GRASS [12] sequences. The chosen flip angle depends on the T1 value of the tissue as well as the TR value used. At short TR values (TR<T1) reduced flip angles can reverse the contrast of short TR images (make lesions hyperintense) and increase S/N as well [24]. Although these images are called T2* weighted, in fact, for water-elevating lesions the hyperintensity of the lesion is achieved on the basis of T1 effects. T2* affects contrast significantly only in gradient echo imaging and where there are magnetic susceptibility differences in the tissue (effects caused by blood, iron, calcium and air, for example). Two-dimensional multislice and three-dimensional sequences of this type are commonly used to perform MRA.

Two tissues A, and B, have relative hydrogen density values reflected by M_{0A} and M_{0B}. After a 90° RF excitation T1 relaxation occurs at different rates, $T1_A$ and $T1_B$ for the two tissues. The choice of the repetition time TR determines the relative amounts of magnetization M_{xyA} and M_{xyB} that become transverse magnetization. M_{xyA} and M_{xyB} decay with relaxation rates $T2_A$ and $T2_B$, respectively. Choice of echo delay time TE determines the relative signal intensities I_A and I_B at the time of readout. It is clear from this example that the final intensity difference is affected by both TR and TE as well as the hydrogen density, T1, and T2 values of the tissues.

Many of the procedures used for imaging blood rely on the inflow of spins, which have received no previous RF excitation, into a volume of stationary tissue that is darkened by frequent RF excitation (short TR value). Inflowing blood behaves as if it experiences an infinite TR. This gives a bright signal from blood while suppressing background signal [20, 28] an effect known as flow-related enhancement. In these techniques TR and flip angle must be selected to give sufficient background suppression while allowing enough time for fresh spins to enter the volume.

These are also referred to as time-of-flight (TOF) effects. Using this mechanism, vascular contrast is generated by creating large differences in longitudinal magnetization between stationary tissue and flowing blood.

It has been shown that the magnetization transfer effect [29] can help to improve vascular contrast in TOF MR angiography (MRA) [27]. Using this method, stationary tissue signal is affected by using an off-resonance RF excitation to reduce the longitudinal magnetization of immobile protons contained in macromolecular structures of the stationary tissue. Through chemical exchange of these immobile protons with the mobile water-based protons the reduced magnetization is transferred to the mobile protons. This reduces the detectable signal since signal comes mainly from mobile protons. The result is a further suppression of stationary tissue signal without a similar suppression of flowing blood's signal. This gives greater vascular contrast.

The other mechanism commonly used to generate vascular contrast uses differences in the phase of flowing and stationary spins. This is performed by using magnetic field gradients to introduce velocity-dependent phase changes. Stationary spins (zero velocity) acquire no phase angle. Moving spins acquire a phase angle that is proportional to their velocity.

Resolution, Signal-to-Noise Ratio, and Imaging Time

Resolution and Field of View

Image quality is affected by its resolution, S/N, and imaging time [3, 17]. Of course, contrast must be present, or these other parameters would not permit any differentiation among tissues. The resolution in MRI is measured by the voxel dimensions used for imaging. It is determined by the frequency bandwidth of the RF excitation and reception and by the strength of the magnetic field gradients. Achievable resolution in a whole-body image is on the order of 0.5×0.5×2 mm. Despite increasing capabilities of the hardware there are other limitations to the minimum voxel dimension. As the voxel size decreases, signal strength decreases in proportion to the reduction in the number of nuclei it contains. The S/N becomes a practical limitation. Even with improvements in noise-reduction techniques, thermal motion and diffusion within a voxel may become a more fundamental constraint. Another consideration is the relationship between resolution, the size of the FOV, and the imaging time. For a fixed matrix size and imaging time the FOV is reduced in proportion to the reduction in voxel size. To maintain FOV at the higher resolution additional measurements would be necessary. If these are taken in the phase-encoding direction, the imaging time increases proportionally.

When the object size exceeds the imaging FOV, a condition known as *aliasing* results, whereby signal from tissue outside of the FOV is interpreted to be overlapping with tissue within the FOV. The result is image wraparound. For example, in a head image for which the FOV in the anterior/posterior direction is smaller than the size of the head, signal from thc anterior of the head that is above the FOV appears at the bottom of the image, overlapping the posterior segment of the image. This can be overcome by increasing the FOV either by increasing the number of samples at the same resolution or by decreasing the resolution for the same number of samples in that direction. An alternative is to eliminate outside tissue by selective excitation or presaturation.

Signal-to-Noise Ratio

The S/N is another important contributor to image quality. Parameters of the imaging sequence such as TR, TE, and flip angle all affect the total signal. Reduction in voxel size provides an improvement in resolution but proportionally reduces the number of signal-generating spins while noise remains the same. If more measurements are taken to provide the resolution, the additional measurements bring back some S/N. Another important determinant of signal is the frequency bandwidth of the voxel's spectrum. Distributing the voxel signal over a larger bandwidth reduces S/N by increasing the noise included in the image. Increasing FOV, total bandwidth, and number of elements by the same factor has no impact on S/N because individual voxel bandwidth does not change.

For a fixed imaging sequence the signal intensity is also affected by the operating frequency of the magnet. Signal increases as the square of frequency, ignoring variations in relaxation times. The noise dependence is not as easily quantified. Theory shows that at high frequency noise increases in proportion to frequency while at low frequency it is proportional to the square root of frequency. The dependence of S/N on operating frequency has been reported experimentally to vary to the first power or less. For a well-tuned system the body itself is the greatest noise source because random currents in the body are picked up as noise by the receiver coil.

Imaging Time

To acquire a full data set, excitation and readout are repeated after time TR for each value of the phase-encoding gradient. Repeated measurements at the same value of the phase encoding gradient may also be obtained to improve the S/N using signal averaging:

$$\text{Total time} = \text{TR}\ N_{pe}\ N_{acq} \quad (5)$$

where N_{acq} is the number of repetitions at each phase-encoding step:

$$\text{S/N} \propto \sqrt{N_{acq}} \quad (6)$$

Thus improving S/N by increasing N_{acq} requires a large increase in imaging time.

In general, the acquisition of multiple slices does not affect the imaging time. *Multislicing* is achieved by using the time between the completion of data acquisition and the start of the next excitation at TR to acquire data at additional slice locations. For example, for a double spin echo sequence with TE values of 30 and 60 ms and a TR value of 2000 ms, generously allowing 100 ms to complete data readout, an interval of 1900 ms is available before the next excitation occurs. During this time 19 additional slices can be acquired by moving the slice selection to a new location. In this way multislicing improves the duty cycle of the acquisition without increasing the total imaging time.

■ Imaging Pulse Sequence

All of the necessary components are now in place to talk about the *pulse sequence*. All of the parameters of the imaging technique are specified with the pulse sequence and are often shown schematically in the pulse timing diagram. The number, strength, timing, and waveform of the RF excitations, the duration and strength of the three magnetic field gradients, and the length and sampling rate of the readout period are all se-

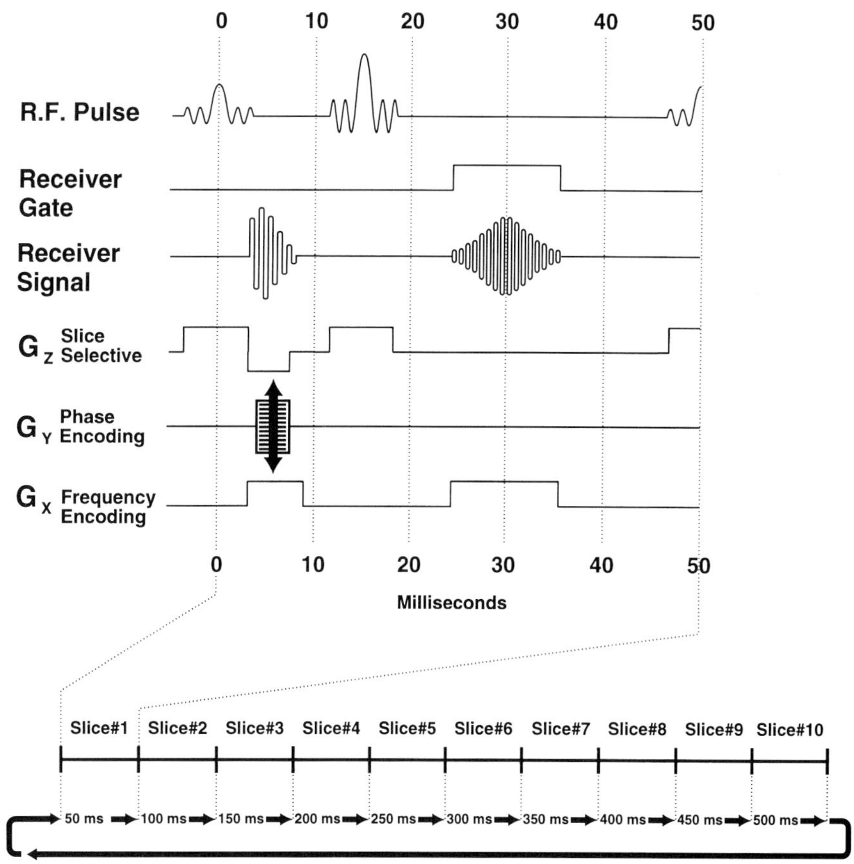

Fig. 7. A pulse timing diagram showing the strengths and timing of transmitted RF excitations, gradients G_x, G_y and G_z, and signal reception for a typical spin-echo data acquisition. In this example data collection is complete in less than 50 ms. This allows excitation and data acquisition to be performed at nine other slice locations before the interval between excitations, TR=500 ms elapses for slice number 1

lected to determine the TR, TE, resolution, FOV, S/N, and contrast for the tissues being imaged. A priori knowledge of the T1 and T2 values helps with the selection of these parameters. Figure 7 presents an example of a pulse timing diagram for a spin-echo pulse sequence with TR=500 ms and TE=30 ms. At the start of the experiment at t=0, a 90° RF pulse is transmitted in the presence of a slice selection gradient along the z-axis. After the pulse is completed, the slice-select gradient is reversed to correct the phase dispersion caused by the slice selection. At the same time the phase-encoding gradient is turned on at its first value. The readout gradient (frequency encoding) also appears. This is a dephasing lobe used to dephase the spins so that a full gradient echo can be measured during readout. At time t=15 ms, a 180° RF pulse is transmitted in the presence of the slice-select gradient to create a spin echo. Because the 180° pulse creates a mirror image of the spin system, the slice-select gradient acts in a positive sense prior to the 180° pulse and in a negative sense afterwards. This is also why the dephasing lobe of the readout gradient is in the same direction as during readout. When the 180° pulse is completed, the readout gradient is turned on, and the signal is sampled symmetrically about the echo time t=30 ms. After time TR the experiment is repeated for each new value of the phase-encoding gradient. In practice, because data acquisition is completed in less than 50 ms, the waiting time can be spent acquiring other slices until it is time to return to the first slice at TR=500 ms.

Many special-function pulse sequences have been developed to address specific imaging needs. The spin-echo pulse sequence has been a standard over the years, but it has some drawbacks. The time spent issuing 180° pulses to correct for field inhomogeneities also serves to prolong the TE value. If the 180° pulse is removed and a shorter TE is used, the loss of signal due to field inhomogeneity can be offset to some extent by the reduced T2 decay. Sequences that create the signal echo by dephasing and rephasing the spins using the readout gradient rather than using 180° pulses are referred to as *gradient-reversal* or *gradient-echo* sequences.

Throughout the development of MRI technology, as methods for signal acquisition and noise reduction have improved, it has become possible to maintain more than adequate S/N while increasing resolution, reducing scan times, and improving contrast.

References

1. Abragham A (1961) The principles of nuclear magnetism. Clarendon, Oxford
2. Bracewell RN (1978) The Fourier transform and its applications. McGraw-Hill, New York
3. Bruner P, Ernst RR (1979) Sensitivity and performance time in NMR imaging. J Magn Reson 33:83–106
4. Carlson JC, Crooks LE, Ortendahl DA, Kramer DM, Kaufman L (1988) Signal-to-noise ratio and section thickness in two-dimensional versus three-dimensional Fourier transform MR imaging. Radiology 166:266
5. Chen J-H, Avram HE, Crooks LE, Arakawa M, Kaufman L, Brito AC (1992) In vivo relaxation times and hydrogen density at 0.063–4.85 T in rats with implanted mammary adenocarcinomas. Radiology 184:427–434
6. Crooks LE, Mills CM, Davis PL et al (1982) Visualization of cerebral abnormalities by NMR imaging: the effects of imaging parameters on contrast. Radiology 144:843–852
7. Curry TS, Dowdey JE, Murry RC (1978) Nuclear magnetic resonance. In: Christensen EE, Curry TS, Dowdey JE (eds) Introduction to the physics of diagnostic radiology. Lea and Febiger, Philadelphia
8. Damadian R (1971) Tumor detection by NMR. Science 171:1151–1153
9. Derby KA, Frankel SD, Kaufman L, Kramer DK, Carlson JW, Mineyev MI, Occhipinti KA, Friedenthal R (1993) Differentiation of Silicone Gel from water and fat in MR phase imaging of protons at 0.064 T. Radiology 189:617
10. Farrar TC, Becker ED (1971) Pulse and Fourier transform NMR. Academic, New York
11. Fukushima E, Roeder ED (1981) Experimental pulse NMR: a nuts and bolts approach. Addison-Wesley, Reading
12. Glover GH, Pelc NJ, Shimakawa A (1987) GRASS movie techniques for gated studies. Proceedings of the 1987 topical conference on fast magnetic resonance imaging techniques. Case Western Reserve University, Cleveland, 15 May 1987
13. Grover T, Singer JR (1971) NMR spin-echo flow measurements. J Appl Phys 42:938–940
14. Haase A, Frahm J, Matthaei D, Hanicke W, Merboldt K-D (1986) FLASH imaging. Rapid NMR imaging using low flip-angle pulses. J Magn Reson 67:258–266
15. Hahn EL (1950) Spin echoes. Phys Rev 80:580–594
16. Herfkens R, Davis PL, Crooks LE, Kaufman L, Price DC, Miller TR, Margulis AR, Watts JC, Hoenninger JC, Arakawa M, McRee RW (1981) NMR imaging of the abnormal live rat and correlation with tissue characteristics. Radiology 141:211
17. Hoult DI, Lauterbur PC (1979) The sensitivity of the zeugmatographic experiment involving human subjects. J Magn Reson 34:425–433
18. Kaufman L (1990) MRI without a magnet. Diagn Imaging 12 (11):197
19. Kaufman L, Crooks LE, Margulis AR (eds) (1981) Nuclear magnetic resonance imaging in medicine. Igaku Shoin, New York
20. Kaufman L, Crooks LE, Sheldon PE, Rowan W, Miller T (1982) Evaluation of NMR imaging for detection and quantification of obstructions in vessels. Invest Radiol 17:554–560
21. Koenig SH, Brown RD (1986) Relaxometry of tissue. CRC handbook on NMR in cells. CRC, Boca Raton
22. Kramer DM, Guzman RJ, Carlson JW, Crooks LE, Kaufman L (1989) Physics of thin-section MR imaging at low field strength. Radiology 173:541
23. Mansfield P, Morris PG (1982) NMR imaging in biomedicine. Academic, New York

24. Mills TC, Ortendahl DA, Hylton NM, Crooks LE, Carlson JW, Kaufman L (1987) Partial flip angle MRI. Radiology 162:531
25. Ortendahl DA, Hylton NM, Kaufman L et al (1984) Analytical tools for magnetic resonance imaging. Radiology 153:479–488
26. Partain CL, Patton JA, Kulkarni MV, James AE (eds) (1988) Magnetic resonance imaging, vol II. Saunders, Philadelphia
27. Pike GB, Hu BS, Glover GH, Enzmann DR (1992) Magnetization transfer time-of-flight magnetic resonance angiography. Magn Reson Med 25 (2):372–379
28. von Schulthess GK, Fisher M, Crooks LE, Higgins CB (1985) Gated MR imaging of the heart: intracardiac signals in patients and healthy subjects. Radiology 156:125–132
29. Wolff SD, Balaban RS (1989) Magnetization transfer contrast (MTC) and tissue water proton relaxation in vivo. Magn Reson Med 10 (1):135–144

Field Strength in Magnetic Resonance Imaging: Its Theoretical Basis

2

L. Kaufman · D. M. Kramer

■ Introduction

The design of medical imaging instrumentation involves complex tradeoffs among sometimes dozens of parameters. No imaging instrument ends up with the "best" of all operating characteristics, as maximizing one such characteristic may unacceptably degrade another. In nuclear medicine, one such parameter is detector thickness in a scintillation camera, and the other is hole spacing and length in camera collimators, both of which trade efficiency vs. resolution. Sizing of these parameters settles out to a narrow range, given enough time. In MRI the parameter that has received the most attention is field strength, and after more than a decade of commercial life there is no indication that this parameter is converging. If anything, it is diverging. While half a decade ago the commercially available choice may have been in the range of 0.08–1.5 T (a range of nearly 20), today the choice ranges from 0.02 to 4 T (a factor of 200). While for any one manufacturer factors of 3 were common (0.5–1.5 T), they are now reaching 7.5 (0.2–1.5 T), so that the trend is towards more divergence in this parameter. A single company may offer products that range over a factor of over 20 in field strength (0.064–1.5 T).

Compare this to the range of detector crystal thickness discussed for scintillation cameras, which ranged from 3 to no more than 30 mm, a factor of 10, and which eventually narrowed to 6 to 12 mm, a factor of 2, with most at 10 mm. What has prevented MRI from following the pattern found in other modalities? If field strength is important technically, then the range should be narrow, and the more important and critical it is, the narrower the range should be. The very fact that it is as large as it is implies that diagnostic performance cannot be strongly dependent on field strength. This being the case, we can only speculate as to the nontechnical reasons to keep field strength as an issue. The most important one is undeniably commercial competition, where companies attempt to differentiate products by field strength, or where companies use field strength as a means of obscuring problems or deficiencies in their equipment. The ability of systems of widely different field strengths to be diagnostically successful is the best indication of the relative unimportance of field strength in MR imaging. There are basic reasons for this assertion.

Imaging

An imaging study can be characterized by measurable properties. These are:

- The size of the volume imaged.
- Spatial resolution, the size of the voxels (in-plane spatial resolution x section thickness), which are directly related to the number of sections, the number of pixels imaged per section and the size of the imaged volume.
- The contrast in the image.
- The amount of structured noise in the image, also called artifact, which may blur or obscure the desired information.
- The signal-to-noise level (S/N), which quantifies how smoothly the information and the structured noise are presented.
- The acquisition time. An object cannot be seen if the contrast is not present, no matter how good S/N is. What this latter parameter does is establish the confidence with which a feature is observed. This confidence factor is given by the product of contrast × S/N [1], which is also equal to the signal difference-to-noise.

Spatial Resolution

Spatial resolution is established in MRI by the strength of the switched magnetic field gradients, the interaction among gradient fields and eddy currents and background field inhomogeneities, and by the available RF power.

Field strength does not enter into these considerations except by three indirect means: (a) The background field inhomogeneity. The value of relevance is in gauss, not ppm. The amount of inhomogeneity in gauss is given by the product of field strength × ppm, so that for equal specifications in ppm the lower field magnet has the higher homogeneity. For instance, a comparatively poor 60 ppm inhomogeneity at 0.05 T is equivalent for imaging purposes to a 2 ppm inhomogeneity at 1.5 T. (b) In general, because lower field magnets have lower costs, these may be produced with weaker gradients, simply because there is an incentive to keep costs down. These can limit resolution. (c) For any one type of pulse sequence, the RF power needed goes up as the square of the field strength. Consequently, a weak RF amplifier can perform better at low field than a much higher power RF amplifier can at high field. For instance, a 1.5-T system would require a 67.5 kW amplifier where a 0.1 T system meets the same needs with a 0.3 kW amplifier.

Eddy currents are the other factor that affects spatial resolution. Eddy current control or suppression is field strength-independent. With the proper engineering this is achievable in any system.

Contrast

The contrast, or relative signal differences among different tissues, results from an interaction between tissue parameters and the imaging sequence. The tissue parameters of interest are many. Typically, imaging depends on the hydrogen density [N(H)], the relaxation times T1 and T2, the state of motion of the tissue (including microscopic motion), and for certain sequences, magnetic susceptibility differences among tissues. There are other tissue parameters that can be exploited, but these are the subject of investigative rather than clinical work. The issue of contrast in MR images is broad and could not be fully covered here. Nevertheless, there are frequent and typical cases that can be used to exemplify the subject.

We discuss here three examples of the behavior of contrast at low and high fields. The first example involves the detection of lesions where water content is increased. This is a typical effect seen in tumors, edema and infarcts, considering the case where there is no blood. For these lesions N(H), T1 and T2 are all elevated [2]. In a spin echo sequence the elevation of N(H) and T2 increases signal, while the elevation of T1 decreases signal. Thus N(H) and T2 effects are diluted by T1 effects. To obtain a lesion that is brighter than background it is necessary to increase TR to the point that T1 effects become unimportant. This results in what is misnamed as a "T2-weighted" image. In fact a more accurate term would be "not T1-weighted." To reliably achieve this condition it is necessary to operate with a TR of at least 2T1, preferably 2.5–3 T1. Since T1 increases with field strength, this means that it is necessary to operate with a longer TR at the higher field. For instance, for brain tissue the increase between 0.064 T and 1.5 T is approximately a factor of 4, from 250 ms to about 1 s for white matter, and from 350 ms to 1.4 s for gray matter. Thus for a spin echo sequence the desired lesion contrast is easier to achieve, and is more reliably achieved, at the lower field (Fig. 1). As we see below, this has significant consequences in terms of S/N as well, since shorter TR values can lead to larger number of data averages for fixed imaging time.

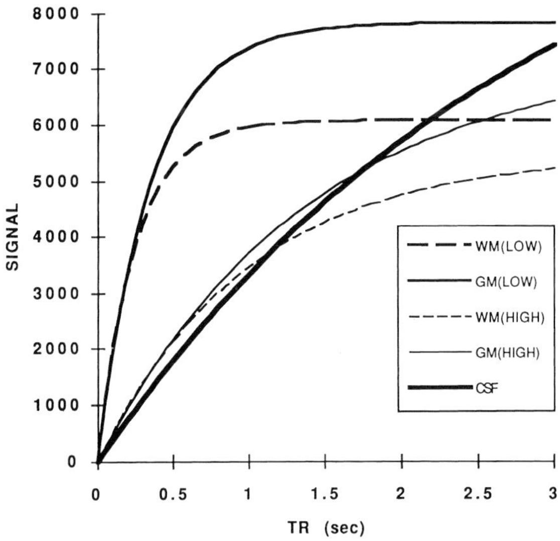

Fig. 1. Signal behavior for gray and white matter and CSF at low and high field. Brain lesions are typically gray matter-like. At low field (*top two curves*), full gray/white differentiation is established at a relatively short TR, and CSF is dark. For high field, reliable differentiation occurs in the same TR range where CSF becomes intense and can mask neighboring lesions. (CSF has a relaxation time that is relatively independent of field strength)

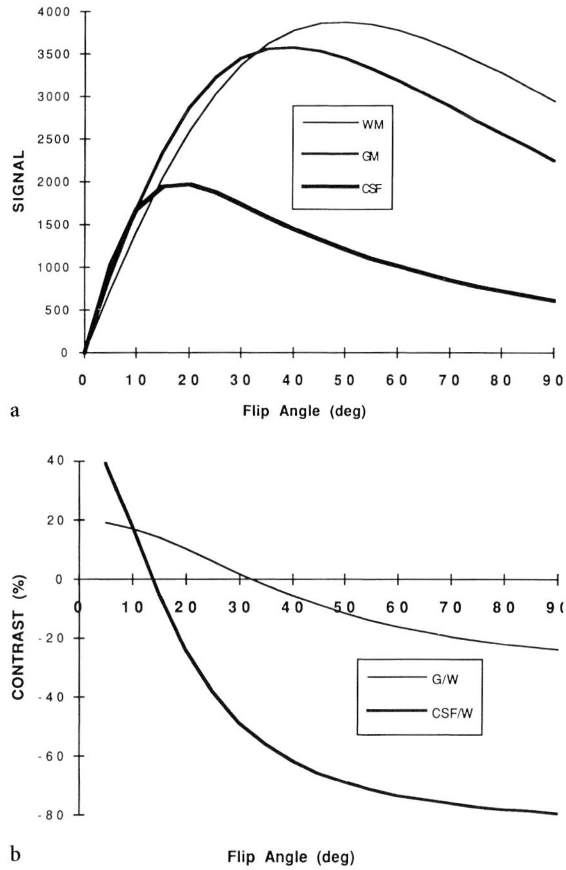

Fig. 2. **A** The ability to reverse contrast by varying flip angle is due to the characteristics of signal behavior for different T1 values. The signal from tissues with longer T1 values peak at smaller angles, and the signal increase in the peak (compared to 90°) is relatively larger. Consequently, relative signal intensities can reverse compared to those at 90°. The example given is for gray and white matter and CSF, with TR = 0.15 s and T1 values typical of middle field. **B** Contrast for two pairs of tissues

For "watery" lesions the ability to use short TR values opens an avenue for imaging with three-dimensional Fourier transformation (3-DFT) sequences. The TR that can be achieved in 3-DFT imaging is limited by practical considerations of time, since this time increases linearly with the number of slices obtained. If gradient echo instead of spin echo imaging is used, an angle smaller than 90° results in a decrease in T1 effects. This occurs because as the angle is made smaller the signal from the tissue with the longer T1 increases (proportionally) more than the signal from the tissue with the shorter TR (Fig. 2A). The peak signal from the longer T1 tissue occurs at a smaller angle than the peak for the shorter T1 tissue. Thus below a certain angle T1 effects can actually result in a reversal of contrast (Fig. 2B). Lowering the angle at fixed TR has the same effect as lengthening TR for a 90° angle. Unfortunately, this cannot be carried to extremes. This process is more effective the larger the ratio TR/T1. Thus from a practical point of view it is only achievable for short T1 values, where it is highly effective. Furthermore, to obtain the desired contrast level it is desirable to operate with a relatively long TE, to take advantage of T2 effects. Gradient echo imaging (used in conjunction for partial flip angles) is highly sensitive to susceptibility and inhomogeneity effects, this sensitivity increasing with TE and with field strength.

Thus, the combination of short T1 and low inhomogeneity and susceptibility effects that accompany low-field operation permit for this application the use of gradient echo 3-DFT imaging, which under these conditions results in S/N levels at low fields comparable to those of middle- and high-field systems when taking into account imaging time and number of sections obtained [3]. More recently a hybrid technique consisting of a multislab two-dimensional Fourier transformation (2-DFT) sequence with two-slice encodings within a slab, coupled with partial flip angle gradient echo imaging has permitted us to develop a sequence that takes advantage of low-field operation characteristics and double the S/N over conventional spin echo [4], as is discussed in more detail in a following section. A significant benefit is derived in low-field operation from the fact that while at low-field solid tissues have shorter T1 values, CSF has a T1 that is constant with field. Consequently, at the short TR where lesion contrast is achieved, the signal from CSF is small. At high field, because TR must be long, CSF signal is large, obscuring lesions that may be contiguous with CSF spaces (Fig. 1). To summarize, low-field strengths offer many advantages for the detection of water-elevating lesions, including increased sensitivity to water changes, ability to operate with relatively short TR values, and the avoidance of confusing effects from bright CSF.

The second example involves MR angiography (MRA). In MRA the clinically most successful techniques take advantage of wash-in effects [5]. The blood entering the volume has not been excited previously and thus produces a great deal of signal following the first one or two excitations [6]. Meanwhile, it is desirable to saturate the signal from stationary tissues by the same repeated excitations that produce signal from blood. This saturation is more effective the longer the T1, since recovery time is longer. Because high-field operation entails long T1 values, high contrast between blood and nonmoving tissues is easier to obtain. This permits more flexibility in trading vessel contrast for depth of penetration (field of view) at high field.

The third example addresses the issue of obtaining contrast on the basis of susceptibility differences. Contrast based on susceptibility occurs in the presence of concentrations of paramagnetic, diamagnetic, or ferromagnetic substances which are sufficient to produce local gradients that dephase the signal from individual nuclei. Typical substances that result in these effects are iron or calcium in the brain, iron in the liver, etc. The signal in the tissues with these elements is reduced. Susceptibility effects are proportional to field strength, being stronger at the higher fields. They also depend on the length of readout windows in spin echo imaging and on TE for gradient imaging. Bulk susceptibility effects also occur at air-tissue interfaces, and this, coupled with field inhomogeneity, limits echo lengths and TE values as the field increases. Even so, because the effect is stronger at the higher field, susceptibility differences are readily observed at high field, independent of whether their observation is desirable or not. At low field, the effect is weaker, but the sequence can be manipulated by using long windows or longer TE values, this making susceptibility effects apparent when desired, for instance, more in a second than a first echo. In any event, in the case of imaging susceptibility changes there is no clear advantage to either low or high-field strengths.

■ Artifacts

Artifacts in MRI arise from many sources. Some of these are field dependent, and these invariably increase with field strength. The most familiar are chemical shift, motion, flow, susceptibility and inhomogeneity artifacts. A great deal of work has gone into ameliorating these artifacts, but in every case reducing the artifacts affects sequence efficiency, either in S/N, number of sections, earliest TE available, or a combination of these.

Chemical shift artifacts are well known and understood. The observed displacement between fat and water increases with field strength and echo window length. Reducing the artifacts involves using a shorter echo window, with consequent loss of S/N. To maintain a constant artifact level entails a S/N penalty of square root of field strength. Other techniques to avoid this problem, such as selective saturations, necessitate doubling of imaging time to obtain a complete image, an equivalent loss of square root of two in S/N per unit time.

Motion and flow artifacts are observed to increase with field strength. A number of mechanisms have been discussed to explain this effect, but none is satisfactory. Nevertheless, the empirical fact is clear. To ameliorate these artifacts techniques have been developed that penalize sequence efficiency in one way or another. Motion compensation by gradient nulling techniques increase TE or reduce echo lengths, both of these resulting in a loss of S/N. Saturation pulses penalize the sequence in terms of loss of slices per unit time, especially so in 2-DFT imaging. Techniques that depend on synchronizing to a pulse or respiratory gate, or to a measure of the position of the body, also give up efficiency in terms of time used for data collection vs. time used for monitoring or gating delays.

Susceptibility effects show up as very smooth borders at air-tissue interfaces, or even as voids bordered by a high intensity region. Inhomogeneity introduces distortions. Both of these artifacts increase with field strength. In spin echo imaging they establish limits to maximum window length (and consequent S/N), and in gradient echo imaging they also force TE to stay short, which is detrimental for obtaining hyperintense lesions or CSF, the contrast of both being improved for longer TE values.

Regarding artifacts, a general rule can be stated as thus: High field has high "intrinsic" S/N and high artifacts. Low field is the opposite. When artifacts are reduced at high field the S/N suffers because the way the artifacts are reduced decreases sequence efficiency. When the S/N is increased at low field, the sensitivity to artifacts also increases, because the ways used to increase S/N makes the sequence more sensitive to artifacts. Thus artifacts and their reduction have the effect of leveling differences in performance across the field strength range, making the variation smaller than would be otherwise predicted.

Another effect needs to be considered which is incidental to field strength. Any one sequence requires RF power that increases with the square of field strength. At high field practical considerations (available peak power, patient heating) force limits on RF power deposition. These limits can indirectly manifest themselves in various ways, for instance, as a loss of number of sections per unit time to keep average power deposition low. A more insidious way to control RF power is to use RF pulse shapes that require less power. These pulses produce poorer section profiles that force operation with gaps between section or loss of signal strength and contrast when no gaps are present [7]. Such effects are avoidable at middle and low fields simply because RF power deposition is not an issue [8]. Irrespective of how the RF power deposition is controlled, it appears as a loss of efficiency (number of sections, signal from the gaps, or signal and contrast from the crosstalk region).

■ Signal to Noise

A perception exists that S/N increases linearly with field strength. The physics of MRI shows that signal increases as the square of the field, and measurements and theoretical considerations (based on certain assumptions about the body) support a linear increase in noise with field, although this latter assumption should be considered with caution. Based on these two factors, "intrinsic" S/N should increase linearly with field. This simplistic view depends on disregarding all the factors that are important in imaging, all of which result in a much smaller increase than presumed [9, 10].

In addition to the "intrinsic" factor, S/N depends on the imaging conditions. Of interest is S/N per unit time for fixed voxel dimensions and imaged volume, as well as constant number of slices. For a 90° flip angle the relative S/N is proportional to $[e^{-TE/T2}(1-e^{-TR/T1}) \times \sqrt{(\text{window length} \times \text{slices}/TR)}]$ for 2-DFT imaging [11]. The reasons for the slices term is that if sequence A yields 10 slices and sequence B yields 20 slices with one excitation, then, to cover the same volume sequence A must be run twice, while sequence B in the same time could be run once with two excitations and gain $\sqrt{2}$ in S/N. Similarly, the TR term comes in because if two sequences provide the same coverage for one excitation, then the sequence with the shorter TR can be run with more excitations and increase S/N accordingly. For 3-DFT there is an additional slices term. For a discussion of the relative merits of 2-DFT vs. 3-DFT imaging the reader is directed to [12]. Based on imaging considerations we an analyze how S/N behaves.

T1. As field strength increases, so does T1 [13]. A longer T1 means smaller signals. For discussion purposes consider T1 varying as the square root of field strength. For a short TR sequence signal decreases linearly with T1, or as square root of field. For a long TR sequence signal does not change much, but for a fixed TR the contrast is lower, or for fixed contrast TR is longer (longer imaging time). In this case the equivalent loss of S/N is smaller, approximately as the fourth root of field strength. Thus T1 effects result in a loss in signal that increases as the fourth root to square root of field.

T2. There is clear evidence that T2 drops with field strength [14]. Between 0.63 and 3 T the T2 of brain drops from about 80 to 58 ms, for muscle from 37 to 30 ms and for liver from 49 to 25 ms. For a TE of 30 ms, this results in signal drops from 16% to 50%, corresponding to a 1/20 to 1/6 power of field for the loss of S/N due to T2. The loss is smaller for shorter TE and bigger for longer TE values.

Window Length. Chemical shift, susceptibility, and inhomogeneity limit window lengths. As discussed above, the artifacts depend linearly on field strength and window length. A shorter window reduces the artifacts, but also decreases S/N as the square root of window length. The net effect is that at constant artifactual level there is a square of field strength term available in the S/N, favoring low-field operation. In some sequences this term is not useable, for instance, where TE is very short, and in others it is not fully useable, but in general it provides relative advantages of factors of 2–3 for low-field operation.

RF power. As discussed above, high-field systems compromise slice profile in the interest of savings in peak and average RF power. At middle and low fields these conditions are not important, and square profiles can be obtained [8]. For a system where a gap of 50% is needed to avoid interslice crosstalk, S/N loss for the slice itself may amount to 20%, and the gap can be considered as an unused potential source of 50% more signal [7]. Thus the full S/N is not being achieved if the slice profile is poor. The loss in 2-DFT imaging is sequence dependent. For 3-DFT imaging there is no difference.

Artifact Reduction. As discussed above, artifact reduction schemes take time away from data collection, either by reducing the echo window length or the number of sections, or by lengthening TE, and result in penalties in S/N per unit time. This loss depends on the particular sequence and can be as small as zero where artifact reduction is not needed and as big as 50% in some extreme cases, such as presaturation in multislice imaging.

Net S/N Change. From the above considerations it can be seen that S/N changes with field in a complex manner, which depends on the clinical purpose of the sequence, the type of sequence used and tissue imaged, on coverage (including gaps) and on artifacts. For a sequence such as MR angiography, a major part of the "theoretical" S/N available from increasing field strength can be obtained. For other sequences the gain is small. An approximate rule is that in many situations the S/N increases as the fourth root of field strength, so that for a 20-fold increase in field, S/N doubles. Some of the loss at low field can be recovered, if needed, by small compromises in operation. For instance, operation with a 1.1 mm resolution instead of the more common 0.9 mm resolution recovers half of this loss. Time is another factor. A typical total patient study time that at high field requires 30–45 min is performed at much lower fields in 45–60 min. These disadvantages must be weighted against the advantages that can accrue from lower field operation.

Discussion

It has been 13 years since the introduction of the first commercially available open MRI unit [15]. Starting in 1988, and accelerating in the past 2 years with the introduction of other open units, open low and middle field MRI systems are obtaining an increasingly larger share of the new equipment market. They combine excellent diagnostic capabilities with sensible economics and the ability to perform studies not possible in closed systems. Not only do these include large subjects, but also claustrophobic patients, motion studies [16] and interventional MRI [17]. These units may offer some particularly attractive features for the latter application, including very low forces on ancillary equipment, and very short T1 values, which aid in real-time imaging [18]. The combination of economic pressures and the advantages of openness will continue to drive the development of new generations of middle and low-field units.

References

1. Rose AA (1974) Vision: human and electronic, chap 1. Plenum, New York
2. Ortendahl DA, Hylton NM, Kaufman L, Watts JC, Crooks LE, Mills CM, Stark D (1984) Analytical tools for MRI. Radiology 153:479
3. Rothschild PA, Schulz M, Kramer DM, Kaufman L (199) Magnetic resonance imaging characteristics of multiple sclerosis plaques imaged with two-dimensional and three-dimensional Fourier transform techniques at low and mid field strengths. J Neuroimaging 1:79
4. Kramer DM, Li A, Kaufman L, Hake K (1989) Two-gradient echo 2-DFT multi-section imaging: comparison with spin echo imaging. J Neuroimaging (in press)
5. Blatter DD, Parker DL, Ahn SS, Bahr AL, Robison RO, Schwartz RB, Jolesz FA, Boyer RS (1992) Cerebral MR angiography with multiple overlapping thin slab acquisition. Radiology 183:379
6. Kaufman L, Crooks LE, Sheldon PE, Rowan W, Miller T (1982) Evaluation of NMR imaging for detection and quantification of obstructions in vessels. Invest Radiol 17:554
7. Kneeland JB, Shimakawa A, Wehrli F (1986) Effect of intersection spacing on MR image contrast and study time. Radiology 158:819
8. Feinberg DA, Crooks LE, Hoenninger JC, Watts JC, Arakawa M, Cheng H, Kaufman L (1986) Contiguous thin multi-section MR imaging by two-dimensional Fourier transform techniques. Radiology 158:811
9. Hoult DI, Chen C-N, Sank VJ (1986) The field dependence of NMR imaging. Magnc Reson Med 3:730
10. Kaufman L (1986) Optimal field strength in proton MRI. Toshiba Med Rev (Int Edn) 16:5–9
11. Kaufman L, Kramer SM, Crooks LE, Ortendahl DA (1989) Measuring signal-to-noise ratios in MR imaging. Radiology 173:265
12. Carlson JC, Crooks LE, Ortendahl DA, Kramer DM, Kaufman L (1988) Signal-to-noise ratio and section thickness in two-dimensional versus three-dimensional Fourier transform MR imaging. Radiology 166:266
13. Koenig SH, Brown RD, Adams D, Emerson D, Harrison CG (1984) Magnetic field dependence of 1/T1 in tissue. Invest Radiol 19:76
14. Chen J-H, Avram H, Crooks LE, Arakawa M, Kaufman L, Brito AC (1992) In vivo relaxation times and hydrogen density at 0.063–4.8 T in rats with implanted mammary adenocarcinomas. Radiology 184:1
15. Kaufman L, Crooks LE, Arakawa M, Hoenninger JC, Watts JC, Winkler ML (1987) Prospects for increasing the accessibility of MRI. Admin Radiol VI (XI):32
16. Carlson JW, Gyori M, Kaufman L (1990) A technique for MR imaging of the knee under large flexing angles. Magn Res Imaging 8:407
17. Gronemeyer DHW, Seibel RMM, Kaufman L (1991) Low-field design eases MR-guided biopsy. Diagn Imaging 13 (3):139
18. Kramer DM, Hawryszko C, Ortendahl DA, Minaise M (1991) Fluoroscopic MR imaging at 0.064 T. IEEE Trans Med Imag 10:358

Open-Magnet Technology for Magnetic Resonance Imaging 3

L. Kaufman · J. Carlson · A. Li · L. Crooks · L. Zha
M. Arakawa · B. Breneman · Y.H. Hsu · K. Matsutani

■ Introduction

Open MRI came to the forefront of commercial activity during 1995, starting with the 1994 annual meeting of the RSNA. Lost in the hype that attends any new trend was the fact that the era of commercially available open MRI started in 1987 with an article describing a low-field permanent magnet MRI system [1] and that the first commercial unit was delivered in middle 1988. The increased interest in open systems is due mostly to the demand by patients for a more comfortable environment and by the economic pressures for lower cost services, both of which are delivered by these systems. The core element that distinguishes an open imager is the magnet. While conventional MRI units developed along relatively common paths (superconducting air-core cylindrical magnets, to which were added ferromagnetic shielding, active shielding, and coolers to decrease cryogen consumption), open MRI systems are based on distinct magnet technologies. We introduce here the basic technologies and discuss the relative merits of various technical alternatives for realizing magnets for whole-body open MRI.

■ Magnet Technology

When considering magnet technology we can focus on two basic components: the driver and the core of the magnet. The driver provides the motive force that establishes the magnetic field. Three kinds of driving technologies are available in the marketplace: resistive, permanent, and superconducting. The earth's magnetic field is a fourth source that has been discussed in the literature but has not become commercially available. The core is the medium upon which the driver acts. Because a patient must be able to be located in the magnet (a prerequisite for reimbursement), all magnets have at least a portion of their field in air. Air core magnets are those where all of the core is air. These may have a return path (the region outside of the core where the magnetic field lines close) that is either air or iron. Iron core magnets have, except for the patient volume, iron paths both for the drivers to act on and as return paths. The relative merits of these approaches to magnet design are discussed below.

Resistive Drivers

In a resistive driver a current is established on a good conducting material, typically copper or aluminum. (During the Manhattan Project silver from the United States reserves was used for huge magnets for uranium separation, since copper and aluminum were needed for armaments.) The conductor is at or near room temperature and therefore offers resistance to the flow of current. This resistance has two effects: power must be used to maintain the current flow and attendant magnetic field, and heat is generated in the conductor through resistive losses, so that water needs to be used to extract this heat. In addition, the stability of the field depends on power supply stability, stability coming at a price.

The advantages of this approach is that the technology is well known and understood, and entry is easy since a great deal of expertise exists or is easily acquired by a company. The disadvantages are high power consumption, large cooling demand, a large conductor mass and its consequent weight. When an iron core is used, the larger mass of conductor forces an increase in the physical size of the core, which then results in further weight increases.

Permanent Drivers

In a permanent magnet the field originates in blocks of permanently magnetized material. Currently available are ferrite magnets for low field operation and Neomax (a rare earth alloy) for higher fields. The attractive aspect of permanent magnet drivers is that they are totally passive, requiring no added services such as electricity, cryogens, or cooling. The disadvantages are that there is a very steep cost/field curve, especially when Neomax is needed for higher fields, and the weight of the permanent magnet material adds to the weight of an iron core.

For the higher field units a potential problem is that the magnet cannot be discharged in an emergency.

Superconducting Drivers

There are materials, generically known as superconductors, that if kept at a sufficiently low temperature, loose all resistance to current flow. In typical magnets for MRI this temperature must be well below 10 K, that is, under 10 °C above absolute zero. A convenient way to achieve this is by the use of liquid helium, which has a temperature of near 4 K. The liquid boils away due to heat leaking into the magnet from room temperature. Because of cost it is desirable to minimize the boil off of the helium. One method used in the early years of commercial MRI is to use a surrounding container with liquid nitrogen, which has a temperature of 77 K, intermediate between helium and room temperatures. This of course adds liquid nitrogen consumption to the services needed for magnet operation. Later, electrical shield coolers were added to magnets to replace the liquid nitrogen "shield," these coolers usually reaching temperatures well below 77 K, thus improving the shielding effect. Also, recirculating coolers which reliquefy vented helium gas were added to some magnets, even though in the United States, because of the relatively low cost of liquid helium, this was not usually economic.

More recently, electrical coolers that reach 4 K have become commercially available. This opens the way to cryogenless superconducting magnets with low power consumption. It is worth noting that the high temperature superconducting materials that a few years were touted as permitting magnets cooled by liquid nitrogen have yet to provide the performance required by MRI magnets but have found use as superconducting leads, which bring current from the outside to the main windings during magnet charging and discharging.

The advantage of superconductors for MRI is relatively higher fields compared to the other technologies, with low weight and modest power consumption. The disadvantage is the need for cryogens (or, more recently, cryocoolers that can replace cryogens) and the technical complexity of these systems compared to other drivers, this making entry more difficult. In terms of cost, at a certain field strength crossover point superconductors become cheaper than other drivers. Once the middle-field range is reached, they have definite advantages in this respect.

Magnet Core

The driver can be shaped so as to obtain the desired imaging field and field return path without the aid of significant amounts of iron, in which case we call this an air-core magnet, or iron can be used for shaping the imaging field and providing a return path, in which case we call the result an iron-core magnet. Some air-core magnets have an iron return path or shield. The advantage of air core magnets is low weight. The disadvantages are inefficient use of conductor, demands on the conductor configuration and manufacturing tolerances (since the homogeneity depends on the conductor), and large fringe fields that require active or passive shielding. All of this of course results in increased costs. Iron core magnets make more efficient use of the driver since the iron provides a medium that offers less "resistance" to the flow of the magnetic field lines. In iron-core magnets fringe fields are relatively small, and homogeneity is determined by the shape of the iron. This places less demands on the driver's configuration and tolerances. The main unavoidable disadvantage of these cores is weight.

There are obviously other nuances about the different drivers and cores that need to be taken into account when designing an MRI system, but the characteristics described above are of a reasonably general nature and not amenable to significant manipulation. Commercially, we have seen the following driver-core combinations become available at one time or another in the dozen years of clinical MRI: resistive, superconducting, and permanent driver air-core, the first two sometimes with iron shielding; and resistive and permanent driver iron-core. The combination that is not currently available is the superconducting iron-core magnet. This will be the subject of further discussion.

■ Open Magnets

The first commercially available open MRI system was delivered in May 1988. It consisted of an iron-core permanent magnet with a field of 640 G. With various improvements these units are still sold today. Half a dozen years passed before other open units followed, after the success of the original one showed that a market existed for the then unusual configuration. This market is not only one of low cost MRI but also includes the imaging of claustrophobic, obese, and seriously ill patients, and more and more, in meeting the demand from patients who, while not necessarily claustrophobic, do not want to be subject to the experience of an MRI study in a narrow, noisy tube. There is also an interest in interventional studies using MRI, and many sites are actively engaged in patient care using this modality to guide biopsies or to treat disks or tumors, as described elsewhere in this book.

The attractiveness of these open units is sometimes limited by perceptions as to what the field range of MRI "should" be. What has been available thus far has fallen into what is generally characterized as "low field." The limitations in the field strength that is practically achievable have to do with the demands that resistive and permanent drivers place on the design. It is in such a case that superconducting drivers can help overcome these limitations. Air core superconducting magnets are not easily configured as open systems. While the central volume can be made relatively accessible, the patient, except for head studies, remains within a bore. In addition to being costly, these systems have large fringe fields.

Iron-core magnets, combined with resistive and permanent drivers, have been the base technology for the commercially available open MRI units, and these result in systems with fields of up to 0.3 T. More recently, iron-core resistive magnets have been introduced for up to 0.6 T operation. Not surprisingly, their weight exceeds the 40-ton level, and power consumption nears 100 kW (excluding cooling). By contrast, combining an iron core with a superconducting driver results in an attractive performance level for middle field operation. Because the field is shaped by the iron, the coils can be quite compact and relatively easy to cool with a single electrical cooler. For 0.35 T operation power consumption is relatively low (comparable to that of an air core superconducting magnet that uses a shield cooler and requires liquid helium consumption in addition), and the magnet is fully cryogen-free. The weight that is achieved is comparable to that of a 1.5-T shielded magnet of the same fringe field. The savings in weight comes from three related factors: (a) the conductor mass is low; (b) given a low mass, the cross-section is small, so that iron is not wasted in spanning the conductor; and (c) the lack of a reservoir for cryogens permits the use of a compact cryostat that further reduces the need for iron mass in the core.

■ Designing a Magnet

Although all magnet designers are confronted by the same physics, the available technology and perceived merits of different characteristics generate sometimes disparate designs. The reason is of course that judgments are made as to the relative merits of different magnet performance parameters, so that the results look very different. Table 1 shows some of the tradeoffs made by the designer. For instance, a higher field strength can be realized by accepting a lower homogeneity or smaller aperture, or larger fringe field, or higher weight, this necessitating physically larger magnets and higher costs. Cost increases with increased field strength, homogeneity, aperture, weight and size, and decreases with increased fringe field.

In open iron-core magnets another design choice is the number of posts used to separate the pole pieces. The magnets are typically supported by either four posts, one at each corner; two

Table 1. Magnet tradeoffs

Increased	Field	Homogeneity	Aperture	Weight	Fringe field	Size	Cost
Field		–	–	+	+	+	+
Homogeneity	–		+	+	O	+	+
Aperture	–	+		+	+	+	+
Weight	+	+	+		–	+	+
Fringe field	+	O	+	–		–	–
Size	+	+	+	+	–		+
Cost	+	+	+	+	–		+

Table 2. Single-variable comparison

Magnet type	Weight (cost/b_0)	Homo-geneity	Fringe field	Mechanical stability
4-post	Lightest	Best	Smallest	Best
2-post	Inter-mediate	Inter-mediate	Inter-mediate	Intermediate
1-post (c-type)	Heaviest	Worst	Largest	Worst

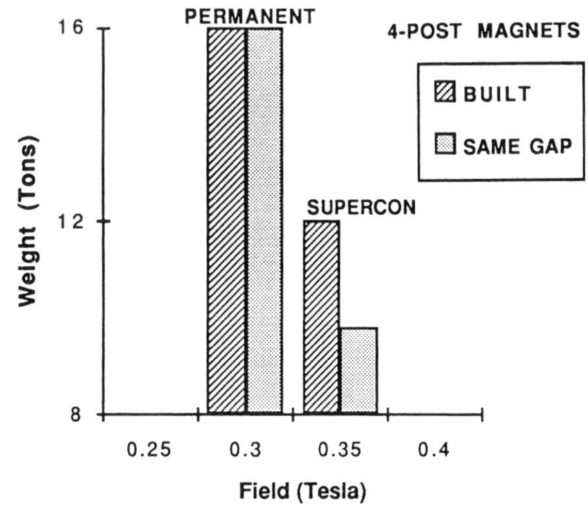

Fig. 1. Comparison of the weight characteristics of permanent and superconducting drivers for open MRI magnets. *Striped bars*, two four-post magnets as built currently, the superconducting one with a larger gap and higher field (0.35 T for the superconducting one vs. 0.3 T for the permanent one); *shaded bars*, the effects of adjusting for gap size. A further correction for field strength would increase the weight difference even more

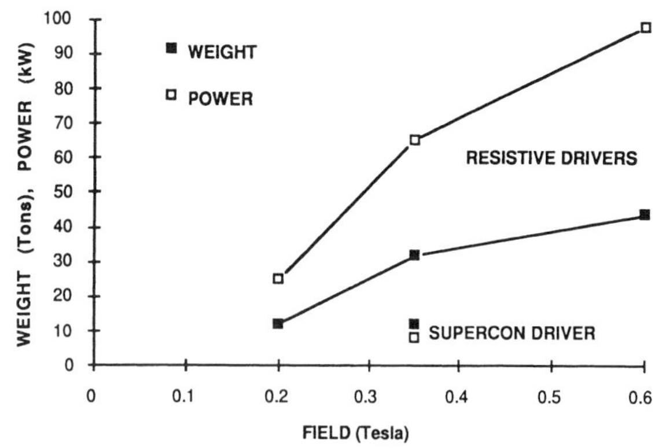

Fig. 2. Comparison of weight and power consumption of resistive open magnets and superconducting ones, based on currently built units. *Lines* connect points for resistive magnets. The differences are dramatic, as demonstrated here

posts, positioned either exactly at 180° from each other or at a somewhat smaller angle; or one post that occupies essentially all of one side of the magnet. these also referred to as C-magnets. If all performance specifications are held the same, for any one kind of driver technology, the four-post magnets offer the lowest weight (and cost per unit field strength) at a given level of mechanical stability. If everything else is held fixed they also offer the best homogeneity, or smallest fringe field, and the highest mechanical stability. The one-post designs offer the least desirable results, and two-post designs are intermediate the other two (Table 2).

The above discussion shows tradeoffs for any one driver technology. To appreciate the difference made by the driver we compare below magnets with permanent and resistive drivers to superconducting ones. Figure 1 shows the effects of moving from permanent to superconducting drivers. The lined bars compare a 0.3-T four-post permanent magnet to a four-post 0.35-T superconducting one of larger gap, the latter weighing approximately 25% less than the former. When the weights are adjusted for gap size, the superconducting magnet weighs 60% less than the permanent one while realizing a 17% higher field (dotted bars). Thus we see that superconducting drivers compared to permanent ones make it possible to obtain larger gaps and stronger fields at much lower weights and lower cost.

Similar effects are noted when comparing superconducting to resistive drivers (Fig. 2). A 35-T middle-field superconducting magnet has the same weight, a third of the power consumption, and a third larger gap than a low field 0.2 T resistive magnet. At the same field strength (0.35 T), the superconducting magnet is almost one-third the weight, uses 12% of the power and has a 15% larger gap than a resistive magnet.

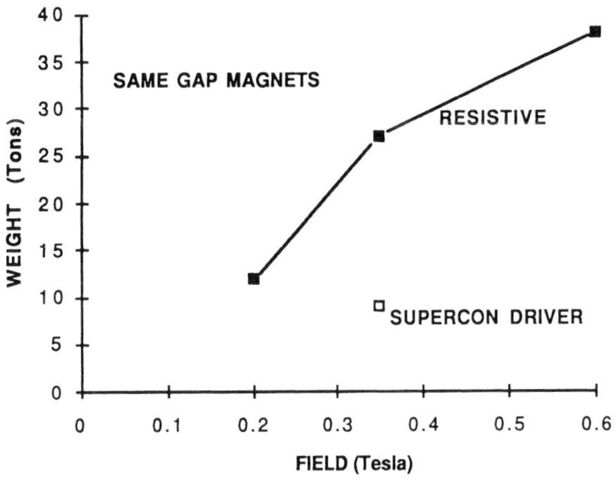

Fig. 3. Comparison of weight by adjusting the data of Fig. 2 for gap size.

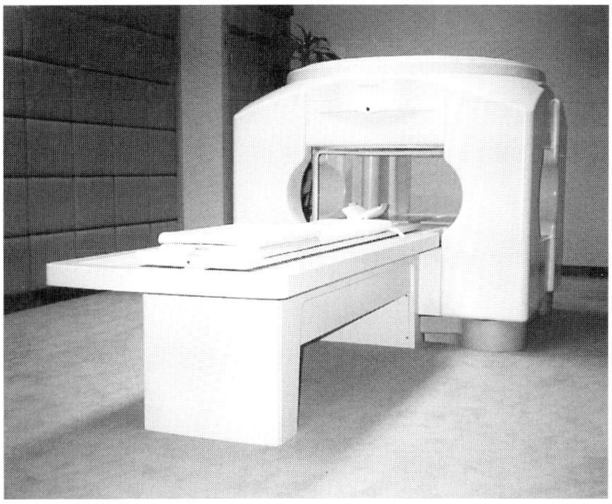

Fig. 4. The 0.35-T superconducting iron-core magnet

While the weight of a higher field superconducting iron-core magnet would increase proportionally, power consumption would stay essentially at the level of that of a 0.2-T resistive magnet. For a resistive driver a doubling of field from the 0.35-T level would result in power consumption levels on the order of 120 kW.

For the same gap and field strength the superconductor offers even more dramatic weight savings (Fig. 3).

Implementing a Superconducting Iron-Core Open Magnet

We have built a 0.35-T superconducting iron-core magnet to explore the marriage of these two technologies. The magnet has a square outside dimension of 170 cm and a gap of 60 cm, of which 55 cm is usable after planar gradient coils are inserted in place. It is open (over 100 cm horizontal opening after covers are accounted for) on all four sides.

The wire used is the conventional niobium-titanium type rather than the higher temperature (and higher cost) niobium-tin. It is cooled by an electrically powered cryocooler using 6.5 kW of power (a two-element quartz room heater typically uses 1.5 kW power). Operation is cryogenless, and cooldown from room temperature is achieved with the single cooler, without the aid of cryogens. The weight of the magnet is 12 tons.

Residual eddy currents are reduced to a fraction of 1% by the use of electrically nonconductive pole tips. The 5-G fringe field of the magnet extends to approximately 2.5 m from its center. The homogeneity achieved is ±15 ppm peak-to-peak over a 30-cm diameter sphere, equivalent for imaging purposes to ±3.5 ppm peak-to-peak at 1.5 T. Measured as a full-width/half-maximum, the homogeneity is better than ±2 ppm. The magnet with its covers is shown in Fig. 4.

Discussion

We have discussed the technological options that realize practical open MRI magnets. While the magnet is the core element, the degree of openness achieved depends also on gradient and RF coils and on the covers for the magnet.

The very early commercially available MRI units used resistive magnets, but by 1983 these had been superseded by air-core superconductive magnets, the "tunnels" or "tubes" that most patients associate with MRI. The technology used in these magnets was fairly uniform, and changes in configuration affected mainly aspects of the unit that the patient was not aware of: cryogen consumption and fringe field.

By contrast, open magnets are available that are fundamentally different in their underlying technology. Iron-core open magnets have definite advantages over air-core ones, at the cost of a higher weight. Permanent magnet drivers are attractive at low field strengths, but cost and weight increase rapidly with field. Superconductive drivers then become the favored technology for middle-field magnets. It is hard to see what the benefits of resistive drivers are, except perhaps for easy entry. Their weight and power consumption and heat dissipation problems are significant.

Reference

1. Kaufman L, Crooks LE, Arakawa M, Hoenninger JC, Watts JC, Winkler ML (1987) Prospects for increasing the accessibility of MRI. Admin Radiol VI (XI):32

Contrast Agents in Magnetic Resonance Interventions 4

H.-J. Weinmann · T. Frenzel · S. Kossler · J. Platzek
B. Radüchel

Introduction

The first reports on the use of paramagnetic ions as contrast modifiers in magnetic resonance imaging (MRI) were published in the late 1970s and early 1980s [1]. The poor tolerance profile of these metallic ions was, however, mentioned as a critical factor, and it was therefore unclear whether administering paramagnetic substances such as ions of the transitional elements and lanthanides or nitroxyl compounds would be feasible for clinical diagnosis. Chelation of these ions led to a dramatic improvement in their pharmacological and toxicological properties [2]. Chelation led to rapid renal excretion after intravenous administration and to elimination of the undesired toxic effects of the free metal ions. The first paramagnetic metal chelate, gadopentetate dimeglumine (gadolinium complex of diethylenetriamine pentaacetic acid, Gd-DTPA) received marketing authorization (Magnevist; Schering, Berlin, Germany) in 1988. Less than two years after the first marketing authorization in Europe, Japan, and the United States, metal chelates became an important tool for routine clinical MRI. Depending on various factors such as indications and clinical experience, some 30% of all clinical MR studies worldwide use a paramagnetic metal chelate. Gd-DTPA is the most widely studied contrast medium, with more than 50% market share.

Because of recent improvements in MR interventional techniques the use of paramagnetic contrast materials became important in this new therapeutic procedure. This chapter reviews the basic properties of extracellular contrast agents used today in routine clinical MR and describes the new specific formulations of these agents that have been studied experimentally. The article also mentions new and more specific contrast agents that may be used in interventional MR techniques.

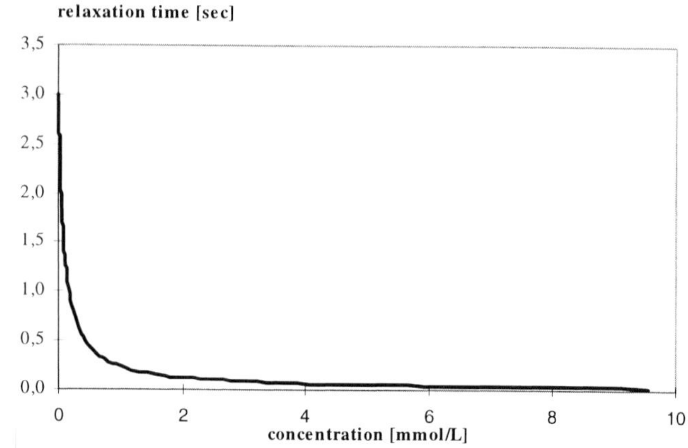

Fig. 1. Effect of a paramagnetic substance on the T1 relaxation time of water

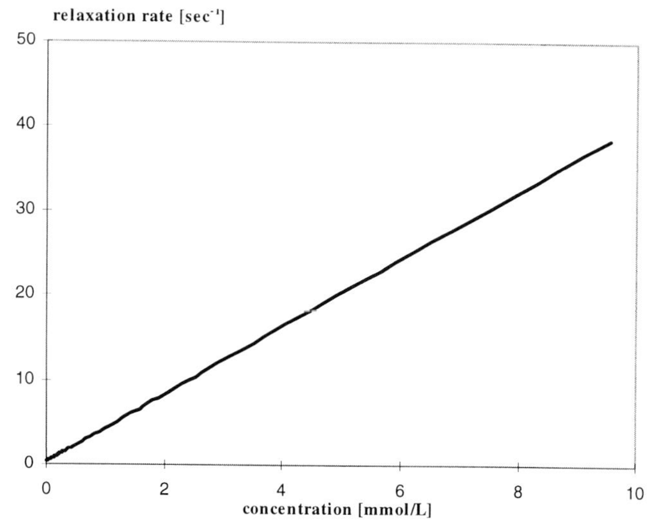

Fig. 2. Reciprocal value of the relaxation time, the relaxation rate, is directly proportional of concentration of a paramagnetic substance. The slope of the graph, the relaxivity, is a measure of the paramagnetic effect

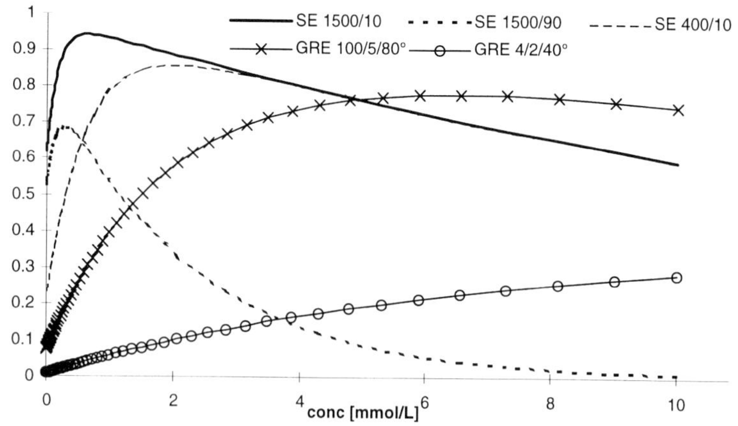

Fig. 3. The brightness or signal intensity of a tissue depends on the relaxation times and the imaging sequence. At higher concentration of a paramagnetic compound and thus shorter relaxation times, T1 and T2, the T2 effect results in a decrease in signal intensity. The computed curves were based on a tissue (plasma) with T1=1500 ms and T2=50 ms, and T1 and T2 relaxivities of 4.0 and 5.0 $l\ mmol^{-1}\ s^{-1}$, respectively

■ Extracellular Agents

The paramagnetic extracellular chelates used in clinical practice are all gadolinium compounds; gadolinium has seven unpaired electrons that provide it with the highest T1-influencing paramagnetic effect of all elements. Also, the atom is not very reactive; gadolinium is relatively inert, and the ion exists only in the three-plus form. Each electron has a magnetic moment about a 1000 times stronger than that of a proton. These electrons cause rapid fluctuation of the local magnetic field at the atomic level and thus facilitate the transfer of energy among the stimulated protons or into their environment (lattice); protons therefore relax faster.

Paramagnetic compounds can only shorten relaxation times – they cannot prolong them. Very small quantities of the gadolinium compounds cause a significant shortening of the relaxation times (Fig. 1). The concentration of the paramagnetic agents is directly proportional to the reciprocal value of the relaxation time, the relaxation rate (Fig. 2). Relaxivity is a measure of the paramagnetic effect and describes how much a given concentration of a compound decreases the relaxation time.

Since all paramagnetic substances decrease both relaxation times, at higher concentrations the shortening of the T2 time predominates and leads to signal decrease (Fig. 3). In most cases paramagnetic agents are used in T1-weighted sequences that positively highlight the contrast effect. However, in special situations one can take advantage of their T2 effect. Gradient echo sequences (GRE) with strong T2 or T2* dependence are used in perfusion studies [3, 4]. This effect is noticeable only during nonhomogeneous distribution of a high concentration of the agent and is not seen after homogenous distribution in the blood or other compartments of the body. Such susceptibility effects occur also with catheters filled with undiluted or only slightly diluted paramagnetic agents. This effect causes signal loss and may produce additional imaging artifacts.

Table 1. Gadolinium complexes used in clinical MRI (Fig. 4)

Generic name	Trade name	Vendor
Gadopentetate	Magnevist	Schering
Gadoterate	Dotarem	Guerbet
Gadodiamide	Omniscan	Nycomed
Gadoteridol	ProHance	Bracco
Gadobutrol	Gadovist	Schering

Note: Not all agents are registered in all countries.

Complex Stability

All gadolinium ions are tightly bound by polycarbonic acids. Five different chelates are used in clinical contrast-enhanced MRI investigations, but not all agents are available in all countries (Table 1, Fig. 4). Chemically these agents can be divided into open-chain and macrocyclic molecules. The dissociation rate of the macrocyclic complexes is extremely slow. The rate constants calculated for gadoteridol and gadobutrol are 2.8×10^{-5} and 2.6×10^{-4} s^{-1}, respectively [5]. These chelates release their metal ions at body temperature very slowly, but they are also almost incapable of rapidly forming the complex again. However, the open-chain compounds have much faster exchange rates, which means that they form the metal ligand bond very quickly. For example, DTPA and Gd^{3+} immediately form the corresponding complex, while DOTA and Gd^{3+} are practically inert. These compounds are so stable that no significant amount of the metal ions is released either in vitro or in vivo (Table 2).

Other substances present in the body, such as magnesium, calcium, zinc, and iron, do not replace detectable amounts of the gadolinium ion. The stability of the chelates also depends on the pH. However, significant lower-binding constants usually occur only at pH values lower than 2. The binding constants and rates vary with different temperatures. At the higher temperatures, used for sterilization (121°) decomplexation and complexation occur much faster.

Table 2. Characteristics of MRI complexes

Generic name	Ligand	Molecular weight	Osmolality (0.5 mol/l) (osmol/kg)	Stability constant log (k_{eff})
Gadopentetate	Open chain	548	1.96	22.2
Gadoterate	Macrocyclic	559	1.35	24.7
Gadodiamide	Open chain	573	0.79	16.9
Gadoteridol	Macrocyclic	559	0.63	23.8
Gadobutrol	Macrocyclic	605	0.56	21.8

The molecular weight does not include the corresponding counter-ions.

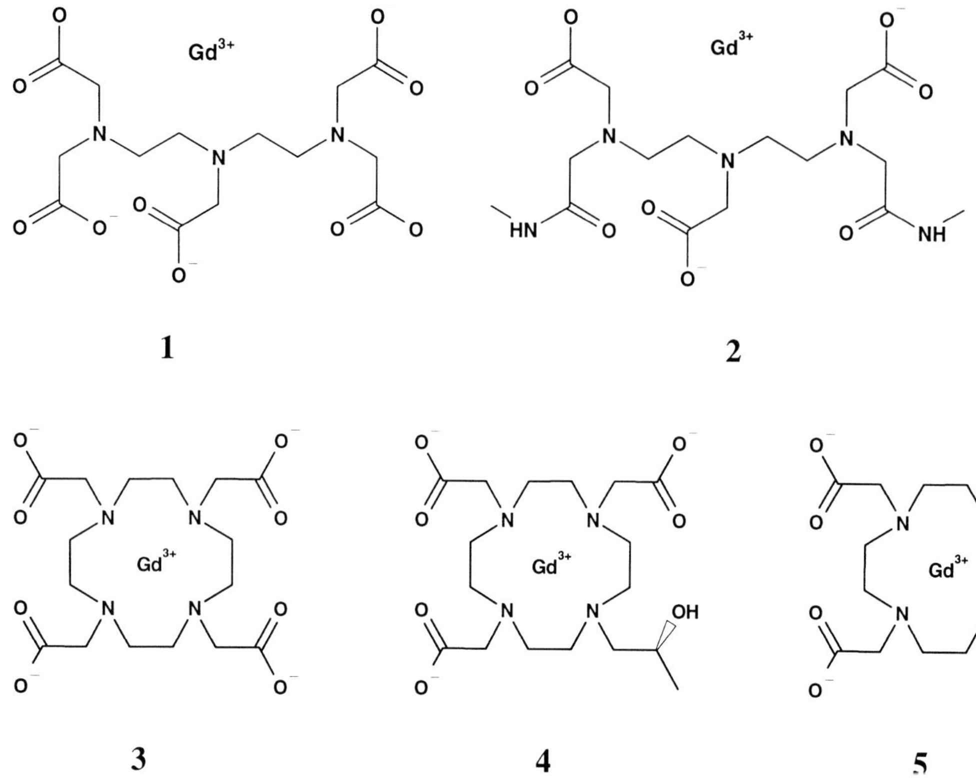

Fig. 4. Chemical structure of clinically used extracellular gadolinium chelates. *1*, Gadopentetate; *2*, gadodiamide; *3*, gadoterate; *4*, gadoteridol; *5*, gadobutrol

A significant decomplexation or transchelation of the paramagnetic ion with naturally occurring anions does not result if higher temperatures are applied to the area of interest (as in hyperthermia and laser induced interstitial thermotherapy). Destruction of the organic ligand occurs at extremely high temperatures (>250°) where practically all organic compounds are combustible. Organic substances produced after laser-thermotherapy are eventually metabolized but may cause some kind of immediate side effects (burning symptoms). In the unlikely event of very high temperature exposure (to the tip of temperature laser with temperatures >250°, for example), small amounts of the rare earth elements may be released. These amounts are so small as to be barely detectable (assuming a local Gd concentration of 0.5 mmol/l, which is equal to 0.5 µmol/ml less than 100 µg of the lanthanides present in this area) and does not result in additional risk to the patient. Since gadolinium is a relatively inert atom with very little tendency to interact with other molecules, this ion does not belong to the class of metals with high toxicity such as cadmium or lead [6, 7].

Toxicity

The acute intravenous toxicity value reflects the osmotic activity of the injection solution. Most of the animals died shortly or within 24 h after dosing without delayed mortality which would give hints for a direct chemotoxic effect. Very large doses of all chelates are required to reach the lethal dose (Table 3) which is roughly 100 times higher than the diagnostic dose providing an excellent margin of safety for all agents. Acute and subchronic toxicity studies with gadopentetate and other commercially available gadolinium chelates do not elicit toxicological findings indicating a significant release of the lanthanide ion. Minor amounts of the metal may be released, however, especially when chelates with less stability (gadodiamide) are used [10]. No significant teratological or genotoxic effects were obvious with any of the commercially available gadolinium contrast agents. A 2-year gadopentetate study conducted in rats did not indicate any carcinogenic potential (data on file at Schering, Berlin). The cardiovascular tolerance of all gadolinium complexes is excellent, no adverse hemodynamic effects were reported in clinical trials after rapid intravenous injection of doses of up to 0.3 mmol/kg.

Table 3. Intravenous acute toxicity (approximate LD_{50}) of contrast media in rats [8, 9]

Generic name	LD_{50} (mmol/kg)
$GdCl_3$	0.5
Gadopentetate	8
Gadoterate	18
Gadodiamide[a]	~25
Gadoteridol	<15
Gadobutrol	~25

[a]Plus excess chelating agent.

In sum, acute and subchronic toxicity studies in various species have demonstrated the inertness of extracellular gadolinium complexes even after intravenous injection in amounts several times higher than clinical doses. Extended clinical experience demonstrated the superb tolerance profile of extracellular metal chelates such as gadopentetate dimeglumine [11, 12].

Pharmacokinetics

Gadolinium complexes are extremely hydrophilic and very soluble in water. After intravenous administration they are rapidly eliminated by the renal route [2]. Highly hydrophilic substances are unable to permeate intact plasma membranes, and their excretion rates are determined by the glomerular filtration rate. The compounds are cleared from the body with a half-life of about 90 min. Distribution and excretion half-lives are determined by their distribution volume and by the glomerular filtration rate. No significant differences among gadolinium chelates have been observed [13–18]. More than 90% of the administered dose is excreted in the urine within the first 24 h after intravenous injection. Extrarenal excretion amounts to less than 1% of the administered dose. In patients with impaired renal function, however, the compound can be removed from the plasma by hemodialysis [19].

■ Special Formulations

As with iodinated contrast agents used in conventional X-ray interventions, paramagnetic substances may be administered in MR interventions. As shown in Table 4, the original formulation must be substantially diluted to achieve concentrations optimal for enhancing signal intensity. Depending on the sequences used, concentrations in the millimolar range produce best results. As a rule of thumb, the original concentration (500 mmol/l) should be diluted 100 times with saline.

A specially prepared hydrogel was developed for interventional applications such as chemoembolizations [20]. The material consists of a protein backbone cross-linked with polyethyleneglycol derivatives to which are attached therapeutic substances such as doxorubicin and a diagnostic label (e.g., Gd-DTPA). Animal studies have verified that the preparation decreased the rate of tumor recurrence. Initial studies have shown that the compound is relatively nontoxic and biodegradable and exhibits good imaging and therapeutic properties.

Transcatheter arterial embolization and percutaneous ethanol injection are widely used in the therapy of primary hepatocellular carcinoma or metastases [21, 22]. MR-guided ethanol administration can be performed by using a gadolinium-doped ethanol formulation. Studies conducted in our laboratories demonstrated that a 90% ethanol solution containing 1 mmol/l Gd-DTPA is easily detectable using T1-weighted imaging techniques [23] (Fig. 5). The gadolinium chelate elicits a remarkably high relaxivity of 26.6 $l\ mmol^{-1}\ s^{-1}$ mainly because of the strong interaction between the paramagnetic center and the hydrogen atom of the hydroxyl group. Unlike the case of an aqueous gadolinium formulation, the contrast was noticeable up to 60 min after injection. The gadolin-

Table 4. Concentration range of optimal signal intensity in blood

Sequence	Concentration range (mmol/l)	Enhancement (%)	Concentration at max. enhancement
SE 1500/90	0.05–1	10–30	0.3
SE 1500/10	0.2–5	30–50	0.5
SE 800/10	0.2–10	60–120	1
SE 400/10	0.2–20	100–250	2
SE 200/10	0.2–30	100–500	3.6
GRE 100/5/60	0.2–60	100–600	6
GRE 20/10/20	0.3–20	100–300	3.5
GRE 10/5/40	0.2–150	100–1800	14

Generally the greatest contrast enhancement occurs in the millimolar concentration range when short echo times are used. If sequences with longer repetition times are favored, the effect is relatively small. T2-weighted spin-echo sequences are of little use in increasing the signal intensities. The values were generated using the T1 and T2 relaxivities (4 and 4.5 $l\ mmol^{-1}\ s^{-1}$) of commercially available extracellular agents.

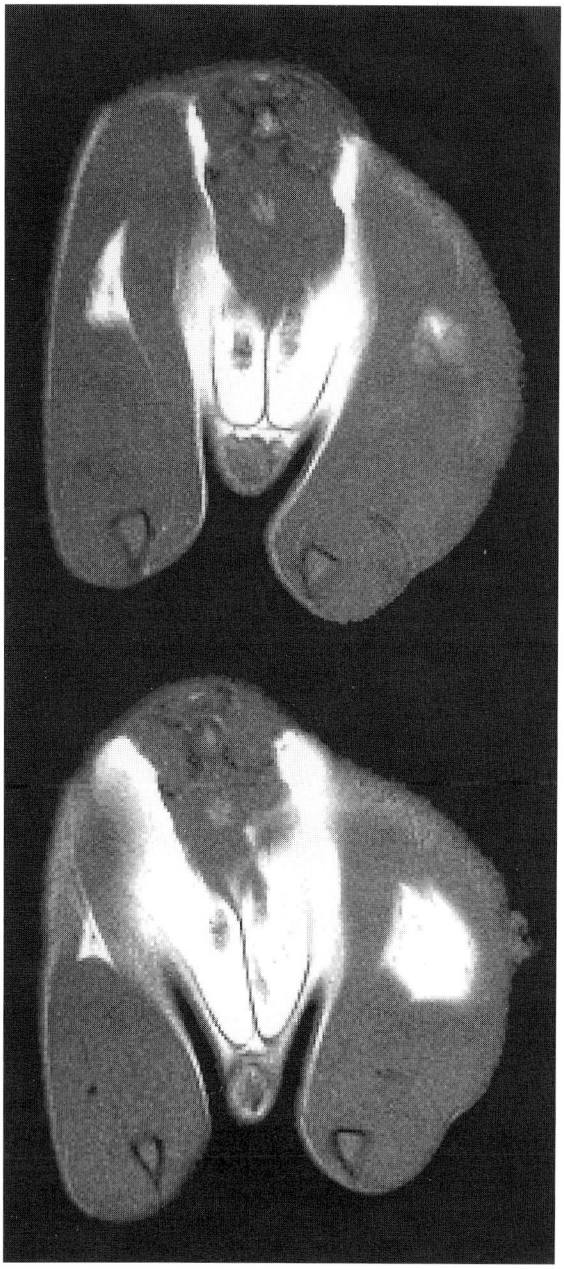

Fig. 5. Injection of a Gd-DTPA (1 mmol/l) doped ethanol solution into an implanted tumor (prostate carcinoma in thigh muscle) of a rat. The T1-weighted (SE 400/15) image was taken before (*above*) and immediately after the injection (*below*) by means of a small-bore MR instrument (SIS 85/310, SISCO, Fremont, CA, USA)

ium chelates are eliminated in an unmodified form by the renal route.

Because of the inertness of Gd-DTPA and other gadolinium chelates they can be widely used in formulations especially prepared for interventional indications. Incompatibility or interaction with pharmaceuticals has not been reported so far.

■ Tissue-Specific Contrast Agents

One of the disadvantages of currently available contrast agents is their relatively nonspecific distribution in the organism. These compounds reach all areas in a more or less homogenous concentration, except for the excretory tissue, the vascular space (shortly after administration only), and certain organs such as the brain. An improvement in diagnostic potential may be possible by directing the paramagnetic molecules to targets of interest and thus achieving locally higher concentrations. This may reduce the dose and lead to improving of the differentiation between the target and the surrounding tissue.

Liver-Specific Contrast Agents

Targeting compounds to liver-specific cells such as hepatocytes or Kupffer cells were the first successful approach to reach tissue specificity. Several compounds with different magnetic properties have been clinically tested. These include water-soluble paramagnetic chelates with hepatobiliary uptake such as Mn-DPDP (mangafodipir; Teslascan, Nycomed, Norway), Gd-BOPTA (gadobenate; MultiHance, Bracco, Italy), Gd-EOB DTPA (Gd-ethoxybenzyl DTPA, gadoxetate; Eovist, Schering, Germany), and superparamagnetic iron particles sequestered by the reticuloendothelial system such as AMI-25 (Feridex, Berlex, USA; and Endorem, Guerbet, France) and SHU555A (Resovist, Schering, Germany).

Mangafodipir is the first manganese complex used as a contrast agent in clinical trials [24–27]. Because of its five unpaired electrons which exhibit optimal correlation times, the Mn^{2+} ion is a powerful T1 relaxation agent. It demonstrates both biliary and renal excretion and has been shown to be a positive and very effective liver enhancer. Its chemical similarity to vitamin B_6 is cited as the reason for uptake by hepatocytes, but it is likely that most of the accumulation of paramagnetic manganese in the liver is due to the metabolism of the parent compound with release of free Mn^{2+} ions, which are known to accumulate in hepatocytes. Pharmacokinetic studies verified that Mn^{2+} is released in the plasma shortly after injection and that the paramagnetic ions accumulate in the liver and other tissues such as pancreas and cardiac muscle [28]. Peak liver enhancement occurs at 15 min and persists for several hours. Since manganese is a powerful relaxation enhancer, a very small amount (5 μmol/kg) is sufficient to significantly enhance the contrast between the liver parenchyma and focal liver lesions. Although general tolerance was favorable, transient facial flushing has been observed. Marketing authorization has recently been granted in Europe for this first manganese-based contrast agent.

The derivatives of the extracellular Gd-DTPA-type compounds exhibit the most useful characteristics [29–31]. The Eovist molecule has a lipophilic residue that targets the agent to a special carrier in the sinusoidal plasma membrane of the hepatocyte (Fig. 6). After entering the intracellular space the gadolinium chelate is sequestered in the bile in a nonaltered form. High hydrophilicity and low protein binding are responsible for the excellent tolerance profile.

The compound is completely eliminated from the body in equal parts by the hepatobiliary and renal routes. Because of the hepatocellular accumulation and high relaxivity, as little as 10 µmol/kg of Eovist is sufficient for an improved detection of liver tumors. Dynamic enhancement shortly after bolus injection was similar to that seen with extracellular agents. During the hepatobiliary phase, which lasts about 2 h, Eovist enhanced images exhibit significant improvement in the detection rate of focal lesions such as metastases, hepatocellular carcinomas, and hemangiomas.

The first clinical experience showed that Eovist not only has an excellent profile for detecting and differentially diagnosing of focal liver lesions but also demonstrated complete excretion and an excellent safety record [30, 32].

Special superparamagnetic iron oxide (SPIO) aggregates are extremely effective T2 relaxation agents [33, 34]. When placed in a magnetic field, they behave as ferromagnetic substances. Outside the magnetic field, however, they do not exhibit the magnetic memory of ferromagnetic materials. The diameter of such particles is in the nanometer range, that is, as large as proteins such as ferritin.

Just 3 µg Fe/g liver causes a signal decrease in 50% in a standard T2-weighted sequence [35]. These iron particles are coated with polysaccharides (e.g., dextrans) and form a mahogany-colored aqueous solution. After intravenous administration, SPIO particles are sequestered by normal phagocytic Kupffer cells, but they are not retained in metastases and no uptake was observed in hepatocytes. SPIO caused a strong susceptibility effect that is especially apparent in T2-weighted sequences. The iron oxides are metabolized into a soluble, and nonsuperparamagnetic form of iron. The solubilized iron is incorporated into the normal iron pool (ferritin, hemosiderin, hemoglobin) within a few days.

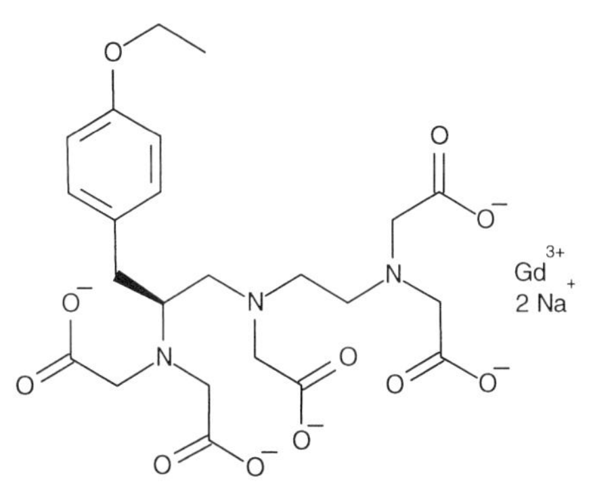

Fig. 6. Chemical structure of the liver-specific complex Gd-EOB DTPA (gadoxetate; Eovist, Schering, Germany). The ethoxybenzyl moiety targets the Gd-chelated residue to carriers located in the plasma membrane of the hepatocyte

With T2-weighted imaging techniques, a dose of about 10 µmol Fe/kg produced excellent clinical results [36, 37]. SPIO-enhanced images of the liver significantly increased the number of hepatic lesions detected and reduced the threshold size for detection to less than 5 mm. While SPIO particles did not accumulate in metastases, some uptake was observed in hepatocellular carcinoma and focal nodular hyperplasia. SPIO-enhanced images during the retention phases offer improved diagnostic accuracy in detecting focal liver lesions. The SPIO tolerance is still under discussion because early preparations caused severe cardiovascular side effects. No clinically relevant adverse reactions or changes in laboratory parameters were observed with the latest formulations, however.

Blood-Pool Agents

MR angiography (MRA) has been revolutionized by the introduction of paramagnetic gadolinium chelates. Extracellular agents permits arterial blood imaging within 30 s or less. However, some indications may require a longer lasting contrast effect, these indications are coronary MRA, high resolution imaging and interventional MR techniques.

A long-lasting enhancement of the blood space is required to permit improved MR angiography. Para- and superparamagnetic agents are in principle both suitable for enhancing the blood signal intensity at low concentrations. Various agents are now in preclinical and clinical development.

Strong protein-binding gadolinium chelates exhibit interesting properties: MS-325 (Epix, Cambridge, USA) [38]. This low-molecular DTPA derivative, binds specifically to albumin, the most common protein in blood. The binding caused

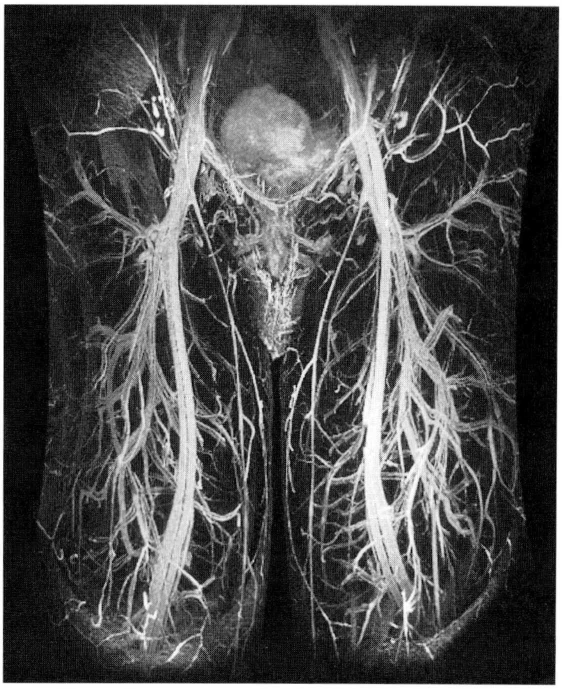

Fig. 7. MRI using MS-325 (0.05 mmol/kg) in healthy volunteers. The image was taken 15 min after intravenous injection. 3D SPGR w/fatsat, 21/2.3/30°; matrix=512×512×128; slice=0.8 mm. (Courtesy of EPIX Medical Cambridge, Mass., USA, and T.M. Grist, F.R. Korosec, D.C. Peters, and C.A. Mistretta, Departments of Radiology and Medical Physics, University of Wisconsin, Madison)

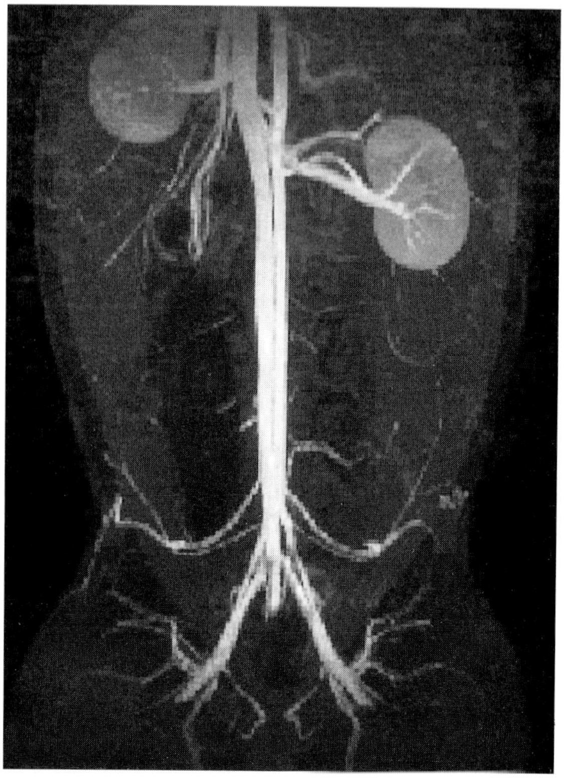

Fig. 8. MRA (3D FISP 20/6/50°, Siemens Vision 1.5 T) in rabbits after intravenous injection of gadomer-17 (50 µmol Gd/kg). (Courtesy of B. Hamm, M. Taupitz, and S. Wagner, Institut fur Röntengendiagnostik, Universitätsklinikum Charité, Humboldt-Universität, Berlin, Germany)

vascular distribution and an increase in the T1 relaxivity to values as high as 48 l $mmol^{-1}$ s^{-1}. Reports from initial clinical studies indicate that the compound may be safe and effective (Fig. 7).

Polymeric gadolinium complexes have been investigated extensively. Such large molecules do not diffuse quickly out of the blood into the interstitial space and elicit a prolonged elimination from the vascular lumen because of the slower glomerular excretion. Significantly higher relaxivities are obtained because of their optimized rotational correlation time.

Several groups tried covalently binding gadolinium chelate to polymeric backbones such as albumin, dextran, polylysine, and novel polymeric structures [39–47].

Polyamidoamine dendrimers are a new class of synthetic polymers with unique structural and physical characteristics. Substantial attention is being focused on gadolinium containing dendrimers such as gadomer-17, a 24 gadolinium atom carrying compound. This molecule has an apparent molecular weight of about 35 kDa, that is, small enough to guarantee renal excretion and large enough to reduce diffusion through the endothelial wall of intact blood vessels. A dose of 12.5–50 µmol Gd/kg body weight is sufficient to produce excellent angiograms shortly after injection (arterial phase) or during a longer-lasting imaging or interventional procedure (Fig. 8). Because of its longer extravasation and elimination time in humans gadomer-17 should allow contrast-enhanced MRA for at least 30 min after bolus injection.

Recently, ultrasmall superparamagnetic iron oxides (USPIOs) have been used as effective T1 blood pool contrast agents. These particles display an improved T1/T2 ratio and thus a lower T2 effect. Using heavily T1-weighted sequence doses of 1–3 mg (15–50 µmol) Fe/kg body weight produced excellent contrast enhancement of the vascular system [48]. The T1-shortening effect and the long intravascular half-life resulted in an improved visualization of vascular anatomy with 3-D gradient-echo sequences. Very short echo times are required to minimize signal loss from T2*-shortening effects, however. As with macrophage-specific SPIOs, these iron oxides are subject to intracellular degradation.

Similar dextran-coated iron-oxide particles have been evaluated as contrast materials for MR lymphography. After intravenous injection, these particles are transported by the lymphatics to the lymph nodes and make possible improved discrimination between neoplastic and unaffected tissue [49–51].

Necrosis-Specific Agents

Although not tumor specific, some metalloporphyrin derivatives (namely, *bis*-Gd-DTPA mesoporphyrin, also called gadophrin-2, Schering Berlin, Germany) accumulates in necrotic tissue (Fig. 9). Between 3 and 24 h after dosing it is possible to identify small infarcts using 25–100 μmol Gd/kg [52]. The porphyrin induced a strong persistent enhancement that remained visible for several days (Fig. 10). This technique may be useful for visualizing spontaneous necrosis such as acute myocardial infarct or necrosis following imaging guided tumor ablation.

■ Temperature Probes

Using MR sequences to locally monitor the temperature has been investigated by several groups [53, 54]. In most cases diffusion-weighted techniques are used for a semiquantitative measurement. Since any kind of movement disturbs the quality of the measurement, these techniques may not always be applicable.

Although the T1 and T2 relaxivities of gadolinium chelates exhibit some temperature dependence, the effects are too small for quantifying the local temperature.

A new lanthanide complex, praseodymium-2-methoxyethyl-DO3 A, was tested as a temperature indicator for ^{1}H-labeled MR spectroscopy [55–57]. The praseodymium complex has a strong chemical shift on the various ^{1}H resonances of the ligand (Fig. 11). The signal of the methoxy group was significantly shifted from the water, allowing easy water suppression and signal identification

Fig. 9. Chemical structure of gadophrin-2 (*bis*-Gd-DTPA mesoporphyrin) a gadolinium complex with affinity to necrotic tissue

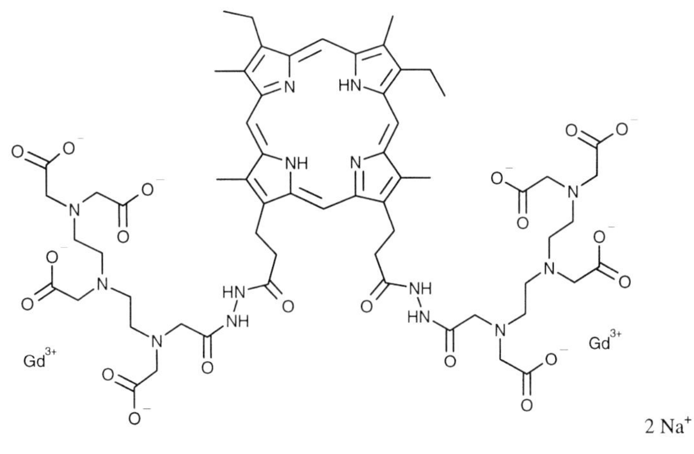

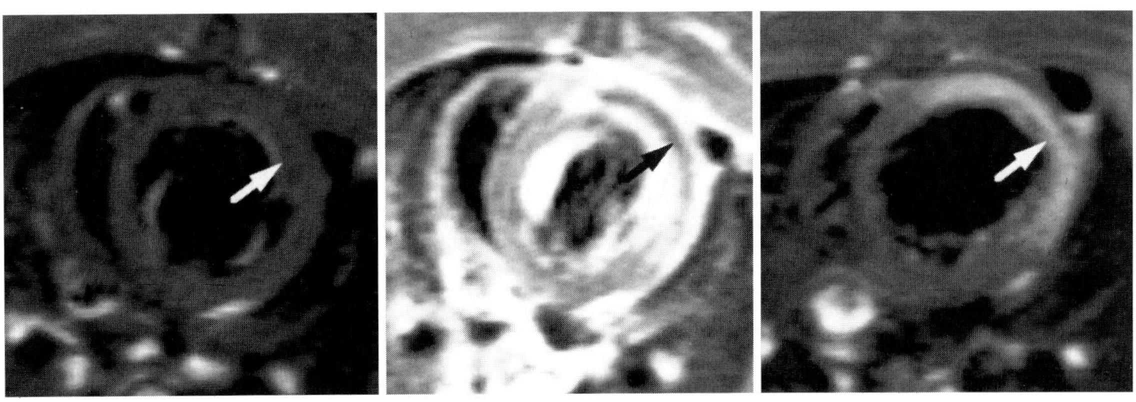

Fig. 10. Detection of a myocardial infarct in rats after intravenous injection of gadophrin-2 (100 μmol Gd/kg) in rats. The enhanced area is correlated with the zone of necrotic tissue verified by triphenyl tetrazolium chloride histochemical staining. The study was performed by means of a small-bore MR instrument (SIS 85/310, SISCO, Fremont, CA, USA)

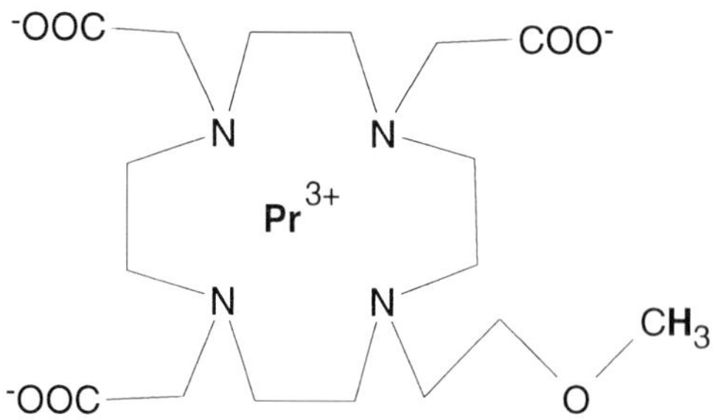

Fig. 11. Chemical structure of the praseodymium 2-methoxyethyl-DO3 A complex. The CH_3 ^1H signal exhibits a strong temperature-sensitive chemical shift well-separated from the water signal

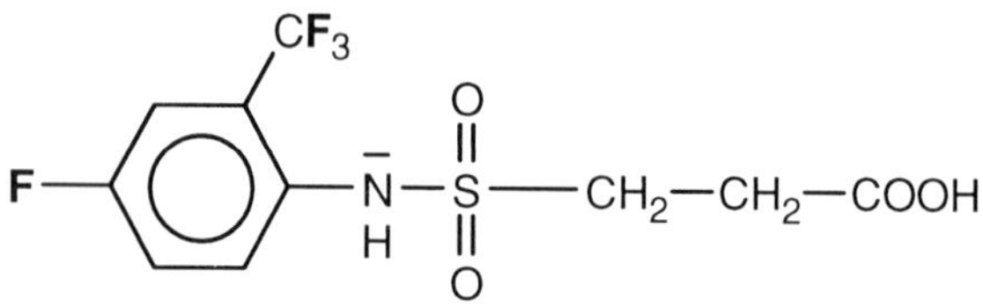

Fig. 12. Chemical structure of 3-[*N*-(4-fluor-2-trifluormethylphenyl)-sulfamoyl]-propionic acid, a ^{19}F-labeled MR spectroscopy probe for pH measurement of the extracellular matrix

both in vitro and in vivo. The shift of the methoxy group displays a sensitive temperature dependence of −0.131 ppm/°C. Using MR spectroscopic techniques, the body temperature of rats could be determined in the liver after intravenous administration of 1 mmol/kg of praseodymium. The calculated MR temperature was correlated with values obtained simultaneously with a thermocouple placed in the rectum of the animals. This technique allows a precise in vivo temperature measurement that is not disturbed by artifacts. However, localized spectroscopy of the chemically shifted ^1H signal is quite difficult.

■ pH Probes

Fluorinated compounds have been synthesized to allow a precise in vivo determination of the extracellular space pH by means of localized ^{19}F MR spectroscopy (Fig. 12) [55, 58, 59]. The resonance frequency of the fluorine nucleus is close to the hydrogen resonance and can be easily measured by conventional spectroscopic techniques (60 MHz at 1.5 T). Current mapping techniques quantify the pH by means of ^{35}P spectroscopy, but this procedure is cumbersome and allows quantification of the intracellular matrix which does not characterize the status of the cell. After intravenous injection the fluorinated compound distributes in the extracellular space. Because of differences in the pH values the two ^{19}F groups display slightly different resonance frequencies that can be easily recognized by MR techniques. The signal from the CF_3 group does not exhibit a significant pH dependence and serves as an internal reference line; the ^{19}F in the *para* position of the phenyl ring, however, displays a strong chemical shift and thus helps quantify the differences in the pH values.

■ Conclusion

Paramagnetic contrast agents have become an integral part of daily MRI not only because of their efficacy but also because of their excellent tolerance profile. It is very likely that the use of extracellular compounds, together with optimized formulation or tissue-specific materials, will expand MRI and in particular MR-guided interventional techniques including percutaneous ethanol injection or laser-induced thermotherapy [60, 61].

■ References

1. Lauterbur PC, Mendonca-Dias MH, Rudin AM (1978) Augmentation of tissue water proton spin-lattice relaxation rates by in-vivo addition of paramagnetic ions. Front Med Biol Eng 1:752–759
2. Weinmann H-J, Brasch RC, Press W-R, Wesbey GE (1984) Characteristics of gadolinium-DTPA complex: a potential NMR contrast agent. Am J Roentgenol 142 (3):619–624
3. Villringer A, Rosen BR, Belliveau JW et al (1988) Dynamic imaging with lanthanide chelates in normal brain: contrast due to magnetic susceptibility effects. Magn Reson Med 6 (2):164–174
4. Rosen BR, Brady TJ (1993) Future uses of MR imaging agents. J Comput Assist Tomogr
5. Toth E, Kiraly R, Platzek J, Radüchel B, Brücher E (1996) Equilibrium and kinetic studies on complexes of 10-(2,3-dihydroxy-(1-hydroxymethyl)-propyl)-1,4,7,10-tetraazacyclodecane-1,4,7-triacetate. Inorg Chim Acta 249:191–199
6. Haley TJ (1965) Pharmacology and toxicology of the rare earth elements. J Pharm Sci 54:663–670
7. Arvela P (1979) Toxicity of rare-earth. Prog Pharmacol 2:71–114
8. Weinmann H-J, Press W-R, Gries H (1990) Tolerance of extracellular contrast agents for magnetic resonance imaging. Invest Radiol 25:S49–S50
9. Vogler H, Platzek J, Schuhmann-Giampieri G et al (1995) Pre-clinical evaluation of gadobutrol: a new, neutral, extracellular contrast agent for magnetic resonance imaging. Eur J Radiol 21:1–10
10. Wedeking P, Kumar K, Tweedle MF (1992) Dissociation of gadolinium chelates in mice: relationship to chemical characteristics. Magn Reson Imaging 10 (4):641–648
11. Niendorf HP, Alhassan A, Geens VR, Clauss W (1994) Safety review of gadopentetate dimeglumine. Extended clinical experience after more than five million applications. Invest Radiol
12. Niendorf HP, Haustein J, Cornelius I, Alhassan A, Clauss W (1991) Safety of gadolinium-DTPA: extended

clinical experience. Magn Reson Med 22 (2):222–228; discussion 229–232
13. Weinmann H-J, Laniado M, Mützel W (1984) Pharmacokinetics of GdDTPA/dimeglumine after intravenous injection into healthy volunteers. Physiol Chem Phys Med NMR 16:167–172
14. Le Mignon MM, Chambon C, Warrington S, Davies R, Bonnemain B (1990) Gd-DOTA. Pharmacokinetics and tolerability after intravenous injection into healthy volunteers. Invest Radiol 25 (8):933–937
15. McLachlan SJ, Eaton S, De Simone DN (1992) Pharmacokinetic behavior of gadoteridol injection. Invest Radiol 27 (1):S12–S15
16. Van Wagoner M, Worah D (1993) Gadodiamide injection. First human experience with the nonionic magnetic resonance imaging enhancement agent. Invest Radiol 28 (1):S44–S48
17. Harpur ES, Worah D, Hals PA, Holtz E, Furuhama K, Nomura H (1993) Preclinical safety assessment and pharmacokinetics of gadodiamide injection, a new magnetic resonance imaging contrast agent. Invest Radiol 28:S28–S43
18. Staks T, Schuhmann-Giampieri G, Frenzel T, Weinmann H-J, Lange L, Platzek J (1994) Pharmacokinetics, dose proportionality, and tolerability of gadobutrol after single intravenous injection in healthy volunteers. Invest Radiol 29 (7):709–715
19. Schuhmann-Giampieri G, Krestin G (1991) Pharmacokinetics of Gd-DTPA in patients with chronic renal failure. Invest Radiol 26 (11):975–979
20. Weissleder R, Bogdanov A, Frank H et al (1993) AUR Memorial Award 1993. A drug system (PDH) for interventional radiology. Synthesis, properties, and efficacy. Invest Radiol 28 (12):1083–1089
21. Tanaka K, Nakamura S, Numata K et al (1992) Hepatocellular carcinoma: treatment with percutaneous ethanol injection and transcatheter arterial embolization. Radiology 185 (2):457–460
22. Sironi S, Livraghi T, Del MA (1991) Small hepatocellular carcinoma treated with percutaneous ethanol injection: MR imaging findings. Radiology 180 (2):333–336
23. Koßler S, Frenzel T, Weinmann H-J (1996) Perkutane Ethanolinjektion (PEI) unter MR-Kontrolle. Rofo Fortschr Geb Rontgenstr Neuen Bildgeb Verfahr 163 (3):316
24. Lim KO, Stark DD, Leese PT, Pfefferbaum A, Rocklage SM, Quay SC (1991) Hepatobiliary MR imaging: first human experience with MnDPDP. Radiology 178 (1):79–82
25. Rofsky NM, Earls JP (1996) Mangafodipir trisodium injection (Mn-DPDP). A contrast agent for abdominal MR imaging. Magn Reson Imaging Clin North Am 4 (1):73–85
26. Padovani B, Lecesne R, Raffaelli C et al (1996) Tolerability and utility of mangafodipir trisodium injection (MnDPDP) at the dose of 5 mumol/kg body weight in detecting focal liver tumors: results of a phase III trial using an infusion technique. Eur J Radiol 23 (3):205–211
27. Schima W, Petersein J, Hahn PF, Harisinghani M, Halpern E, Saini S (1997) Contrast-enhanced MR imaging of the liver: comparison between Gd-BOPTA and Mangafodipir. J Magn Reson Imaging 7 (1):130–135
28. Gallez B, Bacic G, Swartz HM (1996) Evidence for the dissociation of the hepatobiliary MRI contrast agent Mn-DPDP. Magn Reson Med 35 (1):14–19
29. Schuhmann-Giampieri G, Schmitt-Willich H, Press W-R, Negishi C, Weinmann H-J, Speck U (1992) Preclinical evaluation of Gd-EOB-DTPA as a contrast agent in MR imaging of the hepatobiliary system. Radiology 183 (1):59–64
30. Hamm B, Staks T, Mühler A et al (1995) Phase I clinical evaluation of Gd-EOB-DTPA as a hepatobiliary MR contrast agent: safety, pharmacokinetics, and MR imaging. Radiology 195 (3):785–792
31. Reimer P, Rummeny EJ, Shamsi K et al (1996) Phase II clinical evaluation of Gd-EOB-DTPA: dose, safety aspects, and pulse sequence. Radiology 199 (1):177–183
32. Reimer P, Rummeny EJ, Daldrup HE et al (1997) Enhancement characteristics of liver metastases, hepatocellular carcinomas, and hemangiomas with Gd-EOB-DTPA: preliminary results with dynamic MR imaging. Eur Radiol 7 (2):275–280
33. Stark DD, Weissleder R, Elizondo G et al (1988) Superparamagnetic iron oxide: clinical application as a contrast agent for MR imaging of the liver. Radiology 168 (2):297–301
34. Lawaczeck R, Bauer H, Frenzel T et al (1997) Magnetic iron oxide particles coated with carboxydextran for parenteral administration and liver contrasting pre-clinical profile of SH U555 A. Acta Radiol 38:584–597
35. Hahn PF, Stark DD, Weissleder R, Elizondo G, Saini S, Ferrucci JT (1990) Clinical application of superparamagnetic iron oxide to MR imaging of tissue perfusion in vascular liver tumors. Radiology 174 (2):361–366
36. Chachuat A, Bonnemain B (1995) European clinical experience with Endorem. A new contrast agent for liver MRI in 1000 patients. Radiologe 35 [11 Suppl 2]:S274–S276
37. Reimer P, Rummeny EJ, Daldrup HE et al (1995) Clinical results with Resovist: a phase 2 clinical trial. Radiology 195 (2):489–496
38. Lauffer RB, Parmelee DJ, Quellet HS et al (1996) MS-325: a small-molecule vascular imaging agent for magnetic resonance imaging. Acad Radiol 3:S356–S358
39. Schmiedl U, Ogan M, Paajanen H et al (1987) Albumin labeled with GdDTPA as an intravascular, blood pool-enhancing agent for MR imaging: biodistribution and imaging studies. Radiology 162:205–210
40. Schuhmann-Giampieri G, Schmitt-Willich H, Frenzel T, Press W-R, Weinmann H-J (1991) In vivo and in vitro evaluation of GdDTPA-polylysine as a macromolecular contrast agent for magnetic resonance imaging. Invest Radiol 26 (11):969–974
41. Cavagna F, Luchinat C, Scozzafava A, Xia Z (1994) Polymetallic macromolecules are potential contrast agents of improved efficiency. Magn Reson Med 31 (1):58–60
42. Desser TS, Rubin DL, Muller HH et al (1994) Dynamics of tumor imaging with GdDTPA-polyethylene glycol polymers: dependence on molecular weight. J Magn Reson Imaging 4 (3):467–472
43. Frank H, Weissleder R, Bogdanov AJ, Brady TJ (1994) Detection of pulmonary emboli by using MR angiography with MPEG-PL-GdDTPA: an experimental study in rabbits. Am J Roentgenol 162 (5):1041–1046
44. Wiener EC, Brechbiel MW, Brothers H et al (1994) Dendrimer-based metal chelates: a new class of magnetic resonance imaging contrast agents. Magn Reson Med 31 (1):1–8
45. Meyer D, Schaefer M, Chambon C, Beaute S (1994) Paramagnetic dextrans as magnetic resonance blood pool tracers. Invest Radiol 29 (2):S90–S92
46. Adam G, Mühler A, Spuntrup E et al (1996) Differentiation of spontaneous canine breast tumors using dynamic magnetic resonance imaging with 24-gadolinium-DTPA-cascade-polymer, a new blood-pool agent. Preliminary experience. Invest Radiol 31 (5):267–274
47. Loubeyre P, Canet E, Zhao S, Benderbous S, Amiel M, Revel D (1996) Carboxymethyl-dextran-gadolinium-DTPA as a blood-pool contrast agent for magnetic resonance angiography. Experimental study in rabbits. Invest Radiol 31 (5):288–293
48. Anzai Y, Prince MR, Chenevert TL et al (1997) MR angiography with an ultrasmall superparamagnetic iron oxide blood pool agent. J Magn Reson Imaging 7 (1):209–214
49. Tanoura T, Bernas M, Darkazanli A et al (1992) MR lymphography with iron oxide compound AMI-227:

studies in ferrets with filariasis. Am J Roentgenol 159 (4):875–881
50. Taupitz M, Wagner S, Hamm B, Dienemann D, Lawaczeck R, Wolf KJ (1993) MR lymphography using iron oxide particles. Detection of lymph node metastases in the VX2 rabbit tumor model. Acta Radiol 34 (1):10–15
51. Anzai Y, Prince MR (1997) Iron oxide-enhanced MR lymphography: the evaluation of cervical lymph node metastases in head and neck cancer. J Magn Reson Imaging 7 (1):75–81
52. Marchal G, Ni Y, Herijgers P et al (1996) Paramagnetic metalloporphyrins: infarct avid contrast agents for diagnosis of acute myocardial infarction by MRI. Eur Radiol 6 (1):2–8
53. Le Bihan D, Delannoy J, Levin RL (1989) Temperature mapping with MR imaging of molecular diffusion: application to hyperthermia. Radiology 171 (3):853–857
54. Delannoy J, Chen CN, Turner R, Levin RL, Le Bihan D (1991) Noninvasive temperature imaging using diffusion MRI. Magn Reson Med 19 (2):333–339
55. Frenzel T, Roth K, Kossler S et al (1996) Noninvasive temperature measurement in vivo using a temperature-sensitive lanthanide complex and 1H magnetic resonance spectroscopy. Magn Reson Med 35 (3):364–369
56. Roth K, Bartholomae G, Bauer H et al (1996) Pr(MOE-DO3 A), a praseodymium complex of a tetraazacyclododecane: an in vivo NMR thermometer. Angew Chem (Int Ed Engl) 35 (6):655–657
57. Konstanczak P, Wust P, Sander B et al (1997) Thermometry by measuring the chemical shift of lanthanide complex. Strahlenther Onkol 173 (2):106–116
58. Frenzel T, Kossler S, Bauer H, Niedballa U, Weinmann HJ (1994) Noninvasive in vivo pH measurements using a fluorinated pH probe and fluorine-19 magnetic resonance spectroscopy. Invest Radiol 29 (2):S220–S222
59. Miyazawa T, Aoki Y, Akagi K et al (1996) Application of ZK 150 471, a fluorinated pH probe for 19F-magnetic resonance spectroscopy, to in vivo pH measurement after hyperthermic treatment of tumors in mice. Acad Radiol 3 (2):S363–S364
60. Vogl TJ, Weinhold N, Muller P et al (1996) Early clinical experiences with MR-guided laser-induced thermotherapy (LITT) of liver metastases in preoperative care. Rofo Fortschr Geb Rontgenstr Neuen Bildgeb Verfahr 164 (5):413–421
61. Kahn T, Harth T, Bettag M et al (1997) Preliminary experience with the application of gadolinium-DTPA before MR imaging-guided laser-induced interstitial thermotherapy of brain tumors. J Magn Reson Imaging 7 (1):226–229

System and Environment B

The Technology and Potential of Open Magnetic Resonance Imaging

1

J. S. Dworkin

■ Introduction

The innovative designs of open magnetic resonance imaging (MRI) systems have made a significant impact in the practice of diagnostic radiology. First, the unique features of these MRI systems make it possible to bring the diagnostic versatility of MRI to a portion of the population that otherwise could not be scanned due to the physical limitations of narrow-bore MRI scanners. Second, exciting new applications such as MRI-guided tissue biopsy and minimally invasive therapies are enabled by the enhanced ability of technologists to monitor patients and by the increased radiologist accessibility to the patient achieved with open MRI designs. Finally, advances in imaging technology facilitated by hardware and software improvements have already demonstrated the ability of these systems to perform the most sophisticated pulse sequences using different magnet designs over a wide range of field strengths.

■ MRI Technology

The architecture of an MRI system is designed around a magnet, which is the largest and most visible component of the system. This provides the static magnetic field that aligns the proton spins in the patient's body. Less conspicuous are some of the other hardware subsystems depicted in Fig. 1, including shim coils, gradient coils, radiofrequency (RF) transmitter, and receiver coils. These are generally underneath the cosmetic covering, which makes the MRI scanner look sleek, clean, simple, and appealing. It is these critical hardware systems that implement the instructions of the pulse sequence, which controls the physics and tells the spins *how, what, when*, and *where* to do things to create the high-contrast MR images that radiologists all over the world read every day. In fact, the design for each of these MRI subsystems depends on the choice of the system's main magnet. It is thus instructive first to review the way in which they do function in order to better appreciate the technological synergy achieved by the MRI combining these advanced subsystems, and to understand the sensitivity of the images to limitations in their performance.

Fig. 1. MRI architecture

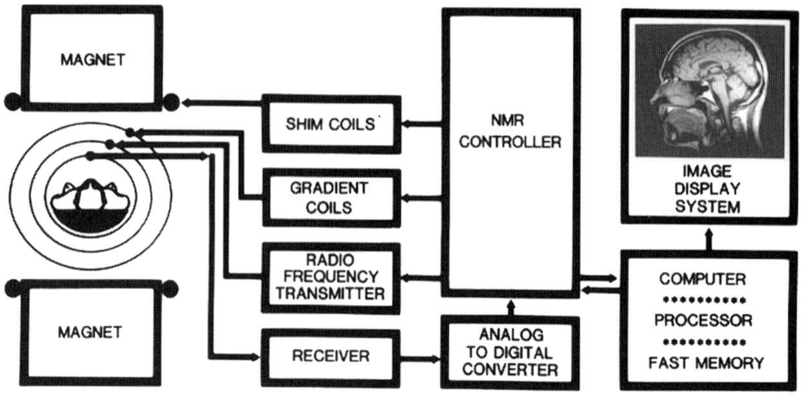

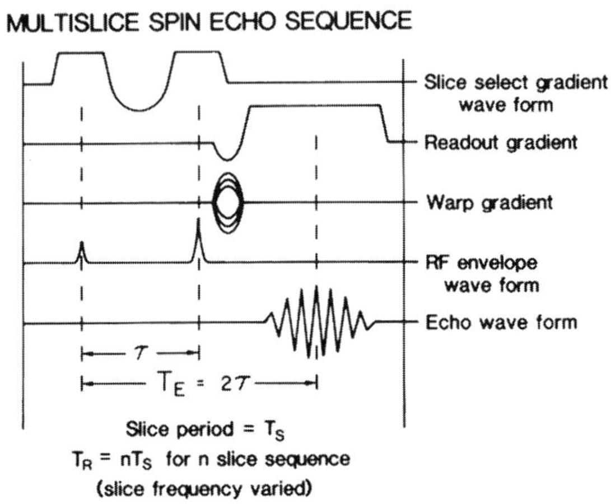

Fig. 2. Spin-echo pulse sequence

We begin with the timing diagram for the ubiquitous spin echo pulse sequence as shown in Fig. 2. Briefly, the steps in the MRI examination depicted are as follows:

- *Transmitting* RF signals at the nuclear magnetic resonance (NMR) resonant frequency of the protons from the transmitting antenna enclosed in the magnet
- Applying and controlling electric currents in a set of three orthogonal *gradient coils* in a way that facilitates measurement of the NMR signal at the location of each pixel in the image
- Tuning into the NMR signals emitted by the resonating protons in the body with a high sensitivity RF *receiver*, and using these detected NMR signals to provide the raw data for the computer reconstruction of the image

The pulse sequence diagram simply illustrates the choreography of the waveforms sent to each individual gradient, the pulses sent to the RF transmitter, and the echo detected by the RF receiver.

Precise timing during these steps is part of the overall computer control and processing function implemented in the MRI system. Tissue contrast is controlled by choosing scan acquisition parameters such as the echo time (TE) and the repetition time (TR). Judicious choices unleash the diagnostic power of the MRI, which originates with the T1 and T2 relaxation time differences between neighboring tissues. The result is the unparalleled soft tissue contrast resolution of MR images. Special hardware processors and a fast memory calculate and store the images, which are finally displayed and manipulated, often with independent microprocessors.

Imaging Requirements

Images require quality performance for the following MRI system specifications: *magnetic field strength*, *field uniformity*, *field stability*, and *pulsed gradient fidelity*. Each of these is in turn influenced by the magnet design chosen as the platform for the MRI system. What happens if any of these requirements is compromised?

A complete analysis of the *field strength* specification is beyond the scope of this discussion (see Kaufman and Kramer, this volume). MRI systems are available for routine clinical use from 640 G (0.064 T) up to 20,000 G (2.0 T). The broad range of magnet systems successfully marketed today (often several by just a *single* manufacturer) is testimony to the tradeoffs faced by potential purchasers. Some countries have established limited reimbursement to users based on field strength, and the American College of Radiology is intending to develop objective performance standards for site accreditation involving spatial resolution, signal-to-noise, and contrast-to-noise [1]. Despite the increase in the signal-to-noise ratio which can be obtained at the higher field strengths [2], there are many compensating factors making lower and middle-field MRI units competitive [3, 4].

MRI magnets are designed to create a *uniform* magnetic field throughout the imaging volume where the patient is positioned. Although field homogeneity requirements are much less stringent for proton imaging than for spectroscopy, the variation of the magnet's main static magnetic field must still be substantially less than the variation superimposed during the application of the pulsed gradients. This guarantees precise pixel definition for every image. Highly homogeneous magnetic fields also provide the only environment in which lower bandwidth pulse sequences can be successfully implemented in clinical MRI protocols. Low-bandwidth techniques improve the image signal-to-noise by employing smaller gradient amplitudes while simultaneously maintaining spatial resolution.

It is also desirable that the main magnetic field change as little as possible during the MR acquisition. As seen in the pulse sequence timing diagram above, an MRI scan is a series of repeated measurements, and *field stability* ensures that there is no miscoding of the spatial information between individual measurements.

Finally, the ability to control the *pulsed gradient magnetic fields* is critical. Several specifications describing the gradients are commonly used as benchmarks. The gradient's *maximum amplitude*, measured in millitesla per meter (mT/m) determines the MRI's minimum achievable field-of-view (FOV). *Linearity* resembles the magnet's uniformity. We want to minimize any deviation from the theoretical linearity of the gradient magnetic fields. *Temporal stability* is important because we depend on the gradient magnetic fields remaining constant over critical times in the application of the pulse sequence, such as when the slice selective radiofrequency pulses are transmitted or during the frequency encoding of the NMR signal. Instabilities can lead to misplaced slices and blurring of the images. Furthermore, we have added flexibility in pulse sequence design if we can reach these gradient amplitudes quickly, and the *rise time* is a good way to gauge the response of the system. The time required for the gradients to reach full amplitude should be less than 1 ms. Finally, the *duty cycle* indicates how long the superimposed magnetic field from the gradients is applied over the duration of the pulse sequence.

Unfortunately, the ever-increasing gradient strength and decreasing rise times required for the development of new pulse sequences is constrained. That is, it is not possible simple to program whatever one wants and expect it to work. A major contributor to this limitation is the effect of *eddy currents*, which result from the application of a magnetic field that changes quickly in time to a conductive metal surface. These eddy currents flow within the metal surface and *oppose* the nearby changing field. Physicists refer to this opposition as Lenz' law. The consequence is that the induced magnetic field distorts the applied gradient field in the imaging volume, causing deterioration in the quality of the MR images.

■ Magnet Designs for MRI Systems

The design of MRI magnets, as with virtually everything in life, is a matter of compromise. Magnet designers make choices among such key specifications as the magnet configuration, type of construction, field strength, physical dimensions, weight, shape, size of the imaging volume, homogeneity, and cost. Benefits and limitations must be evaluated based on the anticipated use of the system [5].

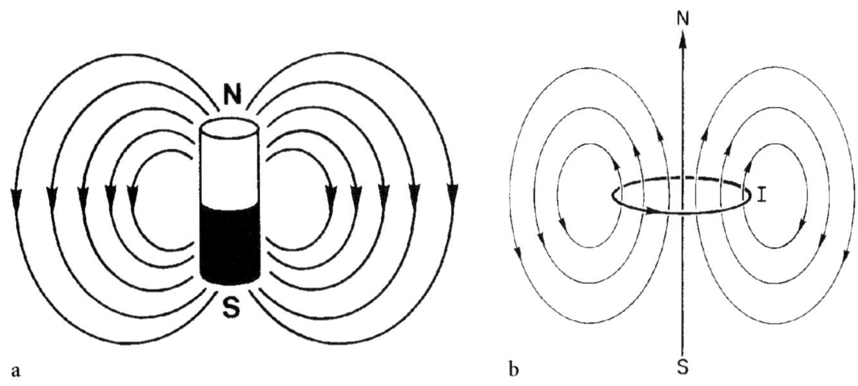

Fig. 3a,b. Creating magnetic fields. **a** Permanent magnet. **b** Current-carrying wire

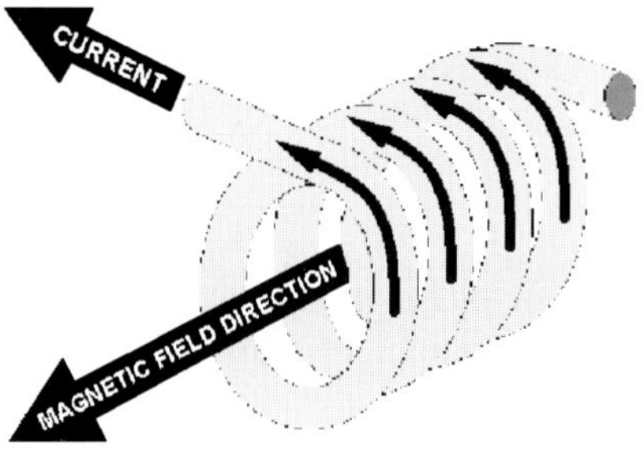

Fig. 4. Solenoid

There are two ways to generate a magnetic field. Most persons are readily familiar with magnetized metal alloys, or permanent magnets (as shown in Fig. 3a). They have gained their experience possibly in school science classes, viewing the patterns of iron filings on a piece of paper, or at home, securing notes for family members to the face of the refrigerator. Permanent magnets have been successfully implemented in many medical systems, including MRI magnets. An alternative means of creating a magnetic field is provided via the laws of physics through Ampere's law of magnetic induction, which describes how a current-carrying wire generates a magnetic field around that wire (Fig. 3b). Any number of possible conductor geometries can be investigated as the basis for a magnet design, and physicists routinely solve Maxwell's equations to understand the magnetic field characteristics for these alternative designs.

For the solenoid design illustrated in Fig. 4, magnet designers build around the magnetic field strength's direct proportional dependence on both the amount of electric current and the number of turns in the conductor in an attempt to navigate the tradeoffs in designing practical MRI magnet systems. Early *air-core resistive magnet designs* required a significant power supply to maintain the current in the solenoid. Field strengths of up to 0.2 T could be reached for practical designs. But there were important limitations, which can be simplistically considered to be caused by the resistance and inductance of the magnet coils. Resistance is the property of a circuit that opposes or limits current. Inductance, however, is the property of a circuit that *opposes any change* in current [6]. The result is that the significant voltage required and the current which is sensitive to voltage modulations translates into magnetic field instabilities. The conducting coils must be water-cooled to remove the heat generated by the wire's resistance, and this takes up more space in the overall magnet design. In addition, the conductor geometry establishes the field uniformity; any motion due to resistive heating and vibration from cooling water turbulence degrades the uniformity and stability of the magnetic field.

Superconductivity was a significant step forward in air-core solenoid design. Immersing the coiled conductor in a bath of liquid helium at the incredibly low temperature of $-268\,^{\circ}C$ made possible large ampere turns and high field strengths with little power because the electrical resistance of the conductor became negligible. The design also desensitized the position of the conductors vis-à-vis field uniformity and stability. During the early 1980s when the first commercial MRI units were being installed some believed that higher magnetic field strengths offered the easiest way to increase image quality [7]. This, and the desire for spectroscopic measurements, drove the market to embrace magnetic fields strengths up to 2.0 T.

The price of this sophistication, however, is another level of cost and complexity. It is necessary to maintain the cryogenic-load environment, and generally a carefully designed evacuated cryostat is required which adds to the size of the magnet (Fig. 5a). There was also a large fringe field which had to be addressed (Fig. 5b); the horizontal flux lines emanating from the superconducting magnet needed to be controlled. One solution was to surround the magnet with magnetic shielding;

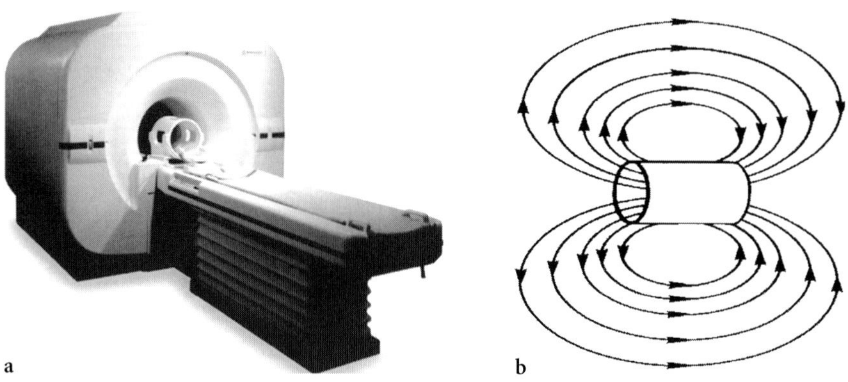

Fig. 5 a, b. Superconducting MRI design. **a** Superconducting magnet. **b** Fringe field otherwise the MRI suite would require substantial space for installation. Recent innovations for ameliorating the fringe field problem include using *active* shielding to reduce the fringe field. In this scheme an *additional* static magnetic field is created by placing coils of *opposite* polarity *outside* the main magnet coils to cancel the field outside the magnet and only partially cancel it inside.

A similar solution evolved to reduce the unwanted *eddy currents* induced in the metal housing containing the magnet coils. These *self-shielded* gradient designs mean more gradient-type coils must be packed cylindrically around the regular gradient coils to undo the distortions eddy currents produce inside the bore of the magnet. The disadvantage is wasted physical space and added power consumption. There are, however, substantial imaging performance benefits. In fact, this area of research has been central in providing the means to successfully implement the faster imaging sequences now used on a routine basis. It also highlights a prime example of changes facilitated by hardware and software improvements yielding new and more powerful imaging applications.

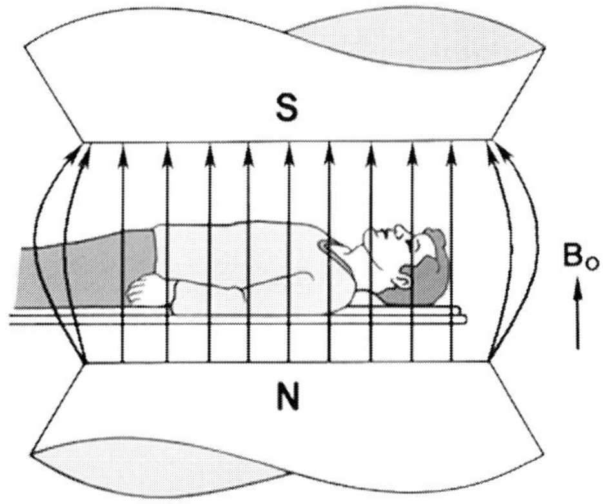

Fig. 6. Vertical magnetic field between two poles

■ Open MRI

Newer MRI systems feature open designs rather than the cylindrical tunnel arrangement in a conventional superconducting MRI system [8]. Economic pressures in the healthcare environment and patient demands for comfort and reduced anxiety in MRI examinations have driven and will continue to drive trends in terms of open MRI products. Cost-effective siting, lower capital and operating costs, easy maintenance, advances in performance enabling a full range of clinical applications, and the unique positioning for investigating interventional MRI procedures have generated enormous enthusiasm on the part of purchasers [9].

A comparison of the open MRI systems on the market today is presented in Table 1. Nonsuperconducting designs are available in a variety of configurations and at different field strengths. These include both permanent magnets and iron-core electromagnets. Various design alternatives exist among the iron-core electromagnets, including both C-arm and four-post configurations. A recent product even utilizes an iron-core superconducting magnet [10]. They all, however, share several significant design advantages. First, an iron-circuit is employed to contain the magnetic flux and channel it between two poles. This creates a vertical magnetic field *transverse* to the patient (Fig. 6), in contrast to the horizontal field orientation along the patient's axis characteristic of the conventional superconducting magnets. Second, the iron flux-return also serves to minimize the fringe magnetic field (Fig. 7), decreasing the amount of space required to install an entire MRI suite and eliminating the need for any additional magnetic shielding. This design approach for open MRI began with the rectangular two-post MRI magnets at 0.3 T manufactured and installed first by Fonar Corporation in the early 1980s. There were two magnet types, one permanent and one electromagnet, both with iron flux returns and a vertical magnetic field orientation (Fig. 8). Similar-looking designs were subsequently introduced by Hitachi and Resonex.

Table 1. Open MRI systems currently on the market

Manufacturer	Field strength (T)	Magnet configuration	Type of construction
Fonar	0.60	Iron-core electromagnet	Four-post
Fonar	0.35	Iron-core electromagnet	Four-post
General Electric	0.20	Permanent	Two-post
Hitachi	0.30	Permanent	Two-post
Picker	0.23	Iron-core electromagnet	C-arm
Siemens	0.20	Iron-core electromagnet	C-arm
Toshiba	0.064	Permanent	Four-post
Toshiba	0.35	Iron-core superconducting	Four-post

Fig. 7 a, b. Iron flux returns. a Permanent magnet flux return. b Iron-core electromagnet design

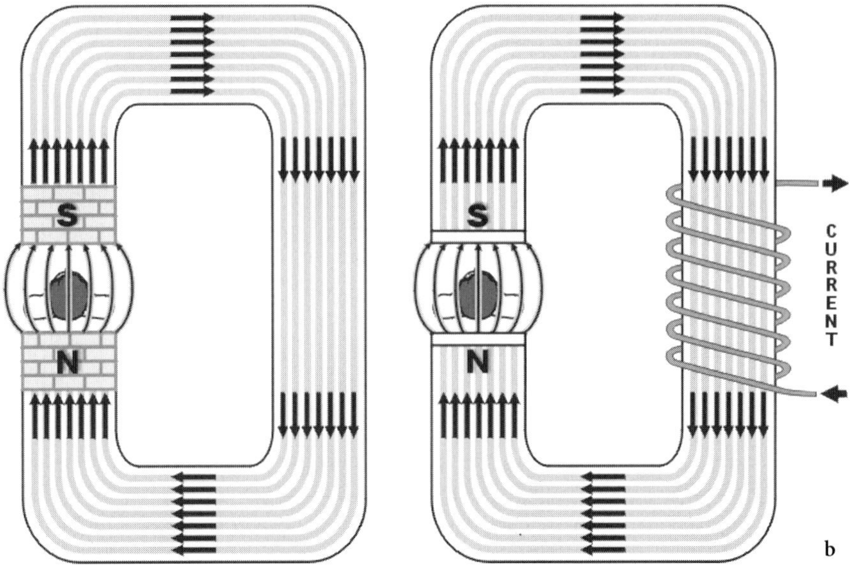

a b

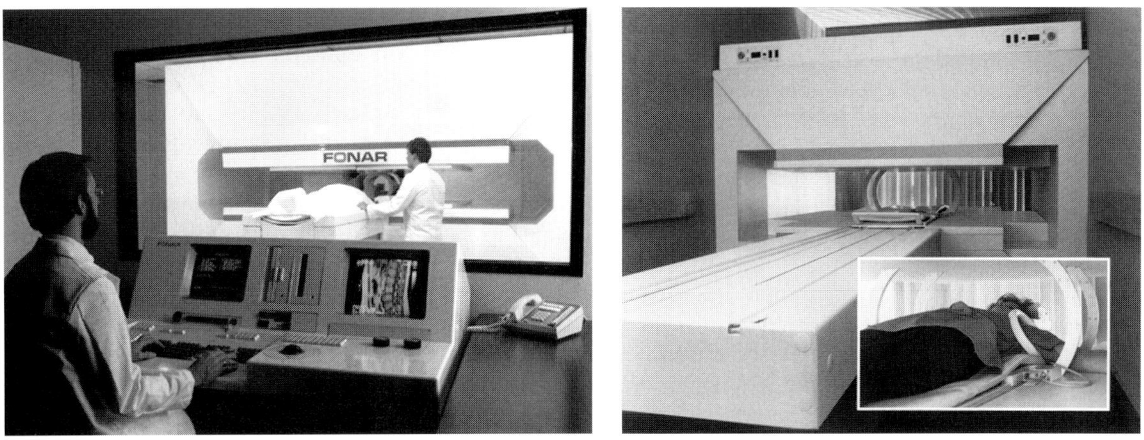

a b

Fig. 8 a, b. Rectangular two-post MRI magnets. **a** Permanent MRI magnet. **b** Iron-core MRI electromagnet

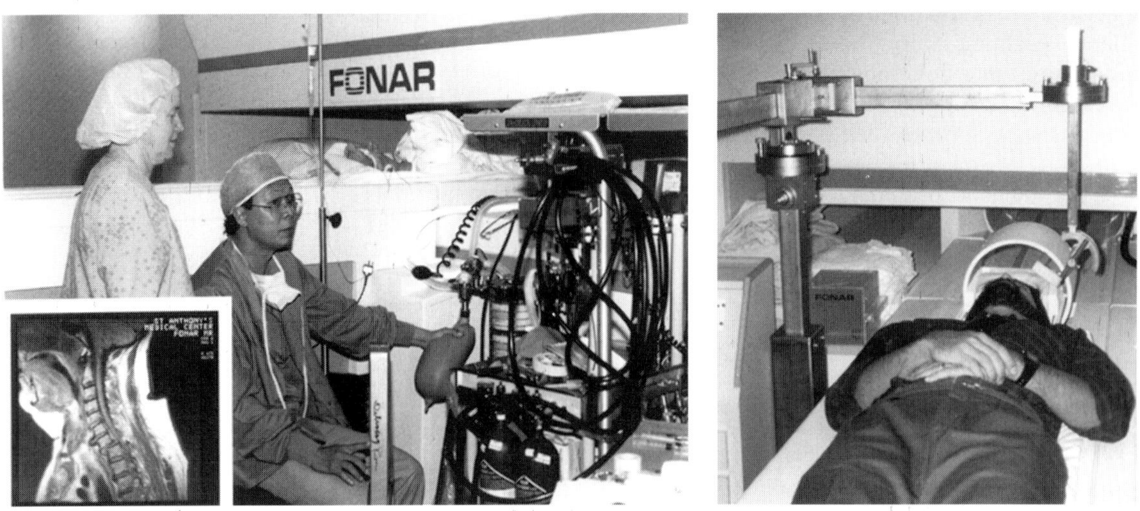

a b

Fig. 9 a, b. Rectangular magnet design advantages. **a** Small fringe field. **b** MR stereotactic system

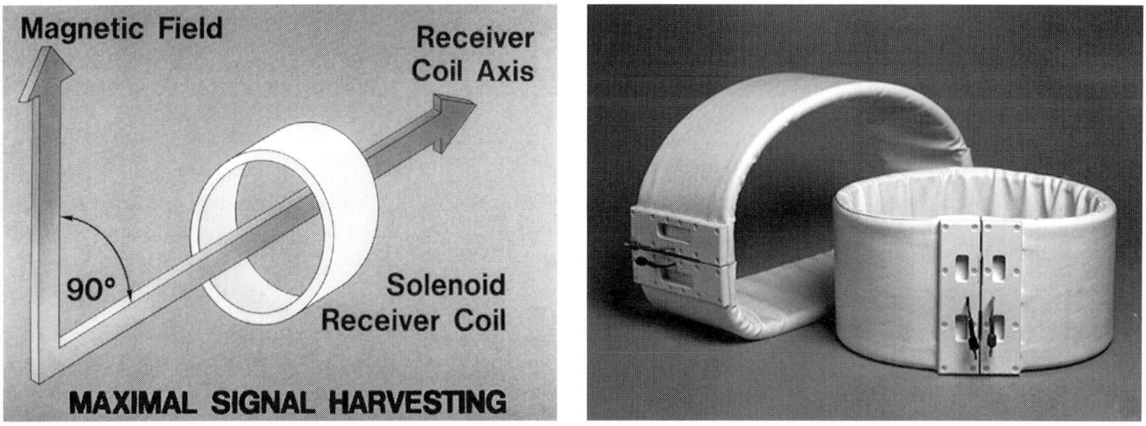

a b

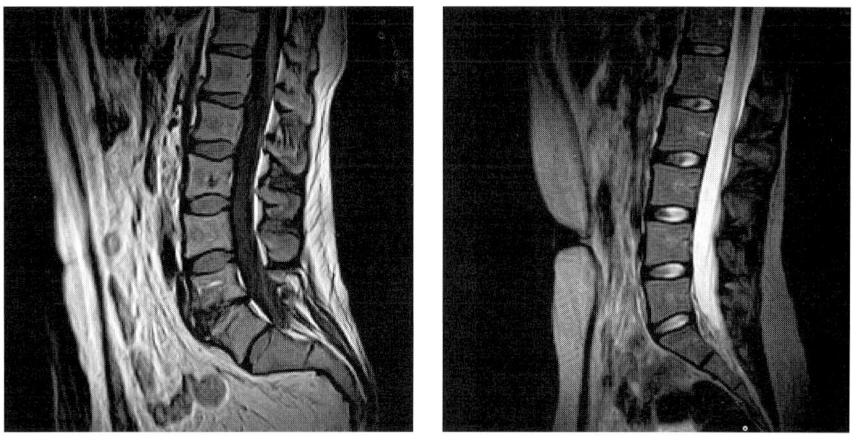

c

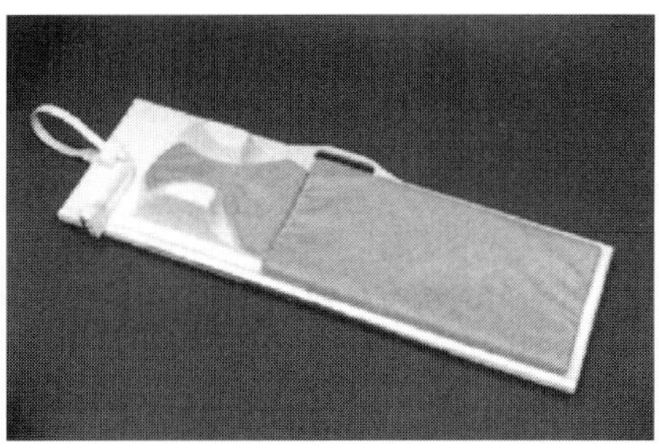

d

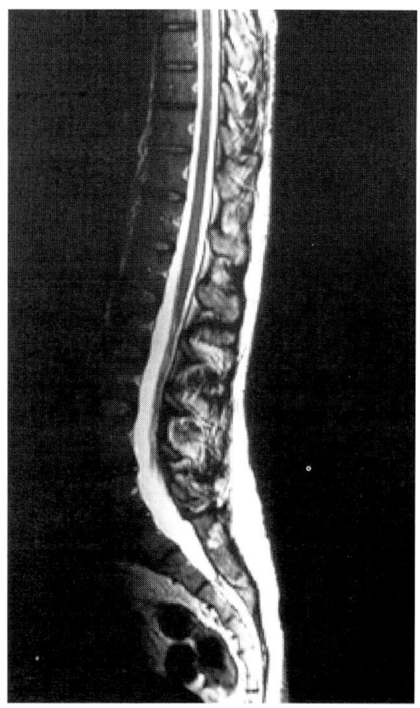

e

Fig. 10 a–e. RF receiver coils and images. **a** Coil alignment requirements. **b** Wrap-around solenoid coils. **c** T1 and T2 images using solenoidal receiver coils. **d** Planar receiver coil. **e** Sample T2 image: planar coil

The initial conception of acquiring orthopedic kinematic studies of the moving shoulder and other joints was derived from this original open MRI magnet design. Notice that there was even enough room for patients to stretch out their arms. These MRI systems were also able to take advantage of the magnet's small fringe field by placing life support equipment directly next to the magnet (Fig. 9a). This is critical for trauma applications. This magnet design also eliminates the dangers of the missile effect, a concern with superconducting MRI systems since loose ferromagnetic objects can be lifted out of the pockets of unsuspecting support personnel and travel along the horizontal field lines into the magnet bore. Other specialized clinical applications performed with these MRI systems included the successful adapting of a CT stereotactic system for use with MR-guided percutaneous procedures (Fig. 9b), as described elsewhere [11].

Compatibility with highly efficient solenoid RF receiver coils is another significant benefit derived directly from the choice of the transverse magnetic field. Remember that MRI physics requires the axis of the receiver coil to be perpendicular to the main magnetic field (Fig. 10a). As persons are cylindrically roughly symmetric, flexible wrap-around single-loop receiving antennas are a simple and elegant approach to MRI surface coil design. High signal-to-noise solenoids can be manufactured in varying circumferences to achieve an optimal filling factor for each region of the anatomy (Fig. 10b). The uniform posterior-anterior signal intensity achieved with this solenoid design, as shown in Fig. 10c, is absent in images acquired with the conventional superconducting system's flat planar coil (Fig. 10d). In this case the images are characterized by an exponential signal intensity falloff (Fig. 10e) [12].

The various open MRI systems summarized in Table 1 do have differences that should be appreciated. In permanent magnet designs magnetic material itself generates the magnetic field instead of electric currents. This concept is illustrated in Fig. 7a. Benefits include the fact that no electricity is needed to generate the magnetic field, and that no water cooling of any conductors is required. However, the temperature of the magnetic material must be maintained within a tight tolerance because there is some thermal sensitivity. It is also impossible to switch off the magnetic field. Examples of permanent MRI magnets are shown in Fig. 11.

The alternative design concept behind the iron-core electromagnet has already been illustrated in Fig. 7b. The open MRI systems shown in Fig. 12

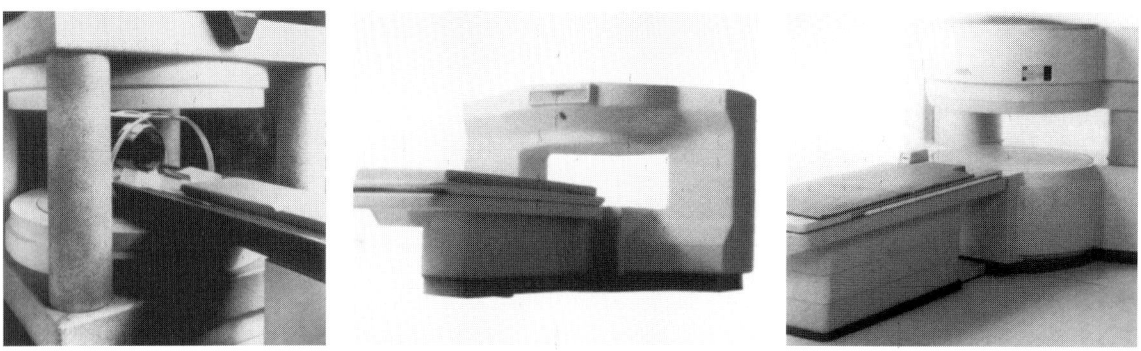

a b, c

Fig. 11 a–c. Permanent magnets. **a** 0.064 T. **b** 0.20 T. **c** 0.30 T

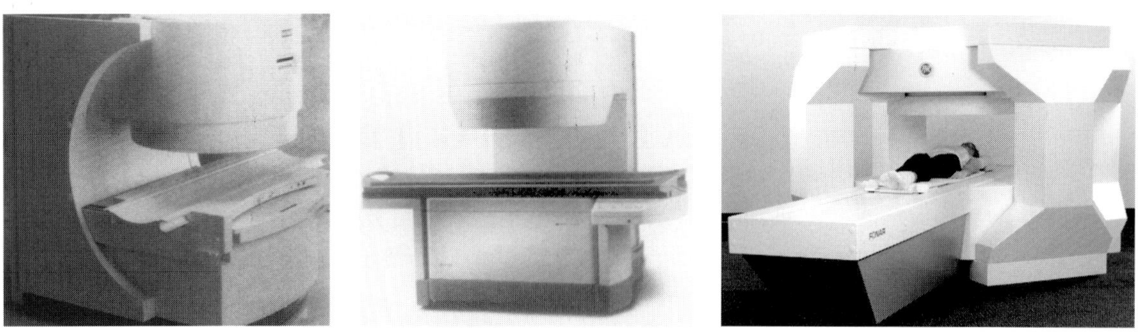

a b, c

Fig. 12 a–c. Iron-core electromagnets. **a** 0.20 T. **b** 0.23 T. **c** 0.6 T

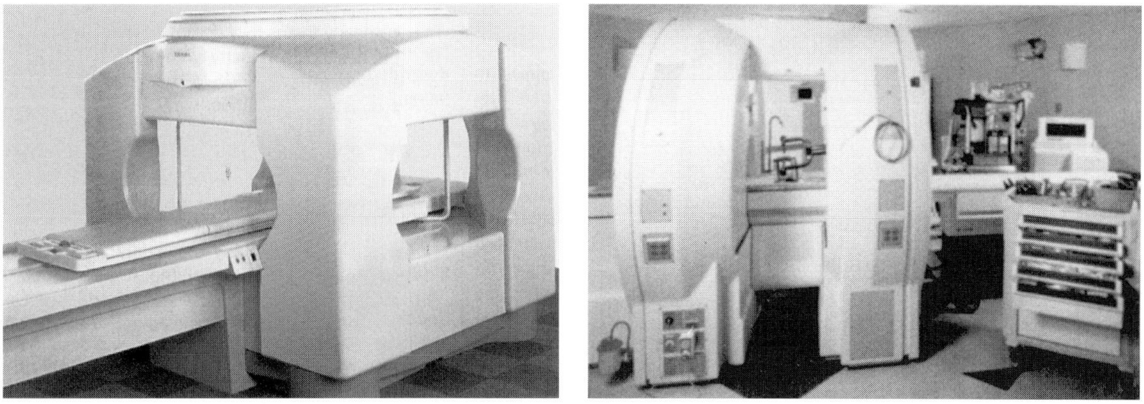

a b

Fig. 13 a, b. Superconducting magnets. **a** 0.35 T. **b** 0.5 T

all overcome the limitations of the air-core resistive magnets described earlier by using iron to concentrate the flux. The principal benefit is that higher magnetic field strengths can be achieved using weaker currents. The field homogeneity is also less dependent on the configuration of the conductors. The single-post designs (Fig. 12), also referred to as C-arms or "clam shells," are available at field strengths of 0.20 and 0.23 T. A four-post construction design creates a more symmetric flux coupling mechanism between the top and bottom poles and also provides enhanced mechanical stability. For a moderate increase in power consumption and weight, field strengths up to 0.6 T can be reached (Fig. 12c).

Superconducting technology has also been used to create open MRI products. An iron-core vertical field open MRI system utilizing a superconducting magnet has recently been introduced. This operates at a field strength of 0.35 T and also offers the benefits of the four-post design (Fig. 13a). Another product utilizes superconducting coils in a split cryostat (Fig. 13b). Here the physician can approach the patient from two sides. This system operates with a horizontal magnetic field orientation at a field strength of 0.5 T and has been designed for the specialized application of MRI-guided interventional procedures (General Electric Medical Systems, Milwaukee, WI) [13].

Another MRI system designed for the specialized application of MR image-guided surgery and minimally invasive therapy is shown in Fig. 14. Here the attending medical team have unrestricted (360°) access to the patient. Two magnetic poles are positioned at the center of a full-size room. The walls and ceiling of the room provide the iron flux return for the magnetic field. The ceiling height is a standard 8 ft, the room width is 14 ft, and the length is effectively unlimited. The iron-core vertical field electromagnet is designed to produce an imaging field strength of 0.6 T (Fonar, Melville, NY).

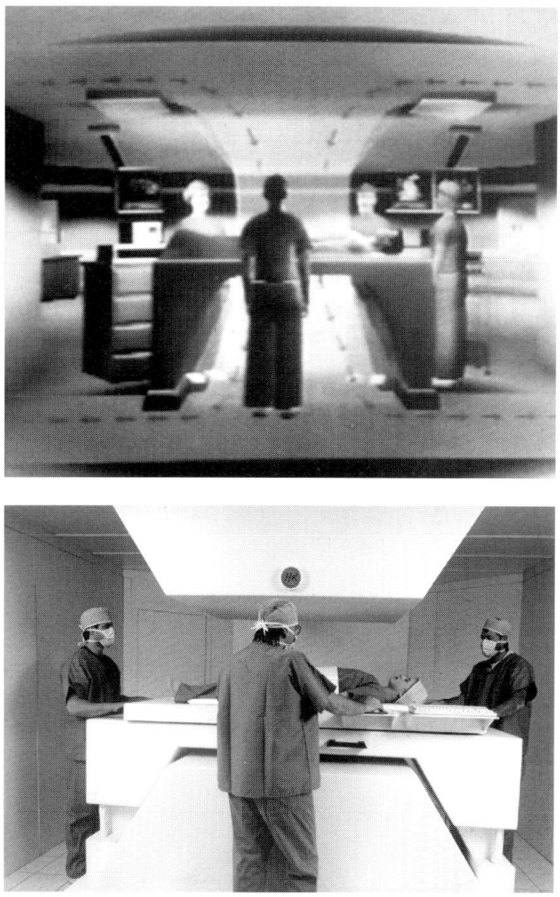

a b

Fig. 14 a, b. Interventional MRI with 360° patient accessibility. **a** Elevation view. **b** Unrestricted access for a surgical team a 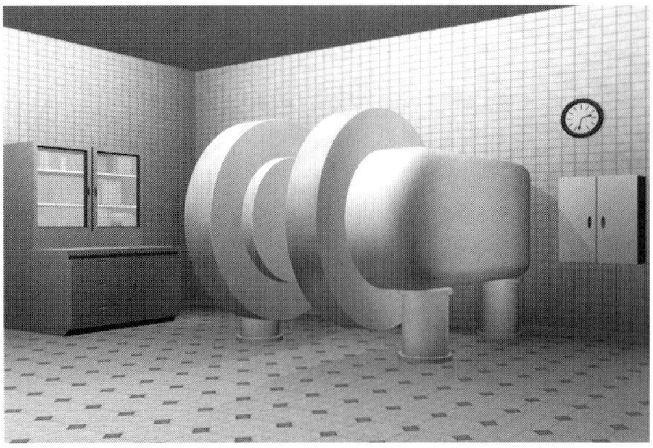 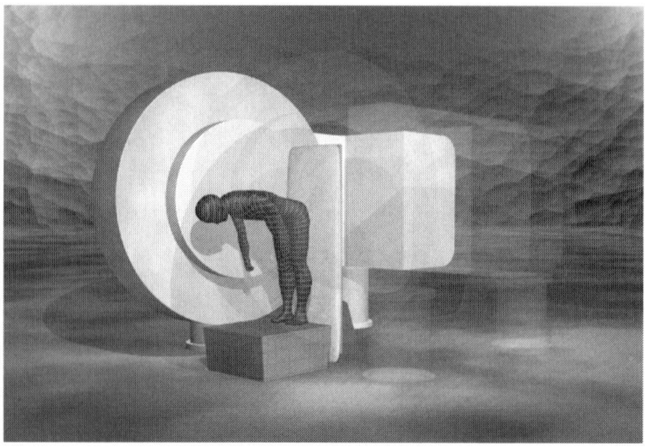 b

Fig. 15 a, b. MRI for weight-bearing imaging studies. **a** Elevation view. **b** Patient positioning

A different MRI design in which the patient can stand upright is shown in Fig. 15. The magnetic field is transverse to the patient (as in the vertical field MRI systems), but in this case the patient can be positioned parallel with the earth's gravitational field. This allows imaging the spine and joints in the weight-bearing state (Fonar).

■ Clinical Applications

The proliferation of numerous open MRI systems incorporating vertical field iron-core technology is a testimony to the inherent flexibility of the design. A planar (flat) gradient geometry is an efficient scheme for generating gradient magnetic fields. In addition, the gradient packages installed in these open MRI magnets are bolted to the immovable poles themselves; this reduces the vibration of the gradient package yielding improvements in stability and reducing the potentially high noise level that so distracts the patient during the examination. Advances in pole design can also improve the field uniformity. Innovations in pole construction have reduced or eliminated eddy currents, a development of significant importance because it obviates the need for installing flat self-shielded gradients on the poles. Un-

a 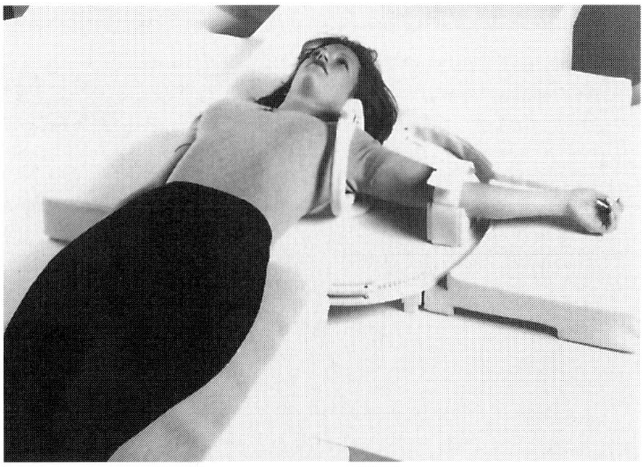

b 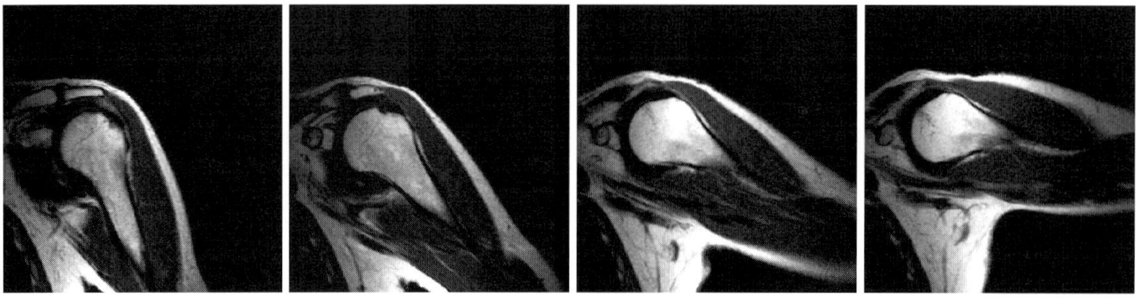

Fig. 16 a, b. a Kinematic shoulder fixture and images. **b** Dynamic shoulder study

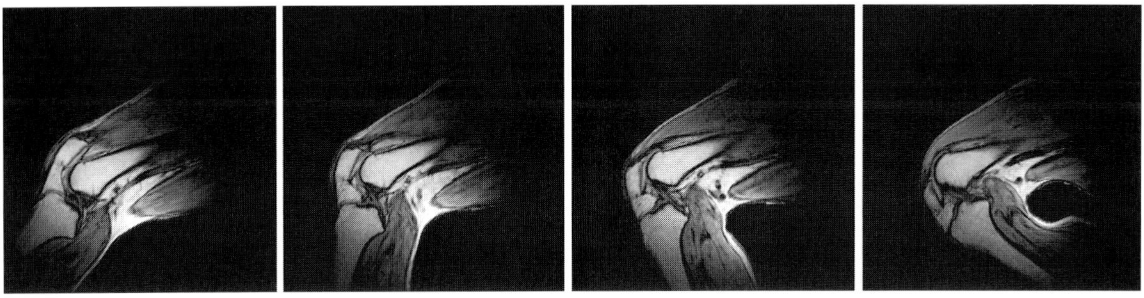

Fig. 17. Kinematic knee study

a 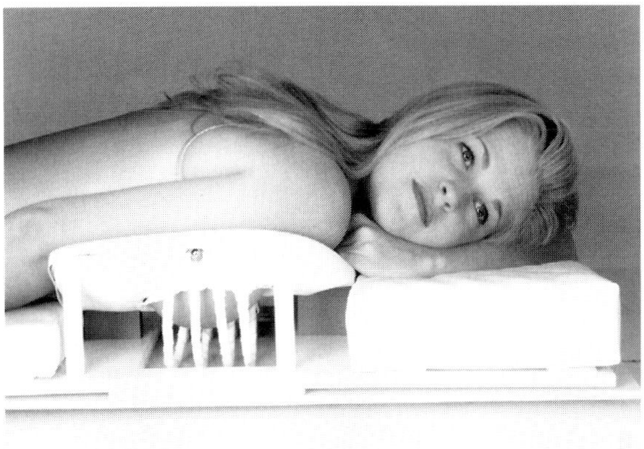

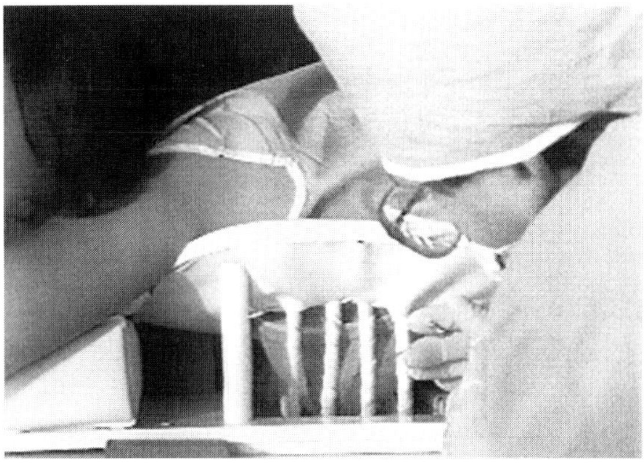 b

Fig. 18 a, b. Bilateral prone dedicated breast coil. a Patient under normal scanning conditions. b Access for MR-guided biopsy

der these circumstances the vertical patient gap dimension can be increased, and the system's overall gradient power consumption is decreased. Indeed, each manufacturer offers a slightly different menu of fast imaging options which can have an impact on both patient throughput and the ability to perform specific clinical exams [14].

The spaciousness of open MRI systems has brought the benefits of MRI to a portion of the population that otherwise could not be scanned, namely anxious, claustrophobic, and very large patients. Family members can stay with the patient and be visible during the scan, providing comfort and relieving patient anxiety. This has become a primary consideration for patients who are requesting open MRI scans.

The spaciousness has other beneficial consequences, including a full range of motion and easy patient positioning for kinematic studies acquired using special orthopedic fixtures. An example of a shoulder fixture which can be moved in fixed increments under computer control, and several images from the resulting dynamic shoulder study, are shown in Fig. 16.

A wide range of motion can also be achieved in a kinematic knee study (Fig. 17), particularly if the vertical gap dimensions permit patients to be scanned on their sides. The potential for lateral decubitus positioning should also enable applications for gravity-dependent MRI which visualizes the impact of fluids moving down and air up within the body cavity.

Specialized receiver coils, such as the bilateral prone dedicated breast coil shown in Fig. 18a, can also be designed. This coil is most effectively utilized with the wide patient bed that only open MRI systems can accommodate. Notice also that the coil has been designed in an open manner to facilitate MRI guidance of tissue biopsy (Fig. 18b), one of many applications envisioned for open MRI units in the future. Such successful intervention will require superior image quality to provide the speed and resolution necessary to minimize interference while targeting a lesion. Minimally invasive surgical procedures under MR guidance will also require maximum flexibility in the ability of physicians to approach the patient based on the degree of access afforded by the open MRI design.

References

1. Pomeranz SJ (1996) Rising to the challenge: a fresh look at open MR. CMRS Vision June 1996, 2(2):1–3
2. Bell RA (1996) Let's be honest about open MRI. Med Imaging Nov 1996:44
3. Stark D (1995) The argument for mid-field MRI. Appl Radiol Feb 1995:9
4. Oldendorf W Jr (1996) MRI: alive and well. Imaging Econ 9 (1):Jan/Feb 1996:77–78
5. Gordon R, Timms W (1984) Magnet systems used in medical NMR. Comput Radiol 8 (5):245–261
6. Capon RJ, Warner D (1988) Electronics fundamentals. Prentice Hall, Englewood Cliffs
7. Jack Jr CR, Berquist TH, Miller GM, Forbes GS, Gray JE, Morin RL, Ilstrup DM (1990) Field strength in neuro-MR imaging: A comparison of 0.5 T and 1.5 T. Journal of Computer Assisted Tomography 14(4):505–513
8. Plymouth Meeting (1995) High field strength vs. low field strength and open MRI. ECRI Health Technology Assessment Information Service
9. Open MRI Maintains Star Status to Produce Impressive Q2 Results. MRI Industry Report, October 1997, p 1–5. Edited by James Brice, Miller Freeman, San Francisco, CA
10. Crooks L (1997) Open Magnets for MRI Medical Electronics, December 1997, published by Measurements and Data Corporation, Pittsburgh
11. Lufkin R, Duckweiler G, Spickler E, Teresi L, Chang M, Onik G (1988) MR body stereotaxis: an aid for MR-guided biopsies. J Comput Assist Tomogr 12 (6):1088–1089
12. Faulkner W Jr (1995) Imaging coil technology. In: Woodward P, Freimarck R (eds) MRI for technologists. McGraw-Hill, New York
13. Schenck JF, Jolesz FA et al (1995) Superconducting open-configuration MR imaging system for image-guided therapy. Radiology 195:805–814
14. Femano P (1995) Jargon jungle revisited: Buyers Beware. Publisher: Miller Freeman, Inc, San Francisco. MR The News Magazine of Magnetic Resonance (Fall 1995):11–13

Instruments and Equipment for Open-Field Magnetic Resonance Imaging 2

A. Melzer

■ Introduction

Interventional MRI procedures have become substantially more feasible with the advent of open-field systems [1, 2] (Table 1). Many new procedures are now possible [3, 4], and several instruments and ancillary equipment for carrying them out have appeared on the market. However, the types of instruments necessary for the carrying out interventional MRI procedures have not yet been clearly defined. We present here our preliminary results evaluating the devices and illustrate their application.

Table 1. Open MRI systems

Manufacturer	Field strength (T)	Magnet configuration	Type of construction
Fonar	0.60	Iron-core electromagnet	Four-post
	0.35	Iron-core electromagnet	Four-post
General Electric	0.20	Permanent	Two-post
	0.50	Superconducting	Two rings, vertical
Hitachi	0.30	Permanent	Two-post
Picker	0.23	Iron-core electromagnet	C-arm
Siemens	0.20	Iron-core electromagnet	C-arm
Toshiba	0.064	Permanent	Four-post
	0.35	Iron-core superconducting	Four-post

■ Ancillary Equipment

The physical nature of MRI instruments and electric equipment affects their use near the magnet. High (radiofrequency, RF) emission from electrical equipment particularly near the Larmor frequency of the open systems can severely reduce image quality (see Fig. 1). Electric shielding and RF filter systems are helpful, but this modification is difficult and cost intensive. Many pieces of equipment can be placed outside the MR suite and controlled via glass fiber and optic coupling. The acquisition system can be used to control electric equipment that emits problematic frequencies so that the devices are switched on and off during the actual image acquisition. These techniques require special software and sequence technology which are now under development.

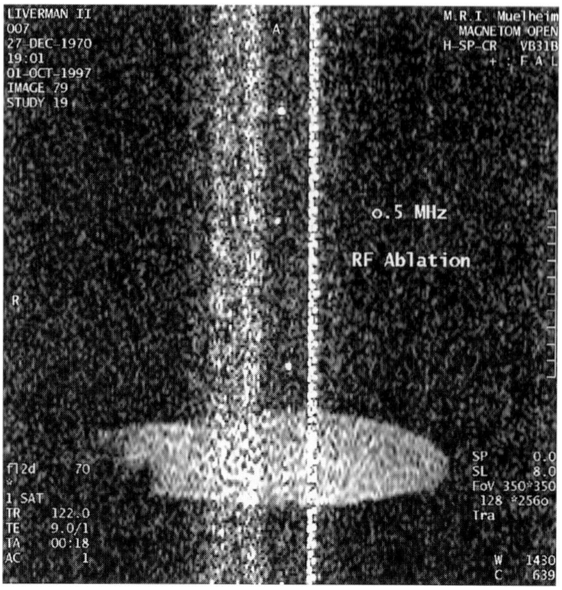

Fig. 1. MR image acquisition (Magnetom Open, Siemens) of an ex vivo liver specimen during RF ablation while the RF generator works with a frequency of 0.5 MHz. The disturbances are caused by RF noise, the range of 8 MHz, and the respective harmonic frequencies

■ Electric Generators

Most electrical generators with axial fans such as light sources, laser, RF, and suction should be placed outside the shielded cabin of the magnet. It is far too costly to modify electric equipment such as RF generators and high power light sources to provide an interference-free use. If an electric coupling is present that runs into the magnet, for example, endoscopic camera and cable and RF needle, these elements function as antennae and may transmit the RF signals from the generator even if it is placed outside the cabin.

RF noise reduction can be achieved in some devices using special RF filters that eliminate the frequencies around 8 MHz and the respective resonance frequencies. However, the sensitivity of MR units and the variance between open and closed magnets with their different RF systems make a general RF compatibility very difficult. Thus for each magnet a special adaptation is required. For the particular purpose of RF ablation techniques it is possible to switch the RF device on and off during the image acquisition. This, however, requires a kind of triggering or synchronization between the RF generator and the acquisition system. The ECG triggering can also be used to provide the acquisition system with a similar signal characteristic as ECG to control the acquisition. This, however, leads to relatively long interruptions of the RF application, and thus effective heating of tissue can be diminished. Further evaluation of RF ablation is required to find the optimal combination of RF generator and MR acquisition system. The cost and effectiveness of tissue ablation RF techniques make them superior to laser techniques. Laser, however, lacks an electric wire for energy supply, which makes it technically safer because there is no antenna transmission between generator and magnet field. Conventional laser generators disturb the image acquisition and need to be placed outside the cabin or switched off during image acquisition. A semiconductor diode laser (Diomed) now allows use inside the MR suite.

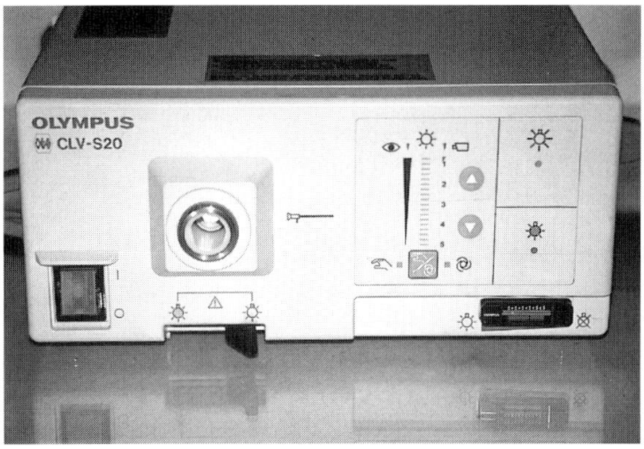

Fig. 2. The light source CLV S20 (Olympus, Tokyo) can be used in the MR suite if it is placed at the ground and in closest proximity to the magnet

■ Light Sources

Siemens has developed a low-power halogen light source with no interference with the imaging system. Unfortunately, this light source can only be used for the magnet illumination. Endoscopy requires higher power and the better color temperature of xenon light [5].

Procedures performed within the magnet and requiring light should be assisted by "cold light." Endoscopic procedures require high-power light sources with daylight quality. The light source (CLV S20, Olympus, Tokyo) (Fig. 2) can be used in the MR suite if it is placed on the floor and in close proximity to the magnet. However, this position is unacceptable from the safety point of view. To avoid this drawback we have collaborated in the development of a 10-m light cable with full MR compatibility (see Fig. 3). It can thus be used throughout the whole procedure, and even when the light cable is within the image plane, it does not cause artifacts. Two types are available, with 3.5 and 5 mm light transmission. The light source can be placed outside the RF cabin and does not interfere with imaging.

Adjustment of the light intensity is achieved through the camera control unit, which can be connected to the light source via a coaxial cable. The camera unit should be place outside the magnet because RF emissions cannot be eliminated completely. However, the line between the chip camera and the control unit should not exceed 5 m to allow optimal image quality. Longer cables decrease the signal to noise ratio (S/N) of the video image.

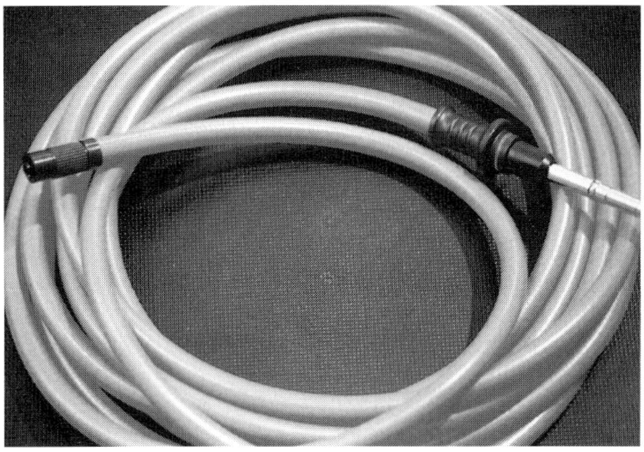

Fig. 3. MR-compatible 10-m light cable for MR-guided endoscopy

■ MR In-Room Monitor and Console

Conventional diagnostic MR procedures can be controlled from outside the MR suite. Interventional MRI requires is a second "in-room" monitor with standard image quality, particularly when fluoroscopiclike sequences are used. Immediate observation of the intraoperative images is mandatory for a safe approach. Achieving a MR-compatible monitor with high display quality entails technological difficulties. The magnetic field leads to image distortion of standard tube monitors. Standard liquid crystal display (LCD) screens do not feature adequate resolution and gray shades. Thin film transistor technology (TFT) active-matrix monitor with analogue control of each pixel provide excellent MR images. A 14″ 1024×768 line display was chosen for the in-room-console. Electric shielding with an ultrathin metal net in front of the screen is required to eliminate high-frequency effects on the MR im-

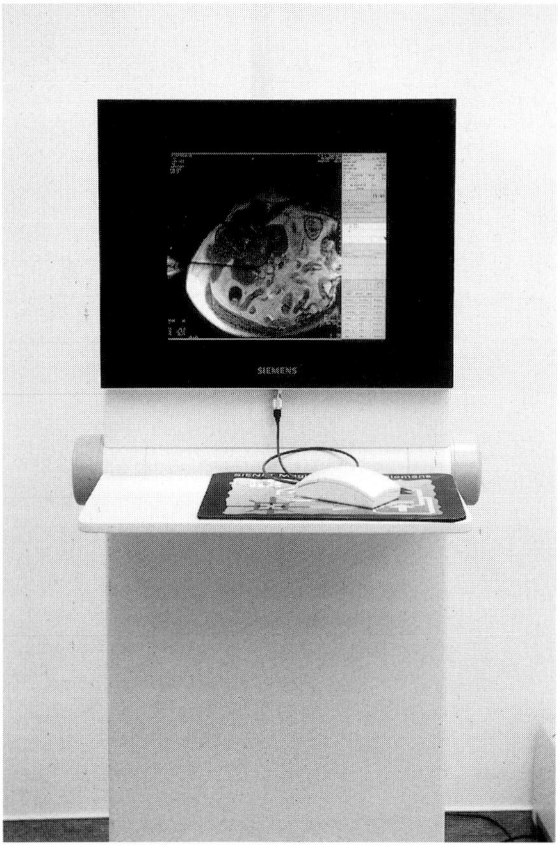

Fig. 4. MR-compatible in-room-console (Siemens, Erlangen, and Pritzel, Prutting, Germany) with analogous TFT active matrix screen

age, and specially developed electric circuits are necessary to provide resistance of the display electronic to the magnetic field. The first prototype, developed by Pritzel, Prutting and Siemens (Erlangen, Germany) has been tested in various in vitro interventions and then clinically approved (Fig. 4). Further development and new improved display technology led to an excellent image that fulfills the diagnostic requirements of MRI. According to our tests the recent design needs some improvement. If the monitor is not moved carefully, it becomes unstable and tends to tilt, because the rear floor wheels do not rotate fully, and the socket is to small. In addition, there is no handle to hold the console firmly, and the rigid supplying line further hampers positioning. The mouse plate is too small and does not allow placement of instruments. An MR-compatible "trackpad" mouse that can be handled under sterile conditions is under development by Siemens.

■ MR-Compatible Materials and Instruments

Instruments and probes inserted in the image plane create a local low signal intensity with two major components: signal elimination due to the displacement of tissue and a susceptibility artifact due to local magnetic field inhomogeneity. If an object is exposed to the field of view, it is represented on the respective image depending on the size of the instruments and the artifact caused by the material. The size of the artifact derives mainly from the material, angle of the probe to B_0, strength of the magnetic field, and sequence type. These parameters cannot simply be changed during the procedure. Field of view, frequency encoding direction, bandwidth, and echo time are secondary effects to the artifact size and allow adjustment during the procedure.

It must be considered that an artifact with a maximum ratio of 1:1 to the instrument is not optimal in all cases. Targets and volumes of interest within the body that contain T1 low-intensity structures such as bone, air, and liquid impede the visibility of the dark gray shades of artifacts. Thus cannulae with larger artifacts are essential for interventions in those areas. In addition, the pixel size of fast gradient echoes is around 2 mm. Thus an instrument smaller than 1 mm and minimal susceptibility artifact ratio of 1:1 may not be easily visualized.

Many interventional procedures require additional T1- and often T2-weighted spin echo and turbo-spin echo controls. As these sequences lack sensitivity to artifacts, smaller instruments can often not be detected. If the needle trajectory is in the direction of the magnet field, the artifact is small and often invisible (Fig. 5). To overcome these drawbacks we developed an adjustable artifact size by simply using different types of stylets. Titanium or nonmagnetic stainless cannulae with mandrins or stylets allow the introduction of different materials. Synthetic stylets are beneficial for the insertion of cannulae larger than 18 G under control of artifact-sensitive sequences, high-field systems, and for precise placement of smaller cannulae. Titanium stylets should be used for puncture with medium-sized cannulae and for insertion into difficult areas with low signal intensity, such as the spine. Cannulae smaller than 20 G require nonmagnetic stainless steel for the stylet to provide optimal visibility of artifacts.

MR-Compatible Materials

Ferromagnetic materials cannot be used in MR tools. Their magnetic field distortion is so great

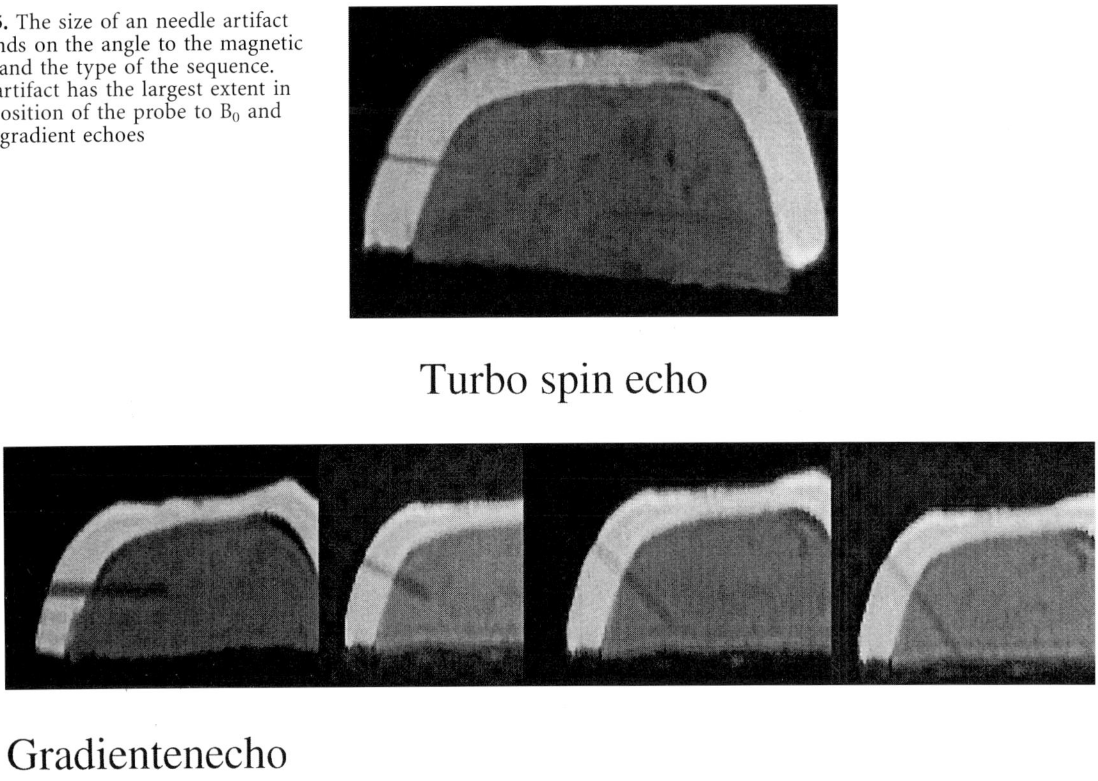

Fig. 5. The size of an needle artifact depends on the angle to the magnetic field and the type of the sequence. The artifact has the largest extent in 90° position of the probe to B_0 and with gradient echoes

that imaging is not possible. Hardened stainless steel provides the best mechanical properties for interventional instruments. Iron-free alloys with high nickel content and nonmagnetic characteristics are appropriate only for interventional instruments smaller than 1 mm in diameter.

Some types of brass, aluminum, and copper are MR compatible and lead to only a 1:1 sized artifact. However, their biocompatibility may not be appropriate for an intracorporeal application. Mechanical characteristics of these alloys are not sufficient for smaller instruments such as cannulae, forceps, baskets. We have found nonmagnetic stainless steel, titanium alloys, and nickel-titanium to be suitable materials.

Ceramic is available in various types, and only some of the recently improved zirconium oxide and aluminum oxide materials are useful for special purposes in interventional instruments. The neurosurgical group of Heidelberg and Brandis (Karlsruhe, Germany) have designed a skull frame made of zirconium oxide ceramic that is fully MR compatible and can be used with in the Magnetom Open device.

Synthetic materials are usually MR compatible, except those that are colored or enriched with para- or ferromagnetic substances. Unfortunately, manufactures seldom provide details of their synthetic materials because this information is often proprietary. We have examined various types of catheter tubing and have obtained information on the contents of the plastic.

We recommend that any material that is planned for use in MR-compatible instruments should be tested for compatibility.

Susceptibility Artifact

Distortion of the magnetic field through paramagnetic effects decreases the relaxation time of the protons encircling the instrument so that their signal is not detected within the respective echo time. The center of a titanium probe is usually dark whereas in the surrounding tissue a bright signal intensive zone is present. This can be interpreted as a T1 effect similar to the signal enhancement of gadolinium. This effect is not seen in gradient echo images (Fig. 6). The bright shadow can theoretically be used to find an instrument which is out of the image plane. However, we found no positive correlation in an examination of 250 clinical cases. If a cannula was out of the image plane we had to use three breathhold slices in any case to find the needle again.

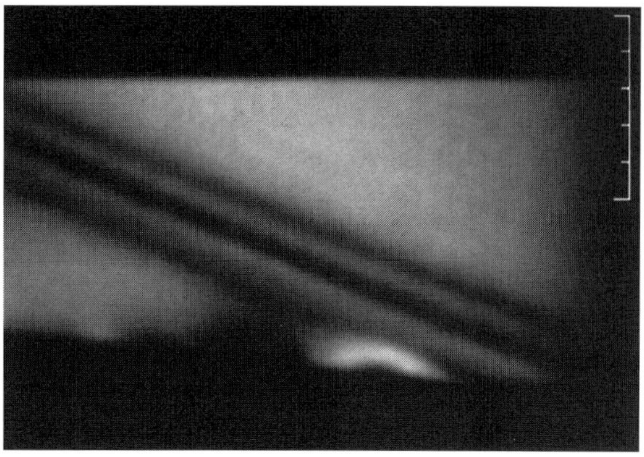

Fig. 6. Signal characteristic of a titanium artifact in T1-weighted spin echo

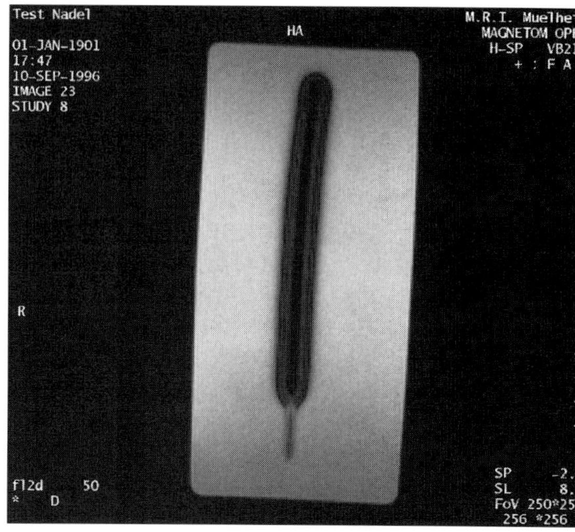

Fig. 7. MR-compatible 20-G titanium puncture needle with variable artifact size

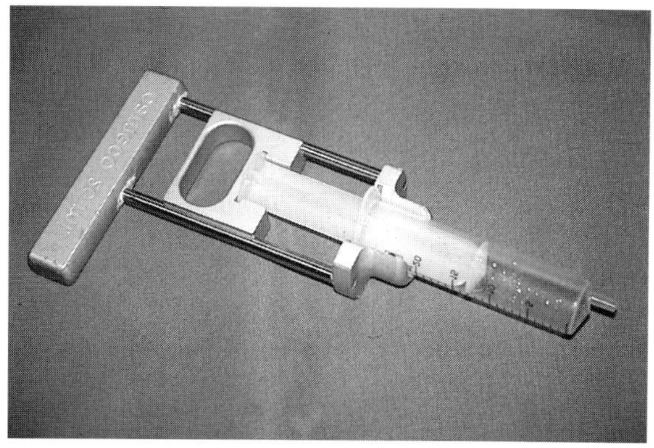

Fig. 8. MR-compatible modified aspiration handle for 20 ml syringes

■ Interventional Devices, Cannulae, and Needles

MR-compatible cannulae have been available for many years from Cook (Denmark; MREye) in sizes ranging from 22 G to 18 G. Similar needles are available from E-Z-EM (Westbury, NY; Lufkin Needle). We have found only the 22-G needles useful for punctures and procedures such as periradicular therapy, ethanol lumbar sympathectomy, intratumoral ethanol injections, and local pain treatment. Larger Cook needles lead to an overly extended artifact for our purposes. For those cases we collaborated in the development of titanium needles (Daum Medical, Schwerin, Germany). Their magnetic susceptibility and artifact size render these cannulae superior to stainless steel items. Disadvantages of titanium cannulae include their relatively rough surface, and low elastic (E) modulus, with a risk of kinking. Needles made of nitinol also feature a low E-modulus but do not kink because of superelasticity. Their precision is excellent and entails a particular advantage: no kinking occurs when the sharp tip of a nitinol needle touches bone.

Variable Artifact Size

Dedicated material selection of either cannula sleeve or internal trocar allows control of the artifact size. The maximum size of the artifact with inserted mandrin and the smallest ratio of 1:1 to artifact is present with the cannula alone (Fig. 7).

Biopsy and Aspiration Cannulae

We prefer aspiration full core biopsy with a modified titanium Menghini cut cannula (Daum Medical). This cannula can be equipped with various types of stylets to allow artifact size to be controlled. For the core biopsy we use a standard aspiration handle for 20-ml syringes (Fig. 8). An automatic biopsy needle is available from Daum that features a light weight handle. On the basis of our tests, an MR-compatible spring has been included in the handle (Fig. 9).

Cannulae for Neurointerventions

Interventional procedures in the CNS require specially designed cannulae that provide mounting with in the bore hole. The neurosurgical groups of the Universities of Heidelberg (Germany) and Zurich (Switzerland) have developed prototypes that allow the use under MRI. Pilling & Weck manufacture MRI-compatible cannulae in Europe. Basically the same aspects are important as with other interventional instruments. The dis-a

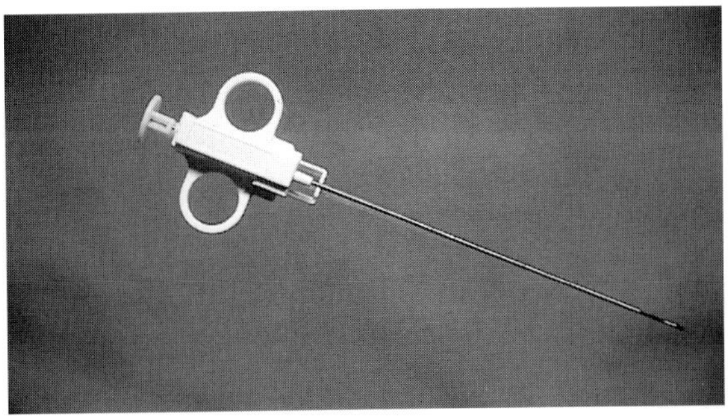

b

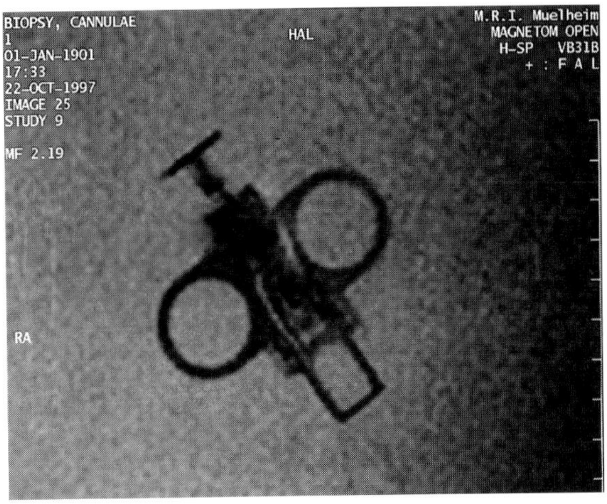

Fig. 9 a, b. Spring-loaded biopsy gun (Daum Medical, Schwerin, Germany)

tal end requires adequate visibility and an artifact size that allows precise placement. The exterior elements for fixation to the skull should not interfere with the imaging but can have an artifact. Thus titanium, ceramic, and plastic are preferable materials.

Tumor Localizer

Tumor localizer should meet the same requirements as other MR tools. The device, including the insertion cannula, should be MR-compatible, and the marker must be visible in the necessary sequences. It is desirable to have a controllable artifact size or variable appearance of the marker to improve differentiation from surrounding tissue. A simple tumor localizer has been evaluated together with Daum that incorporates a nonmagnetic stainless steel wire in a titanium 20-G needle (Fig. 10). Each provides adequate localization of lesions. Other MR-compatible markers are available from Cook and from Mitek (Mama-Lock).

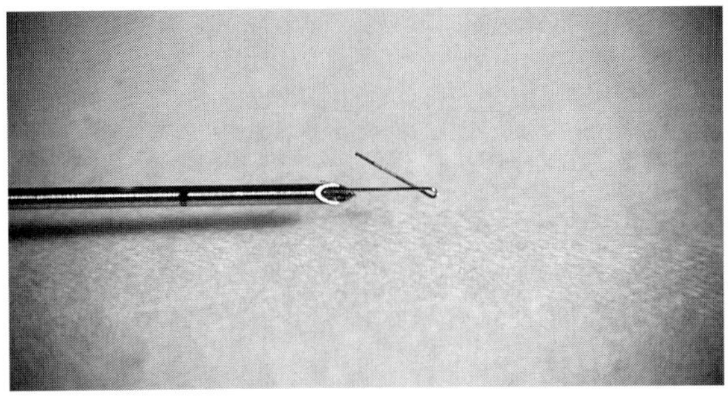

Fig. 10. MR-compatible tumor localizer (Daum Medical, Schwerin, Germany)

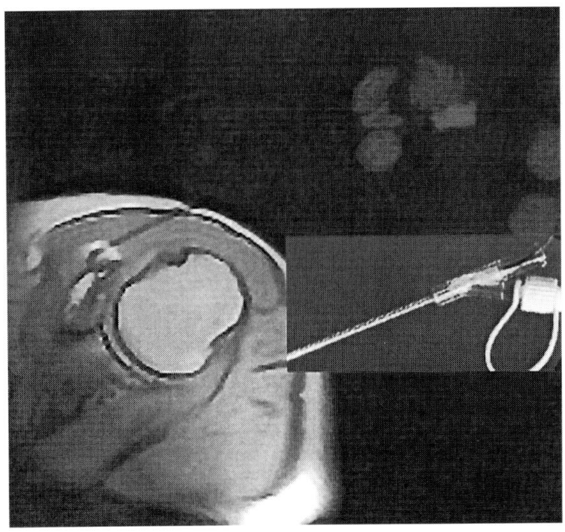

Fig. 11. Y-shaped Luer-Lok facilitates the connection of devices such as syringes and the introduction of laser fibers within the narrow gap of magnet

Deflectable and Superelastic Cannulae

Current designs of open magnets entail spatial limitations for access to the human body. To overcome this limited access we have developed various devices such as Y Luer-Lok, deflectable cannulae, and instruments. The Y-shaped twin Luer-Lok permits connection of syringe and other devices in a variable angle. Introduction of catheters, endoscopes, and laser fibers during the procedure is also facilitated (Fig. 11). This overcomes to some extent the drawback of limited vertical access within the magnet gap. This is not only a practical advantage, but hygiene demands require sufficient distance from sterile instruments and the magnet's surface.

Based on the material examinations and previous experiences with superelastic nitinol, we have developed two different sizes and three lengths of deflectable cannulae (Fig. 12) [6]. The term "nitinol" is derived from "nickel titanium Na-

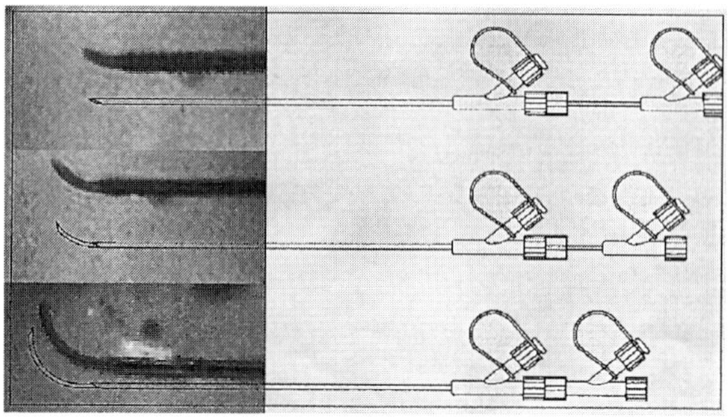

Fig. 12. Deflectable cannula facilitates puncture within the narrow magnet gap (SmartGuide, Daum Medical, Schwerin, Germany)

val Ordinance Laboratory." Nitinol features a thermal and a mechanically stress induced "shape memory." The thermal shape memory entails a shape recovery on heating above a certain temperature threshold between 0 °C and 100 °C. Below the Austenite finish (AF) temperature the material allows plastic deformation (up to 10%) with a low E-modulus. As the AF temperature can be set through a specific temperature treatment above or below, i.e., room or body temperature, the material properties change. Above the AF temperature the material can be deformed up to 10%, but it also recovers its shape elastically when deconstrained. The load required for deformation is relatively constant. This particular characteristic permits several excellent and unique features of instruments and other devices. Self-expanding stents, guide wires, catheters, vena cava filters, and endoscopic instrumentation, in particular, benefit from the superelastic shape memory of nitinol [7].

The deflectable SmartGuide comprises a straight outer sleeve and a superelastic internal precurved cannula that is constrained when introduced into the sleeve. On advancing the internal cannula it gradually recovers its precurvature and creates a puncture "around the corner." From the practical clinical point of view this feature carries two significant benefits. First, it enables the most convenient and the safest approach to operative volume, allowing important anatomical structures such as vessels to be encompassed. Secondly, it increases the accessible volume in accordance with the radius of the curvature of the internal cannula.

■ Catheters

We have evaluated a variety of commercially available catheters of different sizes and materials. All materials and synthetic catheters that we have tested have a more or less 1:1 artifact ratio. Due to the great variety of catheter types we recommend testing the items intended for particular procedures.

Catheters that are marked with metal rings are MR compatible provided that the marker material is also MR compatible. Platinum and gold are MR compatible if appropriate tools have been used for producing the rings. Other materials for MR marking include titanium and nickel alloys. We have evaluated a plating with superparamagnetic iron oxides (SPIOs). A thin film of iron oxide leads to an excellent marking with minimal risk to the patient because these particles are clinically applied as superparamagnetic contrast agents. We have used Endorem (Guerbet, France). The Endorem is dissolved in acrylic lacquer and simply painted on the catheter. The artifact size can be modulated by modifying the concentration.

■ Balloon Catheters

Balloon catheters require the same features as standard catheters for MR compatibility. Usually only the marking rings interfere with MR (Fig. 13). The major aspect of using dilatation balloons is related to the filling of the balloon. Visibility is achieved only if the characteristics of the filling agent significantly differ from those of the signals of the surrounding tissue or liquid (Fig. 14). As filling agents we have evaluated saline, SPIO, gadolinium solutions (1 mmol/l up to pure gadolinium). The indication of the filling depends on the target. If the balloon is used in vessels for PTA and controlled by angiographic sequences, filling with a gadolinium solution of 50 mmol/l saline is required. A higher concentration does not lead to significant differences in signal intensity. If the balloon is controlled by T1-weighted spin or gradient echoes, the filling should be gadolinium with no more than 4 mmol/l concentration to provide the highest intravascular contrast. To provide optimal assess-

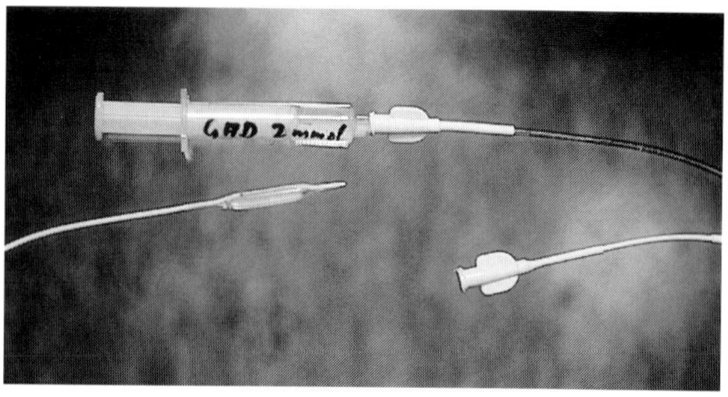

Fig. 13. MR-compatible balloon catheter

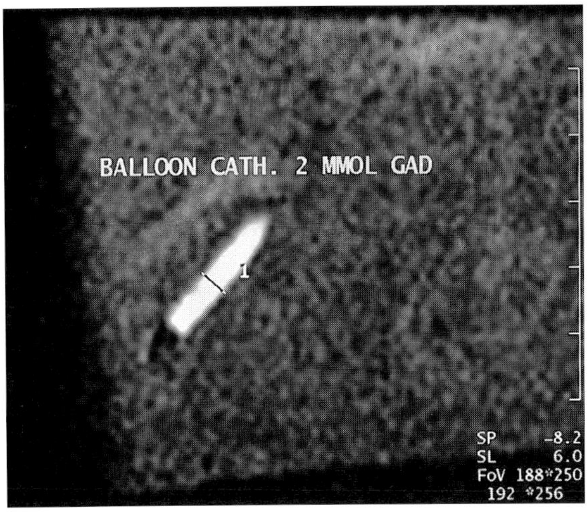

Fig. 14. MR-compatible balloon catheter filled with gadolinium contrast agent

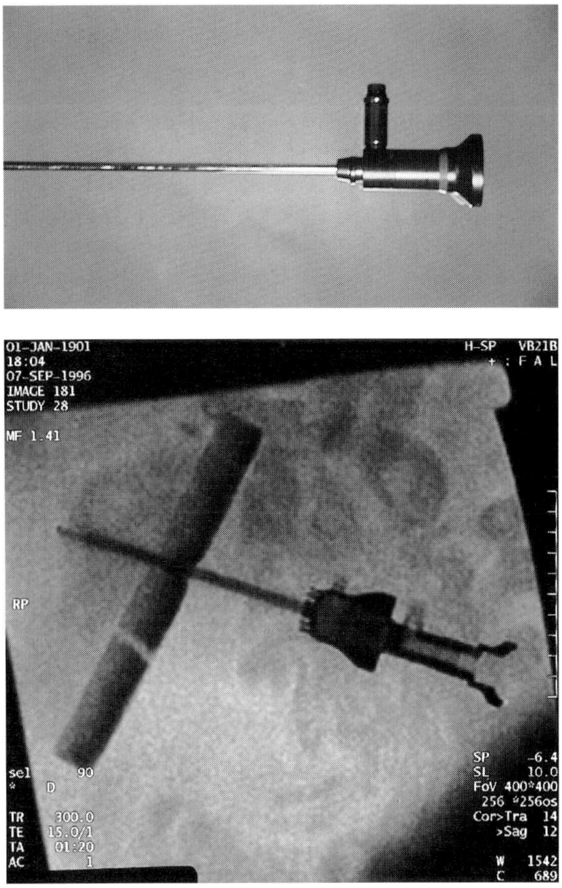

a

b

Fig. 15 a, b. MR-compatible, 4-mm rod lens endoscope (Olympus Winter & Ibe, Hamburg, Germany) introduced in a trocar

ment of the vascular wall (which is not yet possible in low field open systems), filling with saline is appropriate. By washing out the various solutions it is possible to modulate both the signal intensity and the image size of the balloon, which varies from 1:1 with pure saline and 2–4 mmol/l gadolinium concentration filling to 1:3 with 1:10 Endorem solution.

The quantity of 50 mmol/l gadolinium (Magnevist, Schering, Berlin) filling should be useful in cases in which T1-hyperintensive structures surround the balloon (e.g., dilatation of strictures).

MR-Compatible Endoscopes

Rigid rod lens endoscopes contain stainless steel elements and have a stainless steel outer tube. This components create large ferromagnetic artifacts which impede the intramagnetic use. The light transmission takes place via the glass rods, and the air intersections function as lenses. This principle was invented by the English physicist Hopkins. The overall design has been perfected in recent years to provide autoclavable optics, and fully MR-compatible rod lens endoscopes have been elaborated. Replacement of materials and modification of processing techniques are required to achieve optics with adequate reliability, durability, and biocompatibility. In over 100 h of imaging time all components of the endoscope have been evaluated by the following standardized sequence protocol:

- 350-mm diameter water container with 10 l 20 °C saline and 2 mmol gadolinium per liter
- 350-mm FOV body, small 200 FOV multipurpose, large for smaller special items
- 256×256 matrix
- 0 oversampling
- FLASH 2D TR 92, TE 12.7
- FISP 2D TR 32, TE 12

Figure 15 presents versions of prototypes with artifact problems and the items approved finally as being fully MR compatible. We set this requirement for endoscopes because they should remain within the imaging plane during acquisition to allow correlation of endoscopic and tomographic image [8].

Our material examinations in collaboration with Olympus Winter & Ibe have shown adequate alloys and design principles of MRI-compatible endoscopes. The first series of endoscopes have become available in 1998. Telescopes of 4, 5, and 10 mm with straight 0° and 30° view optics produce only a 1:1 size artifact. MR-compatible, lengthened light cables for a cold light source that is placed outside

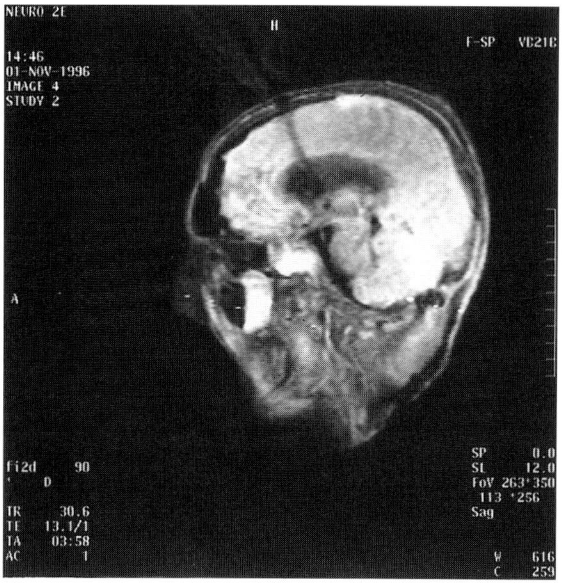

Fig. 16. MR-guided neuroendoscopy of the right ventricle in a cadaver study

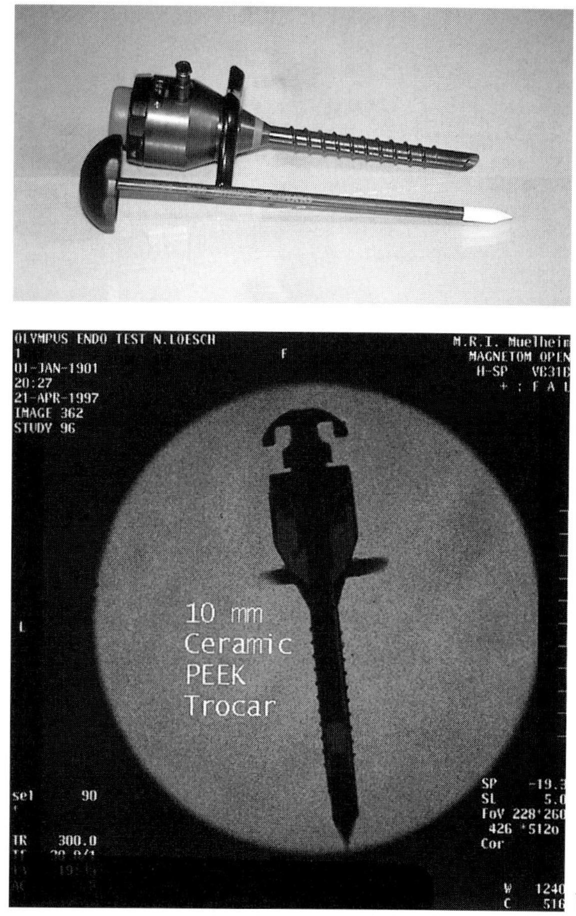

a

b

Fig. 17 a, b. MR-compatible ceramic pointed trocar and plastic cannula for MR-guided endoscopic surgery (Olympus Winter & Ibe, Hamburg, Germany)

the MR unit and a one chip camera (OTV 5 S) have been used for first experimental application in MR-guided neuroendoscopy (Fig. 16). The results are promising. No significant altering of the MR image, endoscopic image, or dysfunction of the electronic camera system have been noted.

Video-Endoscopic Monitoring

Although the image quality is minor compared to the standard tube system, LCD flat screens are marketed for endoscopy. In a comparison of standard digital TFT screen, high-resolution endoscopy monitor (Sony, black matrix) the analogue TFT active matrix display incorporated in the in-room console from Siemens is the only adequate flat screen for endoscopy. For our experimental endoscopic procedures we use an additional in-room monitor. Siemens is preparing a multimedia console with RGB and other video-input interfaces. Future developments will include video inlet technology, whereby the endoscopic image can be overlaid on the MR image and further manipulated to provide optimal tomographic information on the operative volume.

Trocars and Cannulae

To enable operative laparoendoscopic procedures within or close to the magnet, trocar/cannulae are required that feature adequate operative functions and appropriate representation on the MR image. The MRI compatibility of trocar/cannulae was evaluated in vitro. In terms of cannulae sleeves several disposable items made of synthetic and thus MR-compatible materials are available. Trocars are usually produced from hardened stainless steel and are ferromagnetic, which precludes their use in the MRI suite. Some disposable trocars are made of aluminum alloy and are fully MRI compatible. Most disposable trocars are sharp and comprise so-called “safety shield” or trocar stylet retracting mechanisms, and their use therefore requires care and experience. In our view only blunt and cone-shaped trocars should be applied. The most suitable access tool seems to be the Step system (Innerdyne, Sunnyvale, Calif., USA) [9]. We have modified the Veress needle that accompanies Step to a MRI-compatible self-made item. Step enables relatively atraumatic and safe access to the abdominal cavity. Prior puncture with the MR-compatible Veress needle and initial insufflation should be performed under MR fluoroscopic control, which allows the insufflation and distension of the abdominal wall to be observed. Retroperitoneal access can be performed with conventional balloon dissectors [10]. We have found the GSI system (General Surgical Innovations, Portola Valley, Calif., USA) to be appropriate. The balloon should be filled with a 2–3 mmol/l gadolinium/saline contrast agent. Thus the dissection procedure can be observed under MR fluoroscopic control.

Olympus Winter & Ibe has prepared two types of trocars in 5 and 10 mm. One version is equipped with blunt conical trocars and one version with ceramic-pointed sharp trocars (Fig. 17).

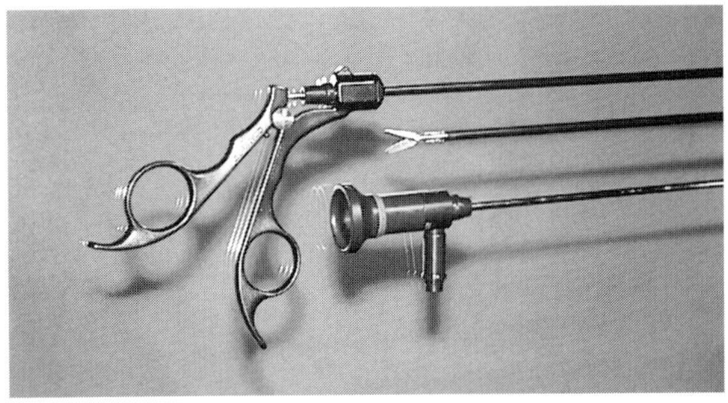

Fig. 18. MR-compatible 5-mm scissors and forceps for MR-guided endoscopic surgery (Olympus Winter & Ibe, Hamburg, Germany)

■ Surgical Instruments

Achieving MRI compatibility in the field of endoscopic instruments such as probes, hooks, forceps, scissors is more difficult because the hinge complex of handles and jaws exclude the use of pure synthetic materials. Ceramics, although MRI applicable, are still too expensive and too difficult to manufacture. Titanium-instruments are available for open neurosurgery because even the microscopic metal filing and debris from ferromagnetic retractor or forceps that come in contact with tissue can lead to significant artifacts in postoperative MRI.

Olympus Winter & Ibe has produced prototypes of MR-compatible titanium instruments. Scissors and forceps of 5 mm are available (Fig. 18). As titanium has poor mechanical properties, new approaches are necessary for designing and producing MR-compatible laparoendoscopic instruments. Instruments with hinges and mechanical articulation entail particular functional drawbacks, such as hysteresis, parts wear, and difficult check of functions and exchange of parts such as insulation. Several gaps and hinges hinder appropriate cleaning. The hinge complex should be substituted to overcome the problems associated with intraoperative MRI [11].

Hingeless instruments (HIT, Menlo Park, CA) have jaws consisting of only a single part. The instruments and jaws open due to the superelastic shape memory of the employed nitinol. Due to the relatively constant load on deformation of superelastic materials an incorporated overload protection permit the adequate grasping of tissues of different thickness and characteristics. The first prototype of a MR-compatible hingeless forceps is shown in Fig. 19.

a

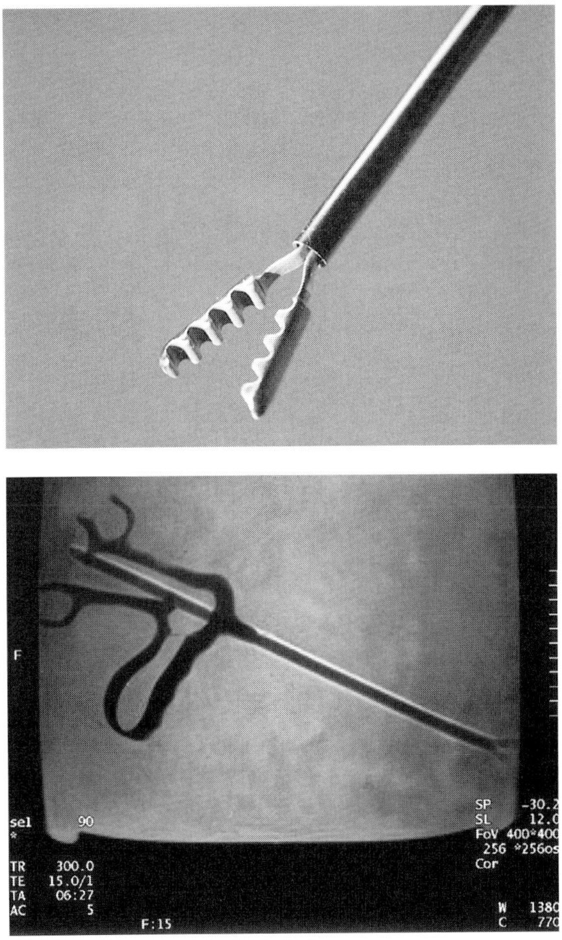

b

Fig. 19 a, b. MR-compatible superelastic and monolithic forceps (HIT, Menlo Park, Ca)

■ In-Room Furniture

Operative procedures require some kind of operating room furniture in the MR suite, including instrument tables, waist bins, and chairs. Usually these items are made of stainless steel. We have a wooden table that is MR compatible and fits the interior of our suite. Wooden tables, however, are not acceptable for use in the operating room. As soon as the surface is scratched, it becomes porous, the wood absorbs liquids, and ceases to provide adequate disinfection. We have collaborated with Veenstra (the Netherlands) in developing fully MR-compatible in-room furniture. Veenstra has now produced a variety of furniture items, such as intravenous stand, instrumentation tables (small and large), trolleys, and waist bins. All items are made exclusively of nonmagnetic components and can therefore be used in closest proximity even into the open magnet (Fig. 20) and at high-field systems.

■ Future Outlook

One of the most important needs is improvement in the instrument display. An artifact with adjustable size and variable "signal intensity" would be optimal. Realization of this technology, however, is far from easy. We have begun to develop active and passive visualization of interventional devices. Early results are promising, but extensive further research is necessary.

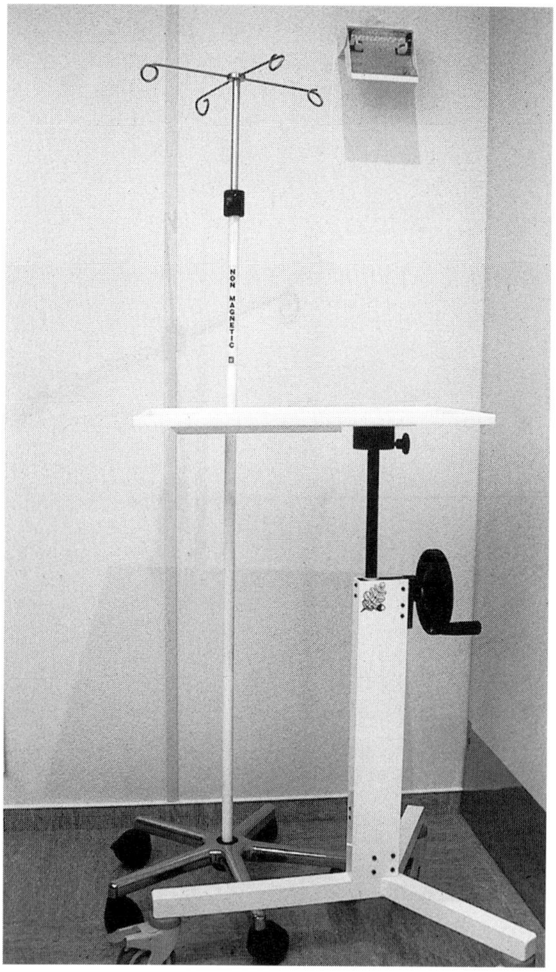

Fig. 20. MR-compatible instrumentation table (Veenstra, The Netherlands)

Image Plane Navigation

The visualization of instruments during MRI-guided procedures is difficult. The interventional tool must be aligned precisely with the orientation of the image plane. If the instrument deteriorates out of the image plane, the search is arduous and time intensive. Inadvertent movements by the patient during insertion can lead to frequent loss of the instrument image. By changing the slice orientation and position detection of the changed needle path can be achieved.

An RF-shielded infrared optical tracking system with three charged coupled device cameras detects multiple light-emitting diodes attached to a handle connected to the interventional or surgical instrument and light-emitting diodes can be mounted at the magnet. The positional information is sent to the MR unit to provide correlation of the instrument with the magnet coordinates. This position can be displayed on the MR screen either to match the previous instrument position or to provide update of the scan plane orientation during fluoroscopic mode. Further electrodes can be attached to the patient or the table so that the navigation system can be used for other procedures (Fig. 21). Images can then be generated according to the position in alignment with the instrument or perpendicular to the distal tip of instrument. The image plane orientation can be changed and redefined without moving the instrument itself. This ensures constant control of a surgical instrument during movement. It must be considered that unattended curvature or bending of the instrument leads to a distortion of the current position of the instrument tip [12].

Tip Tracking

The volumetric nature of the MRI acquisition allows the orientation of specific signal frequencies to be detected in space. Local proton spin signals can be acquired by incorporating a miniature RF coil at the tip of an instrument. The signal source representing the tip of the instrument can then be localized within the coordinate system of the magnetic field and thus within the human body [13, 14]. This technique, known as tip tracking, has been evaluated experimentally. As the instrument

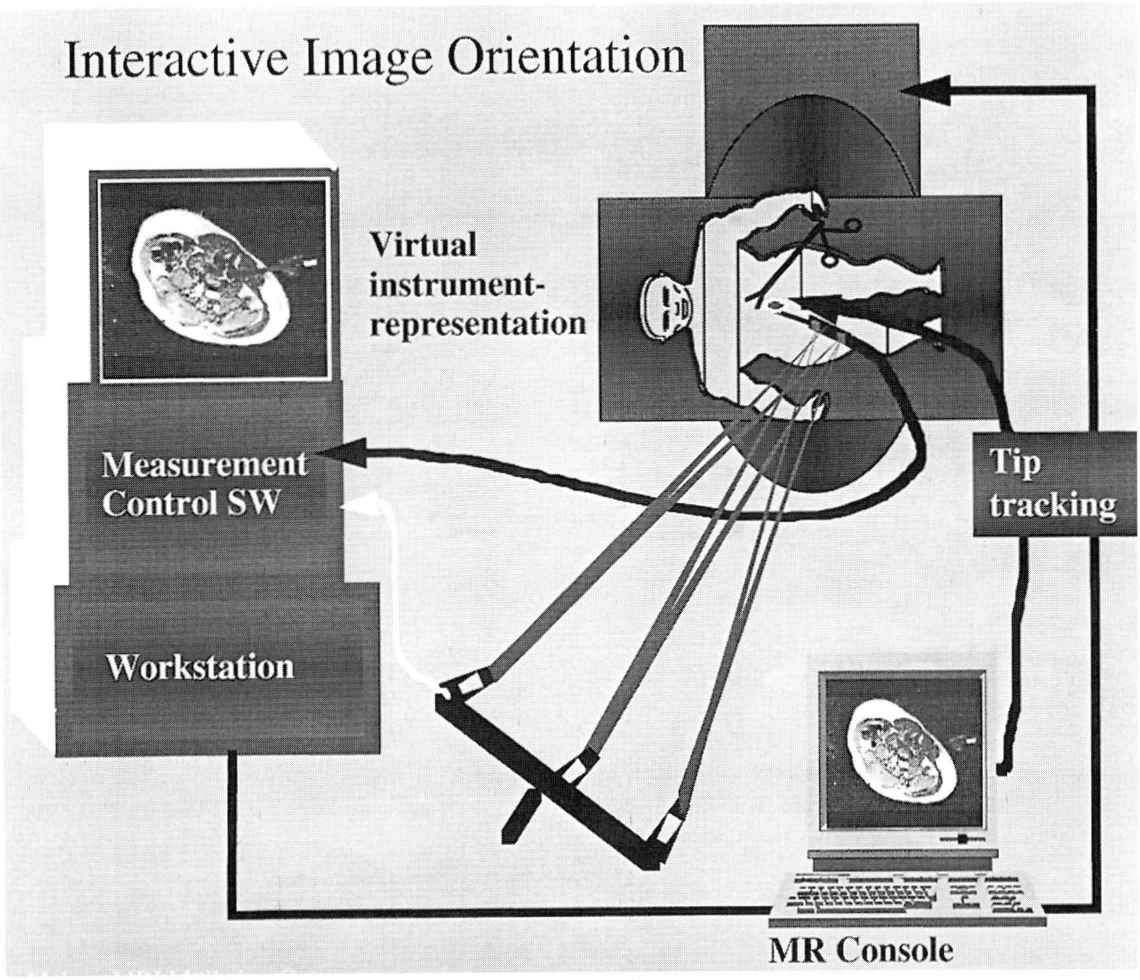

Fig. 21. Schematic principle of interactive slice orientation by means of an optoelectronic navigation system

is moved, the position of the signal moves accordingly and can be tracked. The current approach of tip tracking by Doumulin includes the need for an additional workstation to compute the three-dimensional coordinates of the coil and to display the position as a moving symbol in two planes of a morphological, previously acquired "road map" MR image. Thus direct on-line control is not possible. We have started a project of tip tracking that allows direct display of the instrument signal in a complete MR image, providing interactive slice orientation in axial or perpendicular position in accordance with the instrument. Thus the same function as with optoelectronic navigation is achieved. Extracorporeal tip tracking is less accurate than the navigation, but intracorporeally it functions independently of the bending of instruments.

The new technique is under development in collaboration with the University of Cleveland to image the tip of an interventional device, such as cannulae or catheter, during MRI-guided interven-

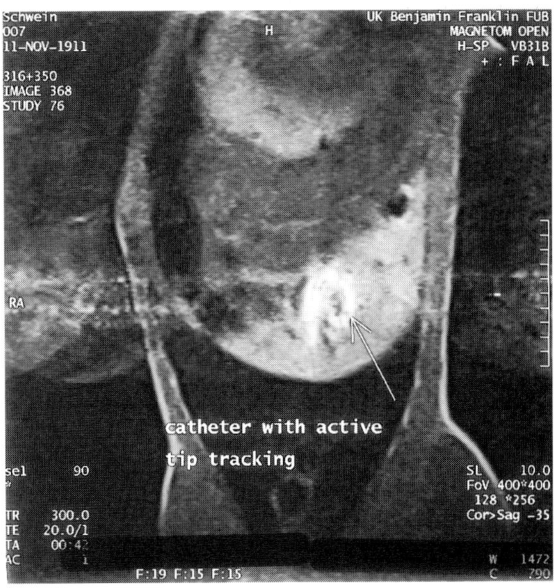

Fig. 22. Tip tracking catheter introduced into the aorta of a pig (Dr. Frank Wacker, Berlin)

tional procedures and with both "real-time" imaging and tip localization. This technique enables localization within a single fluoroscopic-mode sequence, unlike with other techniques [15–17]. A new PHREAK keyhole data capability in combination with a true-FISP sequence provides near "real-time" frame rate [18]. The catheter tip image data acquisition is separated by one TR from the standard coil spin detection. Localization and superimposition of the two images with minimum spatial error is achieved. Misalignment problems associated with patient movement, which may occur between acquisition of the anatomic reference and device localization image data, can be avoided. Initial animal experiments at Benjamin Franklin Hospital, University of Berlin, and Dept. of MRI, CWRU Hospitals, Cleveland, OH, demonstrate the feasibility of this technique (Fig. 22).

Conclusion

Based on our initial experiences with over 250 open-field MRI-guided procedures and the results of examinations of MR-compatible tools and devices we have defined to following basic roles of interventional MR compatibility:

- All instruments and devices to be used an MR suite should be classified and approved according to the open magnet with which they are to be used, for example, 0.067 or 0.5 T, brand name, and manufacturer.
- The manufacturer of the open-field system should provide approval for compatibility of the instrument or device with the MR unit.
- No instrument to be used in an MR suite may be magnetic and or be magnetized by the magnetic field. The degree of magnetism can be determined by the attraction force of a magnet that comes close to the device. This attraction force must be 0 in the horizontal direction. It is important that the device does not become magnetized when exposed to the magnetic field.
- No instrument or part of an instrument that is temporarily used within the human body in approximation to the magnet but not during acquisition may be magnetic (see above).
- No instrument incorporated into the human body and present within the magnetic field during acquisition may cause any relevant distortion of the magnetic field.
- No instrument within the image plane but outside the body may cause any relevant distortion of the magnetic field.
- No instrument within the image plane inside the body and the field of view may cause any relevant distortion of the magnetic field, and all instruments must provide an adequate artifact.

References

1. Lufkin R, Teresi L, Hanafee W (1987) New needle for MR-guided aspiration cytology of the head and neck. AJR 149:380–382
2. Grönemeyer D, Seibel R, Kaufman L (1991) Low-field design eases MRI-guided biopsies. Diagn Imaging 3:161–165
3. Melzer A, Schmidt A, Seibel R, Deli M, Stöckel D, Grönemeyer D (1996) Methodology, technological prerequisites and preliminary clinical results of interventions in a horizontal open MRI unit. Proc ISMRM 2:897
4. Melzer A, Seibel R, Schmidt A, Groenemeyer D (1996) MRI guided neoplasm biopsy/cell aspiration and interstitial drug instillation in an horizontal open MR unit. 13th ESMRB, 12–15 September 1996, Prague
5. Melzer A, Buess G, Cuschieri A (1992) Instruments for endoscopic surgery. In: Cuschieri A, Buess G, Périssat J (eds) Operative manual for endoscopic surgery 1. Springer, Berlin Heidelberg New York
6. Melzer A, Schmidt A, Triebe W, Seibel (1996) Results of experimental and clinical application of a deflectable superelastic cannula instrument guiding sleeve "Smart-guide." 13th ESMRB, 12–15 Sept 1996, Prague
7. Duerig TW, Melton KN, Stoeckel D, Wayman CM (1990) Engineering aspects of shape memory alloys. Butterworth-Heinemann, New York
8. Melzer A, Kipfmüller K, Seibel R, Schmidt A, Groenemeyer D (1996) Techniques and technologies of MRI guided laparo-endoscopic procedures. An experimental study. ESMRB, 12–15 Sept 1996, Prague
9. Melzer A, Kipfmüller K, Groenemeyer D, Seibel R, Bueß G (1995) Ports, trocars/cannulae and other access techniques. Semin Laparosc 2:170–201
10. Melzer A, Buess G, Cuschieri A (1994) Instruments and alled technologies. In: Cuschieri A, Buess G, Périssat J (eds) Operative manual for endoscopic surgery 2. Springer, Berlin Heidelberg New York
11. Melzer A, Stoeckel D (1995) Performance improvement of surgical instrumentation through the use of Ni-Ti materials. Proc SMST 94:401–410
12. Silverman SG, Collick BD, Figueira MR, Khorasani R, Adams DF, Newmann RW, Topulos GP, Jolesz FA (1995) Interactive MR-guided biopsy in an open configuration MR imaging system. Radiology 197:175–181
13. Davis CP, McKinnon GC, Debatin JF, von Schulthess GK (1996) Ultra-high-speed MR imaging. Eur Radiol 6:297–311
14. Leung DA, Debatin JF, Wildermuth S, Heske N, Dumoulin CL, Darrow RD, Hauser M, Davis CP, von Schulthess GK (1995) Real-time biplanar needle tracking for interventional MR imaging procedures. Radiology 197:485–488
15. Dumoulin CL, Souza SP, Darrow RD (1993) Real-time position monitoring of invasive devices using magnetic resonance. Magn Reson Med 29:411–415
16. Leung DA, Debatin JF, Wildermuth S, Schultes GK (1995) Intravascular MR tracking catheter. AJR 164:1265–1270
17. Wildermuth S, Leung DA, Debatin JF (1997) MR imaging-guided intravascular procedures: initial demonstration in a pig model. Radiology 202:578–583
18. Bornstedt A, Busch M, Wendt M, Seibel R, Grönemeyer D (1996) Turbo accelerated asymmetric phase read keyhole (PHREAK) imaging as a method for fast and high contrast MR-guided intervention, 260th ESMRMB, Prague

Graphics Workstations for Interventional Magnetic Resonance Imaging

3

M. L. Williams

Introduction

In the past decade advances in computer technology have revolutionized the processing and display of medical image data. These advances have spurred the development of software systems designed for planning and delivering specific medical treatments. Capabilities that were previously available only in a research environment are now routine in clinical settings.

Stereotactic neurosurgery using magnetic resonance (MR) guidance has benefited greatly from these advances. By their very nature, stereotactic procedures require precise accuracy and reliable targeting. Computer graphics can now offer interactive three-dimensional (3D) visualization to aid the physician for planning and performing a clinical procedure. These capabilities justify the cost of computers dedicated to stereotactic work. This chapter focuses on graphics workstations for MR-guided therapy.

Dedicated planning software is the culmination of numerous developments. The most obvious is the continuing performance gains in speed and processing power per cost for computer hardware. Medical imaging is extremely data intensive. Without the ability to manipulate the data in a timely manner, planning systems would be unfeasible for clinical use. In addition to raw computing power, enormous gains have been made in the graphics capabilities of reasonably priced systems. Computer vendors now supply dedicated hardware and software development packages specifically geared for graphics functionality. Sophisticated color modeling and 3D graphics have become expected features. In parallel with computer developments, advances in the field of medical imaging have provided the data for the software to work with.

With these tools, collaborations between clinicians and computer engineers have produced applications specifically designed for neurosurgical work. This chapter discusses some of the underlying graphics tools and the stereotactic applications that incorporate them.

■ Computer Graphics Techniques

Software planning systems incorporate numerous computer graphics techniques [1] to aid clinicians. Although the graphics are often impressive, in the medical arena it is the information content and how well it is conveyed that are paramount. The flashiest graphics are not always the best or the most accurate in these regards. Another crucial element is how practical the software system is in the context of its intended use. Techniques that require significant processing time might be acceptable for postprocedural analysis. These same techniques would be impractical for stereotactic planning where the time between stereotactic head ring placement and treatment is to be minimized. The ease and flexibility in the ability to manipulate the graphics scene is also an important factor. The planning process usually requires the generation and comparison of multiple plans.

This section presents a basic overview of several important graphics techniques that are encountered repeatedly in medical software. The major steps that the computer takes are outlined for each method. The users do not need to understand the complete details of the algorithms that produce the graphics. Still, it is useful for clinicians to understand the general steps that are taken in producing what appears on the screen. With this knowledge they can better interpret the information that is presented to them. The relative merits of the techniques are discussed with respect to planning requirements.

A discussion of medical imaging is outside the scope of this article. Obviously a significant amount of processing is carried out to acquire and create the two-dimensional (2D) images [2, 3] before they are brought to the planning computer. It is assumed that the data from the medical scanners are correct, and that a goal of the planning system is to maintain the fidelity of the acquired image data as much as possible. Certain graphics techniques "lose" data and others "create" it when compared to the original data set. This is noted in the following discussion.

Image Display

The most basic graphics capability is the display of the 2D image data. Even this simple task warrants some discussion. Most medical scanners are capable of outputting image intensities over a 12-bit range. This means there are a possible $2^{12}=4096$ image intensities. Most clinical images cover only a subrange of these possible intensities; 2800 is a typical intensity range for a cranial computed tomography (CT) image. In MR the ranges tend to vary depending on the pulse sequence employed.

Clinicians are accustomed to viewing film which is capable of capturing many more gray level gradations that a computer monitor. Computer monitors are limited in the number of gray levels they are able to display at given time. Most commercially available displays are capable of displaying a maximum of 256 gray levels. The term "8-bit display" is often used to describe medium capability systems. This means the computer can display up to $2^8=256$ different colors at a time. Simply because a monitor has an 8-bit display does not mean the software display of an image is composed of 256 gray levels. Most often, some of the 256 possible color slots are reserved for non-gray colors needed for image overlays or generic interface functionality. Software images on 8-bit machines are often displayed using 128 gray levels. Trained eyes are able to notice some degradation in image quality between 256 and 128 gray levels.

High end displays are 24-bit with 8 bits each reserved for the red, green, and blue channels used to compose a particular pixel color. This still leads to only 256 possible gray levels because the red, green, and blue components must all be equal to form a gray value. The advantage of 24-bit displays is that the 256 gray levels can be displayed simultaneously with other colors. Even on these high end systems the image display software must be written to take advantage of their capabilities. This can be an important factor when deciding on software to be used in a clinical environment.

From the above discussion it is obvious that for most medical images it is impossible to make a one-to-one mapping between image intensity in the raw data and the pixel gray value on the computer screen. Multiple intensity values in the raw image data must be represented by a single gray level on the computer screen. Window leveling allows for control of how the original image intensities are mapped into the available number of gray levels in the computer. Figure 1 shows two views of a CT slice each with different window leveling. In one view the leveling has been set so the screen gray levels span the intensity levels in the image. In the other view the screen gray levels are centered around intensity levels in the image data that show the tumor definition.

Even though the 2D images of a data set have been acquired in one orientation, it is often desired to view the data set from another orienta-

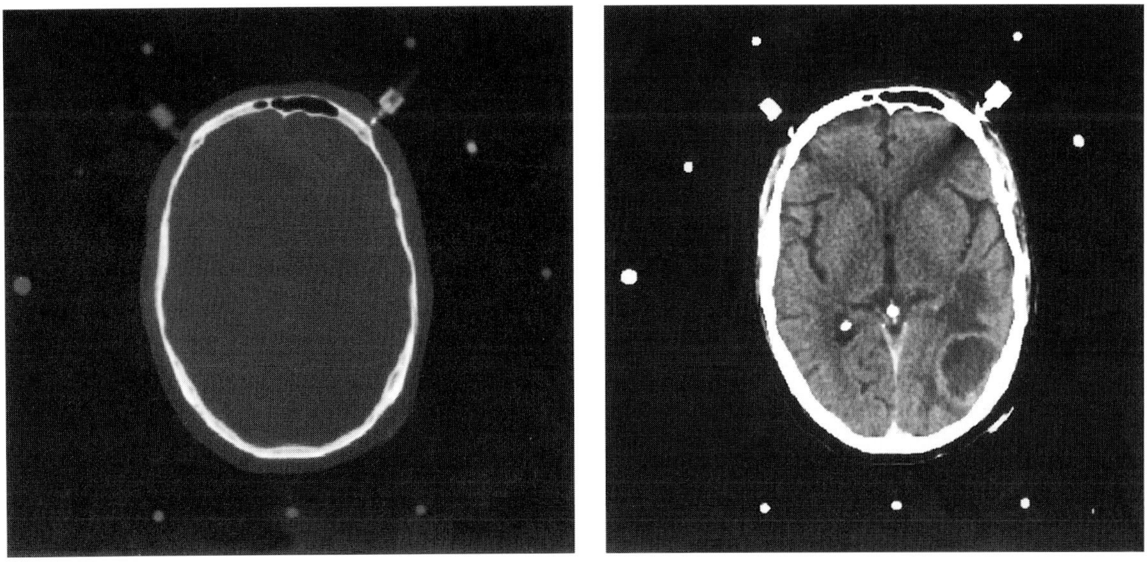

a b

Fig. 1. Two views of the same CT section. a Contrast levels get to span all intensity levels in the image. b Gray levels centered to optimize tumor depiction

tion. To accomplish this the 2D image slices are layered in anatomical order to form a 3D volume. The slice pixel intensities are considered to represent the intensities of 3D voxel volumes determined by the slice pixel size and the slice spacing. This 3D volume can be thought of as a 3D mathematical function of intensities where the values are known only at the centers of the voxels. With no further information the intensity at a point in the volume not coincident with a voxel center is determined by linearly interpolating in all three dimensions between the two closest voxel centers in each direction.

The display of an arbitrarily oriented plane through the image volume is accomplished by first specifying the particular plane. It takes three parameters to specify a plane, two for its orientation and one for its distance from the volume center. A regular grid of pixel locations can be imagined on the arbitrary plane that correspond to the display screen pixels. Once the oblique plane has been specified these screen pixels fall at well defined locations in the image volume but most likely not coincident with voxel center locations. The intensity of each pixel in the display plane is found by interpolating the its neighboring voxel values in the image volume. This process uses the computational resources of the computer for the interpolation process in addition to the graphics display. Computers today are fast enough that the display tracks smoothly as the plane is moved in real-time throughout the image volume. Figure 2 shows several oblique planes through an axially acquire MR data set.

Surface Rendering

It is humanly impossible to simultaneously process all the information contained in a medical image data set. Computers can aid in selecting out and displaying relevant information. The technique of surface rendering is used pervasively in medical software for this purpose. Surface rendering allows 3D viewing of selected anatomical structures and their geometric relationship to each other within stereotactic space.

A surface rendered object is constructed from the original scan data through several simple steps illustrated in Fig. 3. Initially the structures of interest are located on a slice by slice basis. The boundaries of these structures are delineated on each 2D image slice. This 2D segmentation is a whole field of research unto itself. For cases such as the external surface, simple intensity thresholding is sufficient to detect the boundary. Other structures, even those that are easily detected by sight such as the orbital globes, do not lend themselves to segmentation by thresholding. More sophisticated techniques are being actively pursued [4], but no one technique has been found to robustly and accurately segment medical images. The ultimate goal would be a process for automatically segmenting a range of anatomical structures in a short period of time for clinical considerations. The techniques that have presently shown limited success often require prohibitive time requirements for stereotactic planning. For this reason planning systems often fall back on the user manually contouring the anatomy with the computer mouse and display.

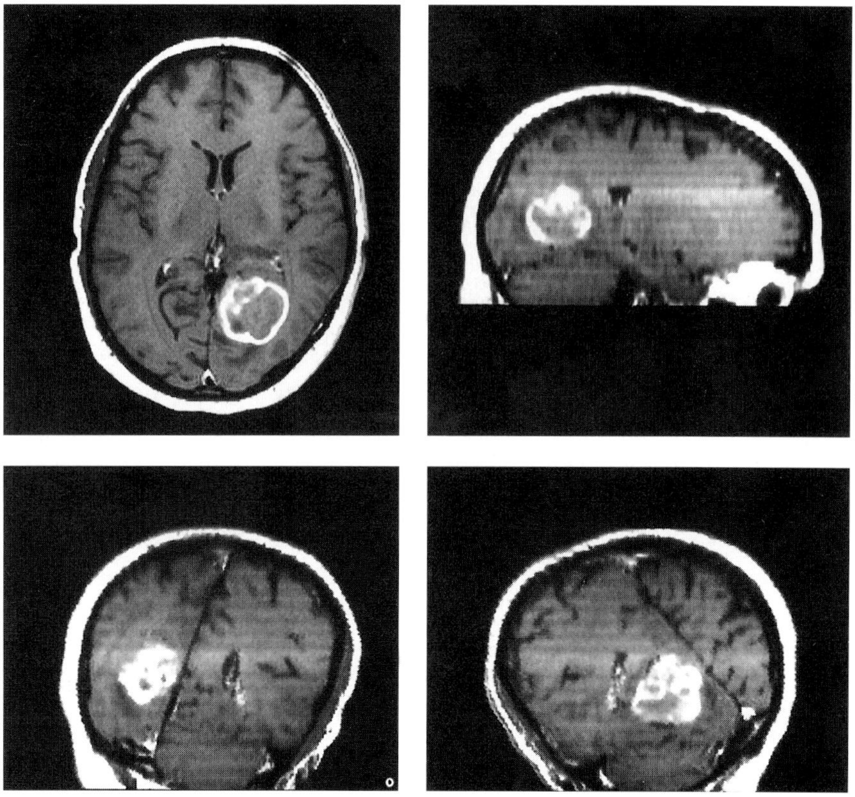

a b c d

Fig. 2a–d. Two oblique planes (**c**, **d**), one sagittal plane (**b**) reformatted from an axially acquired MR data set and one of the original slices (**a**)

At this stage the boundaries of an object are actually pixels on the 2D images. Since the pixels are inherently integral, it is possible to perform some smoothing of the boundary curve. Various smoothing algorithms relax the conditions of integral boundary point locations and slightly move the locations based on neighboring points. To preserve the information content, in medical imaging it is often not desirable to allow the boundary points to move by more than half a pixel size. Especially in stereotaxy, location accuracy should take precedence over prettier pictures. The next step is to convert the boundary points, original or smoothed, to stereotactic space based on the localizer locations appearing on the slices. Obviously, this takes place on a slice by slice basis.

The final step in surface rendering is to create the 3D object from the collection of stereotactically transformed 2D boundary points. The triangle was discovered in ancient times to be ideal as a fundamental building block of architectural structures. The same principle is also true for modern computer graphics. Algorithms exist that automatically connect boundary points on adjacent slices to form triangles. The wire frame diagram in Fig. 3a is an example of this process. The vectors normal to the surface of each triangle are computed and stored. The computer can then display the final 3D representation of the object surface. Various lighting and shading models exist to control the actual display of the object. In particular, objects can be made transparent as illustrated by the external surface in Fig. 5 to display internal structures.

Surface rendering is extremely powerful because computers are very adept at graphically manipulating triangles. Surface rendered objects containing even thousands of triangles can be rotated in real time. This allows the clinician quickly to manipulate and view the 3D patient anatomy with information about stereotactic location. As is be seen below, external objects such as surgical probes or radiation beams can be easily moved within the 3D environment for planning purposes. In many procedures the time taken to construct the surface rendered anatomy is paid for by the information and capabilities gained.

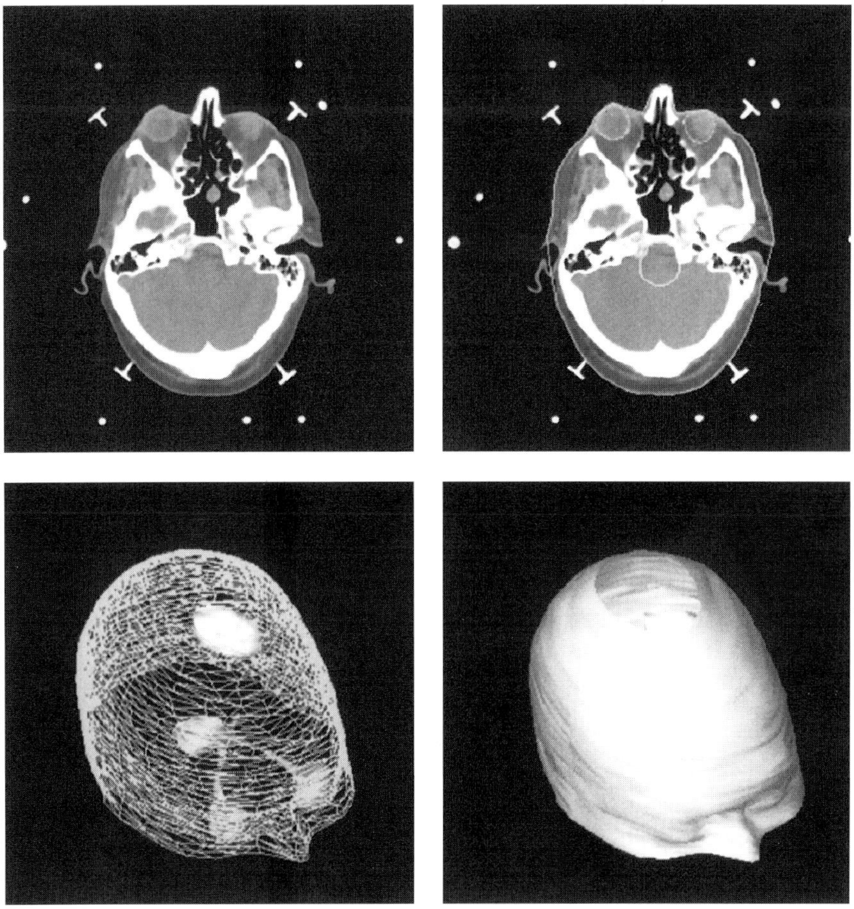

Fig. 3a–d. The steps in surface rendering. **a** An original data slice **b** contouring of anatomical structures **c** wireframe connection between slice layers of anatomical contours. **d** Surface construction with lighting

Volume Rendering

Volume rendering is another graphics technique for viewing objects within a data set. As is seen above, surface rendering views objects within a data set but the objects are extracted from the original data. By contrast, volume rendering attempts at visualization within the context of the complete original data volume. As in the discussion of oblique slicing the 2D image slices are stacked to form a 3D volume. An observation point, usually external to the volume, and a line of sight are chosen based on the desired view of the anatomy. The viewing plane which represents the computer display is imagined on the opposite side of the data volume from the observation point perpendicular to the line of sight. Straight line rays are cast from the observation point through the data volume to the individual pixels in the viewing plane. The value of a pixel in the viewing plane is determined by the voxel intensities its ray intersects on its path from the observation point and the visualization algorithm in use.

Volume rendering can become very sophisticated based on the model used to construct the final scene pixels from the paths and intersection voxel intensities. Varying amounts of information can be stored depending on the model's complexity, as the rays traverse the image volume. Similar to surface rendering, various lighting and shading models can be used to control the final look of the scene. One simple model is to record the first intensity value above a chosen threshold and the distance from the observation point at which it occurred for each ray cast. The scene pixel for each ray is a function of these two parameters with darker values for greater distances to simulate depth. By simply changing the threshold different structures are displayed. Volume rendering using this technique is illustrated in Fig. 4a,b with the threshold parameter set to display the external skin in one view and bone in the other.

a 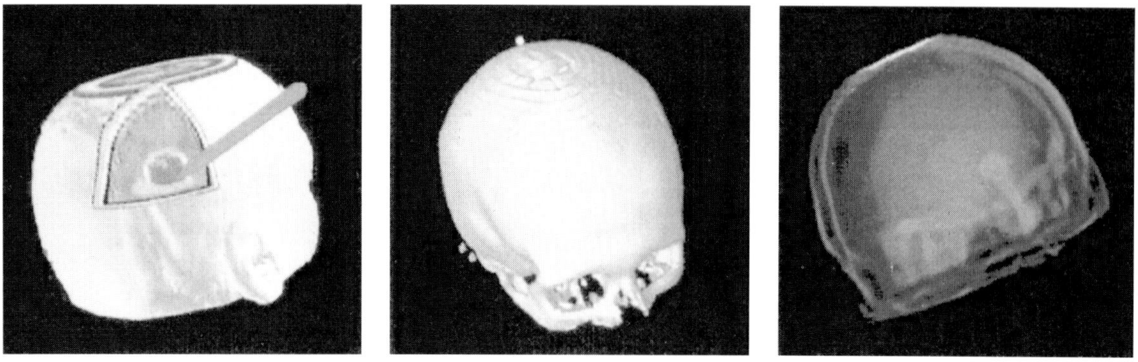 b, c

Fig. 4a–c. Examples of volume rendering. a External skin surface b Skull. c Digitally reconstructed radiograph

Another of example of volume rendering techniques involves digitally reconstructed radiographs. Here a specific algorithm is applied to a CT volume. The intensities of all voxels intersected along a ray's path are summed and normalized. Since a CT image intensity is related to the energy absorbed by an X-ray beam this algorithm simulates the passage of an X-rays through the anatomy. The resultant scene displays a virtual X-ray taken of the anatomy with the source at the observation point. This is illustrated in Fig. 4c. This information is very useful in radiation treatment planning for simulation of port films and the creation of conformal apertures.

Volume rendering has the advantage over surface rendering of requiring no steps in explicitly extracting structures. Once an algorithm has been determined to work it can usually be run over numerous data sets with minor tweaking of parameters. The downside of volume rendering are the computational requirements which result in slower performance. Changing the scene or viewing from another angle involves recasting and recomputing all the rays. Real-time volume rendering is available but on machines whose costs are probably prohibitive for clinical use. Hopefully this will improve, as the history of computer performance has continually proven in the past.

■ Stereotactic Applications

The visualization of image data is important, but this alone would not justify the time, effort, and cost in implementing the graphics previously described. Graphics software is most useful when it is integrated with a complete application that is designed to assist in specific procedures. The software should also model the framework of the specific procedure. This is demonstrated in several examples of 3D planning systems.

Surgical Planning

Stereotactic neurosurgery has always required the accurate connection of the image data to the patient in the operating room. The purpose of stereotactic equipment is to allow the surgeon to target a specific location and to confidently achieve this target. Traditionally this has been a 2D exercise. Information on trajectories is obtained on a slice-by-slice basis in conjunction with the physician's anatomical knowledge. It is very difficult to accurately integrate data from multiple imaging modalities from films alone.

3D software applications for stereotactic neurosurgery have advanced the planning of such procedures to a new plateau [5, 6]. StereoPlan (RSA, Burlington, Mass.) is a software planning system used in conjunction with the CRW stereotactic hardware (Radionics, Burlington, Mass.). Once the fiducials have been detected in the image data, all work is carried out in stereotactic coordinates. The software provides for viewing of the 2D image data in conjunction with 3D surface renderings of the patient anatomy. A surgical probe is manipulated in the 3D anatomy and if desired the stereotactic arc system is displayed. Numerous methods in both 3D and 2D are available for choosing targets and trajectories. Information from multiple image modalities are handled simultaneously in the common stereotactic space. The software supports data from CT, MR, and angiographic films.

The software automatically determines stereotactic coordinates of any chosen target. The physician is able easily to investigate various trajectories to a target through manipulation of the graphics and the software's integrated user interface. The strength of the system is the coupling of the graphics to the modeling of the stereotactic hardware. Targeting also does not depend on which modality a structure came from.

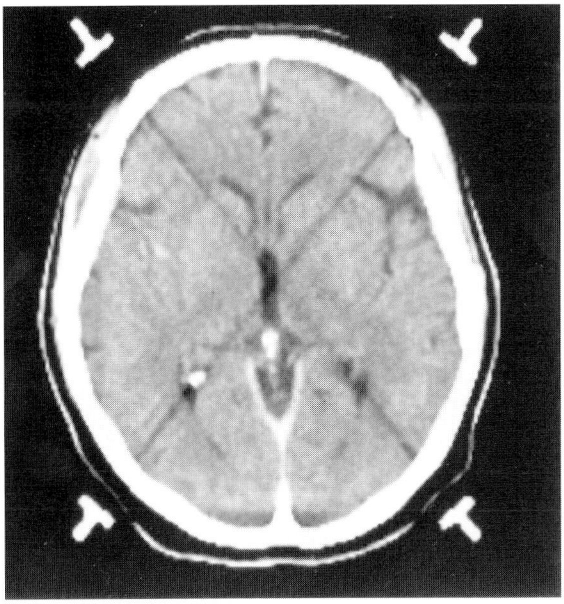

a

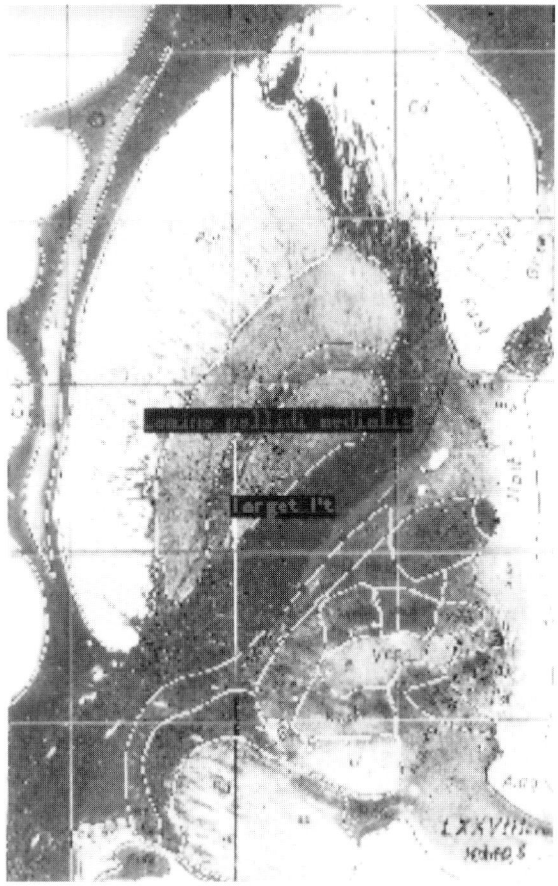

b

Fig. 5 a, b. Functional atlas for neurosurgical planning. **a** Patient data. **b** Atlas data

Planning of functional neurosurgical procedures benefits by the inclusion of a surgical atlas [7] in the software. The atlas consists of photographs of regularly spaced stained brain slices. The nuclei of the slices are meticulously contoured, and this information is stored in the computer. Positioning and scaling the atlas data to the patient is handled by locating the anterior and posterior commissars in the patient data. Further scaling in the lateral direction is possible through identification of common landmarks in both the atlas and the patient data sets. After the patient and atlas data are correlated, the planner may target off the atlas where the nuclei are better delineated. The corresponding point in the patient data set (and 3D view) is updated automatically along with the frame information necessary to target the desired location. Conversely, a target in the patient data selected and the corresponding point in the atlas is indicated. Figure 5 displays the atlas slice and the corresponding CT slice.

Frameless Stereotaxy

The discussion above focuses on exploiting the computer workstation for planning purposes. Entering the realm of frameless stereotaxy, the computer is now employed during the actual procedure. Removing the frame requires other methods for achieving stereotactic localization. The computer workstation coupled with the imaging data provides this fundamental capability throughout the procedure.

The design of the user interface and the inclusion of the graphics into the software become even more important when they are used in the operative environment. Unlike a planning process, the computer is no longer the prime focus of attention of the clinicians. The use of the software must be as self-evident as possible. Simplicity should take precedence over functionality that would possibly confuse the operation of the system.

Interactive Operating Digitizers

When performing a frameless neurosurgical procedure and accurate localization is still de-

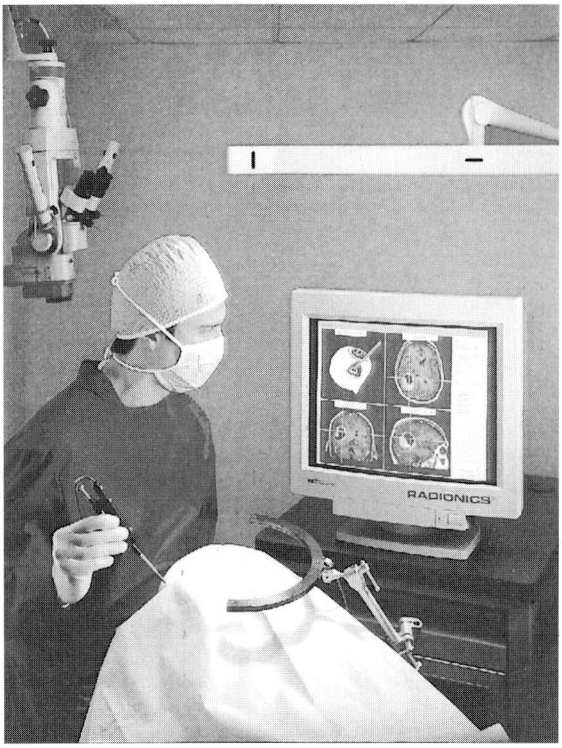

Fig. 6. Operating Arm System mechanical digitizer

sired, the stereotactic information must come from another source. One method coming to prominence is the use of a 3D digitizer in conjunction with a previously acquired image volume [8, 9]. The digitizer is a device that is able to supply information about its position in 3D space. A number of digitizers have been developed based on various physical principles for geometric tracking. These include mechanical, optical, ultrasonic, and electromagnetic systems.

The minimum requirements are the ability to determine the location and orientation of a handheld instrument and to relay this information to a computer. Localization is achieved by tracking the digitizer's position and displaying the corresponding point in the image data on a computer display. The Operating Arm System (OAS; RSA, Burlington, MA; Fig. 6) is an example of a system that uses a mechanical digitizer for frameless stereotactic neurosurgery

Each digitizer possesses its own internal coordinate system. This system must be correlated with the patient anatomy. Prior to surgery the patient is scanned with fiducial markers placed around the anatomical area of interest. These may be skin staples or specially made adhesive markers. The markers must remain in place from scanning through the duration of the procedure. After the images are loaded onto the computer, the fiducials are identified in the images and their image locations are stored. Figure 7 shows the OAS interface for fiducial selection. Notice the simplicity of the interface and the size of the components for easy recognition.

The goal is to correlate the 3D space of the digitizer which the patient anatomy resides in to the coordinate system of the image data. This is carried out by touching each fiducial on the patient with the digitizer and passing the location of the fiducial in digitizer coordinates to the computer. Mathematically at least three noncollinear points are needed but, it is desirable to use more for self-consistency checks. The computer is able to calculate the transformation necessary to go from digitizer space to image space.

Subsequent to the calibration process, when the digitizer moves within the patient anatomy, the computer is able to calculate the corresponding location in the image volume and display the appropriate images. The displayed images can be slices composing the original data volume or slices reformatted in other planes. Figure 8 contains a triorthogonal set of image slices intersecting at the digitizer location. The data were acquired axially while the sagittal and coronal views were reformatted from the axial data set. In this viewing mode the images are updated in real time.

In Fig. 9 the slices are reformatted based on the digitizer orientation. In addition to the standard axial slice, one slice is cut perpendicular to the probe direction, and the other is a vertical slice containing the plane of the probe. This display also contains a volume rendered anatomy with sections removed to show the probe location. There is more information in this mode than can be updated and real-time. The view is updated through a foot pedal controlled by the surgeon.

In general, frameless stereotaxy is not as accurate as frame-based examination. It is assumed in forming the data volume that all slices are parallel. Patient movement during the scanning process and the ability to localize the fiducials on the patient and in the image set contribute to system errors. When accuracy on the order of 2–5 mm is acceptable, the digitizing systems provide a power localization tool through graphics visualization.

Interventional Magnetic Resonance

The recent introduction of MR scanners that allow access to the patient have spurred the development of interventional MR systems. These open

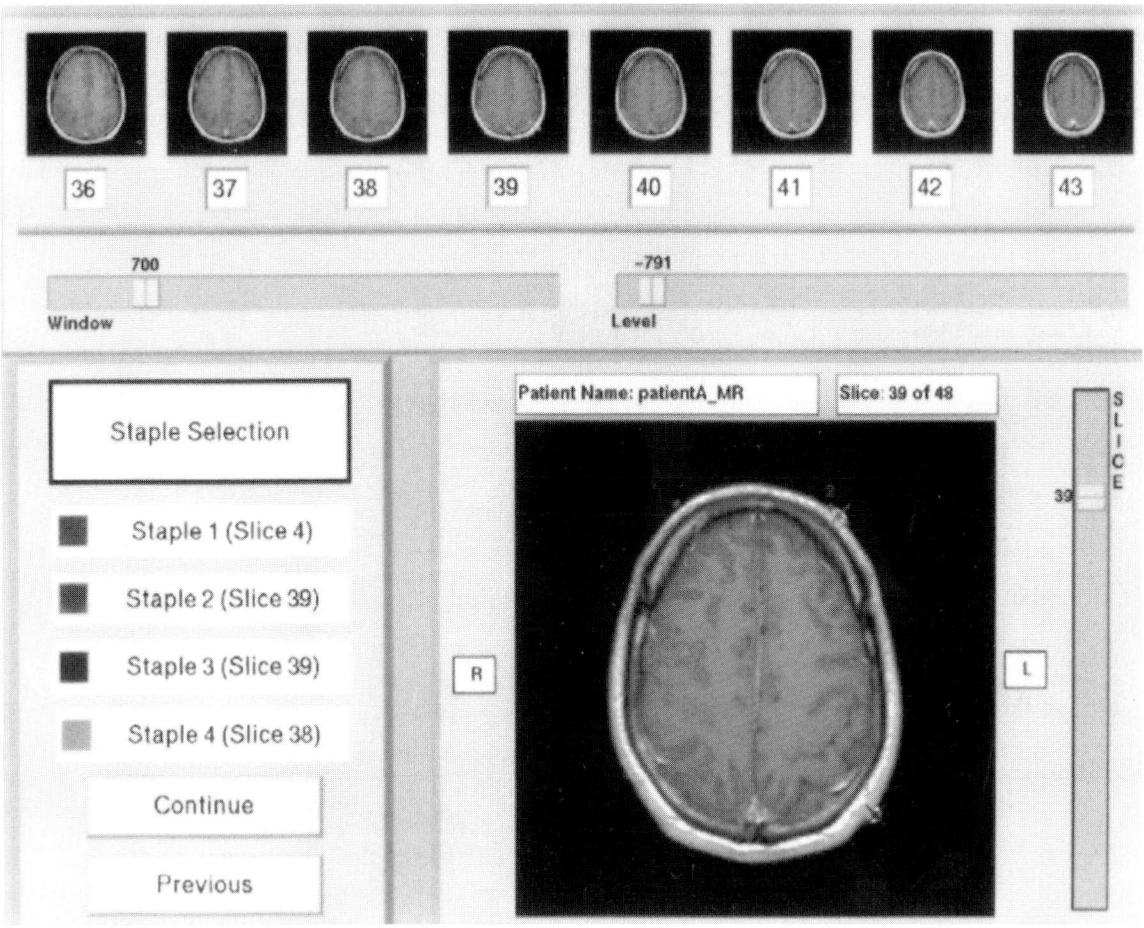

Fig. 7. Operating Arm System fiducial selection panel

scanners have provided for a new type of frameless stereotaxy. The previously discussed digitizing systems work with a historical data set for targeting. Interventional MR systems work with images that are acquired throughout the procedure. This gives greater control and flexibility to the physician which hopefully leads to better accuracy.

To achieve their full potential as interventional systems, the open scanners are interfaced with a computer workstation and a digitizing device. The computer works as interface between the digitizer and the scanner. In this domain the digitizing device is calibrated not to the patient but to the scanner's internal coordinate system. When the digitizer moves in the magnet bore (where the patient resides), the computer knows the digitizer location in scanner coordinates. The computer is able to request image slices to be acquired in the coordinates the scanner understands. The described system allows the physician to control what part of the anatomy the scanner is imaging by moving the digitizer to desired locations.

Through the workstation software the physician can also be given control over what types of images are acquired. The scanners are capable of directly acquiring oblique slices. Thus views dependent on probe orientation do not require reformatting of historical data. Nearly real-time image acquisition controlled by the physician provides a powerful tool for accurate and reliable probe insertions. This can be thought of as real-time planning.

The images from the scanner are sent back to the workstation. The workstation knows both what slices are acquired and the location and orientation of the probe. This information together with the computational power of the computer can be harnessed to perform image processing in addition to simple image display. Currently software is being developed to aid specific procedures.

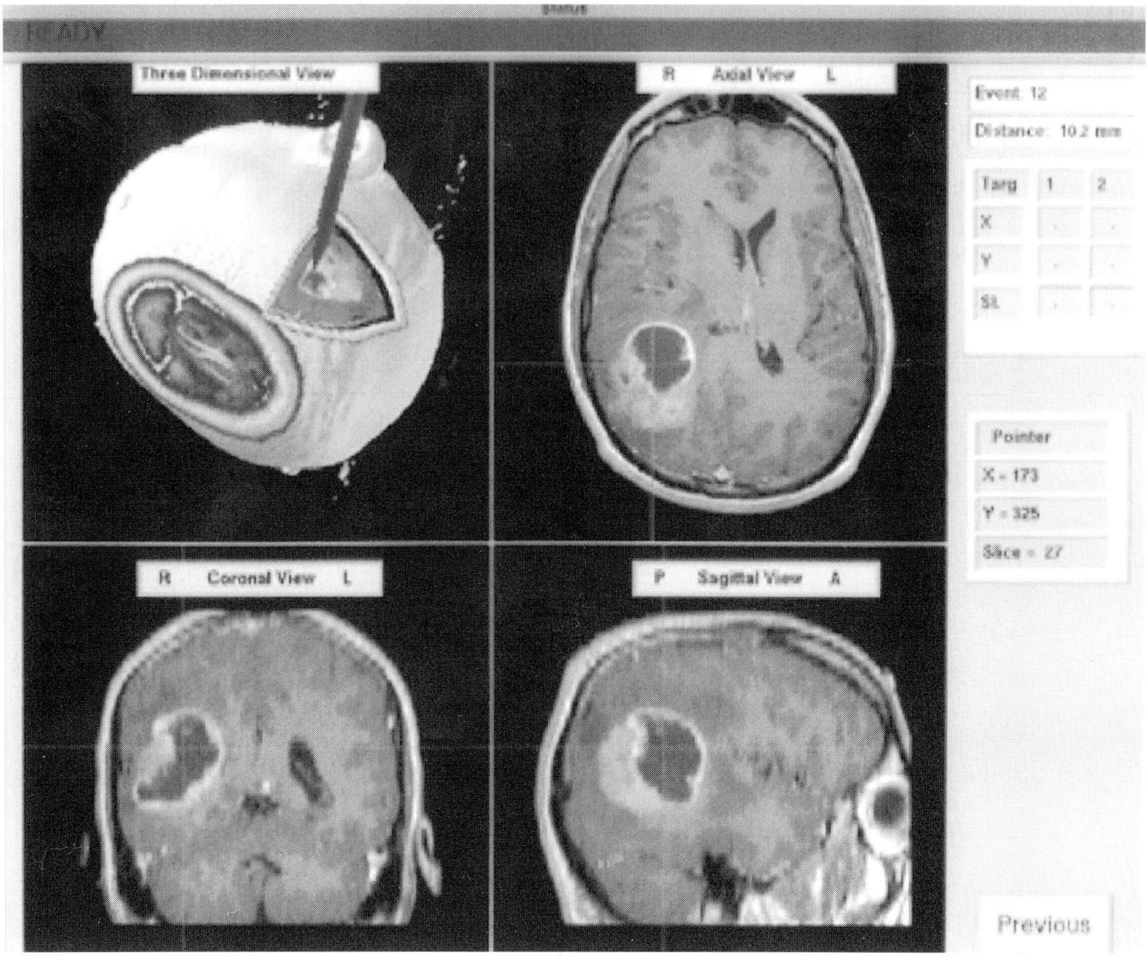

Fig. 8. Operating Arm System viewing slices: standard triorthogonal slices

As an example, radiofrequency lesioning is an active area of research in minimally invasive therapy [10]. The interventional system can help not only in guiding the probe to the target location but also in determining the treatment delivery parameters. Predictive temperature profiles can be overlaid on the acquired images in color. Thus the clinician can possibly plan treatment based on the actual probe location within the anatomy. Studies are investigating how well physiological changes can be visualized in MR during actual radiofrequency delivery. The workstation is able to store a starting image and compare it to incoming images through image subtraction (Fig. 10). These capabilities would not be possible without the workstation as a component of the interventional system.

■ Conclusion

Computer technology has already proven its value in neurosurgical planning and intraoperative support. Advances will surely continue in Both the hardware and software arenas. Computational and graphics performance gains are inevitable and will become available at even lower cost. Algorithmic development in areas such as automatic segmentation and customized atlas registration will provide powerful tools to the physicians. Success has been greatest when the sophisticated graphics and algorithms are integrated into software that is designed for specific procedures. The technology must always be grounded in applications that are capable of delivering better treatment to the patient. This requires the continued close collaboration between the clinicians and computer engineers.

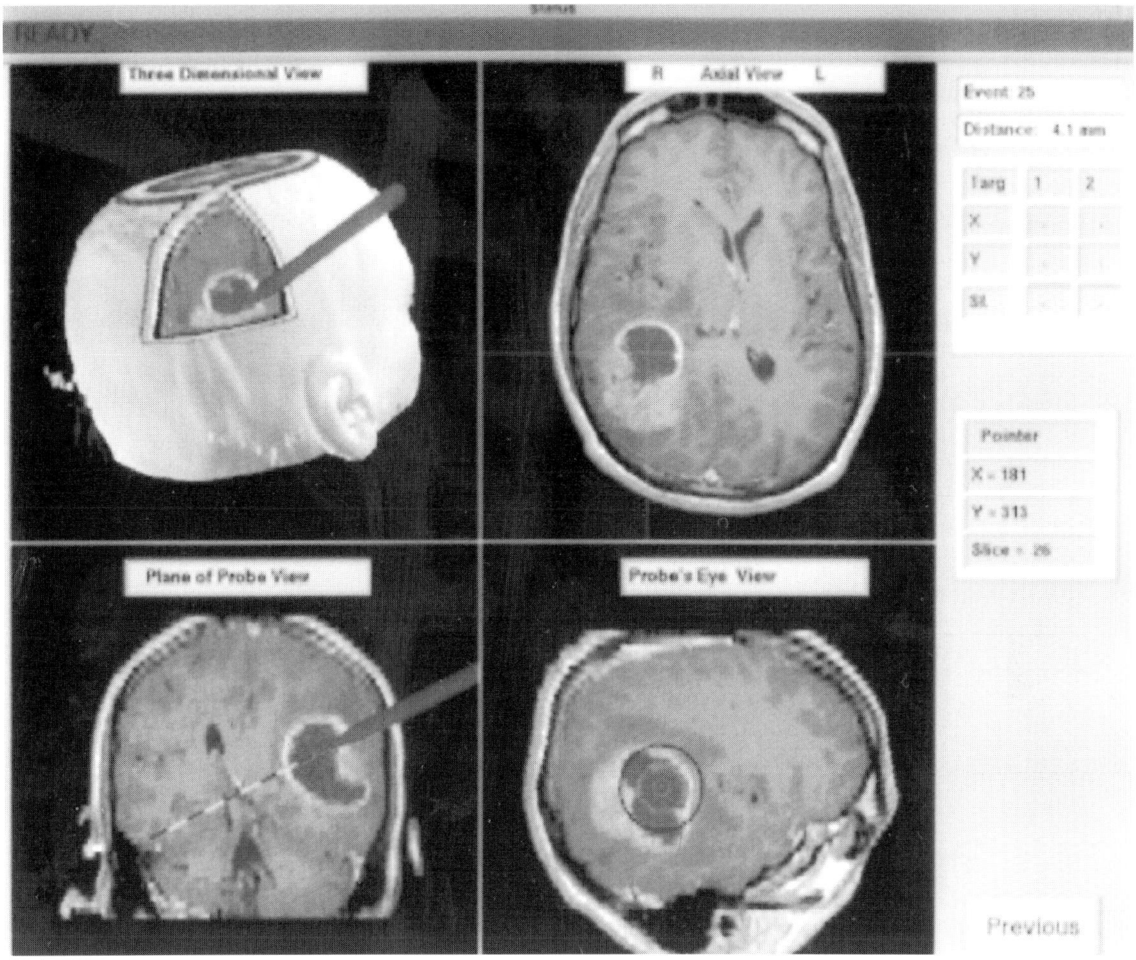

Fig. 9. Operating Arm System viewing slices: probe's-eye-view and plane of probe

a

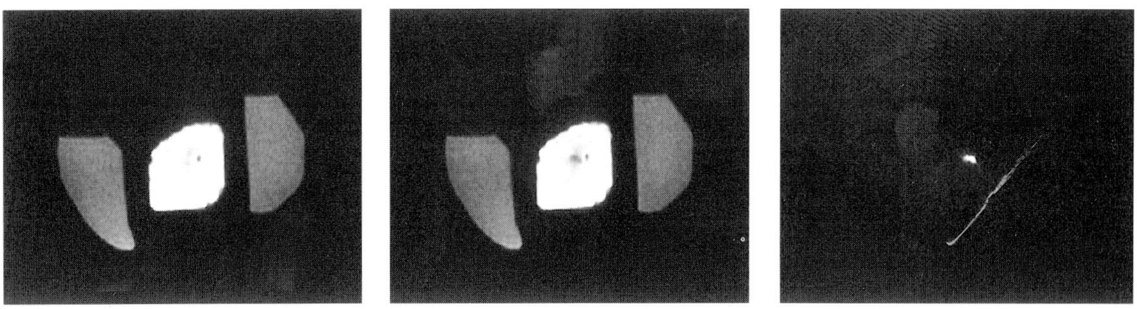

b, c

Fig. 10a–c. Image subtraction during lesioning of a sheep brain. a Prior to lesioning. b During lesion formation. c Subtracted image

■ References

1. Foley JD, van Dam A, Feiner SK, Hughes JF (1990) Computer graphics principles and practice, 2nd edn. Addison-Wesley, Reading
2. Webb S (1988) The physics of medical imaging. Hilger, Bristol
3. Lufkin RB (1997) The MRI manual, 2nd edn. Mosby, St. Louis
4. Clarke LP, Velthuizen RP, Camacho MA (1995) MRI segmentation methods and applications. Magn Reson Imaging 13:343–368
5. Kelly PJ, Kall BA (eds) (1992) Compuers in stereotactic neurosurgery. Blackwell, Oxford
6. Pillay PK, Phavichitr P (1993) Computer workstation stereotaxis. Proceedings of the XIth Meeting of the World Society for Sterotactic and Functional Neurosurgery
7. Schaltenbrand G, Wahren W (1977) Atlas for stereotaxy of the human brain. Year Book, Chicago
8. Guthrie BL, Adler JR Jr (1992) Computer-assisted preoperative planning interactive surgery and frameless stereotaxy, Clin Neurosurg 38:112–131
9. Maciunas RJ (ed) (1993) Interactive image-guided neurosurgery. American Association of Neurological Surgeons,
10. Anzai Y, Lufkin R, DeSalles A, Hamilton DR, Farahani K, Black KL (1995) Preliminary experience with MR-guided thermal ablation of brain tumors. Am J Neuroradiol 16:39

Interventional Operation Theaters

4

D. H. W. Grönemeyer, A. Gevargez, R. Seibel, A. Melzer, M. Deli

■ Introduction

More and more radiology departments are organizing their computed tomography (CT) or magnetic resonance imaging (MRI) suites for interventional procedures [1]. For semisterile procedures this can normally be carried out very easily; for sterile procedures the scanners must be installed in conventional operation rooms (OR) or in newly developed operation theaters. The special equipment must be defined by an interdisciplinary team, but the basics are imaging and navigation systems, electronic equipment for ablation techniques or hyperthermia, monitors for all imaging modalities [including those for three-dimensional (3D) imaging], patient couch, and special instruments [2–4].

■ Scanner Technology

The key to all access techniques is the combination of imaging systems: CT, MRI, ultrasound, X-ray, and endoscopy [5]. One of the new access techniques is a combined interventional procedure: for this technique an X-ray C-arm is placed directly at the CT or the ultrafast electron beam tomography (EBT) scanner, but can also be combined with MRI. By combining a mobile fluoroscope with or without digital subtraction angiography (DSA) and CT/EBT, the structures to be punctured can be visualized in 3D with excellent morphological differentiation in real time.

Another possibility is to use an open MRI scanner for guidance technology. With the addition of CT, EBT, and MRI all interstitial and bone structures can be defined with high accuracy. Therefore the treatment and the approach to the region of therapy can be planned and controlled precisely. The thickness and extension size of

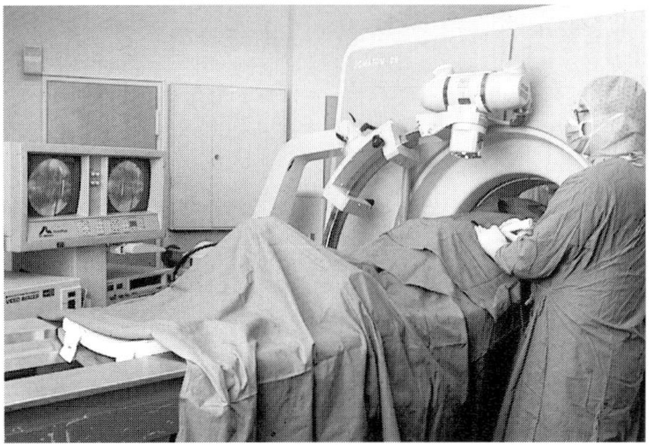

Fig. 1. Interventional CT: suite

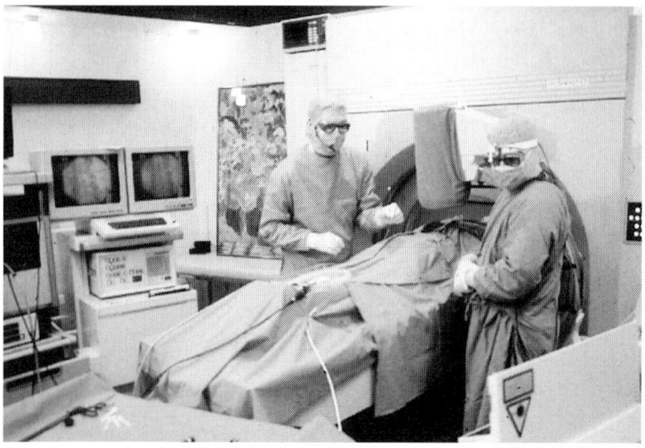

Fig. 2. Hybrid EBT unit (Imatron, Siemens). The fluoroscopy unit is installed near the gantry and the surrounding

muscles, fat, lymph nodes, and tendons are also visible as well as risk areas such as nerves, vessels, and dural sack. Complications can be detected at an early stage and therapeutic effects documented interactively.

■ Hybrid Scanner: Computed Tomography and Fluoroscopy

Minimally invasive treatments require CT scanners with gantry openings for the patient of more than 60 cm. Our treatments are performed in a spiral CT scanner with a 70-cm gantry (Somatom Plus S and Plus 4; Siemens, Erlangen, Germany; Fig. 1). The distance between patient couch and gantry requires between 0.5 and 1.0 m, so that a fluoroscopic unit can be installed close to the gantry with optimal space for the therapist in all directions. The table must be moved to defined positions in- and outside the gantry to the operative field. Monitors, laser systems, endoscopy, and ultrasound units are placed close the gantry.

■ Hybrid Scanner: Electron Beam Tomography and Fluoroscopy

The recent revolution in advanced digital imaging technologies widens the field for interventional scanners. Ultrafast EBT has been developed for noninvasive calcification screening [6] in coronary arteries (Imatron, Los Angeles, CA, USA; Fig. 2). One important requirement for minimally invasive procedures is that the gantry opening have diameter of at least 80 cm. This is important for minimally invasive guidance procedures with long instruments such as endoscopes and forceps. We initially reported this technique in 1989 [7], and currently we are combining a C-arm for fluoroscopy unit with EBT (Fig. 2) to achieve a 3D view of the operative field. During scanning mode an electron beam is focused to a 1- to 2-mm focal spot that is deflected across a series of four semicircular tungsten targets around the patient. Each target can produce an X-ray beam. Frame rates up to 34 images per second are possible (simultaneous multilevel scan acquisition in 50 ms). Two detector rings are installed above the patient so that a pair of EBT images can be obtained each time that any one of the tungsten rings is "swept" by the electron beam. Thus up to eight levels can be scanned at the same time without moving the patient table. Scans can be acquired at two, four, six, or eight levels during a single acquisition. Instruments can be followed through several planes at the same time.

Also, ultrafast scanning and fast 3D reconstruction will be helpful in the future for virtual endoscopy examination of the alimentary tract. This ultrafast imaging is not significantly degraded by moving organs and can be carried out within seconds.

■ Open MRI

The advantage of MRI guidance using an open system for interventional procedures is the nonionizing image, high soft-tissue contrast, multiplanar imaging, and the possibility of operating with fast MRI-fluoroscopic modes inside the magnet. An early ultralow-field MRI scanner [8] (Access, Toshiba MRI, San Francisco, USA) utilized a permanent magnet with a field strength of 0.064 T (Fig. 4). The vertical field magnets of this scanner permit circumferential open access at the four lateral sides similar to the 0.3- and 0.6-T

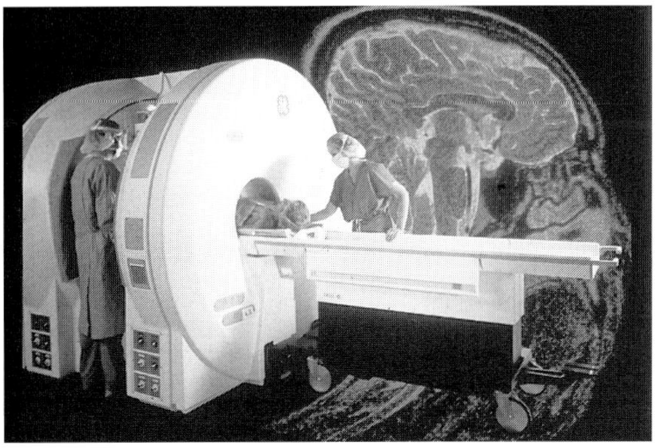

a

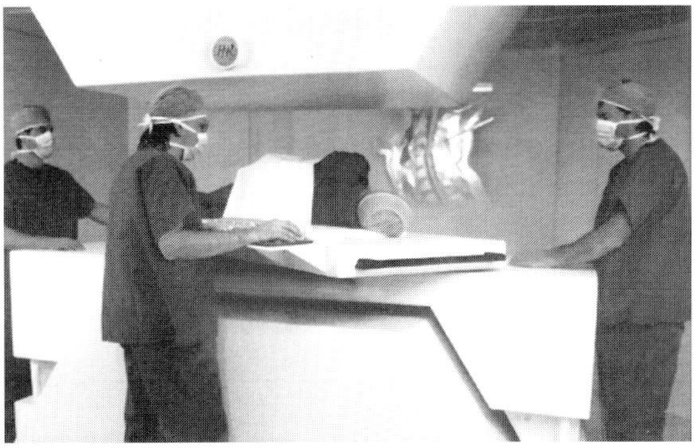

b

Fig. 3 a, b. Open MRI unit. a GE (USA), 0.5 T. b Proposed design for new open unit. (Fonar USA)

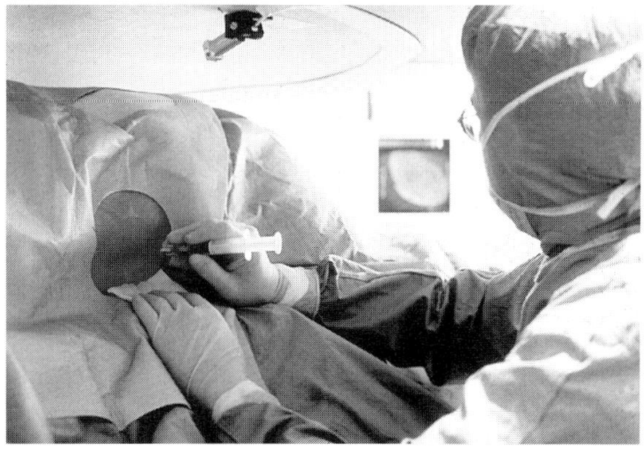

Fig. 4. Minimally invasive surgery performed inside the magnet: Access Toshiba (Japan), 0.064 T

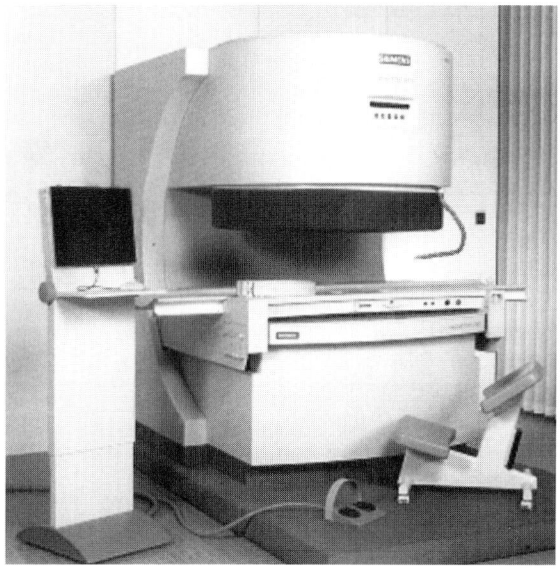

Fig. 5. Magnetom Open (Siemens, Germany) for interventional procedures

units from Fonar. Since the early 1990s other open MRI unit configurations have been developed with various field strengths (U-shaped 0.2 T: Siemens (Fig. 5), Picker; Mid-field: 0.5 T, GE Medical Systems; 0.3 T Hitachi, Fonar (Fig. 3); Tables 1, 2).

The efficiency and possibilities of open magnets and low-field MRI are currently undergoing extensive research. Open systems for MRI are generally more comfortable than the narrow, tube-like scanners, and patients therefore tend to be more cooperative and amenable to diagnosis and percutaneous procedures. Additionally, it is easier to examine "claustrophobic" and frightened patients.

■ Electronic Equipment, Software, and Instruments

A special development of shielding the electronic equipment for MRI allows the use of lasers, endoscopic systems, monitors, light boxes, etc. close to the magnets. Because flat liquid crystal display monitors are not sensitive to magnetic distortion, they can be used for screening MRI scans and for endoscopy, ultrasound, or other imaging. To avoid projectile effects and artifacts in MRI, mechanical instruments and endoscopes are being developed by using special nonferromagnetic materials such as titanium, platinum, stainless steel, special plastics, and superelastic nitinol [9].

A positioning device (Picker, Cleveland, Ohio, US; Micromed, Bochum, Germany) can transfer the given entry point and puncturing angle automatically to the skin. The laser light is projected directly onto the hub end of the instruments and is so positioned that the crosshairs of the laser beam are projected onto the target surfaces of the endoscopes, forceps, cannulae, etc. Speech control enables the patient couch in EBT to be moved in all directions.

Table 1. MRI units for interventional procedures (in ascending order of field strength)

System	Field strength (T)	Magnet system	Design	Interventional capability
Toshiba Access	0.064	Permanent	Open 4-sided	Open system with (360°) vertical "temple" access, fluoroscopy, general interventions
InnerVision	0.14	Permanent	Open 3-sided	Dedicated system for head and extremities, restricted vertical access
Siemens Open	0.2	Resistive	C form	Open system, open 3-sided suitable for "Big Mac" intervention, fast imaging possible, restricted vertical access
GE Open	0.2	Permanent	Open 2-sided	Open system, suitable for intervention, fast imaging possible, restricted vertical access
Picker Outlook	0.23	Resistive	C form	Open system, open 3-sided suitable for intervention, fast imaging possible, restricted vertical access
Fonar	0.3	Hybrid permanent	Open 4-sided	Open system, suitable for interventions
Magnalab	0.3	Permanent	C form	Dedicated open 3-sided system for extremities
Hitachi Airis	0.3	Permanent	270° access	Open system, suitable for intervention, fast imaging possible, restricted vertical access
Toshiba	0.35	Hybrid	Open 4-sided	Open system with (360°) vertical "temple" access, fluoroscopy, general interventions
GE "Double Donut"	0.5	High-temperature superconductor	Full vertical, restricted horizontal access	Developed especially for treatments in standing position, fast imaging
Picker Asset	0.5	Superconducting tube	2-sided system	Suitable as tube system with limitations
Philips NT 5	0.5	Superconducting tube	2 sided system	Suitable as tube, combination with DSA integrated LCD monitor
Fonar	0.6	Hybrid permanent	Open 4-sided open system	Suitable for interventions
Siemens	1.0	Superconducting, tube	2-sided system	"Harmony" suitable with limitations, in room monitor
Siemens	1.5	superconducting, tube	2-sided system	"Symphony" suitable with limitations, in room monitor
Bruker	2.0	Superconducting, tube	2-sided system	Suitable with limitations, food pad guidance in OR

Table 2. Equipment suite preference by procedure (from [11])

		Best imaging suite	Good suite(s)	Poor suite(s)
Spine	Percutaneous nucleotomy (acute herniation)	CT	EBT	MRI
	Sequestrectomy	CT	EBT	MRI
	Periradicular therapy (chronic herniation)	CT	EBT	MRI
	Facet joint therapies (C/T spine: high-risk areas)	CT	EBT	MRI
	Facet joint therapies (L spine: low-risk areas)	MRI	CT	EBT
	Iliosacral joint	MRI	CT	EBT
Biopsy	Biopsies (thorax, heart, abdomen)	EBT	CT	MRI
	Biopsies (low-risk areas)	MRI	EBT/CT	
	Biopsies (high-risk areas)	CT	EBT	MRI
Cancer	Local cancer therapy (low-risk areas)	MRI	CT/EBT	
	Local cancer therapy (high-risk areas)	CT	EBT	MRI
Neurolysis	Sympathectomies	EBT	CT	MRI
Endoscopy	Thorax, heart, abdomen	EBT	CT	MRI
	Joints	MRI	EBT	CT
	Spine	CT	EBT	MRI
	Ear, nose, throat (sinus, ear, throat, soft tissue)	MRI	CT	EBT
	Brain (guidance)	CT	MRI	EBT
	Brain (treatment, documentation)	MRI	CT/EBT	
Vascular	Tip tracking	EBT	MRI	CT
Open surgery	Brain, neck, spine, thorax, abdomen, joints	MRI[a]	MRI/EBT[b]	CT

[a] Dedicated system
[b] Outside gantry

Tabelle 3. Comparison of open MRI scanners

	Access (Toshiba)	Open (Siemens)	Open MRI (General Electrics)
Field strength	0.064 T	0.2 T	0.5 T
Magnet	Permanent	Resistive	Superconducting
Design	Sandwich "Temple"	C-arm "Big Mac"	Open tube "Double donut"
Gantry opening	60×110 cm	41 cm	55/56 cm
Table centering	Manual	Manual	Automatic
Projectile effect (ferromagnetic instruments)	–	++	+++
Problems with conventional electronic equipment near the gantry	– to +	++	+++
Gradient noise	(+)	++	+++
TV Monitor in OP room	Yes	Yes	Yes
Endoscopic monitor in OP room	No	No	Yes
Fluoroscopy/keyhole imaging	Yes (>2 s)	Yes (>4 s)	Yes (>4 s)
3D localizer	Yes	No	No
MR angiography	No	Yes	Yes
Interactive 3D guidance	No	Yes	Yes
Laser in OP room	Yes	No	Yes
Mouse guidance in OP room	No	Yes	No
Foot pad guidance in OP room	No	Yes	No
Conventional operation inside the magnet possible	Limited	(No)	Yes
Weight	7 tons	12 tons	4.9 tons
Cooling	No	Water: 17–40 l/min	Cryogens
Electrical power	10 kVA	29 kVA	60 kVA

■ 2D Versus 3D Imaging for Interventional Procedures

All of today's cross-sectional imaging modalities allow 3D reconstructions in the postprocessing mode and more and more virtual endoscopy as well as 4D possibilities. Real-time processing is under development. The advantage of 3D imaging over 2D is the rapid recognition of anatomic regions, especially for inexperienced physicians. Transparent surfacing and several processing options enable the physician to examine organ structures such as surfaces or individual vessels and nerves. Also, more and more 3D reconstructions of inner surfaces of intestinal organs for virtual endoscopy are under development.

For access and guidance techniques the therapist requires high resolution for tip tracking and if possible also ultrafast or real-time imaging. Tissue changes such as regional edema, bleeding, and lesions caused by thermal treatments (laser, RF, cryotherapy, etc.) between operating manipulations can be controlled only by high-resolution imaging [17–24]. For this reason 3D or virtual guidance must be combined interactively with actual and not with prescanned slices.

3D imaging is also an important tool for postprocessing documentation of therapeutic effects such as drug distribution (e.g., percutaneous ethanol instillation for cancer therapy or sympathectomy), laser-induced tissue changes or implantations. 3D models are very helpful for operation planning and for education and training, especially if animal studies can be avoided [10].

■ Minimal Access Technique for CT, EBT, and MRI Guidance

The patient is positioned to provide best access to the lesion. Premedication is seldom required due to the minimal trauma from the microinstruments and the use of local anesthesia. The procedure is performed as following. First CT, EBT, or MRI of the region of interest is performed. In CT/EBT injection of intravenous contrast medium is required in those regions where vascular structures (e.g., in the mediastinum) are not visible in soft tissues (for MRI contrast media are used only for tumor and scar tissue differentiation). Then the entry point, the puncture angle, and the distance to the therapeutic region are determined electronically and visualized at the monitor. After disinfection local anesthesia of 1% mepivacaine is administered using a special guidance coaxial set (EZEM, USA; Cook, Denmark; EFMT or Daum, Germany). The direction and position of the cannulae are checked with CT, EBT, or MRI.

All instruments, including lasers, endoscopes, and forceps, are introduced through the guidance cannula. The distance from the skin level to the structure which must be reached, can always be determined through the centimeter scale at the instrument's shaft. Injury to high-risk structures such as lung, nerves, and vessels in the path of the instruments is avoided by injecting local anesthesia and saline solution during the advancing, which helps to push these structures away from the cannula's tip (so-called "hydraulically assisted cannula insertion" [9–10]). Percutaneous procedures using open-field MRI system can be approached in similar manner as with either fluoroscopically or sonographically guided techniques. After imaging the patient can be treated inside the gantry or removed from the center of the magnet for performing major interventional procedures where greater access is needed. For biopsies specially reduced artifact instruments are available from Somatex (Germany), Daum (Germany), and EZEM (USA). Therapeutic sets for cancer therapy are also available from Somatex. Before intratumoral drug instillation, diluted contrast media in CT and MRI (gadolinium) must be injected for documentation of drug extent. In CT or EBT the patient couch must be moved out of the gantry for the treatments several times.

■ Therapy Phases [11]

There are four major therapy phases for each procedure, which require different imaging modalities:

1. Localizing: slice definition and electronic measurement (high resolution)
2. Guidance: introduction of instruments (fast imaging, low resolution)
3. Treatment: controlling of therapeutic effects (high resolution, 3D imaging)
4. Documentation: of treatment (high resolution, several planes, 3D imaging)

■ CT or MRI for Guidance Techniques?

Although computed tomography has in the past been the gold standard for interstitial instrument guidance, MRI is gaining in importance with the newly developed open systems. In contrast to CT, MRI does not produce X-rays. This is important not only for the therapist but also for the patient. In addition imaging in three planes can be gained almost in real time.

Also, without contrast media, arteries and veins can be documented, as well as changes in tissue contrast after heating with laser or cooling with cryotherapy or using hyperenergetic ultrasound for tissue ablation. The use of this patient-friendly open device is advantageous not only to corpulent persons but also to children and persons suffering from claustrophobia; parents, relatives, or medical staff are thus able to accompany anxious patients.

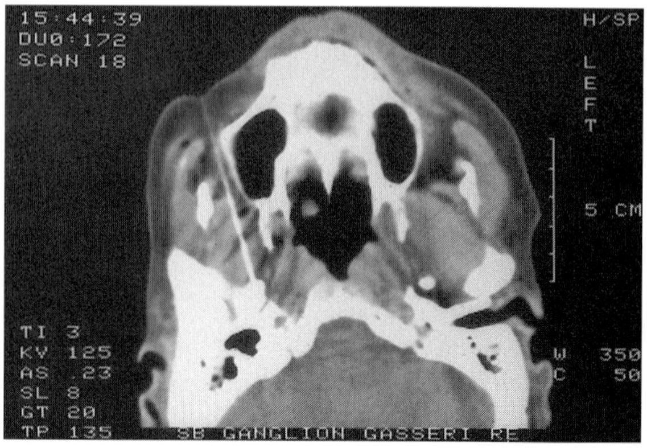

Fig. 6. Preparing a CT guidance to the gasserian ganglion. The entry point, distances, and angle are measured electronically on the monitor

In open MRI systems, operations can be carried out quite comfortably inside the gantry without the patient being moved, with nearly real-time guidance using fast keyhole sequences [10, 11].

When there are vital structures such as nerves and vessels in the target region (Figs. 6–10), CT is our gold standard for guidance technology [12]. The tip guidance precision with CT is 1 mm^3, the edges of the instruments are sharply displayed, and the tip can be defined to ± 0.2 mm. In many cases correct and safe access can be gained by CT/EBT for interstitial therapy such as drug injection or placement of prostheses and implants (Fig. 11). Other applications are drilling and fixation with the correct angle for osteosynthesis, hybrid tomographic systems for balloon dilatation, laser treatments, and stent implantation. With this kind of tracking technique for intravascular catheter guidance the tip can also be placed very exactly inside the vessel in precise relation to the wall of the artery or vein.

As pointed out above, EBT has the largest gantry (90 cm) and the fastest acquisition time, but current computer processing is to slow.

Best access for treatment has been found in the open MRI systems with nearly real-time guidance of the instruments by using especially fast keyhole sequences. This technique is faster than CT, but with a lower quality image. For high-quality scans the total scan time is much longer than in CT. For high-resolution documentation T1- and T2-weighted sequences must be acquired after

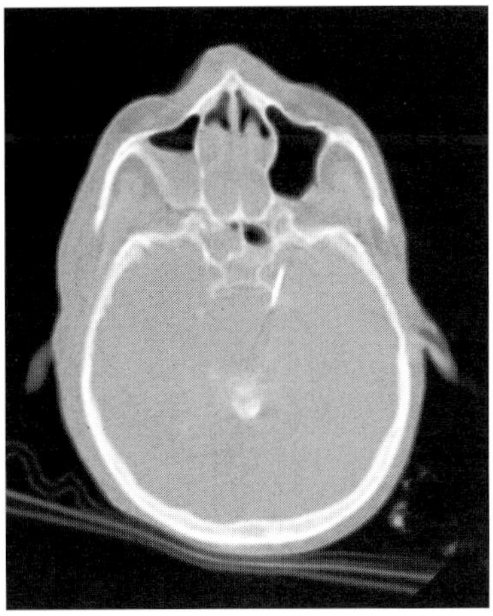

Fig. 7. The guidance cannula (18 G) is directed through the foramen ovale into the brain. The tip is positioned 1 mm inside Meckel's space without damaging the bone (EBT): cadaver study

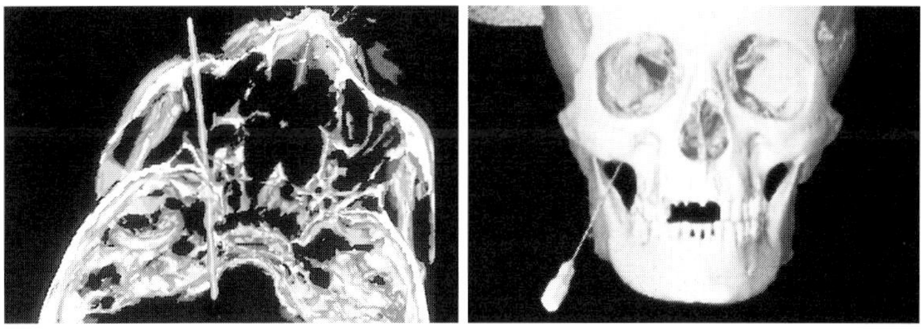

a b

Fig. 8. a 3D reconstruction of EBT scans for access to the gasserian ganglion. b Volume reconstruction of the bone

fluoroscopy mode in a single plane in additional minutes. Special materials are required for the instruments because conventional instruments cause artifacts in the displayed scans. Some special nonferromagnetic cannulae are available today for interventional MRI. However, the major drawback is that the resolution of tip and longitudinal edges of the instruments is only ±3.5 mm [10].

Open MRI is useful in low-risk areas. Organs affected by breathing should be penetrated during breath holding. Furthermore, it is possible to start with CT for safety of the guidance procedure and then change to MRI for visualization of treatment effects such as laser ablation. Other advan-

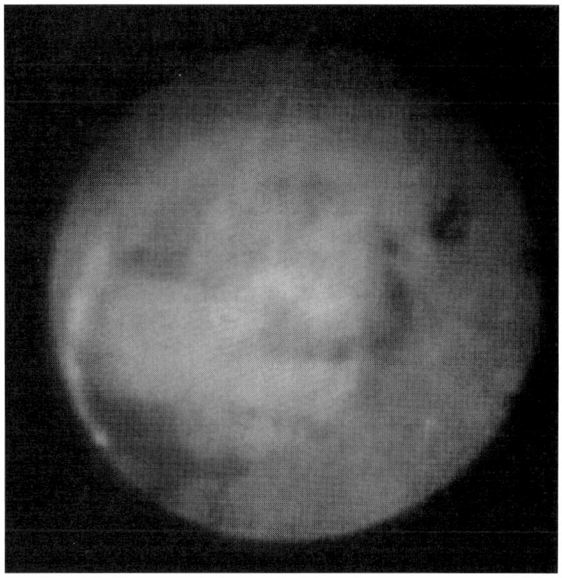

Fig. 9. A view of the gasserian ganglion and the vessels with a 0.6-mm microendoscope (Micromed) guided through the 18-G cannula

a 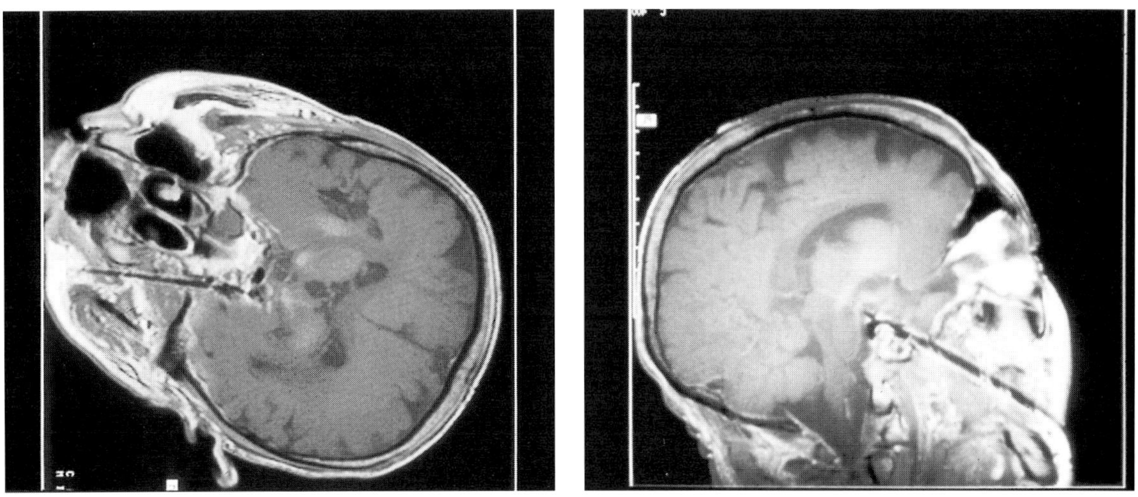 b

Fig. 10. The same study as in Fig. 9 but inside the MRI scanner. Note that the tip and edges of the nonferromagnetic cannula are not as precisely defined as in EBT

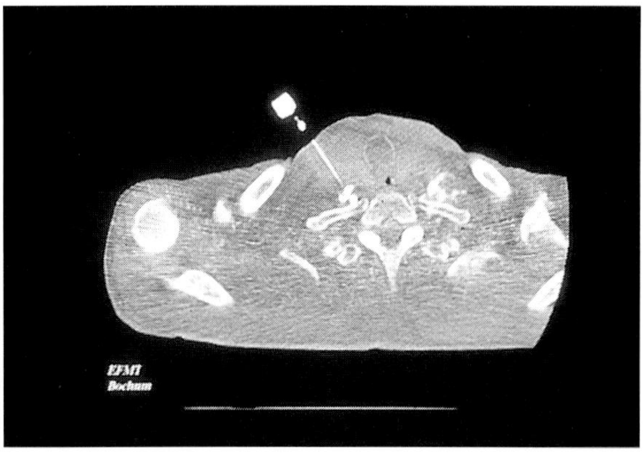

a

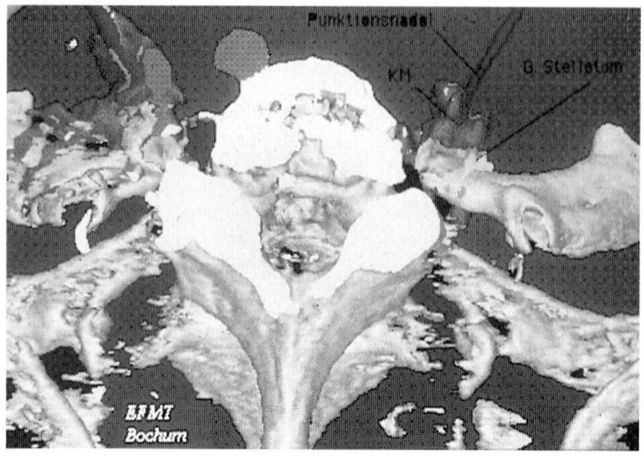

b

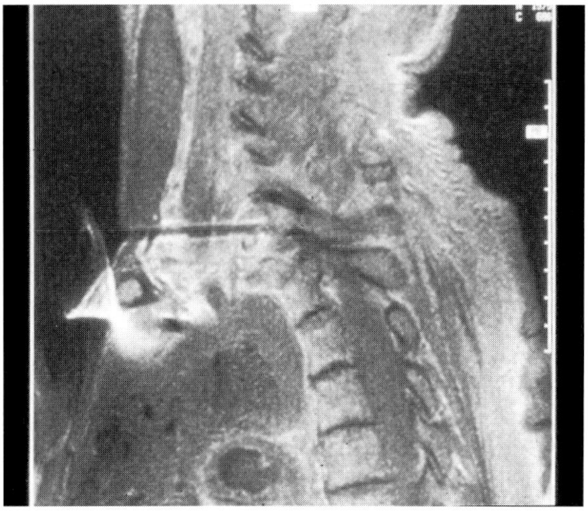
c

Fig. 11 a–c. Comparison of interventional studies in MRI, CT, and EBT for preparing pain therapy of ganglion stellate with local anesthesia and endoscopic treatments. **a** EBT. Guidance with instillation of contrast media. **b** 3D reconstruction. **c** MRI guidance of the same case

tages of MRI over CT/EBT is temperature mapping [13] and the possibility of measuring metabolic changes with imaging or spectroscopy mode in high-field (1.5–2 T) systems. Preoperative planning in all tomographic systems is also possible as well as 3D-reconstruction before and after the treatment.

We believe that these tomographic systems (CT, EBT, and MRI) will soon exist in many operating theaters in combination with endoscopy or ultrasound, x-ray units and microtherapeutic workstations [14] (see chapter C4). The conventional X-ray devices that provide only a shadowy image of the body structures will disappear. At the same time, prices of high-tech systems will be comparable to those of classical X-ray units due to the widespread installation of tomographs. In the future, dedicated CT/EBT [10, 11] or MRI systems should be available for all diagnostic or microinvasive procedures.

References

1. Grönemeyer DHW, Seibel R, Melzer A (1996) Editorial: Radiological imaging modalities revolutionize surgical and therapeutic procedures. Minimally Invasive Therapy and Allied Technologies 5:224–225
2. Lufkin R (1999) Interventional MRI. Mosby
3. Jolesz FA, Bleier AR, Jakob P et al. (1988) MRI imaging of laser tissue interactions. Radiology 168:249–253
4. Melzer A, Schmidt AM, Kipfmüller K, Deli M, Stöckel D, Grönemeyer DHW, Seibel RMM (1996) Prerequisites for magnetic resonance image guided interventions and endoscopic surgery. Minimally Invasive Therapy and Allied Technologies 5:255–262
5. Grönemeyer DHW, Seibel RMM, Melzer A, Schmidt A, Deli M, Friebe MH, Busch M (1995) Future of advanced guidance techniques by interventional CT and MRI. Minimally Invasive Therapy and Allied Technology 4:251–259
6. Boyd D, Gold R, Quinn J, Sparks R, Stanley R, Hermannsfeldt W (1979) A proposed dynamic cardiac 3D densitometer for easy detection and evaluation of heart disease, IEEE Trans Nucl Sci NS 26:2724
7. Jaschke W, Grönemeyer DHW, Seibel RMM, Boyd DP (1989) Perspektiven für CT-gesteuerte Punktionstechniken durch Ultra-Fast-Cine-CT, in Grönemeyer DHW, Seibel RMM (eds) Interventionelle Computertomographie. Ueberreuter Wissenschaft, Berlin, pp 291–295
8. Kaufmann L, Crooks L, Mitsuaki A, Hoenninger J, Watts J, Winkler M (1987) Admin Radiol 6:32–38

9. Melzer A, Kipfmüller K, Grönemeyer DHW, Seibel R, Buess G (1995) Ports, Trocars/Cannulae, and access techniques. Seminars in Laparoscopic Surgery 2:179–204
10. Grönemeyer DHW, Seibel RMM, Melzer A, Schmidt A (1995) Image-guided access techniques. Endoscopic Surgery 3:69–75
11. Grönemeyer DHW, Seibel RMM, Erbel R, Schmidt A, Melzer A, Plaßmann J, Schmermund A, Baumgart D, Welsch R, Ge J, Görge G (1996) Equipment configuration and procedures: Preferences for interventional microtherapy. Journal of Digital Imaging 9:81–96
12. Grönemeyer DHW (1989) Interventionelle Computertomographie. Ueberreuter Wissenschaft, Berlin
13. Knuettel B, Juretschke HP (1986) Temperature measurements by nuclear magnetic resonance. Recent Results Cancer Res 101:109–118
14. Grönemeyer DHW, Gevargez A, Möhlenkamp S, Deli M, Kriener P, Schmermund A, Melzer A, Erbel R (1998) Workstation for tomographic microtherapy. Min Invas Ther and Allied Technol 7/5:433–442

Technical Procedures for Diagnosis and Intervention

C

Temperature-Sensitive Magnetic Resonance Sequences

U. Sinha · S. Sinha · T. Oshiro

■ Introduction

The introduction of the open-magnet configuration with wide-angle accessibility to the patient and real-time monitoring of images within the scanner room has sparked considerable interest in magnetic resonance (MR) guided interventional procedures. Such procedures, including MR-guided biopsies, hyperthermia, cryoablation, and ablation using laser, radiofrequency (RF), and focused ultrasound (FUS), have been performed both in conventional 1.5-T scanners (closed configuration) and at low fields (open and closed configurations) [1–6]. A critical part of MR-guided ablation procedures is the ability to monitor spatially localized changes in temperature using heat-sensitive MR pulse sequences. An important area of MR-guided interventional procedures is the thermal ablation by laser-induced thermotherapy (LITT), FUS, and RF techniques. MR imaging is unique in its ability noninvasively to measure the distribution of spatial temperature through the effect of temperature on MR parameters (T1, diffusion, and proton chemical shift). The demands on temporal resolution are high, although not necessarily requiring real-time frame rates as in tracking of MR-guided procedures. The ablations typically are in the range of 20–40 s for FUS, 1–2 min for RF, and 10–20 min for LITT. In order to monitor temperature with sufficient temporal resolution in FUS and RF ablations it is necessary to be able to acquire temperature maps at least every 5–10 s. This chapter introduces the reader to the MR parameters that are sensitive to temperature and to the pulse sequences used to measure temperature with emphasis on the temporal requirements of the ablation procedures, followed by a brief overview of general scan methodologies for reducing scan times that are also applicable to temperature monitoring.

High temporal resolution is required to monitor RF and high-intensity FUS ablation procedures whereas the requirements for LITT and hyperthermia applications are more relaxed. The temperature dependency of three MR tissue parameters have been used for MR thermometry: spin-lattice relaxation (T1), the apparent diffusion coefficient (ADC), and the proton resonance frequency. There are relative merits and drawbacks to using any of these parameters for MR thermometry. The temperature sensitivity of the diffusion coefficient is 2.4%/°C, higher than the temperature sensitivities of T1 (0.8%–2%/°C) and proton resonance frequency (–0.0107 ppm/°C for pure water and a range of –0.007 to –0.009 ppm/°C for in vitro muscle and other organ tissues) [9, 17, 18]. The T1 dependence on temperature varies in various tissues and tissue physiological and metabolic changes during thermal therapy cause deviations from linear behavior. The temperature sensitivity of the diffusion coefficient is high, but diffusion imaging requires the application of large magnetic field gradients for rapid imaging. Recent investigations at high field strengths have established the proton resonance frequency method to be more suitable for MR thermometry than the measurement of diffusion and T1. However, to maintain an overall perspective, we present all three methods below.

Temperature from a Measurement of T1 or from T1-Weighted Sequences

The spin-lattice relaxation time T1 for tissues exhibits a linear dependence which can be expressed by the relationship:

$$\mathrm{T1_T} = \mathrm{T1_{ref}} + \mathrm{S}(\mathrm{T} - \mathrm{T_{ref}}) \qquad (1)$$

where $\mathrm{T1_{ref}}$ is the spin-lattice relaxation time at a reference temperature $\mathrm{T_{ref}}$, and S is the temperature sensitivity of T1. T1-weighted images using fast two-dimensional (2D) spoiled grass (SPGR) or 2D fast spin echo (FSE) sequences have been used to monitor temperature changes at 1.5 T during ultrasonic heating [7]. The temporal resolution of these scans has been measured as 4 s for the SPGR sequence and 5–16 s for the FSE sequences. A linear variation in the signal intensity of the T1-weighted images with temperature has been verified for porcine liver samples and gel phantoms (temperature change 36°–66 °C). However, these measurements were confined to correlating signal intensity changes to temperature changes and did not involve an explicit calculation of T1 values. Thus a separate calibration study is in general required for each type of tissue and imaging sequence. However, a recent investigation has revealed nonlinear signal intensity variations with temperature using a T1-weighted FSE for thermometry during interstitial laser photocoagulation in vivo in rabbit livers [8]. The latter study showed that changes in the tissue alter the MR imaging signal intensity and confound the intensity changes due to temperature.

The changes in signal intensity of a T1-weighted image may arise from sources other than changes in T1 with temperature alone. A more accurate method of T1-based MR thermometry would be to calculate T1 at each temperature point rather than merely to use the signal intensities of T1-weighted images. MR temperature mapping has been performed during FUS surgery using T1 values calculated from an optimized fast SPGR sequences using the following signal intensity relationship and Eq. 2:

$$\mathrm{S_T M_o} \propto \frac{(1 - \exp(-\mathrm{TR}|\mathrm{T1_T}))\sin(\theta)}{1 - \cos(\theta)\exp(-\mathrm{TR}|\mathrm{T1_T})} \qquad (2)$$

where $\mathrm{S_T}$ is the signal intensity at a temperature T, $\mathrm{M_0}$ is the equilibrium magnetization, θ is the flip angle, TR is the repetition time and $\mathrm{T1_T}$ is given by Eq. 1. An independent calibration study calculated the temperature coefficients [9]. In this and other earlier studies the T1 value at each temperature was calculated using the signal intensity of a reference image at ambient temperature [9, 10]. However, the equilibrium magnetization, $\mathrm{M_o}$ in Eq. 2, is also inversely dependent on the absolute temperature. The effect of this term may be significant, as shown in a hyperthermia investigation on the calves of human subjects. This study confirms the need for two-point measurements at each temperature to preclude the effects of proton density variations in order to obtain accurate values of T1 [11].

Two-point measurements involve the acquisition of two sequences at each temperature point, which obviously decreases the temporal resolution. High temporal resolutions can, however, be maintained using an inversion-prepared turbo fast low-angle shot (turbo-FLASH) sequence. Images with two or more values of TI can be acquired at the rate of one image per second, so that temporal resolutions of 2 s can be easily achieved. T1 values can be calculated by a linear fit to the following signal intensity relationship for images acquired with different values of TI (TR and flip angle remain fixed):

$$\mathrm{S_T} \propto (1 - 2\exp(\mathrm{TI}|\mathrm{T1_T})) \qquad (3)$$

where the symbols have the same meaning as in Eq. 2, and TI is the effective time of inversion. The linear relationship between T1 and temperature was verified in a gel phantom using a single-shot sequentially ordered inversion prepared turbo-FLASH sequence at 1.5 T using five values of

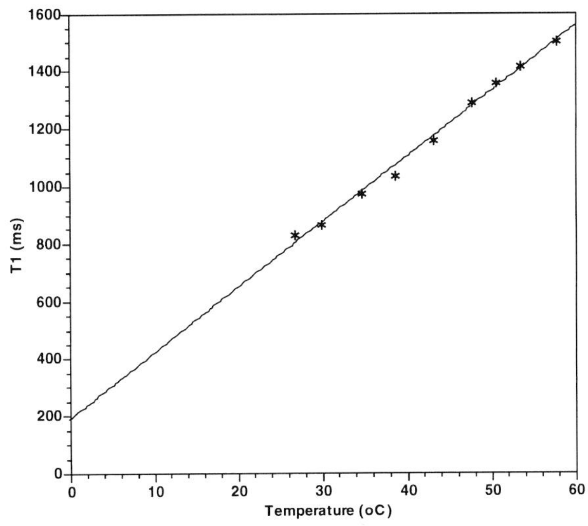

Fig. 1. Variation in T1 with temperature measured in a gel phantom at 1.5 T. T1 was calculated by a least squares fit to a signal intensity variation in the form given by Eq. 3 where TI_{eff} is the effective TI when the low order k-space lines were collected (five values of TI_{eff} at 676, 876, 1076, 1476, and 1776 ms were used). A sequentially reordered turbo-FLASH sequence with scan parameters: TE/TR/FA 3.9/8.9/12° was used to acquire images every 1.15 s. A linear temperature dependence of T1 with a sensitivity of 1.5%/°C was estimated in the temperature range 27°–58°C

TI at each temperature (Fig. 1) [12]. Similar measurements in an open configuration system at 0.2 T also confirmed the linear relationship, but problems relating to the lower signal to noise ratio (SNR) at 0.2 T (leading to high standard deviations) must be addressed before in vivo implementation [13].

In order to increase the SNR at low field strengths we have investigated alternate methods of modest reduction in acquisition. Parametric T1 maps were generated using gradient echo and turbo inversion recovery sequences (phase-sensitive reconstruction). Temporal resolution of the image acquisition was increased by keyhole and/or reduced field-of-view (FOV) techniques.

The choice of sequence depends on the specific requirements of the procedure: temporal resolution, temperature resolution, and spatial resolution.

■ Apparent Diffusion Coefficient

The temperature dependence of the diffusion coefficient is given by the relationship:

$$(1/T) = (1/T_o) - (k/E_a) \times \ln(D/D_o) \quad (4)$$

where k is Boltzmann's constant, E_a (0.18 eV) is the activation energy for translational molecular diffusion, D_o is the diffusion coefficient at room temperature, T_o (in K), and D is the diffusion coefficient at temperature T (in K). The diffusion coefficient, D, can be calculated from a two-point measurement at each temperature using the relationship:

$$\ln\left(\frac{S_g}{S_o}\right) = D(b_g - b_o) \quad (5)$$

where S_g is the signal intensity for an applied gradient g with b value b_g. (The b value is a term that is proportional to the square of the applied diffusion gradient strength, g, and to the cube of the separation of the diffusion lobes). The accuracy of the temperature measurements can be improved by a linear fit to signal intensities at more than two values of the diffusion gradients, but this would result in an increase in the scan times for each temperature measurement. The measurement of the diffusion coefficient, especially with a high temporal resolution, is fraught with difficulties. The long acquisition times and the motion sensitivity of spin-echo diffusion-weighted sequences precludes their use in vivo temperature monitoring. Single-shot diffusion-weighted echo-planar sequences have been used to measure temperature to monitor hyperthermia procedures [14]. It is possible to determine 0.5°C changes in 1 cm^3 volumes in less than 10 s using the diffusion-weighted echo-planar sequence. However, this technique has been implemented at 1.5 T in a closed-configuration system, and echo-planar upgrades are currently not available on any of the commercial open systems. We have investigated an alternate single-shot diffusion-prepared turbo-FLASH sequence as a possible candidate for MR thermometry (Fig. 2). The linear dependence of the diffusion coefficient with temperature in a gel phantom was verified at 1.5 T with this sequence (Fig. 3) [15]. The temporal resolution of the sequence is 2 s/diffusion-weighted image, which is adequate for temperature monitoring.

We have implemented a diffusion prepared turbo-FLASH sequence and obtained preliminary data on diffusion-weighted imaging of the liver and kidneys at 0.2 T. The ADC values obtained in regions of interest placed in the various tissues agreed with those reported in the literature, but the SNR of the images was not sufficiently high to generate meaningful ADC maps. However, initial experience with measuring temperature at 0.2 T using this sequence revealed problems arising

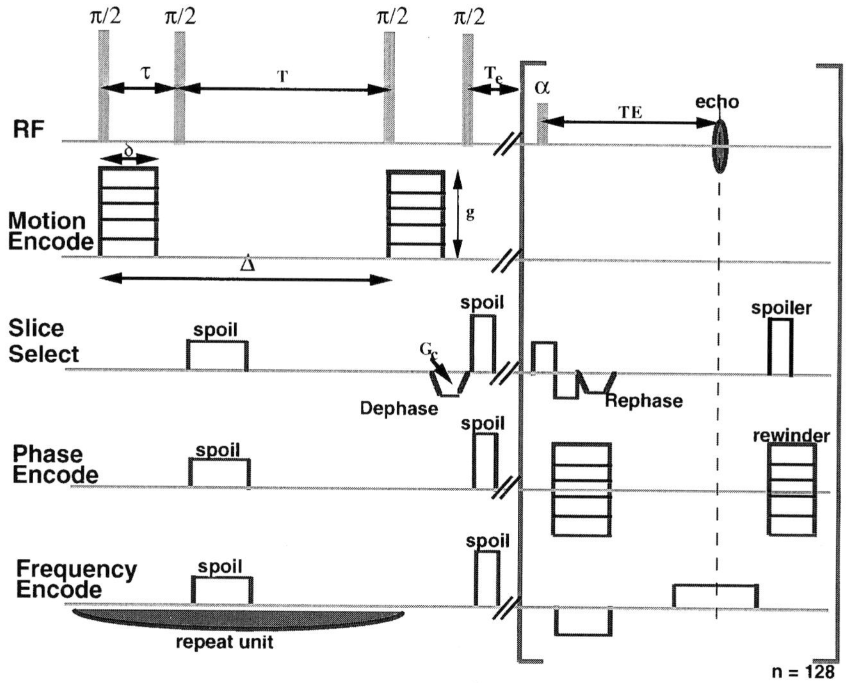

Fig. 2. A diffusion-weighted, centrally reordered turbo-FLASH sequence which is relatively insensitive to the effects of eddy currents. The diffusion gradients are applied during the magnetization preparation period which has four broadband 90° RF pulses and two diffusion gradients, g (t=24.6 ms, d=20 ms, T=165 ms, T_e=90 ms). The repeat unit of the sequence (*square brackets*) is applied before any RF pulse is applied. The crusher gradient G_c, is applied along the slice select direction (duration: 1 ms; amplitude: 1 mT/m). Spoiler gradients are applied along all the three axes during the two longitudinal evolutions to dephase remnant transverse magnetization

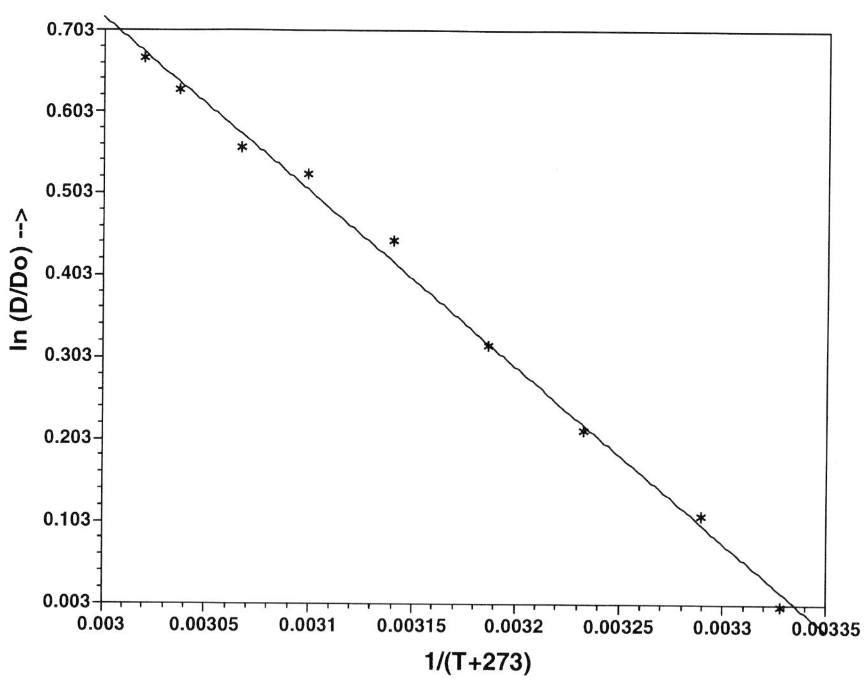

Fig. 3. Variation in ln(D/Do) with 1/(T+273) in a gel phantom (at 1.5 T) for the sequence shown in Fig. 2. Measurements of the diffusion coefficient D were made by an exponential fit to the signal intensity variation at three values of the diffusion gradient strength. A temperature sensitivity of 2.9%/°C was obtained for the diffusion coefficient with this sequence

from lower SNR and artifacts from residual eddy currents [16].

The long acquisition times of spin echo diffusion-weighted sequences do not provide the temporal resolution required to monitor an ablation procedure. Further, these sequences are motion sensitive and thus difficult to implement under in vivo conditions. We have incorporated navigator echo correction to reduce the effects of view-to-view phase shifts due to motion. Scans were acquired at a temporal resolution of 43 s/diffusion-weighted image. The error in temperature estimation using a spin echo diffusion-weighted sequence was approx. 10° with a five-point acquisition. Further work is required before this sequence can be used for temperature monitoring. Reduction in acquisition times can be accomplished by sampling a reduced FOV using slab excitation (see below).

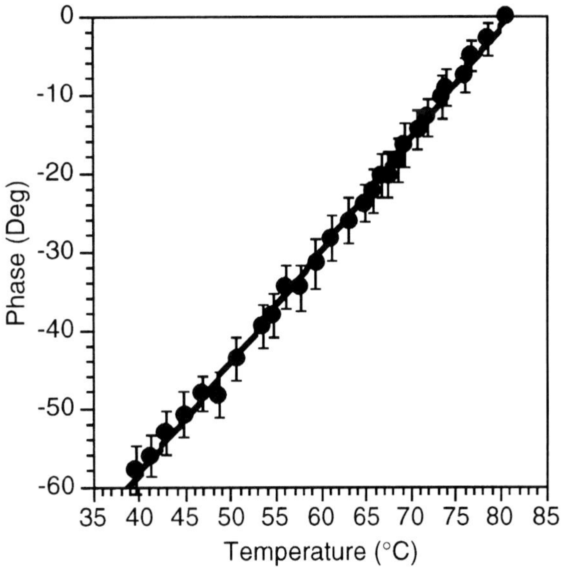

Fig. 4. Phase changes due to temperature differences in a gel phantom. Scan parameters: gradient echo, TE 30 ms, TR 100 ms, 128×128 matrix, slice thickness 10 mm

■ Proton Resonance Frequency from Gradient Echo Phase Images

Recent investigations of MR thermometry based on the temperature-dependent proton resonant frequency have confirmed it to be an accurate method which may prove clinically viable. This technique has been applied very successfully to map temperature using phase images of gradient echoes. Most of the measurements have been performed at high fields (1.5 T or greater) in closed configuration systems [17–21]. Phase change images are calculated by subtracting either the phase or complex images acquired at higher (or lower) temperatures from a corresponding image at a reference image [27, 29]. Phase unwrapping and phase drift correction must be performed before a temperature map can be generated using the relationship:

$$\left(\frac{d\Phi(x_{||}y)}{dT(x_{||}y)}\right) = C * \gamma * B_{ext} * TE_{||} \tag{6}$$

where $d\Phi(x_{II}y)$ is the phase difference induced by a temperature change of $dT(x_{II}y)$ at a pixel location (x,y), γ is the gyromagnetic ratio of proton, C is the constant of proportionality, B_{ext} is the external magnetic field flux, and TE is the echo time of the gradient echo sequence [29]. The sensitivity of phase change with temperature is linearly proportional to the main magnetic field (Eq. 6). Thus in order to achieve an equivalent sensitivity at low field strengths the TE of the gradient echo must be increased. This implies a concomitant increase in TR, resulting in longer acquisition times. Our investigations show that temperature changes can be measured with a standard deviation of 1.03 °C using a navigator-echo corrected gradient echo sequence with a TE/TR: 60 ms/100 ms at 0.2 T (Fig. 4) [22]. The navigator echoes are used to correct for view-to-view phase variations that may result in high standard deviations of the measured phase. The temporal resolution of these scans (100 ms×128=12.8 s) are not sufficiently high to monitor RF ablation procedures which last 1–2 min.

We have successfully implemented a keyholing method in which only the central lines of k-space are collected, thereby reducing scan times by 50%. Simulation experiments showed that contrast and size distortions of a simulated heat lesion were within 10%–15% for a keyhole size up to 4 (keyhole size is defined here as the number of levels in the high-resolution image/number of levels in the keyholed image; Fig. 5). This sequence has been used to monitor the temperature profile of a heat lesion generated by a RF probe in a gel phantom (Fig. 6). Some aspects of phase imaging relevant to imaging in an open magnet configuration are the larger phase drifts and higher likelihood of view-to-view phase variations from coupling to external magnetic field perturbations. However, the first problem can be overcome by correction using a reference phantom maintained at ambient temperature and the second by incorporation of navigator echoes.

Fig. 5. a Image of a lesion simulated in a phase image, seen as a rectangular region of hyperintensity. **b–e** Images of the lesion reconstructed using 192 (**b**), 128 (**c**), 64 (**d**), and 32 (**e**) raw data lines of the image and the remaining high-resolution lines from an image without the simulated lesion. A zoomed region of the phase image centered on the rectangular lesion is shown here. **f–k** Three-dimensional temperature profiles corresponding to the lesions in **a–e**

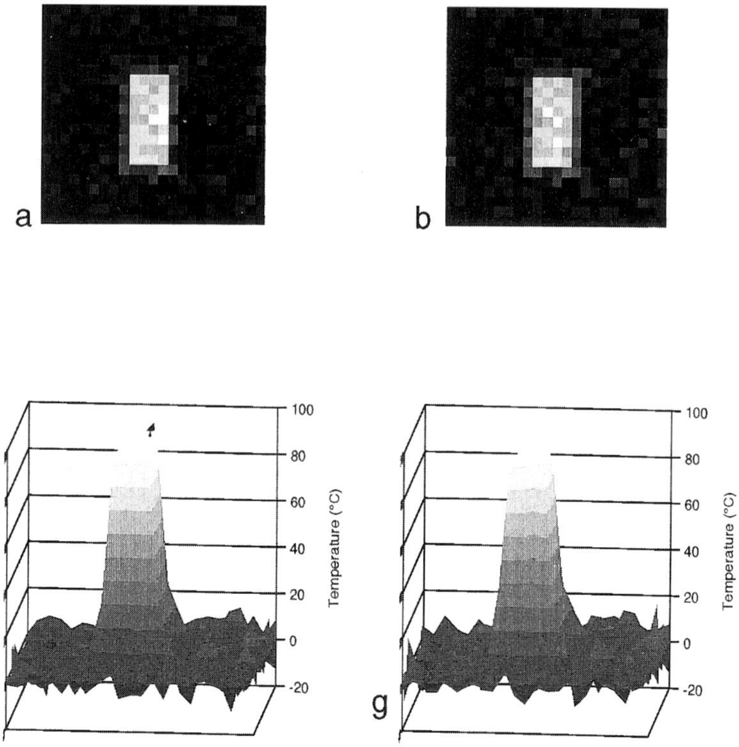

Echo-Shifting Methods

The conflicting requirements of long TE for maintaining temperature sensitivity and high temporal resolution for monitoring ablation procedures has lead to the idea of echo-shifted sequences [23]. The rationale for echo shifting is that TE is greater than TR accomplished by a special design of the gradient waveforms (Fig. 7a). Crusher gradients are included along one of the three orthogonal axes with sufficient strength to dephase any gradient-recalled echo of spins excited in the same TR, but the phase of the crusher gradient is alternated so that it rephases spins excited by the RF pulse of the previous TR interval. Spins are completely rephased along the read direction within a TR interval, and phase encode gradients are applied at the end of each TR period. The slice gradient rephases the spins excited by the $(n-1)$th RF pulse during the nth TR interval (Fig. 7a). Thus the spins excited by the $(n-1)$th RF pulse are refocused in the nth TR interval, resulting in a TE greater than TR. An ultrafast version of this sequence termed PRESTO involves acquisition of multiple gradient echoes per TR reducing acquisition times to 144 ms for a 64×64 matrix (Fig. 7b). The echo-shifted and PRESTO sequences have been shown to measure temperatures accurately at 4.7 T [23]. However, considerable work is still required before either of these sequences can be established as suitable for thermometry at low fields in open systems.

■ General Schemes for Reduction in Scan Times

Reduction in FOV

The techniques discussed in this subsection rely on scan speed reduction by imaging a reduced FOV. The method is specially applicable to MR therapeutic interventional procedures in which dynamic changes are limited to a small portion of the total FOV. One of the earlier methods proposed was to acquire a base image with the full FOV and subsequent dynamic images with a reduced FOV [24]. This is accomplished by sampling densely in the phase encoding direction for the full FOV and sparsely for the reduced FOV images. The increase in temporal resolution is equal to the ratio of phase lines in the full FOV to the reduced FOV. The dynamic images cannot, however, be directly Fourier-transformed since this would result in an image with wrap-around artifacts from outside the reduced FOV. Difference images formed by subtracting corresponding lines of the base and dynamic data can be Fourier-transformed without aliasing artifacts. A phase correction must be applied (for proper positioning) before superposing this dynamic image on

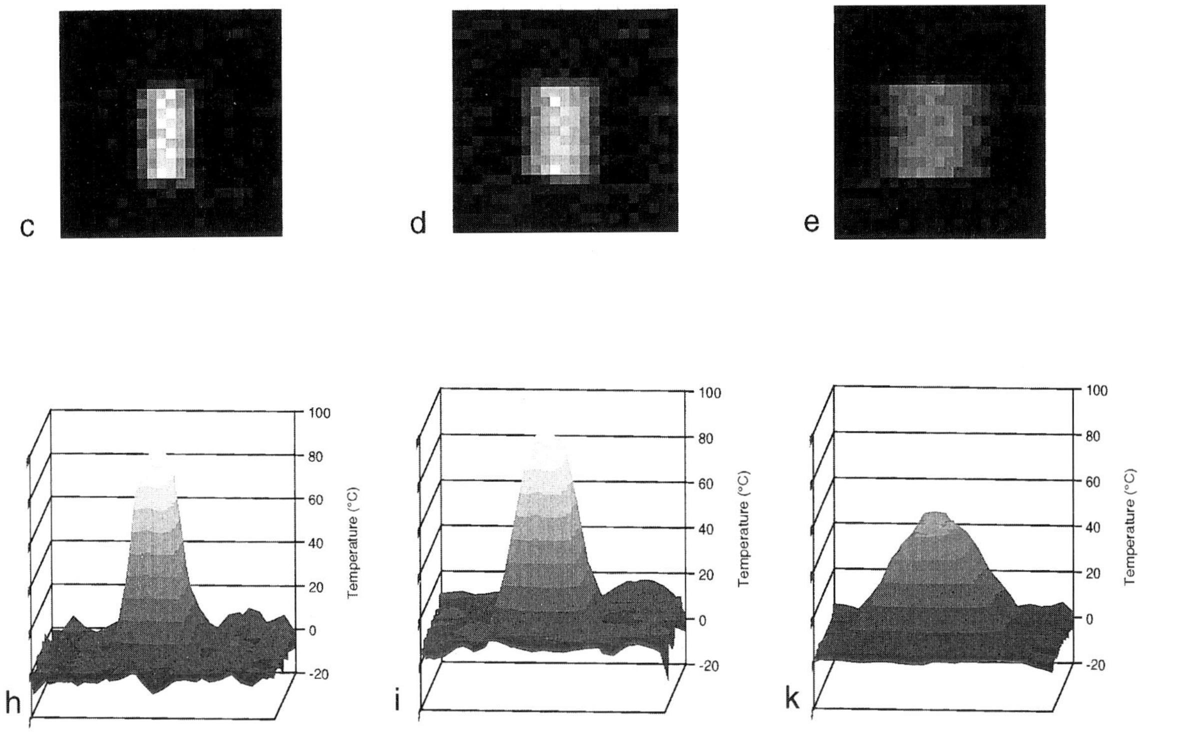

Fig. 5 (*cont.*)

the base image. The chief drawback of this system is that changes outside the reduced FOV alias back in the subtracted image resulting in artifacts, and prior knowledge of the location of the change within the larger FOV is required. This method has been shown to be successful in tracking the position of a moving finger images at 1.5 T. It remains to be seen whether the technique is applicable on a clinical basis. An alternate method of preventing aliasing in the reduced FOV images is to excite a strip rather than the entire slice as proposed in the localized look (LoLo) method [25]. A strip is excited by application of orthogonal gradients during the slice excitation (90°) and slice focus (180°) RF pulse durations.

A locally focused MR technique has been proposed to image selectively with high resolution in the region of interest [26]. These images require much less scan time than those with which the entire image is acquired at high resolution. The technique permits user-specified spatial resolution in user-defined portions of the FOV. The user identifies regions of high and low resolution and other regions of no signal intensity in the image. This is used to synthesize a set of training images from which an orthonormal basis set spanning the image reconstruction space is determined. The locally focused images are then reconstructed by utilizing a small number of acquired phase-encoded signals to calculate image projections onto these basis functions. This method affords greater flexibility in terms of multiple user-specified regions of high resolution than does the reduced FOV discussed above, but the method suffers from being computationally intensive.

Keyhole Strategies

Keyhole techniques were initially suggested to improve temporal resolution of dynamic MR imaging to monitor contrast agent uptake [27, 28]. The simplest keyhole strategy is to acquire a reference image at full resolution and only the central k-space lines for the dynamic images. The dynamic images are then reconstructed after substituting the higher k-space lines from the reference high-resolution image. Simulation of the keyhole technique has shown that spatial and contrast distortions of the dynamic images are less than 10% up to a keyhole factor of 4 [29]. The temporal resolution is greater than the reference image since only a subset of the k-space is acquired.

The drawback of conventional keyhole imaging is that the higher spatial frequencies are never updated, and this can result in significant blurring and loss of information when attempting to apply keyholing for tracking objects (such as a biopsy

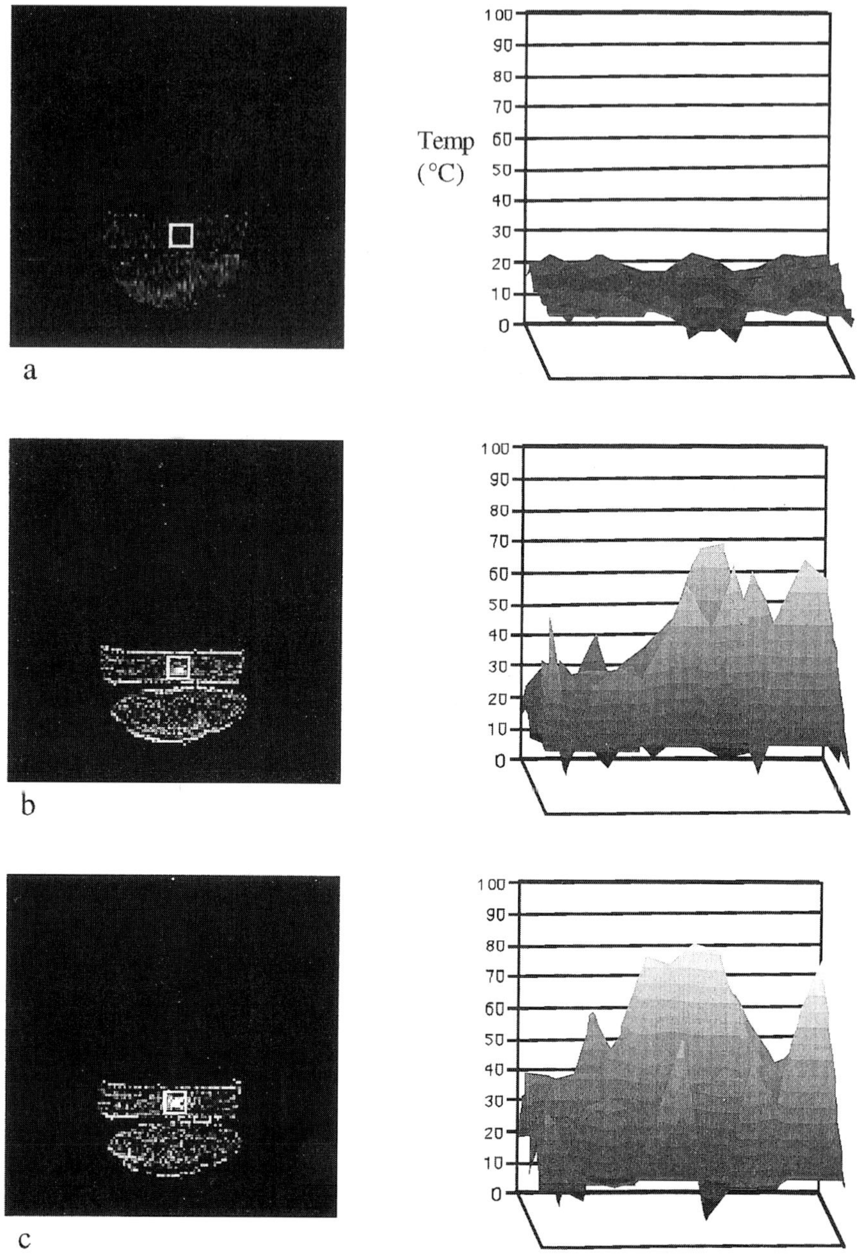

Fig. 6 a–f. Gel phantom images at various time points of an RF ablation procedure. Images shown here have been phase unwrapped and corrected for drifts. Images acquired while the RF power is increased (**a–c**) and after the RF generator is powered down (**d–f**). The three-dimensional temperature profiles are shown (to the *right* of each image) for the ROI (*white rectangle*) shown superposed on the subtracted phase image

needle tip) which are spatially small. A number of methods have been suggested to ensure that all k-space data are eventually refreshed [30, 31]. One technique is based on a random encoding of the phase lines, as opposed to the linear update approach of conventional keyholing. In this method, termed continuous update with random encoding, a random ordering of the phase encode lines is used with the low k-space lines acquired more frequently [30]. An ultrafast gradient echo sequence with a TR of 6.5 ms is used to acquire images using the phase encode order dictated by the random table. Data are acquired continuously with the same random phase table used repeatedly. An image at any time point is reconstructed by searching the data outward from that time point until all the phase line information is available. If two low k-space data are located in the

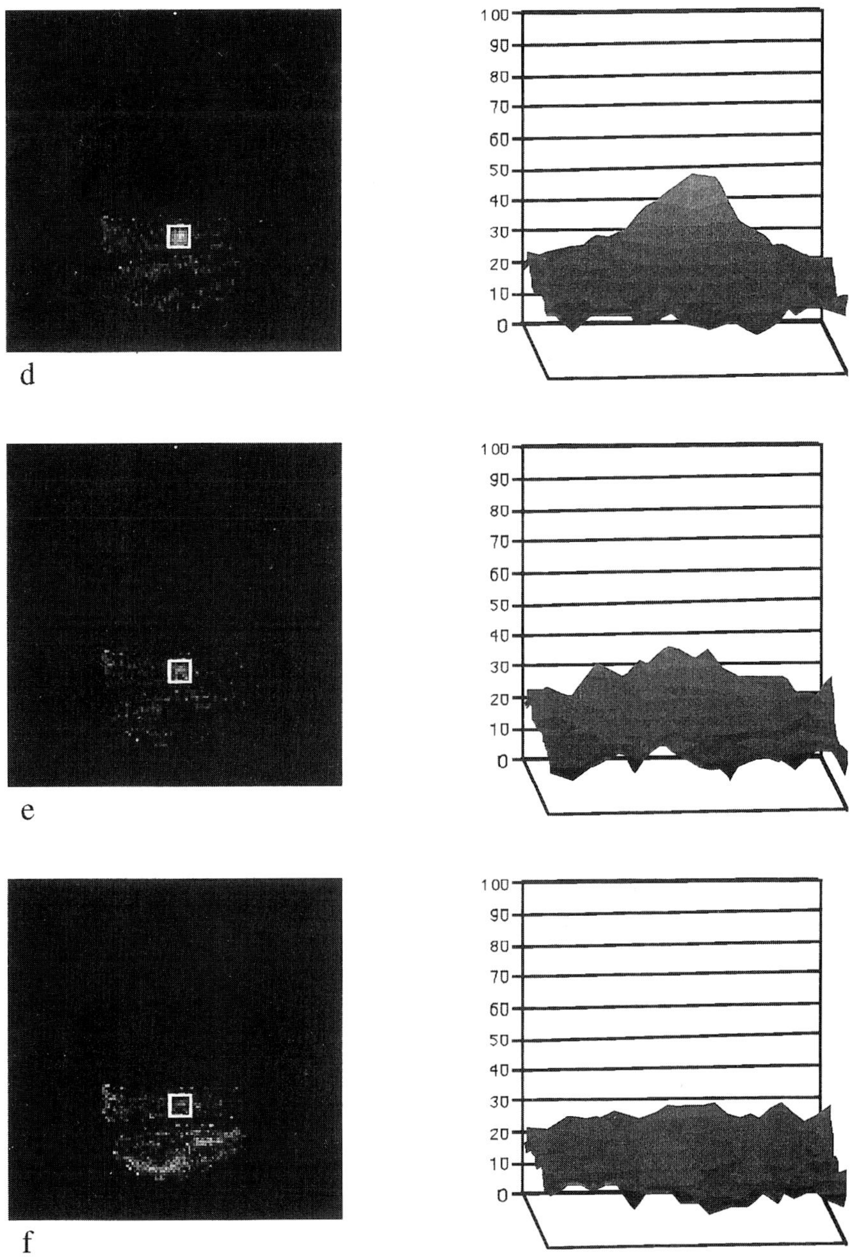

Abb. 6d–f

search, the line closer to the desired time point is included. Images of the human heart and a flexing lower leg reconstructed every 90 ms demonstrate the feasibility of the technique. This technique could potentially be employed in interventional MR applications if the image reconstruction can also be implemented in real time as opposed to off-line reconstruction. An alternate keyhole strategy, termed striped k-space scanning, has been proposed in which eight strips each rotated 22.5° cover the whole of k-space, and each dynamic scan acquires one strip. The sequence was implemented on a 0.064-T MR system with open access and shows potential for interventional applications [32].

A simulation study compared the efficacy of various keyhole strategies in tracking a biopsy needle [33]. All the simulations were performed

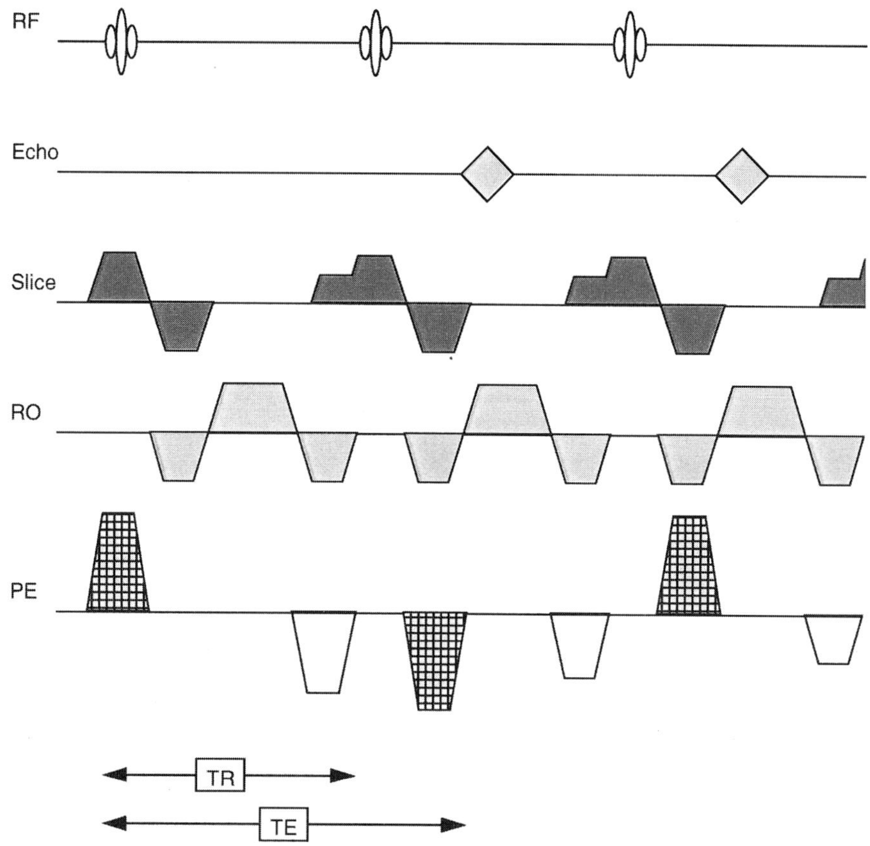

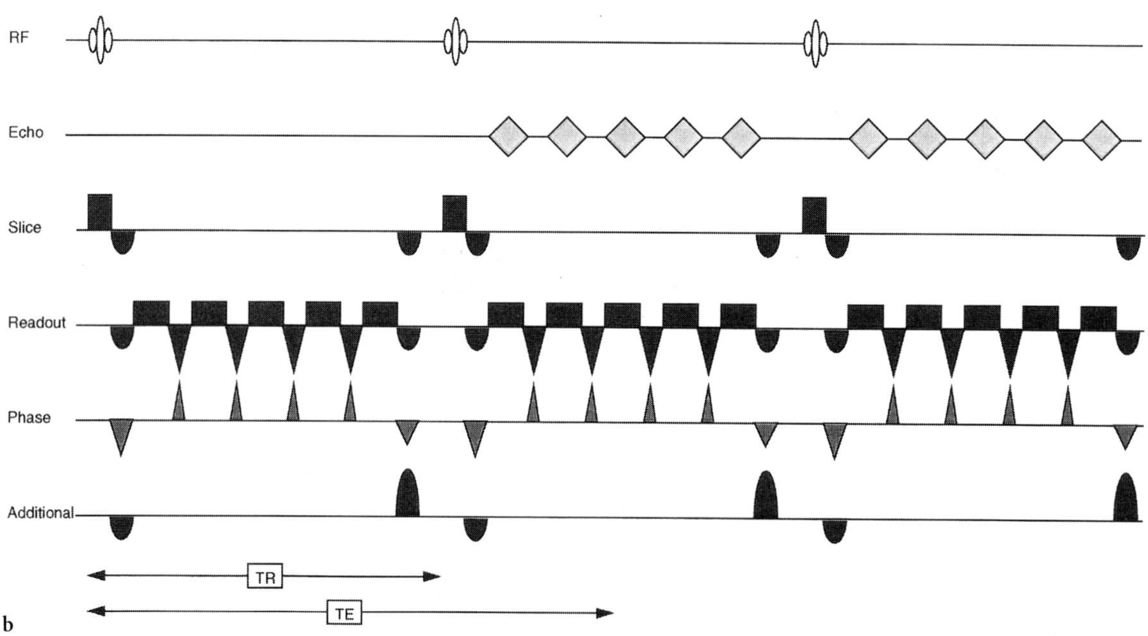

Fig. 7. a Schematic of the pulse sequence to generate an echo-shifted image. The gradient waveforms are manipulated to cause the spins excited in the (n–1)th TR interval to be focused in the nth TR interval. *Cross-hatched alternating gradients* (along the phase direction), crusher gradients. These are shown applied along the phase direction but can be applied along any one of three axes. The first three TR periods shown here illustrate the method by which the spins excited by any RF pulse are collected in the following TR interval leading to TE greater than TR. **b** Schematic of the PRESTO pulse sequence which is a fast version of the echo-shifted sequence. Here five echoes are collected every TR interval, reducing the scan time by a factor of five compared to the echo-shifted sequence shown in **a.** The effective TE is still maintained greater than TR

with 25% of the phase encode lines acquired every segment and with the needle traversing parallel and perpendicular to the phase encode axis. The standard keyhole which repeatedly acquired the central 25% phase lines was found to be inadequate for needle localization due to lateral blurring of the needle when the phase axis was perpendicular to needle path. When the needle was parallel to the phase encode axis, there was no lateral blurring, but the needle tip was poorly defined. This simulation study showed the best scheme to be that in which the central one-eight of phase lines were always collected with the remaining lines ranked and sequentially acquired. Ranking was performed based on the order of maximum to minimum magnitude of the 2D Fourier transform of the needle image projected onto the read axis.

Keyhole techniques specifically applied to open-access magnets include conventional keyhole scheme in conjunction with phase imaging for temperature monitoring during RF ablation studies [22]. A keyhole diffusion-weighted spin echo sequence has also been investigated for low-field (0.064 T) MR thermometry [23]; a weighted k-space acquisition was implemented in which the outer lines were sampled sparsely and inner lines in the normal way.

References

1. Cline HE, Hynenen K, Hardy CJ, Watkins R, Schenk JF, Jolesz FA (1994) MR temperature mapping of focussed ultrasound surgery. Magn Reson Med 31:628–636
2. Hathout G, Lufkin R, Jabour B, Andrews J, Castro D (1992) MR guided aspiration cytology in the head and neck at high field strength. J Magn Reson Imaging 2:93–94
3. Matsumoto R, Oshio K, Jolesz FA (1962) Monitoring of laser and freezing-induced ablation in the liver with T1-weighted MR imaging. J Magn Reson Imaging 2:555–562
4. Cline HE, Schenck JF, Hynynen K, Watkins RD, Souza SP, Jolesz FA (1992) MR-guided focused ultrasound surgery. J Comput Assist Tomogr 16:956–965
5. Jolesz FA, Silverman SG, Kikinis R et al (1994) Interactive image-guided interventions in an Open-configuration MR imaging system (abstract). Radiology 193(P):252
6. Chung YC, Duerk JL, Lewin JS (1996) Generation and observation of radiofrequency thermal lesion ablation for interventional magnetic resonance imaging (abstract). In: Book of Abstracts. International Society for Magnetic Resonance in Medicine. New York, p 1743
7. Matsumoto R, Mulkern RV, Hushek SG, Jolesz FA (1994) Tissue temperature monitoring for thermal interventional therapy comparison of T1-weighted MR sequences. J Magn Reson Imaging 4:65–70
8. Fried MP, Morrison PR, Hushek SG, Kernahan GA, Jolesz FA (1996) Dynamic T1-weighted magnetic resonance imaging of interstitial laser photocoagulation in the liver. Observations on in-vivo temperature sensitivity. Lasers Surg Med 18:410–419
9. Cline HE, Hynynen K, Hardy CJ, Watkins RD, Schenck JF, Jolesz FA (1994) MR temperature mapping of focused ultrasound surgery. Magn Reson Med 31:628–636
10. Dickinson RJ, Hall AS, Hind AJ, Young IR (1986) Measurement of changes in tissue temperature using magnetic resonance imaging. J Comput Assist Tomogr 10:468–472
11. Young IR, Hand JW, Oatridge A, Prior MV, Forse GR (1994) Further observations on the measurement of tissue T1 to monitor temperature in vivo by MRI. Magn Reson Med 31:342–345
12. Sinha S, Sinha U (1994) Comparison of MR Pulse Sequences. Presented in the Society for Magnetic Resonance Workshop on Interventional MRI Program, Marina Del Rey, Calif., 13–14 August
13. Oshiro T, Sinha U, Sinha S, Lu D, Atkinson D, Lufkin R (1997) Comparison of temperature measurements using phase shift and T1 imaging at 0.2 Tesla. Presented at the 5th Annual Meeting of the International Society for Magnetic Resonance in Medicine, Vancouver
14. MacFall J, Prescott DM, Fullar E, Samulski TV (1995) Temperature dependence of canine brain tissue diffusion coefficient measured in vivo with magnetic resonance echo-planar imaging. Int J Hyperthermia 11:73–86
15. Sinha U, Sinha S (1996) High speed diffusion imaging in the presence of eddy currents. J Magn Reson Imaging 6
16. Sinha S, Oshiro T, Sinha U, Lufkin RB (1996) Temperature monitoring with single shot diffusion imaging on a 0.2 T scanner. Proceedings of the International Society for Magnetic Resonance in Medicine, vol 3, pp 1753
17. Chung AH, Hynynen K, Colucci V, Oshio K, Cline HE, Jolesz FA (1996) Optimization of spoiled gradient-echo phase imaging for in vivo localization of a focused ultrasound beam. Magn Reson Med 36:745–752
18. De Poorter J, De Wagter C, De Deene Y, Thomsen C, Stahlberg F, Achten E (1994) The proto-resonance-frequency-shift method compared with molecular diffusion for quantitative measurement of two-dimensional time-dependent temperature distribution in a phantom. J Magn Reson 103:234–241
19. De Poorter J, De Wagter C, De Deene Y, Thomsen C, Stahlberg F, Achten E (1995) Noninvasive MRI thermometry with the proton resonance frequency (PRF) method in vivo results in human muscle. Magn Reson 33:74–81
20. Ishihara Y, Calderon A, Watanabe H et al (1995) A precise and fast temperature mapping using water proton chemical shift. Magn Reson Med 34:814–823
21. Vitkin IA, Moriarty JA, Peters RD, Kolios MC, Gladman AS, Chen JC, Hinks RS, Hunt JW, Wilson BC, Easty AC, Bronskill MJ, Kucharczyk W, Sherar MD, Henkelman RM (1997) Magnetic resonance imaging of temperature changes during interstitial microwave heating A phantom study. Med Phys 24:269–277
22. Sinha S, Oshiro T, Sinha U, Lufkin R. Phase Imaging on a 0.2 tesla MR scanner application to temperature monitoring during ablation procedures. J Magn Reson Imaging
23. de Zwart JA, van Gelderen P, Kelly DJ, Moonen CTW (1997) Ultra fast MRI thermometry. In: Proceedings of the Society for Magnetic Resonance in Medicine vol 1720
24. Hu X, Parrish T (1994) Reduction of field of view for dynamic imaging. Magn Reson Med 31:691–694
25. van Vaals JJ, van Yperen G, de Boer R (1994) Real-time MR imaging using the LoLo method for interactive and interventional MRI at 0.5 T and 1.5 T. Presented at the Second Annual Meeting of the Society for Magnetic Resonance, San Francisco. Proceedings, p 421
26. Cao Y, Levin DN, Yao L (1995) Locally focused MRI. Magn Reson Med 34:858–867

27. Van Vaals J, Brummer ME et al (1993) Keyhole method for accelerating imaging of contrast agent uptake. J Magn Reson Imaging 3:671–675
28. Jones RA, Haraldseth O, Muller TB et al (1993) K-space substitution a novel dynamic imaging technique. Magn Reson Med 29:830–834
29. Spraggins TA (1994) Simulation of spatial and contrast distortions in keyhole imaging. Magn Reson Med 31:320–322
30. Parrish T, Hu X (1995) Continuous update with random encoding (CURE). A new strategy for dynamic imaging. Magn Reson Med 33:326–336
31. Busch M, Friebe M, Lerchner H, Hellwig S (1994) Striped k-space. An extension of the keyhole technique for rapid imaging with high contrast differentiation. Presented at the Second Annual Meeting of the Society for Magnetic Resonance, San Francisco. Proceedings, p 347
32. Duerk JL, Lewin JS, Wu DH (1996) Application of keyhole imaging to interventional MRI. A simulation study to predict sequence requirements. J Magn Reson Imaging 6:918–924
33. Friebe M, Busch M (1994) Low-field NMR thermometry with diffusion sensitized keyhole and weighted k-space sequencing schemes. Presented at the Second Annual Meeting of the Society for Magnetic Resonance, San Francisco

Wavelet Encoding for Interventional Magnetic Resonance Imaging

2

M. WENDT · M. BUSCH

■ Introduction

This chapter introduces a new encoding technique, wavelet transformation, and its use for tracking interventional tools [2–6]. Use of wavelet transformation is a technique similar to keyhole imaging [2–9] and permits the visualization of an interventional device in space and time. Minimizing the redundancy of the acquired magnetic resonance (MR) data by updating only a locally limited region of the image data improves temporal resolution of MR images for interventional applications.

■ Background

As in fast Fourier transformation (FFT), discrete wavelet transformation (DWT) is a linearly invertable operation. The integral wavelet transformation $F_g(a,b)$ of a real-valued finite-energy function, f(x), is defined as:

$$F_{g_{s,w}}(a,b) = \frac{1}{\sqrt{a}} \int f(x) \cdot g_{s,w}\left(\frac{x-b}{a}\right) dx \qquad (1)$$

where a is scale, b is translation, g_w is wavelet function, g_s is scaling function, f(x) is the original function to be wavelet transformed, and $F_g(a, b)$ is the wavelet transform of f(x). The term f(x) can be reconstructed from the signal $F_g(a,b)$ using an inverse DWT [3, 4].

Both FFT and DWT can be seen as a rotation in function space, i.e., from the input space domain to an alternative domain. For the FFT this new domain has basis functions that are the familiar sines and cosines. In the wavelet domain the basis functions are more complicated and are called the scaling function (g_s) and the wavelet function (g_w). What makes these wavelet basis functions so interesting for imaging is that, unlike sines and cosines, individual wavelet basis functions are localized in space. Their localization in space is described by the translation, b. Simultaneously, as with sines and cosines, individual wavelet functions are localized in frequency or, to be more precise, they are of characteristic scale, a.

When using a two-dimensional Fourier transform, all data samples are typically ordered in an equidistant frame, i.e., k-space. The wavelet transform is comparable to the central idea of a multiresolution analysis with hierarchically ordered subspaces. A low-resolution approximation subspace, $V_{-\xi}$ ($\xi \in N$, e.g., $\xi=4$), is spanned by a family of scaling functions which can be compared to the low-pass filters found in multiresolution analysis. The detail spaces W_{-4}, W_{-3}, etc. are spanned by a family of wavelet functions comparable to the band-pass filters of the multiresolution analysis with increasing high-pass characteristics according to the scale a. Therefore the acquired wavelet coefficients represent a detail, or difference, signal corresponding to their scale that is not contained in the approximation space spanned by the scaling function of the same

Fig. 1. a Raw data space for one-dimensional Fourier and one-dimensional wavelet-encoded data sets. **b** Raw data space in which only a spatially selective part is updated

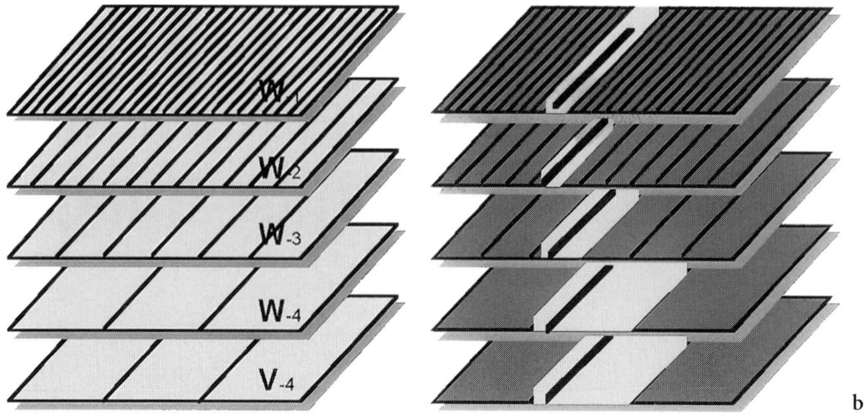

scale. adding the detail space W_{-4} to the corresponding approximation subspace V_{-4} created a new approximation subspace V_{-3} with the same shape but an increased resolution (Fig. 1a). This offers the possibility of images with a scaled resolution. By acquiring only a few neighboring coefficients of the detail spaces a *zoom-in* effect can be achieved. The high-resolution area V_{hi} within an image is reconstructed by considering the coefficients of all detail spaces (e.g., four level wavelet-encoded: $V_{hi}=V_{-4}+W_{-4}+W_{-3}+W_{-2}+W_{-1}$). For the low-resolution areas, V_{lo}, the coefficients with a high spatial localization are not acquired and therefore set to zero (e.g., two level wavelet-encoded: $V_{lo}=V_{-4}+W_{-4}+W_{-3}$). In contrast to the coefficients of a Fourier transform, individual wavelet coefficients refer to a specific area of the encoded image according to their translation b. More detailed descriptions of wavelet theory can be found elsewhere [10, 11].

■ Wavelet Encoding in MR Imaging

Figure 1a illustrates a wavelet raw data space as it is used in MR imaging, with one dimension being wavelet encoded (phase encoding direction in standard sequences) and one dimension being frequency encoded (readout direction). When implementing wavelet encoding on an MR scanner, the radiofrequency (RF) pulse profile is the Fourier transform of the scaling or wavelet basis function. The dilation a of the excited region can be changed by varying the duration of the RF pulse or by making use of the fact that a is proportional to the strength of a simultaneously applied gradient (e.g., G_x). Increasing this gradient also increases a and thereby decreases the expansion of the excited object stripe. The desired translation b is achieved by varying the central frequency of the RF pulse.

New techniques make use of the spatial localization of the wavelet basis functions and the hierarchically ordered subspaces of the wavelet transformation to image the movement of an interventional device; these minimize the total MR imaging acquisition time without loss of information. This is achieved by taking into account that only a small part of the previously imaged volume changes over time during the tracking of an interventional device (e.g., biopsy needle, catheter, RF probe, laser/fiber-optic catheter). Therefore only this changing part of the image requires periodic updates.

In planing an interventional procedure, the point of entrance, the target, and hence the direction of the movement of the interventional device are well known before the actual procedure begins. This information can be used to plan the wavelet-encoded data acquisition so that the interventional device (e.g., biopsy needle) is moved forward predominantly in the readout direction by orienting the readout direction parallel to the predicted needle movement. Now only those wavelet coefficients mainly affected by the invasive device, i.e., the spatial regions of the images expected to change during the interventional procedure, are updated (Fig. 1b). This approach allows a zoom-in effect of the wavelet transformation by using only the limited amount of acquired wavelet encoded data sets to reconstruct a new image.

Figure 1b shows an image with only the central part being acquired at all wavelet-encoding scales. This area has a resolution of 1 mm/pixel (field of view=256 mm). The boundary region of the image in the wavelet encoding direction has a resolution of 2 mm/pixel (Fig. 2). Figure 3 presents an ex vivo bovine flank muscle during the simulation of an interventional procedure while tracking an interventional device. Here the data acquisi-

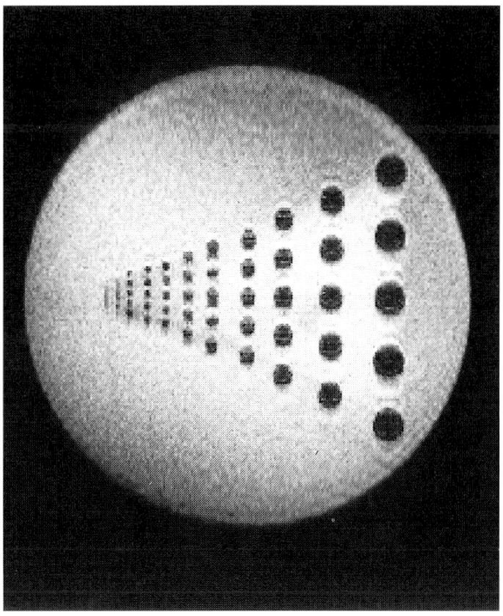

Fig. 2. Final image, using all acquired coefficients for the reconstruction. The final resolution in the center part is 1 mm × 1 mm and 1 mm × 2 mm in the upper and lower part

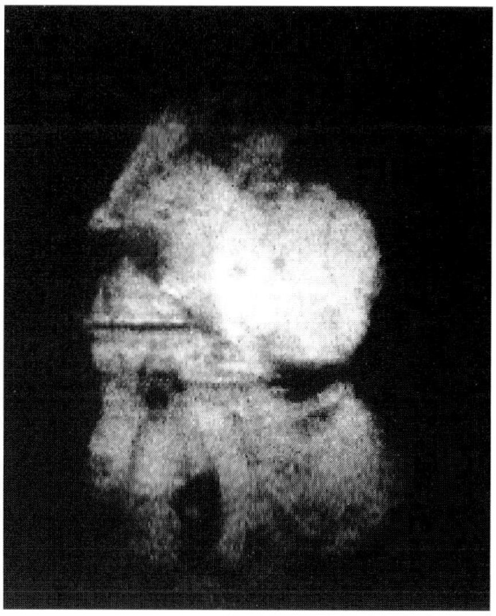

Fig. 3. Ex vivo bovine flank muscle imaged with our new data acquisition strategy showing the movement of an interventional device

tion is limited to the region of the movement of the device (one-seventh field of view). Under these conditions a reduction can be achieved in the total acquisition time by a factor of seven over a conventional two-dimensional fast low-angle shot acquisition with identical resolution and comparable TE/TR.

Discussion

Apart from the lower signal to noise ratio due to the reduced excited region and therefore reduced signal amplitude, wavelet encoding can be used to show all necessary information to monitor the tracking of an interventional device. These sequences can make use of the spatial localization of the encoded stripes, as only those regions affected by the movement of the interventional device require an update. The motion can be tracked perpendicular to the movement of the interventional device as suggested in [6], or parallel to the movement as described here, allowing a "real-time analysis" of the interventional procedure that is not limited by the velocity of the interventional device. Furthermore the band-pass characteristics of the wavelet functions could be used to create a filter to search for specific structures (e.g., needles) within the object.

In conclusion, despite the disadvantages of low signal-to-noise ratio wavelet-encoding sequences are feasible for rapid imaging on currently available systems. This can allow imaging strategies to be tailored to specific clinical applications, with variable spatial resolution at various locations within the imaging volume, especially when the contrast between tissues is not the major imaging objective but rather following the change within a limited region of interest (i.e., image guidance of an interventional device or flow quantification).

References

1. Grönemeyer DHW, Seibel R, Melzer A, Schmidt A (1995) Image-guided access techniques. Endosc Surg 1:369–75
2. van Vaals JJ, Brummer ME, Dixon WT, Tuithof HH, Engels H, Nelson RC, Gerety BM, Chezmar JL, den Boer JA (1993) Keyhole method for accelerating imaging of contrast agent uptake. J Magn Reson Imaging 3:671–675
3. Healy DM, Weaver JB (1992) Two applications of wavelet transforms in magnetic resonance imaging. IEEE Trans Inf Theory 38:840–860
4. Healy DM, Weaver JB (1995) Adapted waveform encoding for magnetic resonance imaging. IEEE Eng Med Biol Mag 5:621–638
5. Panych LP, Jakob PD, Jolesz FA (1993) Implementation of wavelet-encoded MR imaging. J Magn Reson Imaging 3:649–655
6. Panych LP, Jolesz FA (1994) A dynamically adaptive imaging algorithm for wavelet-encoded MRI. Magn Reson Med 32:738–748
7. Peters RD, Wood ML (1993) Practical Considerations for the implementation of wavelet encoding in MRI. Presented at the 12th Annual Meeting of the Society for Magnetic Resonance in Medicine, New York. Abstract 1212
8. Wendt M, Lenz G, Baetz L, Busch M, Bornstedt A, Groenemeyer D (1995) Dynamic tracking algorithm for interventional MRI using wavelet-encoding. Presented at the Annual Meeting of the International Society for Magnetic Resonance, Nice, p 1162

9. Wendt M, Busch M, Lenz G, Bornstedt A, Seibel R, Groenemeyer D (1996) Dynamic tracking algorithm for interventional MRI using wavelet-encoding in 3D gradient echo sequences. Presented at the International Society for Magnetic Resonance, New York. Abstract 49
10. Mallat SG (1989) A theory for multiresolution signal decomposition: the wavelet representation. IEEE Trans Pattern Anal Machine Int 2:674–693
11. Benedetto JJ (1994) Wavelets – mathematics and applications. CRC, Boca Raton
12. Hinshaw WS (1976) Image formation by nuclear magnetic resonance: the sensitive-point method. J Appl Phys 47:3709–3721
13. Panych LP (1993) Adaptive magnetic resonance imaging by wavelet transform encoding. Thesis, Massachusetts Institute of Technology

Fast "Real-Time" Imaging with Various k-Space Update Strategies for Interventional Procedures

3

M. Busch, M. Wendt, A. Bornstedt, D. H. W. Grönemeyer

■ Introduction

Open magnetic resonance (MR) systems are used to guide interventional procedures. They need to deliver acceptable tissue contrast as demanded by diagnostic or therapeutic considerations and voxel sizes of about 1×1×5 mm (typical) to display interventional devices with a diameter of about 1 mm. Secure tracking of the interventional tool requires an acquisition time (including online reconstruction and display) of less than 3 s for three adjacent slices. Especially on low-field systems, however, the amount of high-speed acquisition schemes is limited. One technique for increasing the image frame rate is the keyhole acquisition scheme, which is discussed in this chapter.

■ General Keyhole Imaging

Using standard imaging techniques the acquired data are stored in a raw data space called k-space. This is two- or three-dimensional and contains all necessary information to reconstruct the images using a fast Fourier transformation (FFT). The center of k-space is referred to as the "keyhole" of the raw data set and contains the most import information on the images. Here all low-frequency changes are stored that define the image contrast, all major object features, and the signal to noise ratio. The boundary regions, on the other hand, define the edges and contain all information about the resolution of the images.

The fundamental idea behind "keyhole" techniques [1, 2] is to increase the image frame rate for sequences running in a fluoroscopic mode by frequently updating those lines of k-space "running" through the keyhole (Fig. 1). Using this data acquisition strategy only a central fraction (e.g., one-fourth or one-eighth) of the entire raw data matrix is updated, and an image reconstruction is performed using the newly acquired data combined with "old" data contained in the reference data set. Reconstructing new images after collection of the keyhole lines leads to a faster image update (e.g., by a factor of 4 or 8) with fair image quality as long as there are no essential changes in the content of the image. However, the amount of high-resolution data, normally stored in the outer parts of k-space, is not updated using this basic keyhole version, and the images tend to become blurry after only a few update cycles.

The demand of fluoroscopic sequences with high resolution led to extended keyhole techni-

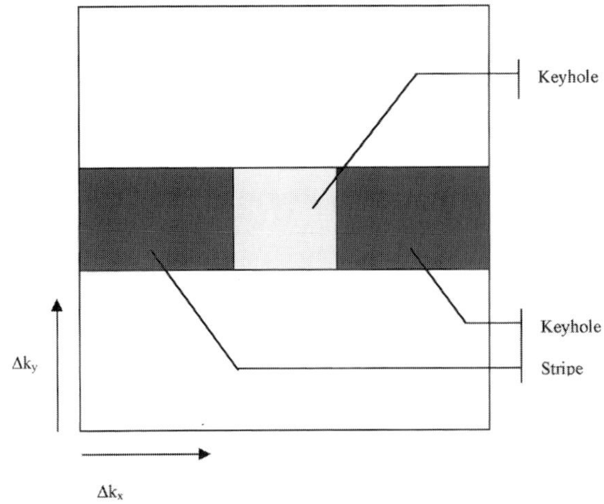

Fig. 1. Keyhole with keyhole slice inserted into the reference image. *White area*, the nonupdated part of the entire raw data set

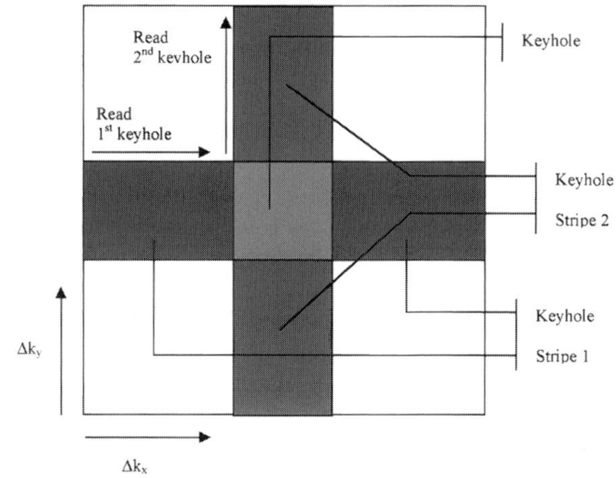

Fig. 2. Keyhole with two orthogonal keyhole slices (PHREAK). *White area*, the nonupdated part of the entire raw data set

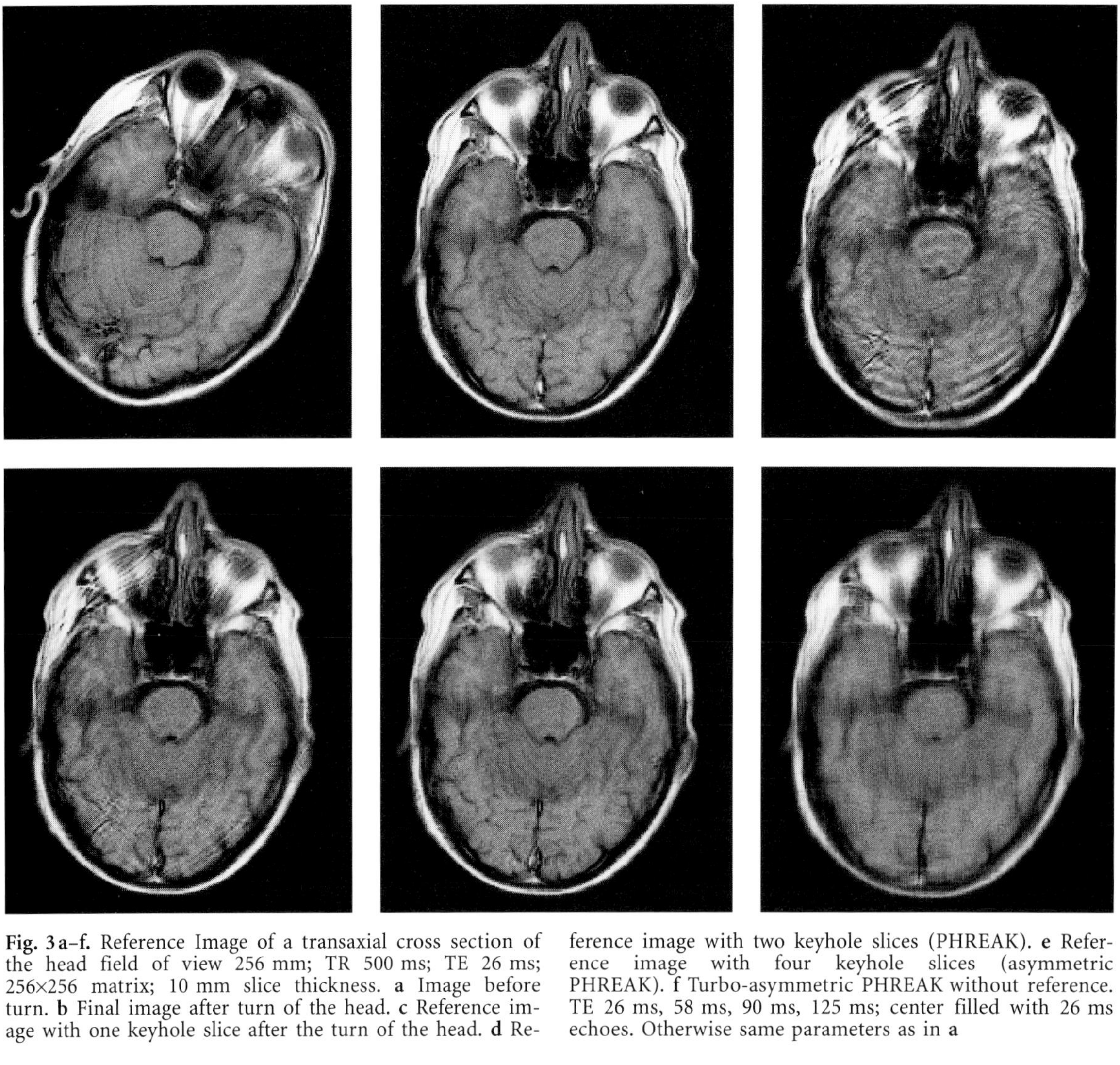

a b, c d e, f

Fig. 3 a–f. Reference Image of a transaxial cross section of the head field of view 256 mm; TR 500 ms; TE 26 ms; 256×256 matrix; 10 mm slice thickness. **a** Image before turn. **b** Final image after turn of the head. **c** Reference image with one keyhole slice after the turn of the head. **d** Reference image with two keyhole slices (PHREAK). **e** Reference image with four keyhole slices (asymmetric PHREAK). **f** Turbo-asymmetric PHREAK without reference. TE 26 ms, 58 ms, 90 ms, 125 ms; center filled with 26 ms echoes. Otherwise same parameters as in **a**

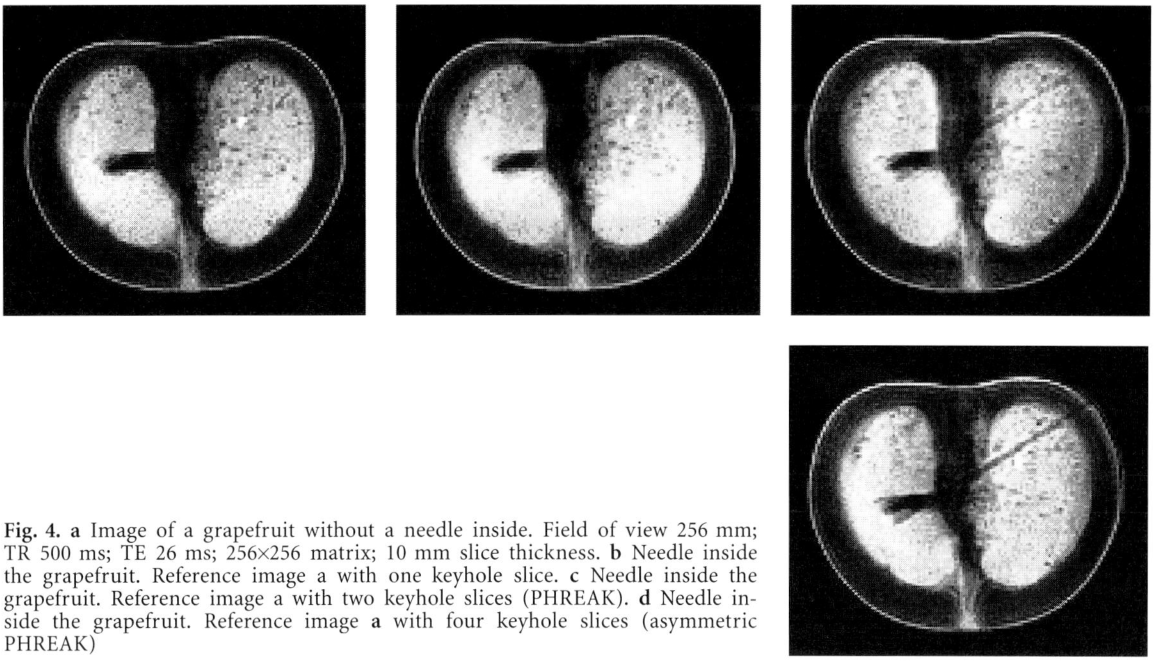

a b, c d

Fig. 4. **a** Image of a grapefruit without a needle inside. Field of view 256 mm; TR 500 ms; TE 26 ms; 256×256 matrix; 10 mm slice thickness. **b** Needle inside the grapefruit. Reference image a with one keyhole slice. **c** Needle inside the grapefruit. Reference image a with two keyhole slices (PHREAK). **d** Needle inside the grapefruit. Reference image **a** with four keyhole slices (asymmetric PHREAK)

ques such as phase read exchange keyhole (PHREAK) [3].

■ Phase Read Exchange Keyhole

The concept of the PHREAK technique is very similar to the keyhole technique itself [4–9]. Obtaining fast image updates with good image quality and good tissue contrast requires that a larger portion of the raw data space be covered. To achieve this the keyhole slices updated in a fluoroscopic sequence are switched with regard to their phase- and read-encoding direction after every update. This increases the amount of higher frequency data sets, as illustrated in Fig. 2.

The basis for implementing PHREAK are symmetric sequences with a constant Δkx and Δky, and for reasons of symmetry most of them have a square matrix size. Furthermore, it is advantageous to form the echo of every readout interval at the center of the sampling time. This simplifies the insertion of the newly acquired data slices after being switched into the already existing k-space, as with respect to a perfect MR system the single data points can be copied directly into k-space. However, a postprocessing algorithm is needed to correct for the resulting data variation due to the imperfect scanner hardware, i.e., small differences in the gradient strength in different orientations caused by nonlinearities unique to each physical gradient axis. This algorithm reduces artifacts arising from mismatching Δkx and Δky values and shifted echoes by determining the "hot spot," i.e., the data point with the maximum amplitude in the raw data set, in each acquired raw data slice. The "hot spot" of every newly acquired data striped is adjusted to superimpose at the center of k-space by shifting the matrices. Prior to applying the inverse FFT in the phase-encoding direction a phase correction of the acquired data is performed to match the superimposed data sets.

Figure 3 shows some images using a PHREAK technique based on a spin echo sequence. Instead of an interventional procedure, with normally small changes in the image content due to the motion of the interventional device, a drastic movement of a head is shown. After the acquisition of a reference image with a matrix size of 256×256, the head is turned. The following keyhole slices were acquired with 64 phase encoding cycles (one-fourth of the entire matrix size). Figure 3a shows the reference image acquired with the base sequence. Figure 3c illustrates an image reconstructed after superimposing the newly acquired data slice with the readout direction parallel to that of the reference raw data set. Updating both keyhole slices, parallel and perpendicular to the reference data set, improves the image quality with respect to the resolution, as illustrated in Fig. 3d. Figure 4 shows a simulation of an interventional procedure. After acquiring a reference image of a grapefruit without a needle inside the fruit the various slices acquired with the needle inside the fruit are inserted into the reference image. Figure 4c shows the improvement of PHREAK over the normal keyhole imaging (Fig. 4b)

Overall the data acquisition using PHREAK is as fast as with standard keyhole sequences as both reconstruct an image after the acquisition of n lines, with n being the number of lines in every keyhole slice. With respect to the reconstruction of PHREAK images a pure raw data set must be kept in memory to allow direct storage of the new keyhole data slices. However, it is obvious that after a dramatic change in the image content, as illustrated in the example given here, the image reconstructed from a PHREAK sequence after updating two keyhole slices contains more detailed information than a standard keyhole sequence. This is because a larger part of the k-space data set in the boundary regions is updated, as is seen by comparing Fig. 3c and Fig. 3d.

■ Asymmetric PHREAK

An asymmetric extension of the PHREAK method is illustrated in Fig. 5 [5–7]. Asymmetric PHREAK acquires four instead of two update keyhole slices. Here the newly acquired slices are not placed symmetrically about the center of k-space but rather are shifted to either side in the phase-encoding direction (Fig. 5). As in the PHREAK technique, the "hot spots" must be contained in every raw data slice to ensure correct alignment of all four data slices. To implement asymmetric PHREAK the number of slices is increased to expand the updated region of k-space with the same time resolution as offered by keyhole or PHREAK sequences. This offers higher resolution (a larger portion of the boundary regions of k-space are updated) without decreasing the image frame rate offered by the standard keyhole or PHREAK technique as long as an image reconstruction is performed after the acquisition of each slice.

As this acquisition scheme can cover a large part of the entire k-space (depending on the number of lines forming a keyhole slice) no reference raw data set is required. After the acquisition of all four keyhole slices characterized by asymmetric PHREAK the image quality is comparable to an image reconstructed from an entirely filled raw data space using standard data acquisition schemes. Figure 3e presents an example of a transverse slice through a head, and Fig. 4d shows a simulation of an interventional procedure. Note that this image is comparable to that in Fig. 3a, acquired with the base sequence

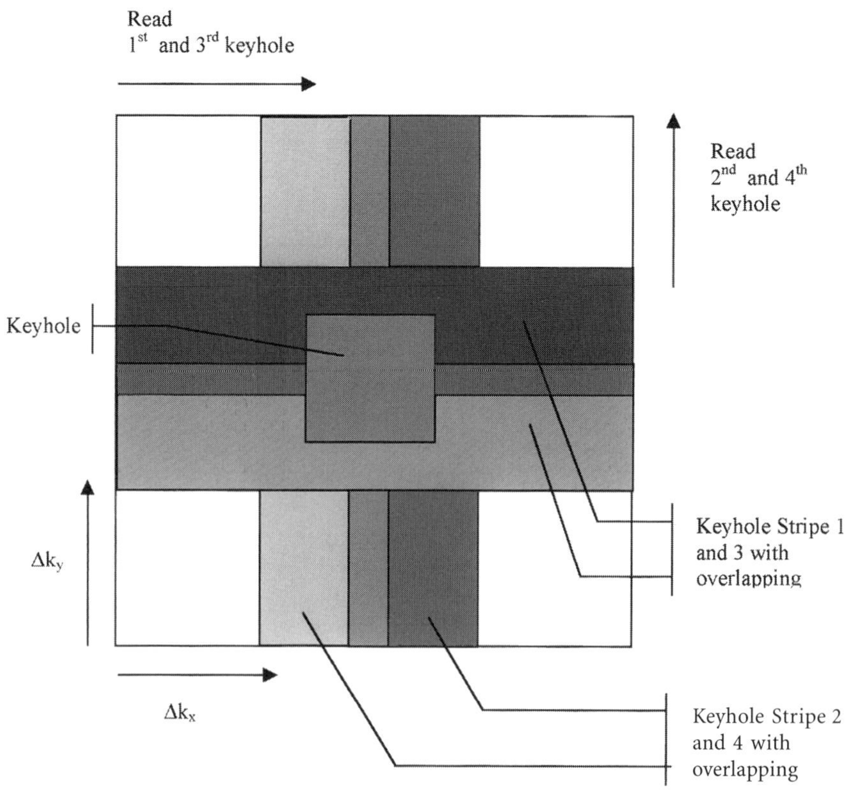

Fig. 5. Keyhole with four keyhole slices. Asymmetric PHREAK. *White area*, the nonupdated part of the entire raw data set

used to implement asymmetric PHREAK. As in the PHREAK technique, a pure raw data set must be stored to superimpose the newly acquired data sets. A phase correction and alignment of the "hot spots" needs to be performed prior to reconstructing an image using a two-dimensional FFT.

Using PHREAK or its extension with asymmetric slices increases the image frame rate by a factor of n/N with n being the number of lines in the keyhole slice and N the number of lines needed for a conventional scan. To obtain even shorter acquisition times "turbo asymmetric PHREAK" has been developed. Here, as in standard multiecho sequences, multiple echoes are acquired after every excitation with a different phase encoding. Figure 3f shows an image reconstructed from a four-echo asymmetric PHREAK sequence. Depending on the TR, the acquisition time can be shortened proportional to the number of echoes acquired after one excitation.

■ Rotating Sliced k-Space

The basic concept of the rotating sliced k-space data acquisition scheme is to extend the PHREAK technique and update the entire k-space in a fluoroscopic sequence mode [8, 9]. To achieve this the updated keyhole slices are rotated in "arbitrary" angles about the center (hot spot) in k-space rather than flipped by 90°. Four orientations of the updating slices running through the center of k-space match the rectangular pattern of data points in k-space and therefore do not require an interpolation algorithm to match the newly acquired data points and the initial standard raw data space. These slices are aligned with kx or ky or are at an angle of 45° to kx and ky.

However, this technique cannot yet cover the entire k-space, as unfilled gaps remain between the overlapping rotated slices. Sequences rotating the slices by 22.5° after every update instead of the former rotation of 45° can be used to reduce this effect. Unfortunately, with a 22.5° rotation some of the acquired data points do not match the perpendicular data grid of k-space. Therefore interpolation is needed prior to reconstruction by a two-dimensional FFT to "force" the keyhole data points onto the perpendicular k-space data grip of the initial matrix. As described above, the hot spots of the various keyhole slices must be matched at the center of k-space, and a phase correction is necessary to eliminate errors due to system imperfections.

Using this acquisition scheme the whole k-space is covered in a starlike manner, with the outermost data points of k-space being updated within every eighth cycle and the center part, containing the more important data (as discussed above) being updated with every update slice. Acquired images using this technique have already been published, but major problems related to this technique still prevent its routine use. The most striking difficulties are the sensitivity of this technique to system imperfections (gradients, receive channels, field inhomogeneities, etc.) and the misregistration of data points with regard to the rectangular reference k-space, requiring difficult grid interpolation algorithms.

■ Discussion

Without major changes in the object space, the image quality with PHREAK or any of its extensions is satisfying for interventional procedures, even when using a commercial open low field strength MR system. When imaging minor changes in the object space (e.g., movement of an interventional device), the fast update of the low spatial resolution frequencies allows a fast image update illustrating the position of the interventional tool. However, limiting the update to the low spatial frequencies and not updating "enough" boundary regions of k-space, as it in the basic keyhole scheme, leads to problems. After essential changes of the object (e.g., a movement of the patient), artifacts resulting from inconsistency between the old and new data sets lead to decreased image "quality."

None of the strategies described in this chapter require especially strong gradient systems for fast imaging and can be used with almost any sequence type (e.g., spin echo, gradient echo, two-dimensional, three-dimensional). In particular, with very fast scanners and a powerful reconstruction unit one could conceptually implement these schemes within fast sequences (e.g., echo planar imaging) to obtain image rates higher than 20 frames per second. In addition to guiding and visualizing interventional procedures, this would allow a variety of different medical applications, such as functional brain imaging and contrast-enhanced breast imaging.

References

1. van Vaals JJ, Engels HE, Boer JA et al (1992) Accelerated Dynamic MR Imaging. Presentation #451, RSNA, Chicago
2. Pike GB, Fredrickson JO, Glover GH, Enzmann DR (1992) Partial fourier space dynamic contrast imaging. Presentation #452, RSNA, Chicago
3. Riederer SJ, Tasciyan T, Farzaneh F, Lee JN, Wright RC, Herfkens JR (1988) MR fluoroscopy: technical feasibility. Magn Reson Med 8:1–15
4. Korin HW, Farzaneh F, Wright RC, Riederer SJ (1989) Compensation for effects of linear motion in MR-imaging. 12:99–113
5. Bornstedt A, Busch M, Wendt M, Seibel R, Grönemeyer D (1996) Turbo accelerated asymmetric phase read keyhole (PHREAK) imaging as a method for fast and high contrast MR-guided intervention. Presentation #260, European Society for Magnetic Resonance in Medicine and Biology, Prague, 12–15 September
6. Bornstedt A, Busch M, Wendt M, Seibel R, Grönemeyer D (1996) Acceleration of 3D imaging sequences through keyhole k-space acquisition techniques. Presentation #1503, International Society for Magnetic Resonance in Medicine, New York
7. Busch M, Friebe M, Hellwig S, Lerchner H, Seibel R, Grönemeyer D (1994) Acceleration of arbitrary sequences through different k-space updating strategies for interventional monitoring. Presented in the Society for Magnetic Resonance Workshop on Interventional MRI, Marina del Rey, Calif. 13–14 August, p 106
8. Busch M, Friebe M, Hellwig S, Lerchner H (1994) Keyhole sequence in 2 dimensions for high speed fluoroscopic imaging (PHREAK). Presented at the Society for Magnetic Resonance Imaging, Dallas
9. Duerk JL, Lewin JS, Wu DH (1996) Application of keyhole imaging to interventional MRI: a simulation study to predict sequence requirements. J Magn Reson Imaging 6:918–924

Magnetic Resonance Imaging for Microtherapy and Surgery

4

D. H. W. Grönemeyer · F. Jolesz · R. B. Lufkin
R. M. M. Seibel · R. Kikinis · A. Melzer

■ Introduction

Magnetic resonance imaging (MRI), computed tomography (CT), and electron beam tomography (EBT) units are constructed for radiological diagnosis. They are being used with increasing frequency for interventional procedures and in open surgeries. All scanners can be combined with various imaging modalities such as endoscopy and electronic equipment which are normally used in conventional operation rooms. There are presently limitations on the use of MRI for therapy in magnet designs, electronic equipment, and instruments. However, MRI affords multiplanar localization and imaging without X-ray exposure and open access, and fluoroscopic imaging allows nearly real-time guidance of instruments and real-time documentation of therapeutic effects.

In surgery the physician can see only structures directly in front of his eyes or in front of his extended eyes by using endoscopes, whereas tomographic imaging provides a transparent picture of the entire operative field. Analogous to microscopy, which obtains a transparent view of cells, the use of tomography during operations can be defined as "tomographic macroscopy" [1] because the therapist has a transparent view of the operation field.

The first steps using MRI for tomographic therapy were carried out by several groups between 1986 and 1989 [2–8]. In the past few years MRI-guided access techniques have become more popular because of the availability of open scanners [1, 9, 10] and faster imaging sequences [11].

■ MRI Systems

The advantage of MRI guidance using an open system is that the patient can be scanned by

Table 1. MRI units for interventional procedures (in ascending order of field strength)

System	Field strength (T)	Magnet system	Design	Interventional capability
Toshiba Access	0.064	Permanent	Open 4-sided	Open system with (360°) vertical "temple" access, fluoroscopy, general interventions
Siemens Open	0.2	Resistive	C form	Open system, open 3-sided suitable for intervention, fast imaging possible, restricted vertical access
GE Open	0.2	Permanent	Open 2-sided	Open system, suitable for intervention, fast imaging possible, restricted vertical access
Picker Outlook	0.23	Resistive	C form	Open system, open 3-sided suitable for intervention, fast imaging possible, restricted vertical access
Hitachi Airis	0.3	Permanent	270° access	Open system, suitable for intervention, fast imaging possible, restricted vertical access
Toshiba	0.35	Hybrid	Open 4-sided	Open system with (360°) vertical access, fluoroscopy, general interventions, restricted access
GE "Double Donut"	0.5	High-temperature superconductor	Full vertical, restricted horizontal access	Developed especially for treatments in standing position, fast imaging
Philips NT 5	0.5	Superconducting tube	2-sided system	Suitable as tube, combination with DSA integrated LCD monitor
Bruker	2 T	Superconducting tube	2-sided system	Suitable as tube system, food pad guidance in OR

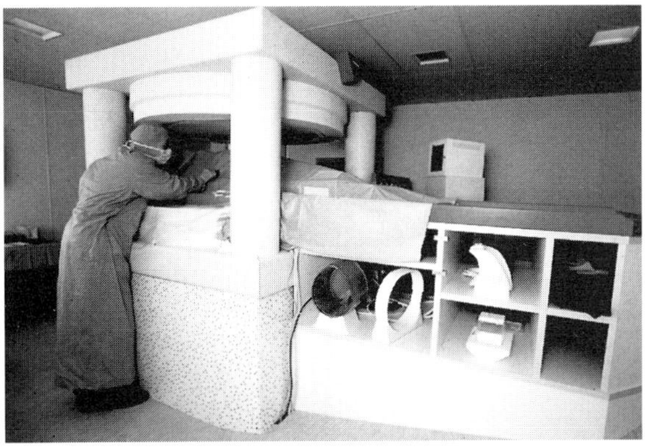

Fig. 1. Open MRI (0.064 T): Access (Toshiba)

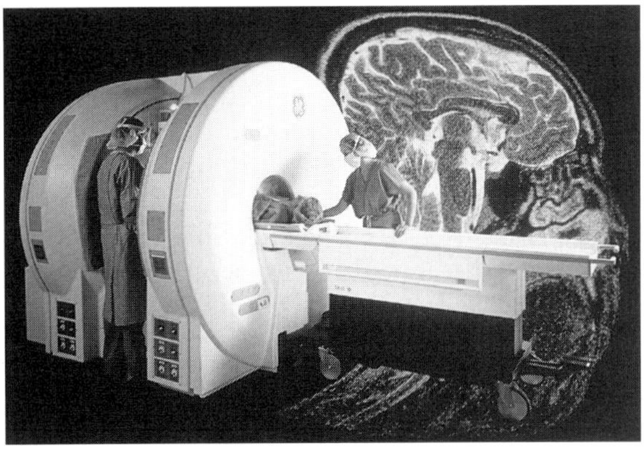

Fig. 2. Open MRI (0.5 T): MRT (General Electric)

means of a so-called fluoroscopic mode inside the magnet. The ultra-low-field MRI scanner developed by Kaufman et al. [12] in 1987 was the first open MR system. This MRI unit (Access, Toshiba MRI, San Francisco, CA, USA) utilizes a permanent magnet with a field strength of 0.064 T (Fig. 1). The vertical field magnets of this scanner permit circumferential open access at the four lateral sides. Since 1993 other open MRI unit configurations with various field strengths have been developed (Table 1).

Open systems are generally more comfortable for patients than the narrow, tube-like MRI scanners, and patients therefore tend to be more cooperative and amenable to percutaneous procedures. Additionally, "claustrophobic" and frightened patients can be examined more easily, and the open structure of the system allows continuous observation with the ability to administer medications during the procedures.

One dedicated MRI system (GE Signa SP) developed especially for intraoperative and interventional imaging consists of a 0.5-T unit with two vertically oriented magnetic poles, so that the therapist can stand inside the magnet for the access procedure, therapy, and documentation without moving the patient [13] (Fig. 2). This system has excellent vertical but more limited horizontal access. An interactive guidance system for defined imaging in nearly real-time and in several planes along the instruments is connected with the acquisition mode of the MRI system. Also, a workstation for three-dimensional (3D) imaging and pre- and postprocessing modalities is directly connected. A MR-compatible anesthesia delivery system (XL10-MRI Compatible Anesthesia Sta-

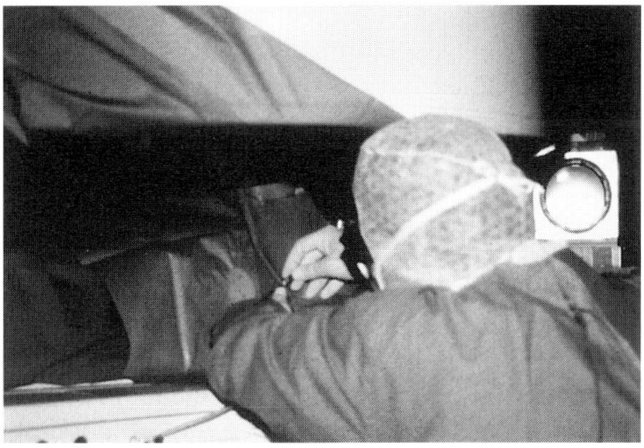

Fig. 3. Open MRI (0.2 T): Magnetom Open (Siemens)

tion, Ohmeda, Madison, Wis., USA) and a patient monitoring system (MagLife ODAM, Bruker, Wissembourg, France) is installed beside the magnet.

The 0.2-T Magnetom Open (Siemens; Fig. 3) and the 0.064-T Access (Toshiba) units have horizontally orientated magnets. For treatments inside the magnet the physician must lean into the magnet, or for optimizing especially operative procedures the table must moved out of the gantry, but not as far as in closed tube systems.

All systems have integrated monitors for imaging in the MRI room. A second monitor for other imaging modalities such as endoscopy (Storz, Germany) is installed ahead from the operative in the dedicated system as well as five controlling monitors outside. In both other systems a portable endoscopy system (Micromed, Bochum, Germany) can be used.

The patient couch of the dedicated system is disconnectable, and the patient can be moved in and out of the room without changing position. The Siemens system is connectable with an especially developed bed, which is mobile and can be precisely connected with the fixed installed patient couch.

The projectile effect of the 0.064-T low-field system is minimal in comparison to higher field strength. If necessary, ferromagnetic instruments such as scalpels can be used without any risk of projectile effect in the 0.064-T field strength. Therefore the scans must be obtained subsequent to the procedure to avoid ferromagnetic artifact in the images. Additionally, it is possible to use emergency life-support equipment in close proximity. There is sufficient space inside the magnet to ventilate a patient [1].

Interactive image processing inside the room can be performed by the therapist or an assistance only in the Magnetom Open. Here a mouse and a foot pad are available within the therapeutic field for starting, processing, and stopping the acquisition mode.

■ Microtherapeutic Workstation

In the future all electronic equipment for image post-processing, navigation, treatment with energetic systems, such as laser, RF, fluid or air support , etc. and couch positioning, could be integrated into an equipment tower, placed close to the therapist. The best solution would be to manage the different electronic devices via a single computer platform. This would reduce the number of key-pads needed to manage each individual component. Virtual guidance, such as voice control, which we developed for table movement, would simplify procedures: e.g. measurements of impedance, activation energy, changing image modalities, 3D view, movement of navigation systems or positioning systems, activating or closing operation lights onto the skin etc. Each procedure also has to be documented on the screen and must be archived on CD. At the end of every procedure, a protocol has to be printed for documentation.

Preplanned surgical images, as well as prescanned images, must be available during the procedure. For intra-operative image fusion, interactive or real time 3D imaging, or post-processing of temperature-sensitive sequences, a member of the team has to work backstage on an image workstation, which is connected to both the archive and the therapeutic workstation in the OR.

■ Imaging

There are four major therapy phases for each procedures, which acquire different imaging modalities [14]:

- Localizing: slice definition and electronic measurements (high resolution)
- Guidance: introduction of instruments (fast imaging, low resolution)
- Treatment: controlling of therapeutic effects (low and high resolution, three-dimensional)
- Documentation: of treatment (high resolution, several planes, 3D)

The image quality of fluoroscopic guidance procedures is virtually the same in all systems. The fastest mode at present is available at the 0.064-T Access system (Table 3 (Chapter B4)).

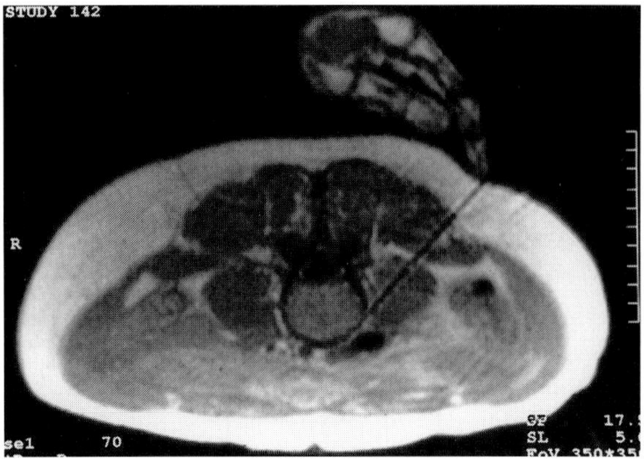

Fig. 4. MR-guided RF lumbar sympathectomy. FLASH (66/9) image of electrode placement at a lower level. The physician's hand is visible over the electrode

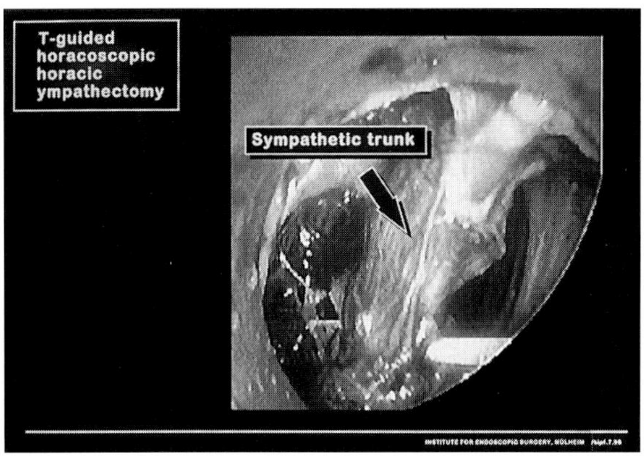

Fig. 5. Tomographically guided endoscopy of sympathetic trunk

■ Microtherapy

Minimally invasive techniques using endoscopes for image-guided therapy are common in the surgical field and in internal medicine. Interventional procedures in the past were generally performed with fluoroscopy, ultrasound guidance, or CT. MRI guidance is new. With the help of cross-sectional tomography (macroscopy) the risk of complications of minimally invasive procedures can be significantly reduced by minimizing access techniques [1, 14] and the size of instruments. Reducing the diameter of the instruments below 1 mm and tomographic guidance of these probes leads to the field of microtherapy [1, 14]. This is leading increasingly to the change from general to local anesthesia and to the performance of therapeutic procedures on an outpatient basis.

Imaging techniques allow the visualization of therapy effects. Temperature-induced signal changes [15–19], flow in vessels, changes in metabolism, diminishing soft tissue in tumor ablations [14], and shrinking of disk herniations can be directly identified [20]. Even high-risk structures such as nerves or vessels which may not be visible during endoscopic procedures when they are hidden behind the tissue can be visualized and protected. Neuroscopic (Fig. 4 and 5), arthroscopic, thoracoscopic, and other endoscopic operations will be facilitated by the increased transparency of the patient's individual anatomy and pathology. Overall, within the same tomographic guidance procedure a combination of open surgery, interventional procedure, and endoscopic operation is possible as well as drug instillation, prosthesis/stent implantation, tissues activation (e.g., photoablation), and physiological measurements. Microtherapeutic tomographic treatments will be helpful in all medical disciplines in the near future.

Spine

The major indications of tomographic guidance include the treatment of acute and chronic disk herniation, postdiskectomy syndrome, and scar tissue after open surgery. Different treatments are possible in MRI:

Facet Joints. Generally the facet anesthesia is used for acute radicular pain caused by functional disorders and for diagnosis before ethanol injection. Percutaneous ethanol instillation for lysis is important for chronic pain caused by spondylarthrosis or chronic prolapse. Pain caused by postdiskectomy syndrome can also be treated very easily with facet anesthesia and/or iliosacral joint therapy [14, 21].

Iliosacral Joints. Acute and chronic pain caused by sterile inflammation (sacroiliitis) is treated with 10–40 mg crystalline cortisone. This therapy technique is very helpful in combination with facet joint therapy, periradicular and epidural treatments, and nucleotomy/diskectomy [14].

Chronic Disc Herniation. Instillation of 40–80 mg crystalline cortisone for chronic disk herniation and scar tissue after operation up to eight times every 3 weeks directly in proximity to the herniated disk (Fig. 6) [14, 22].

Acute Disk Herniation. Nd-YAG or Hol-YAG laser treatment can be used for acute more than for chronic medial or lateral disk herniation after 6 weeks of unsuccessful conservative therapy

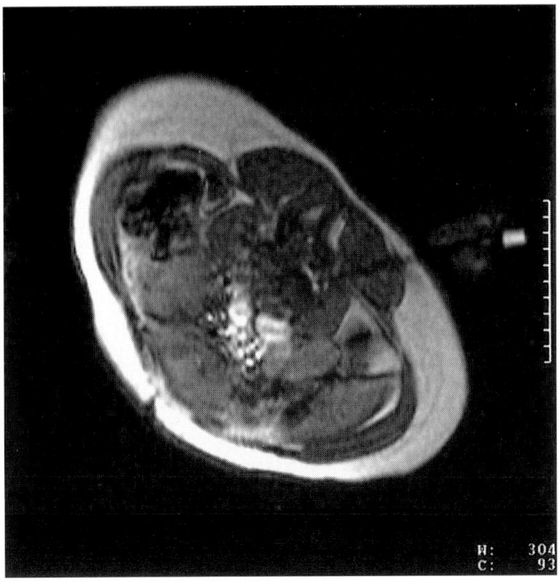

Fig. 6. Periradicular therapy (PRT) for chronic disk herniations (Magnetom Open, Siemens, 0.2 T)

(Fig. 7) [1, 14, 23]. This technique must be combined with endoscopy.

Sinus Surgery

Endoscopic sinus surgery was introduced in United States over 10 years ago [24, 25] and is now the most common sinus technique there. MRI can be a very important tool for avoiding complications by losing depth perception and for precise and fast guidance techniques in several planes [26].

Oncology

There are a wide spectrum of possibilities using MRI for cancer treatments in all medical disciplines; biopsies are only one step in a complex surgical planning and treatment concept. Percutaneous microtherapeutic therapy techniques were developed from fine-needle biopsy. CT-guided biopsies developed out of fluoroscopy- and ultrasound-guided techniques and have now been have been standard procedure in radiology for many years in all regions [27–30]. The major advantages of tomographic over ultrasound guidance are that less training is needed to understand the image, and that the system itself is not moved. Consequently an exact reproduction of the scan level is possible for each physician. When using ultrasound for biopsy, more time is needed to place the transducer over the area of pathology, especially in cases of repeated examinations.

Biopsies

There are various concepts of guidance techniques. Normally physicians are accustomed to performing biopsies with frameless devices. This technique can be performed in all MRI systems in virtually the same manner as in CT scanners [31–33]. Another approach has long been known in neurosurgery using stereotactic frames for guid-

a

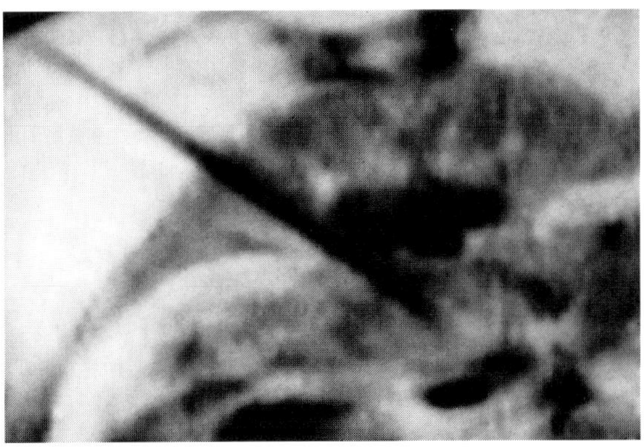

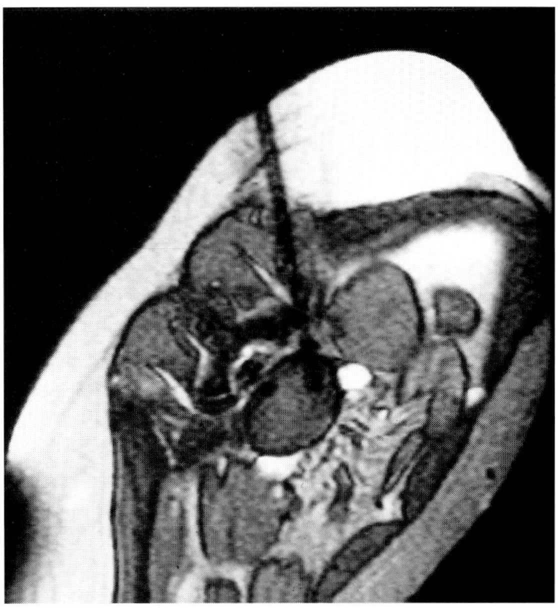

b

Fig. 7. a Percutaneous laser diskectomy using Nd-YAG laser (experimental, Access, Toshiba). **b** Clinical (Magnetom Open, Siemens)

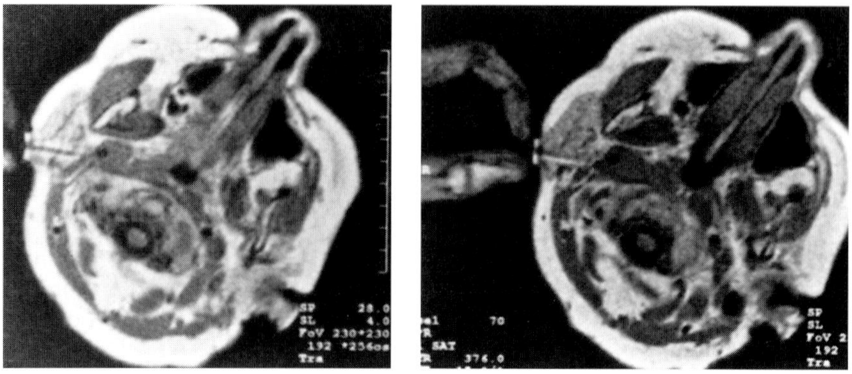

a b

Fig. 8a,b. MR-guided aspiration cytology of retropharyngeal mass on 0.2 T system. a Rapid MR "fluoro" images during needle placement. b Documentation: with the needle in place for aspiration (Clinical, Siemens)

ance procedures in predefined virtual image environments [34, 35]. Interactive guidance systems are also in use which are connected with the instruments via robotic arms (e.g., Viewing Wand, ISG, Toronto, Canada) or directly with the instruments [36] (e.g., Radionics, Mass., USA). These are stand-alone systems and are helpful in all MRI units by the installation of a separate workstation. The guidance procedure is possible only with prescanned images in a virtual volume. The best interactive concept is that in the dedicated open MRI system of GE. Here the image plane is automatically referenced to a hand-held or a fixed probe over the region of therapy. The position of the probe is constantly identified, and the radiologist can interactively define up to three orthogonal image planes that are related to the axis of the probe [31, 32] (Fig. 7).

Cancer Therapy

Cancer and metastatic disease, especially to bone, often worsens the situation of patients due to immobilization caused by intractable pain and/or neurological deficits. Tumors inside the brain cause constant headache, and infiltration into bone causes one of the most intense types of pain that exists [37]. Effective tumor therapy must therefore deal with three important parameters: fast pain relieve, effective reduction in tumor growth, and stabilization of bone or of the vertebral body to prevent paralysis. New and effective concepts are now available with less traumatic treatments by image guidance for these patients.

Virtually all treatment modalities that have been used under CT or ultrasound guidance are possible in MRI. Today, however, only few instruments and electronic devices are commercially available for artifact-free guidance. The easiest means of percutaneous cancer therapy is the local administration of concentrated ethanol (percutaneous ethanol instillation, Fig. 9) or chemotherapeutic agents (percutaneous drug instillation) [38–40]. The disadvantage of this technique is that the controlling fluid spreading inside tissue is not exactly assignable, but ethanol instillation is helpful for fast pain relief and for calcification and stabilization of infiltrated bony structures [14, 40].

Other possibilities are intratumoral hyperthermia or vaporization such as in the liver, neck, or brain using the Nd-YAG laser [41–43] (Fig. 10), radiofrequency (RF) ablations [44], cryotherapy [45], hyperenergetic ultrasound [46], and brachytherapeutic treatments. Imaging of temperature change in tissues is possible only in MRI, and the therapist can control exactly the depth of the temperature infiltration. New imaging modalities in the dedicated MRI system using temperature-sensitive sequences and interactive image subtraction are being developed and are helpful in controlling the predefined treatment area.

Also, percutaneous sympathectomies at all levels of the spine are helpful as a first step in pain therapy using CT or ultrafast EBT either with or without combination of endoscopy and RF ablation or 96% ethanol instillation [14, 47].

■ Open Surgery

Carrying out open surgery in the traditional standing position directly ahead of the therapeutic field is possible only in the dedicated MRI system (Fig. 11). In all other units the physicians must approach the patient from the side. For the sake of safety the interactive supervision of operative results without moving the patient and without changing instrument positions – especially by combining open surgery and microtherapeutic procedures – is of major interest.

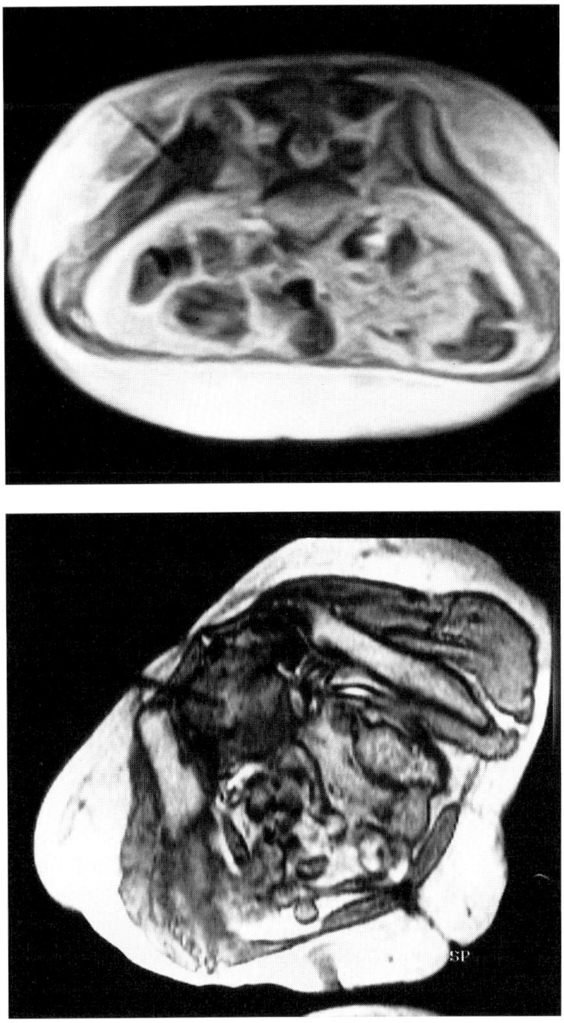

a

b

Fig. 9a,b. Percutaneous ethanol instillation for cancer therapy (96% ethanol). a Metastasis of os ilium (ethanol; signal decreasing in T1; Access, Toshiba). b Metastasis of os sacrum (after contrast media instillation; diluted Gd-DTPA in plasma concentration; Magnetom Open, Siemens)

This kind of technique also makes it possible to detect residual tumor tissue, disk fragments in spinal micro-operations, and conventional prosthesis implantation, for example, in orthopedic or traumatic cases. Also, combinations with endoscopy and interactive radiotherapy are possible.

■ Three-Dimensional Imaging for Tomographic Procedures

All cross-sectional imaging modalities such as ultrasound, CT, MRI, EBT, positron-emission tomography, and single photon emission computed tomography allow 3D reconstruction in the post-

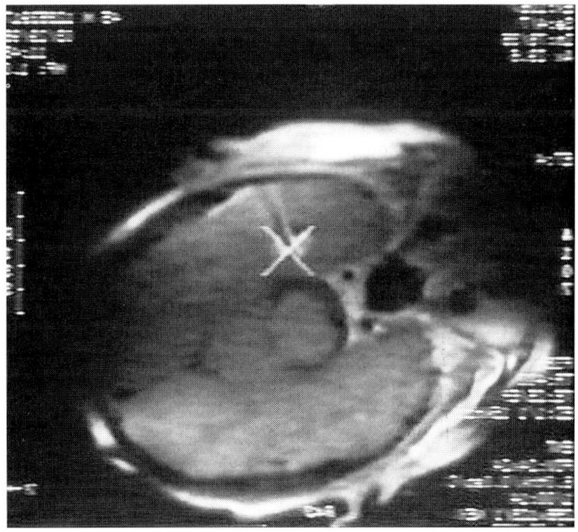

Fig. 10. Laser therapy with Nd-YAG inside a brain tumor (Dedicated system, GE)

processing mode. Real-time processing is not yet possible. The advantages of 3D over 2D imaging is the fast comprehension of anatomic regions, especially by nonspecialized physicians, and the ability to match images from different systems. Transparent surfacing in- and outside of tissue structures and several processing modalities enable the physician to examine organ structures such as surfaces, vessels, and nerves etc. Also, ever more 3D reconstruction are being developed for virtual endoscopy [26].

Regional and density resolution is better than in cross-sectional 2D slices. For access and guidance techniques the therapist needs high-resolution for tip tracking and, if possible, ultrafast or real-time imaging. Tissue changes such as regional edema, bleeding, and lesions caused by energy treatments (laser, RF, cryotherapy, etc.) between surgical manipulations can be controlled only by high-resolution imaging. For this reason 3D or virtual guidance must be combined interactively with current and not with prescanned slices.

3D imaging is also a wonderful tool for post-processing documentation of therapeutic effects such as drug distribution (e.g., percutaneous ethanol instillation for cancer therapy or sympathectomy), laser-induced disk shrinking, and implantations. 3D models are very helpful for surgical planning and for education and training, especially if animal studies can be avoided [48] (Fig. 12).

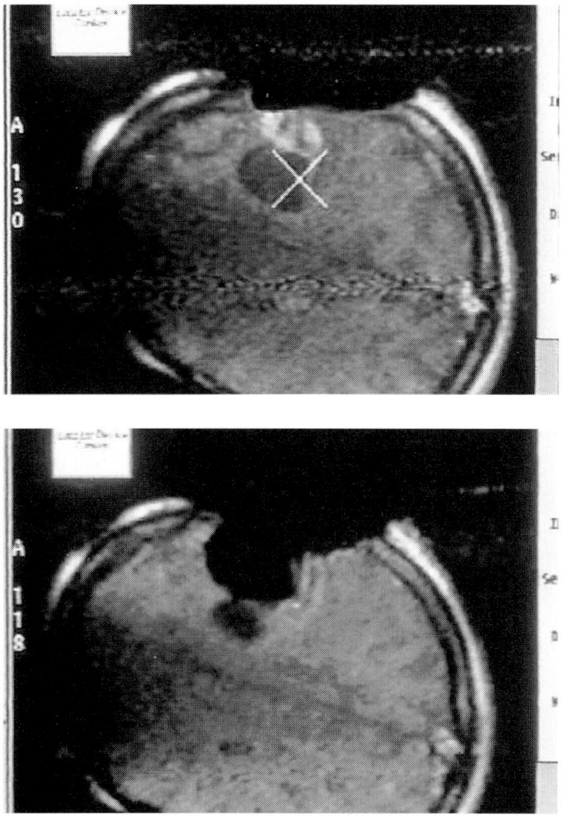

a

b

Fig. 11. Open surgery of a brain tumor. a Before therapy of tumor mass beside the ventricle. b After resection of the tumor

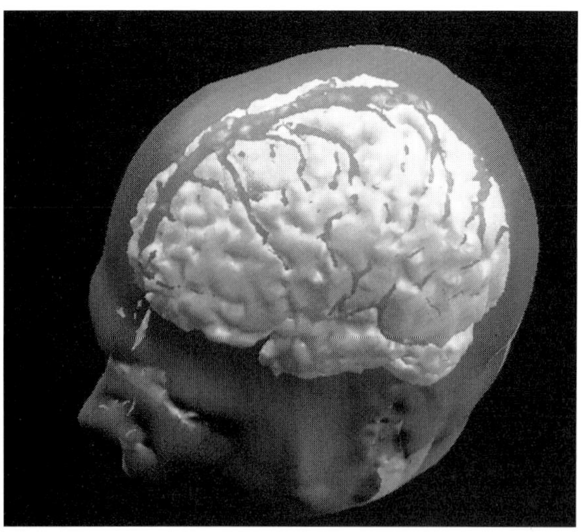

Fig. 12. Postprocessed 3D imaging for documentation and educational work

■ Future Possibilities

In the near future all medical disciplines will very likely be using tomographic scanners increasingly for operative procedures, not only for minimally invasive or microtherapy but also for open surgery inside the magnet and as a 2D/3D imaging modality for controlling treatment any time before, during, and after therapy. Also, tip tracking of catheters in vessels is now being developed [14]. These catheter-guidance procedures may prove possible inside MRI as well as in combination with digital subtraction angiography and MRI such as the 1.5-T unit which Philips is now developing, or without electronic tip tracking in combined X-ray units of digital subtraction angiography and spiral CT or ultrafast EBT.

Flow measurements of arteries can be carried out using MRI or EBT and in MRI without contrast media. Other fields will include tomographic balloon dilatation, intravascular laser treatment, and stent implantation. With this kind of technique the tip of the catheter can be placed very precisely inside the vessel at the exact location from the artery or venous wall.

Additional advantages of MRI include the lack of radiation, temperature mapping [15–17], and the possibility of measuring metabolic changes with the spectroscopy mode in high-field (1.5-T) systems. Correct access can also be gained also by tomographic guidance for interstitial therapy such as special drug injection, for example, in pain therapy. The philosophy behind this is administering a high concentration of drugs in the region of therapy and very low or no concentration in other areas of the body. Also possible are the placement of gene-technological implants [1, 14] and the drilling and fixation with the correct angle for osteosynthesis.

MRI, CT, and EBT offer safe access in conjunction with minimal risk for vital structures. When there are vital structures such as nerves and vessels in the target region ("high-risk area"), CT, and – inside vessels and in lung or heart – EBT are our preferred techniques of guidance-technology. The puncture precision with CT is down to 1 mm^3. Open MRI is useful in "low-risk areas" of every part of the body, because of tip artifacts produced by instruments. There is a great need for artifact-free and "intelligent" instruments such as trocars, cannulae, scissors, forceps, and deflectable instruments with superelastic alloys as well as MRI-compatible electronic equipment [14, 49]. Only a few are now available or are under development. Furthermore, it is possible to approach structures which are located behind or in front of other organs by special puncture techniques without damaging these organs by interactive real-time 3D guidance with oblique planes in open MRI or virtually in CT/EBT.

Because the transparency of the patient gained by MRI, CT, or EBT adds important information about the spatial configuration of anatomical structures, image-guided access techniques may help to avoid complications and reduce risks and side effects. The combination of endoscopy with tomographic scanners, fluoroscopy units, or intravascular ultrasound and preoperative 2D/3D images of any desired system allows every structure in the body to be visualized, defined, and treated. In addition, the small diameter of instruments (<1 mm; Fig. 12) reduces the risk of accidental injury to vital structures such as vessels and nerves, and it is important that the therapeutic effect be visible at once within the surgical procedure (e.g., open tumor surgery, shrinking of the disk). These microinvasive techniques increasingly permit the change from general to local anesthesia and the carrying out of treatment on an outpatient basis.

Transparent real-time 3D guidance in the future would be helpful for inexperienced therapists and to provide more safety. Also, by learning a new procedure all physicians must begin with an easy procedure such as biopsies in low-risk areas and with CT guidance. MRI guidance high risk treatments are the next steps in the learning curve. Biopsies are very helpful for learning because the target region must be reached precisely.

Future therapeutic procedures will have to be conducted in interdisciplinary groups. For the health of the patient an experienced physician with a conventional therapeutic method is much better than a less experienced physician with a new method: "The right procedure at the right time by the right physician for the right indication" [50]. Bearing this in mind, this is a wonderful prospect for patients in the new century of medicine. An effective change is possible from treatments inside hospitals to safe image-guided procedures with reduced complications and side effects on an outpatient basis. This also has the potential to dramatically reduce costs in health care systems worldwide [1].

■ References

1. Grönemeyer DHW, Seibel RMM, Melser A, Schmidt A (1995) Image guided access techniques. Endosc Surg Allied Technol 1:69–75
2. Thomas DG, Davis CH, Ingram S, Onley JS, Bydder GM, Young IR (1986) Stereotaxic biopsy of the brain under MR imaging control. Am J Roentgennol 7:161
3. Mueller PR, Stark DD, Simeone JF, Saini S et al (1986) MR-guided aspiration biopsy: needle design and clinical trials. Radiology 161:605
4. Herman SD, Friedman AC, Radecki PD, Caroline DF (1986) Incidential prostatic carcinoma detected by MRI and diagnosed MRI/CT-guided biopsy. Am J Roentgenol 146:351
5. van Sonnenberg E, Hajek P, Baker L et al (1986) Materials for MR-guided interventional radiology procedures: laboratory and clinical experience (abstract). Radiology 161:121
6. Lufkin R, Teresi L, Hanafee W (1987) New needle for MR-guided aspiration cytology of the head and neck. AM J Roentegenol 149:380
7. Jolesz FA, Bleier AR, Jakob P et al (1988) MR imaging of laser tissue interactions. Radiology 168:249
8. Grönemeyer DHW, Seibel RMM, Kaufman L et al (1990) Interventional procedures in low field magnetic resonance imaging. Diagn Imaging Int 11/12:321
9. Jolesz FA, Shtern F (1992) The operating room of the future. Invest Radiol 27:805
10. Grönemeyer DHW, Seibel RMM, Melzer A, Schmid A, Deli M, Friebe MH, Busch M (1995) Future of advanced guidance techniques by interventional CT and MRI. Minim Invas Ther 4:251
11. Riederer SJ, Tasciyan T, Farzaneh F, Lee JN, Wright RC, Herfkens RJ (1988) MR fluoroscopy: technical feasibility. Magn Reson Med 8:1
12. Kaufman L, Crooks L, Arakawa M, Hoenninger J, Watts J, Winkler M (1987) Admin Radio VI(XI):32
13. Schenck JF, Jolesz FA, Roemer PB et al (1993) Superconducting open-configuration MR imaging system for image-guided therapy. Radiology 195:805
14. Gronemeyer D, Seibel R, Erbel R, Schmidt A, Plasmann J, Deli M, Melzer A, Schmermund A, Baumgart D, Welsch R, Ge J, Goerge G (1996) Equipment configuration and procedures – preferences for interventional microtherapy. J Dig Imaging 9(2):81
15. Le Bihan D, Delannoy J, Levin R (1989) Non-invasive temperature mapping using magnetic resonance imaging of molecular diffusion: application to hyperthermia. Radiology 171:853
16. Goldhaber DM, Deli M, Gronemeyer DHW, Kramer DM, Avram HE, Seibel RMM, Kaufmann L (1993) Measurement of tissue temperature by MRI. IEEE Nucl Sci Med Imaging 3:1702
17. Young I, Hand J, Oatridge A, Prior M, Forse G (1994) Further observations on the measurement of tissue T1 to monitor temperature in vivo by MRI. Magn Reson Med Magn Reson Med 31(3):342
18. Cline H, Schenck J, Hynynen K et al (1992) MR-guided focused ultrasound surgery. J Comput Assist Tomogr 16(6):956
19. Anzai Y, Lufkin RB, Saxton RE et al (1991) Nd: YAG interstitial laser phototherapy guided by magnetic resonance imaging in an ex vivo model: dosimetry of laser-MR-tissue interaction. Laryngoscope 101:755
20. Grönemeyer DHW, Seibel RMM, Schmidt A, Kremer G, van Leeuwen P (1993) A traumatic CT-controlled percutaneous laser nucleotomy. Minim Invas Ther 2:247
21. Seibel RMM, Grönemeyer DHW, Grumme T (1990) New possibilities for treatments of chronic disk herniationof. In: Seibel RMM, Grönemeyer DHW (eds) International Computed Tomography. Blackwell Science, Oxford
22. Grönemeyer D, Seibel R, Schindler O, Schattauer K, Lange S, Schmidt A (1995) Microinvasive CT guided periradicular therapy for treatment of chronical disk herniation. Wien Med Wochenschr 145:129
23. Seibel RMM, Grönemeyer DHW (1994) Technique for CT guided microendoscopic dissection of the spin. Endosc Surg Allied Technol 12:313
24. Kennedy DW, Zinreich SJ, Rosenbeim AE, Johns ME (1985) Functional endoscopic sinus surgery: theory and diagnostic evaluation. Arch Otolarygol 111:576
25. Maniglia AJ (1991) Fatal and other complications of endoscopic sinus surgery. Laryngoscope 97:1270

26. Fried MP, Hsu L, Topulos GP, Jolesz F (1996) Image-guided surgery in a new magnetic resonance suite: preclinical considerations. Laryngoscope 106(4):411
27. Nordenström B (1967) Paraxiphoid approach to the mediastinum for mediastinography and mediastinal needle biopsy: a preliminary report. Invest Radiol 2:141
28. Göthlin JH (1976) Post-lymphographic percutaneous fine needle biopsy of lymph nodes, guided by fluoroscopy. Radiology 120:205
29. Haaga JR, Alfidi RJ (1976) Percise biopsy localization by computed tomography. Radiology 118:603
30. Grönemeyer DHW, Seibel RMM, Arnold WH et al (1990) Atlas of CT-guided biopsies. In: Seibel RMM, Grönemeyer DHW (eds) Interventional computed tomography. Blackwell, Oxford, p 3
31. Silverman SG, Collick BD, Figueira et al (1995) Interactive biopsy in an open configuration interventional MRI system. Radiology 197:175
32. Silverman SG (1996) Percutaneous abdominal biopsy: recent advances and future directions. Semin Interv Rad 13(1):3
33. Schmidt AM, Melzer A, Seibel RMM, Gronemeyer DHW (1996) Tomographic guided biopsy and cell aspiration of neoplasms. Min Invas Ther Allied Technol 5:249
34. Lunsford L, Martinez A, Latchaw R (1986) Stereotaxic surgery with a magnetic resonance- and computerized tomography-compatible system. J Neurosurg 64:872
35. Leksell L, Leksell D, Schwebel J (1985) Stereotaxis and nuclear magnetic resonance. J Neurol Neurosurg Psychiatry 48:14
36. Fried MP, Kleefield J, Taylor R (1999) A new armless image guidance system for endoscopic sinus surgery. Otolaryngol Head Neck Surg (in press)
37. Bonica JJ (1953) The management of cancer pain. In: Zimmerman M, Irings P, Wagner H (eds) Pain in cancer patients. Springer, Berlin Heidelberg New York (Recent results in cancer research, vol 83)
38. Livraghi T, Festi D, Monti F et al (1986) US-guided percutaneous alcohol injection of small hepatic and abdominal tumors. Radiology 16:309
39. Sheu J Ch, Huang GT, Chen D Sh et al (1987) Small hepatocellular carcinoma: intratumor ethanol treatment using new needle and guidance systems. Radiology 163:43
40. Grönemeyer DHW, Seibel RMM (1993) Microinvasive CT-guided cancer therapy of soft tissue and bone metastases. Wien Med Wochenschr 12:313
41. Anzai Y, Lufkin R, Castro D et al (1991) MR imaging-guided interstitial ND: YAG laser phototherapy: dosimetry study of acute tissue damage in an in vivo model. JMRI 1(5):553
42. Vogl TJ, Muller PK, Hammerstingl R et al (1995) Malignant liver tumors treated with MR imaging-guided laser-induced thermotherapy: technique and prospective results. Radiology 196:257
43. Kahn T, Bettag M, Ulrich B et al (1994) Mr-imaging guided laser-induced interstitial thermotherapy in cerebral neoplasm. JCAT 18:519
44. Matsumoto S, Shima F, Hasuo K et al (1992) MR imaging of stereotactic thalamotomy using radiofrequency methods. Nippon Igaku Hoshasen Gakkai Zasshi 52:1559
45. Matsumoto R, Oshio K, Jolesz J (1993) Monitoring of laser and freezing-induced ablation in the liver with T1 weighted MR imaging. J Magn Reson Imag 3:770
46. Cline HE, Hynyunen K, Watkins RD et al (1995) A focused ultrasound system for MRI guided ablation. Radiology 195:176
47. Grönemeyer DHW, Seibel RMM, Melzer A, Schmid A, Deli M, Friebe MH, Busch M (1995) Future of advanced guidance techniques by interventional CT and MRI. Minim Invas Ther 2:251
48. Kikinis R, Gleason PL, Moriarty TM et al (1996) Computer-assisted interactive three-dimensional planning for neurosurgical procedures. Neurosurgery 38(4):640
49. Melzer A, Schmidt AM, Kipfmueller et al (1996) Perequisites for magnetic resonance image-guided interventions and endoscopic surgery. Min Invas Ther Allied Technol 5:255
50. Grönemeyer DHW, Seibel RMM, Melzer A (1996) Radiologic Imaging modalities revolutionize surgical and therapeutical procedures. Min Invas Ther Allied Technol 5:224 (editorial)

Magnetic Resonance: Safety, Bioeffects, and Patient Monitoring

5

F. G. Shellock

Introduction

During the performance of magnetic resonance imaging (MRI) the patient is exposed to three different forms of electromagnetic radiation: a static magnetic field, gradient magnetic fields, and radiofrequency (RF) electromagnetic fields. Each of these may cause significant bioeffects if applied at sufficiently high exposure levels.

Numerous investigations have been conducted to identify potentially adverse bioeffects of MRI [1–83]. Although none of these have determined the presence of any significant or unexpected hazards [1–83], the data are not comprehensive enough to assume absolute safety. In addition to bioeffects related to exposure to the electromagnetic fields used for MRI, there are several areas of health concern for both the patient and health practitioner with respect to the use of clinical MRI.

This chapter: (a) discusses the safety and bioeffects of static, gradient, and RF electromagnetic fields with an emphasis on the data that pertains to MRI and (b) provides an overview of other safety considerations and patient monitoring aspects of this imaging technique.

Bioeffects of Static Magnetic Fields

General Bioeffects of Static Magnetic Fields

There is a paucity of data concerning the effects of high-intensity static magnetic fields on humans. Some of the original investigations on human subjects exposed to static magnetic fields were performed by Vyalov [84, 85], who studied workers involved in the permanent magnet industry. These subjects were exposed to static magnetic fields ranging from 0.0015 T to 0.35 T and reported feelings of headache, chest pain, fatigue, vertigo, loss of appetite, insomnia, itching, and other, more nonspecific ailments [84, 85]. Of note is that exposure to other potentially hazardous environmental working conditions (elevated room temperature, airborne metallic dust, chemicals, etc.) may have been partially responsible for the reported symptoms in these study subjects. Because this investigation lacked an appropriate control group, it is difficult to ascertain whether there was a definite correlation between the exposure to the static magnetic field and the reported abnormalities. Subsequent studies performed with more scientific rigor have not substantiated many of the above findings [86–89].

Temperature Effects

There are conflicting statements in the literature regarding the effect of static magnetic fields on body and skin temperatures of mammals. Reports have indicated that static magnetic fields either increase or both increase and decrease tissue temperature, depending on the orientation of the organism in the static magnetic field [19, 66]. Other articles state that static magnetic fields have no effect on skin and body temperatures of mammals [55, 61, 88, 90].

None of the investigators who identified a static magnetic field effect on temperatures has proposed a plausible mechanism for this response, nor has this work been substantiated. In addition, studies that reported static magnetic field induced skin and/or body temperature changes used either laboratory animals that are known to have labile temperatures or instrumentation that may have been affected by the static magnetic fields [19, 66].

A recent investigation indicated that exposure to a 1.5-T static magnetic field does not alter skin and body temperatures in humans [90]. This study was performed using a special fluoroptic thermometry system demonstrated to be unperturbed by high-intensity static magnetic fields. Therefore skin and body temperatures of human subjects are believed to be unaffected by exposure to static magnetic fields of up to 1.5 T [55, 61].

Electric Induction and Cardiac Effects

Induced biopotentials may be observed during exposure to static magnetic fields and is caused by blood, a conductive fluid, flowing through a magnetic field. The induced biopotential is exhibited by an augmentation of T-wave amplitude as well as by other, nonspecific waveform changes that are apparent on the electrocardiogram and have been observed at static magnetic field strengths as low as 0.1 T [86, 91, 92].

The increase in T-wave amplitude is directly related to the intensity of the static magnetic field, such that at low static magnetic field strengths the effects are not as predominant as those at higher field strengths. The most marked effect on the T-wave is felt to be caused when the blood flows through the thoracic aortic arch. This T-wave amplitude change can be substantial enough to falsely trigger the RF excitation during a cardiac-gated MRI examination.

Other portions of the electrocardiogram may also be altered by the static magnetic field, and this varies with the placement of the recording electrodes. Alternate lead positions can be used to attenuate the static magnetic field induced electrocardiographic changes in order to facilitate cardiac gating studies [93]. Once the patient is no longer exposed to the static magnetic field, these EKG voltage abnormalities revert to normal.

Because there are no circulatory alterations that appear to coincide with these electrocardiographic changes, no biological risks are believed to be associated with the magnetohydrodynamic effect that occurs in conjunction with static magnetic field strengths of up to 2.0 T [86, 91, 92].

Neurological Effects

Theoretically, electrical impulse conduction in nerve tissue may be affected by exposure to static magnetic fields. However, this is an area in the bioeffects literature that contains contradictory information. Some studies have reported remarkable effects on both the function and structure of those portions of the central nervous system that were associated with exposure to static magnetic fields, whereas others have failed to show any significant changes [14, 20, 34, 68, 69, 76–79, 94–99]. Further investigations of potential unwanted bioeffects are needed because of the relative lack of clinical studies in this field that are directly applicable to MRI. At the present time, exposure to static magnetic fields of up to 2.0 T do not appear to significantly influence bioelectric properties of neurons in humans [97–99].

In summary, there is no conclusive evidence of irreversible or hazardous biological effects related to acute, short-term exposures of humans to static magnetic fields of strengths up to 2.0 T. However, as of 1999 there are several 3.0-, 4.0-T, and one 8-T whole-body MR systems operating at various research sites around the world. A preliminary study has indicated that workers and volunteer subjects exposed to a 4.0-T MR system have experienced vertigo, nausea, headaches, a metallic taste in their mouths, and magnetophosphenes (which are visual flashes) [50]. Therefore considerable research is required to study the mechanisms responsible for these bioeffects and to determine possible means, if any, to counterbalance them.

■ Bioeffects of Gradient Magnetic Fields

MRI exposes the human body to rapid variations of magnetic fields due to the transient application of magnetic field gradients during the imaging sequence. Gradient magnetic fields can induce electrical fields and currents in conductive media (including biological tissue) according to Faraday's law of induction. The potential for interaction between gradient magnetic fields and biological tissue is inherently dependent on the fundamental field frequency, maximum flux density, average flux density, presence of harmonic frequencies, waveform characteristics of the signal, polarity of the signal, current distribution in the body, and electrical properties and sensitivity of the particular cell membrane [97–99].

For animals and human subjects the induced current is proportional to the conductivity of the biological tissue and the rate of change of the magnetic flux density [98–101]. In theory, the largest current densities are produced in peripheral tissues (i.e., at the greatest radius) and diminish linearly towards the body's center [98–101]. The current density is enhanced at higher frequencies and magnetic flux densities and is further accentuated by a larger tissue radius with a greater tissue conductivity. Current paths are affected by differences in tissue types, such that tissues with low conductivity (e.g., adipose and bone) change the pattern of the induced current.

Bioeffects of induced currents can be due either to the power deposited by the induced currents (thermal effects) or to direct effects of the current (nonthermal effects). Thermal effects due to switched gradients used in MRI are negligible and are not believed to be clinically significant [96, 98, 99].

Possible nonthermal effects of induced currents are stimulation of nerve or muscle cells, induction of ventricular fibrillation, increased brain mannitol space, epileptogenic potential, stimulation of visual flash sensations, and bone healing [98–103]. The threshold currents required for nerve stimulation and ventricular fibrillation are known to be much higher than the estimated current densities that are induced under routine clinical MRI conditions [96–100].

The production of magnetophosphenes is considered to be one of the most sensitive physiological responses to gradient magnetic fields [96–99]. Magnetophosphenes are supposedly caused by electrical stimulation of the retina and are completely reversible with no associated health effects [96–99]. These have been elicited by current densities of roughly 17 $\mu A/cm^2$. In contrast to this level, the currents that are required for the induction of nerve action potentials are roughly 3000 $\mu A/cm^2$, and those required for ventricular fibrillation induction of healthy cardiac tissue are calculated to be 100–1000 $\mu A/cm^2$ [96]. Although there have been no reported cases of magnetophosphenes for fields of 1.95 T or less, magnetophosphenes have been reported in volunteers working in and around a 4.0-T research system [50]. In addition, a metallic taste and symptoms of vertigo seem also to be reproducible and associated with rapid motion within the static magnetic field of these 4.0-T systems [50].

Time-varying, extremely low-frequency magnetic fields have been demonstrated to be associated with multiple effects, including clustering and altered orientation of fibroblasts, as well as increased mitotic activity of fibroblast growth, altered DNA synthesis, and reduced fentanyl-induced anesthesia [49, 64, 99]. Possible effects in multiple other organisms, including humans, have also been mentioned [99]. While no studies have conclusively demonstrated carcinogenic effects from exposure to time-varying magnetic fields of various intensities and durations, several reports still suggest that an association between the two is plausible [104–106].

■ Bioeffects of Radiofrequency Electromagnetic Fields

General Bioeffects of Radiofrequency Electromagnetic Fields

RF radiation is capable of generating heat in tissues as a result of resistive losses. Therefore the main bioeffects associated with exposure to RF radiation are related to the thermogenic qualities of this electromagnetic field [96–99, 108–116]. Exposure to RF radiation may also cause athermal, field-specific alterations in biological systems that are produced without a significant increase in temperature [108–114]. This topic is somewhat controversial due to assertions concerning the role of electromagnetic fields in producing cancer and developmental abnormalities, along with the concomitant ramifications of such effects [108–114]. A report from the United States Environmental Protection Agency claimed that the existing evidence on this issue is sufficient to demonstrate a relationship between low-level electromagnetic field exposures and the development of cancer [106]. To date there have been no specific studies performed to study potential athermal bioeffects of MRI. Those interested in a thorough review of this topic, particularly as it pertains to MRI, are referred to the extensive article by Beers [113].

Regarding RF power deposition concerns, investigators have typically quantified exposure to RF radiation by means of determining the specific absorption rate (SAR) [108–112, 116–119]. SAR is the mass normalized rate at which RF power is coupled to biological tissue and is indicated in units of watts per kilogram. Measurements or estimates of SAR are not trivial, particularly in human subjects, and there are several methods of determining this parameter for RF energy dosimetry [108–112, 119].

The SAR that is produced during MRI is a complex function of numerous variables including the frequency (which, in turn, is determined by the strength of the static magnetic field), type of RF pulse (e.g., 90° or 180°), repetition time, pulse width, type of RF coil used, volume of tissue within the coil, resistivity of the tissue, configuration of the anatomical region imaged, as well as other factors [96–99]. The actual increase in tissue temperature caused by exposure to RF radiation is dependent on the subject's thermoregulatory system (e.g., skin blood flow, skin surface area, sweat rate) [97–99].

The efficiency and absorption pattern of RF energy are mainly determined by the physical dimensions of the tissue in relation to the incident wavelength [108–112]. Therefore, if the tissue size is large relative to the wavelength, energy is predominantly absorbed on the surface; if it is small relative to the wavelength, there is little absorption of RF power [108–112]. Because of the above relationship between RF energy and physical dimensions, studies designed to investigate the effects of exposure to RF radiation during MRI that are intended to be applicable to the clinical setting require tissue volumes and anatomical shapes comparable to that of human subjects. Of additional note is that there is no laboratory animal that sufficiently mimics or simulates the thermoregulatory system or responses of man. For these reasons, results obtained in laboratory animal experiments cannot simply be "scaled" or extrapolated to human subjects [110–112, 119].

MRI and Exposure to RF Radiation

Few quantitative data have been previously available on thermoregulatory responses of humans exposed to RF radiation prior to the studies performed with MRI. The few studies that existed did not directly apply to MRI because these investigations either examined thermal sensations or therapeutic applications of diathermy, usually involving only localized regions of the body [108–110, 114].

Several studies of RF power absorption during MRI have been performed recently and have yielded useful information about tissue heating in human subjects [28, 58–60, 62, 63, 65]. During

MRI tissue heating results primarily from magnetic induction with a negligible contribution from the electric fields, so that ohmic heating is greatest at the surface of the body and approaches zero at the center of the body. Predictive calculations and measurements obtained in phantoms and human subjects exposed to MRI supports this pattern of temperature distribution [58–60, 115, 116].

Although one paper reported significant temperature rises in internal organs produced by MRI [65], this study was conducted on anesthetized dogs and is unlikely to be applicable to conscious adult human subjects because of factors related to the physical dimensions and dissimilar thermoregulatory systems of these two species. However, these data may have important implications for the use of MRI in pediatric patients since this patient population is typically sedated or anesthetized for MRI examinations.

An investigation using fluoroptic thermometry probes that are unperturbed by electromagnetic fields [117] demonstrated that human subjects exposed to MRI at SAR levels up to 4.0 W/kg [i.e., ten times higher than the level currently recommended by the United States Food and Drug Administration FDA)] have no statistically significant increases in body temperatures and elevations in skin temperatures that are not believed to be clinically hazardous [62]. These results imply that the suggested exposure level of 0.4 W/kg for RF radiation during MRI is too conservative for individuals with normal thermoregulatory function [62]. Additional studies are needed, however, to assess physiological responses of patients with conditions that may impair thermoregulatory function (e.g., elderly patients; patients with underlying health conditions such as fever, diabetes, cardiovascular disease or obesity; and patients taking medications that affect thermoregulation such as calcium blockers, beta-blockers, diuretics, vasodilators, etc.) before subjecting them to MRI procedures that require high SARs.

Temperature Sensitive Organs

Certain human organs that have reduced capabilities for heat dissipation, such as the testis and eye, are particularly sensitive to elevated temperatures. Therefore these are primary sites of potential harmful effects if RF radiation exposures during MRI are excessive. Laboratory investigations have demonstrated detrimental effects on testicular function (e.g., a reduction or cessation of spermatogenesis, impaired sperm motility, degeneration of seminiferous tubules) caused by RF radiation-induced heating from exposures sufficient enough to raise scrotal and/or testicular tissue temperatures up to 38° to 42 °C [118].

Scrotal skin temperatures (i.e., an index of intratesticular temperature) were measured in volunteer subjects undergoing whole-body MRI averaged SAR of 1.1 W/kg [63]. The largest change in scrotal skin temperature was 2.1 °C, and the highest scrotal skin temperature recorded was 34.2 °C [63]. These temperature changes were below the threshold known to impair testicular function. However, excessively heating the scrotum during MRI could exacerbate certain preexisting disorders associated with increased scrotal/testicular temperatures (e.g., acute febrile illnesses, varicocele) in patients who are already oligospermic and lead to possible temporary or permanent sterility [63]. Therefore additional studies designed to investigate these issues are needed, particularly if patients are scanned at whole-body averaged SARs higher than those previously evaluated.

Dissipation of heat from the eye is a slow and inefficient process due to its relative lack of vascularization. Acute near-field exposures of RF radiation to the eyes or heads of laboratory animals have been demonstrated to be cataractogenic as a result of the thermal disruption of ocular tissues if the exposure is of a sufficient intensity and duration [108, 110]. An investigation conducted by Sacks et al. [53] revealed no discernable effects on the eyes of rats produced by MRI at exposures that far exceeded typical clinical imaging levels. However, it may not be acceptable to extrapolate these data to human subjects, considering the coupling of RF radiation to the anatomy and tissue volume of the laboratory rat eyes compared to those of man.

Corneal temperatures have been measured in patients undergoing MRI of the brain using a send/receive head coil at local SARs up to 3.1 W/kg [59]. The largest corneal temperature change was 1.8 °C and the highest temperature measured was 34.4 °C. Since the temperature threshold for RF radiation-induced cataractogenesis in animal models has been demonstrated to be between 41° to 55 °C for acute, near-field exposures, it does not appear that clinical MRI using a head coil has the potential to cause thermal damage in ocular tissue [59]. The effect of MRI at higher SARs and the long-term effects of MRI on ocular tissues remain to be determined.

RF Radiation and "Hot Spots"

Theoretically, RF radiation "hot spots" caused by an uneven distribution of RF power may arise whenever current concentrations are produced in association with restrictive conductive patterns. There has been the suggestion that RF radiation "hot spots" may generate thermal "hot spots" under certain conditions during MRI. Since RF radiation is mainly absorbed by peripheral tissues, thermography has been used to study the heating pattern associated with MRI at high whole-body SARs [57]. This study demonstrated no evidence of surface thermal "hot spots" related to MRI of human subjects. The thermoregulatory system apparently responds to the heat challenge by distributing the thermal load, producing a "smearing" effect of the surface temperatures. However, there is a possibility that internal thermal "hot spots" develop from MRI [59].

■ United States Food and Drug Administration Guidelines for MR Devices

In 1988 MR diagnostic devices were reclassified from class III, which requires premarket approval, to class II, which is regulated by performance standards, as long as the device(s) are within the "umbrella" of defined limits addressed below [107]. Subsequent to this reclassification new devices had only to demonstrate that they were "substantially equivalent" to any class II device that was brought to market using the premarket notification process (510 [k]) or, alternatively, to any of the devices described by the 13 MR system manufacturers that had petitioned the FDA for such a reclassification.

Four areas relating to the use of MR systems have been identified for which safety guidelines have been issued by the FDA. These include the static magnetic field, gradient magnetic fields, RF power of the examination, and acoustical considerations. Excerpts from the wording of the FDA Safety Parameter Action Levels are as follows [107]:

Static Magnetic Field. Static magnetic field strengths not exceeding 2.0 T are below the level of concern for the static magnetic field. Should the static magnetic field strength exceed 2.0 T, additional evidence of safety must be provided by the sponsor.

Gradient Magnetic Field. Limit patient exposure to time-varying magnetic fields with strengths less than those required to produce peripheral nerve stimulation or other effects. There are three alternatives:

- Demonstrate that the maximum dB/dt of the system is 6 T/s or less.
- Demonstrate that for axial gradients, dB/dt <20 T/s for p>120 ms, or dB/dt<(2400/p) T/s for 12 ms<p<120 ps, or dB/dt <200 T/s for p<12 ps (p equals the width in microseconds of a rectangular pulse or the half period of a sinusoidal dB/dt pulse). For transverse gradients, dB/dt is considered to be below the level of concern when it is less than three times the above limits for axial gradients.
- Demonstrate with valid scientific evidence that the rate of change of magnetic field for the system is not sufficient to cause peripheral nerve stimulation by an adequate margin of safety (at least a factor of three).

  The parameter dB/dt must be lower than that either of the two levels of concern by presentation of valid scientific measurement of calculational evidence sufficient to demonstrate that the time rate of magnetic field change (dB/dt) is of no concern.

RF Power Deposition. Options to control the risk of systemic thermal overload and local thermal injury caused by RF energy absorption are as follows:

- If the specific absorption rate is 0.4 W/kg or less for the whole body and 8.0 W/kg or less spatial peak in any 1 g of tissue, and if the specific absorption rate is 3.2 W/kg or less averaged over the head, it is below the level of concern.
- If exposure to RF magnetic fields is insufficient to produce a core temperature increase of 1 °C and localized heating to no greater than 38 °C in the head, 39 °C in the trunk, and 40 °C in the extremities, it is considered to be below the level of concern.

  The parameter RF heating must below either of the two levels of concern by presentation of valid scientific measurement or calculational evidence sufficient to demonstrate that RF heating effects are of no concern.

Acoustic Noise Levels. The acoustic noise levels associated with the device must be shown to be below the level of concern established by pertinent federal regulatory or other recognized standards-setting organizations. If the acoustic noise is not below the level of concern, the sponsor must recommend steps to reduce or alleviate the noise perceived by the patient [107].

■ MRI and Acoustic Noise

The acoustic noise produced during MRI represents a potential risk to patients. Acoustic noise is associated with the activation and deactivation of electrical current that induces vibrations of the gradient coils. This repetitive sound is enhanced by higher gradient duty cycles and sharper pulse transitions. Acoustic noise is thus likely to increase with decreases in section thicknesses, decreased fields of view, repetition times, and echo times.

Gradient magnetic field-related noise levels measured on several commercial MR scanners were in the range of 65–95 dB, which is considered to be within the recommended safety guidelines set forth by the FDA [107]. However, there have been reports that acoustic noise generated during MRI has caused patient annoyance, interference with oral communication, and reversible hearing loss in patients who did not wear ear protection [9, 120]. A study of patients undergoing MRI without earplugs resulted in temporary hearing loss in 43% of the subjects [9]. Furthermore, the possibility exists that significant gradient coil-induced noise may produce permanent hearing impairment in certain patients who are particularly susceptible to the damaging effects of relatively loud noises [9, 120].

The safest and least expensive means of preventing problems associated with acoustic noise during clinical MRI is to encourage the routine use of disposable earplugs [9, 120]. The use of hearing protection has been demonstrated to successfully avoid the potential temporary hearing loss that can be associated with clinical MRI examinations [9, 120]. MR-compatible headphones that significantly muffle acoustic noise are also commercially available.

An acceptable alternative strategy for reducing sound levels during MRI is to use an "antinoise" or destructive interference technique that not only effectively reduces noise but also permits better patient communication [122]. This technique consists of a real-time Fourier analysis of the noise emitted from the MR system [122]. A signal possessing the same physical characteristics but opposite phase than the sound generated by the MR system is produced. The two opposite-phase signals are then combined resulting in a cancellation of the repetitive noise, while allowing other sounds such as music and voice to be transmitted to the patient [122]. An investigation demonstrated no significant degradation of image quality when MRI is performed with MR systems that utilize this "antinoise" method [122]. While this technique has not yet found widespread clinical application, it has considerable potential for minimizing acoustic noise and its associated problems [123].

■ Investigations of MRI Safety and Bioeffects

Over the years there have been many investigations performed specifically to study the potential safety and bioeffects of MRI [1–83]. The results of these MRI-related bioeffects studies research have been predominantly negative, supporting the widely held view that there are no significant health risks associated with the use of this imaging modality. Experiments that yielded positive results either identified possible, nonspecific biological responses, determined short-term biological changes that were not considered to be deleterious, or found bioeffects that require further substantiation.

When perusing these studies, the reader should note that the dosimetric aspects of the exposure(s) to static, gradient, and/or RF electromagnetic fields are quite variable and include those that exceed clinical exposures, simulate clinical exposures, or involve low-level, chronic exposures. In certain cases the effects of only one of the electromagnetic fields used for MRI was evaluated. Theoretically there is a possibility that the combination of static, gradient, and RF electromagnetic fields may produce some unusual and/or unpredictable bioeffects that are unique to MRI.

"Window" effects are often present with respect to biological changes that occur in response to electromagnetic radiation. "Window" effects are those biological changes associated with a specific spectrum of electromagnetic radiation that are not observed at levels below or above this range [108, 119]. Both field strength and frequency "windows" have been reported in the literature [108, 119]. Virtually all of the experiments conducted to date on MRI biological effects have been performed at specific "windows" and the results cannot be assumed to apply to all of the various field strengths or frequencies used for clinical MRI.

A variety of different biological systems were also used for these experiments. As mentioned above, the coupling of electromagnetic radiation to biological tissues is highly dependent on organism/subject size, anatomical factors, duration of exposure, sensitivity of the involved tissues, and a myriad of other variables, and therefore studies performed on laboratory preparations may not be extrapolated or seen as directly applicable to human subjects nor for the clinical use of MRI. Therefore caution is advisable in interpreting the results of these studies.

■ Electrically, Magnetically, or Mechanically Activated Implants and Devices

The FDA requires labeling of MR systems to indicate that the device is contraindicated for patients who have electrically, magnetically, or mechanically activated implants because electromagnetic fields produced by the MR system may interfere with the operation of these devices [107]. Therefore patients with internal cardiac pacemakers, implantable cardiac defibrillators, cochlear implants, neurostimulators, bone-growth stimulators, implantable electronic drug infusion pumps, and similar devices that could be adversely effected by the electromagnetic fields used for MRI should not be examined by this imaging technique [120, 124–127]. Prior ex vivo testing of certain of these implants and devices may indicate that they are, in fact, MR safe.

The associated risks of scanning patients with cardiac pacemakers are related to the possibility of movement, reed switch closures or damage, programming changes, inhibition, or reversion to an asynchronous mode of operation, electromagnetic interference, and induced currents in lead wires [120, 124, 125, 127–130]. At least one patient with a pacemaker has been scanned by MRI without incident [126]. A letter-to-the editor indicated that a patient who was not pacemaker dependent underwent MRI by having his pacemaker "disabled" during the procedure [126]. Although this patient sustained no apparent discomfort, and the pacemaker was not damaged, it is inadvisable to perform this type of maneuver routinely on patients with pacemakers because of the potential to encounter the aforementioned hazards. Of note is the fact that there has been an MRI-related death of a patient with a pacemaker [99].

Of particular concern is the possibility that the pacemaker lead wire(s) or other similar intracardiac wire configuration could act as an antenna in which the gradient and/or RF electromagnetic fields may induce sufficient current to cause fibrillation, a burn, or other potentially dangerous event [99, 120, 124, 125, 125]. Because of this theoretically deleterious and unpredicted effect, patients referred to MRI with residual external pacing wires, temporary pacing wires, Swan-Ganz thermodilution catheters, and/or any other type of internally or externally positioned conductive wire or similar device should not undergo MRI because of the possible associated risks [99, 120, 131].

Some types of cochlear implants employ a relatively high-field strength cobalt samarium magnet used in conjunction with an external magnet to align and retain a RF transmitter coil on the patient's head, while other types of cochlear implants are electronically activated [132]. Consequently MRI is strictly contraindicated in patients with these implants because of the possibility of injuring the patient and/or damaging or altering the operation of the cochlear implant [133, 134].

Because there is a potential for demagnetizing implants that involve magnets (e.g., dental implants, magnetic sphincters, magnetic stoma plugs, magnetic ocular implants, and similar devices) that may necessitate surgery to replace the damaged implant, these implants should be removed from the patient prior to MRI, if possible [132, 135, 136]. Otherwise MRI should not be performed on a patient with a magnetically activated implant or device. A patient with any other similar electrically, magnetically, or mechanically activated implant or device should be excluded from examination by MRI unless the particular implant or device has been previously demonstrated to be unaffected by the magnetic and electromagnetic fields used for MRI [120].

■ Patients with Metallic Implants, Materials, and Foreign Bodies

MRI is contraindicated for patients that have certain ferromagnetic implants, materials, or foreign bodies, primarily due to the possibility of movement or dislodgment of these objects [97–99]. Other problems may also occur in patients with ferromagnetic implants, materials, or foreign bodies that undergo MRI including the induction of electrical current in the object, excessive heating of the object, and the misinterpretation of an artifact produced by the presence of the object as an abnormality [97, 99, 137–141]. These potentially hazardous situations, however, are infrequent or are insignificant in comparison with movement or dislodgment of a ferromagnetic implant or foreign body by the magnetic fields of the MR system.

Numerous investigations have evaluated the ferromagnetic qualities of a variety of metallic implants, materials, or foreign bodies by measuring deflection forces or movements associated with the static magnetic fields used by MRI [140, 142–160]. These studies were conducted to determine the relative risk of performing MRI on a patient with a metallic object with respect to whether the magnetic attraction was strong enough to produce movement or dislodgment.

A variety of factors require evaluation when establishing the relative risk of performing an MR procedure in a patient with a ferromagnetic implant, material, device, or foreign body, such as: the strength of the static and gradient magnetic fields, relative degree of ferromagnetism of the object, mass of the object, geometry of the object, location and orientation of the object in situ, and length of time that the object has been in place [98, 99]. Each of these should be considered before allowing a patient that has a ferromagnetic object to enter the electromagnetic environment of the MR system.

While it may be acceptable to perform MRI using an open-field MR system in a patients with certain bioimplants or devices that are unsafe when using a high field strength MR system, to date this has not been documented (the exception is a patient undergoing an MR procedure using a dedicated extremity MR system (Artoscan, Esaote, Milan, Italy) for which preliminary tests have indicated that it is safe for patients to undergo procedures with ferromagnetic aneurysm clips, cardiac pacemakers, and implantable cardiac defibrillators). Therefore the information contained below pertains to all patients without regard to the specific type of MR system being used for the examination.

Aneurysm and Hemostatic Clips. Of the various aneurysm and vascular clips studied and reported in the literature, many of the aneurysm clips and none of the vascular clips were found to be ferromagnetic [161]. Therefore only patients that definitely have nonferromagnetic aneurysm clips should be exposed to the magnetic fields used for MRI, while any patient with one of the previously tested hemostatic clips may safely undergo MRI.

Carotid Artery Vascular Clamps. Each of the carotid artery vascular clamps evaluated for ferromagnetism exhibited deflection forces. However, only the Poppen-Blaylock clamp was considered to be contraindicated for patients undergoing MRI because of the significant ferromagnetism shown by this object. The other carotid artery vascular clamps are believed to be safe for MRI because of the minimal deflection forces relative to their use in an in vivo application (i.e., the deflection forces are insignificant, and therefore there is little possibility of significant movement or dislodgment of the implant).

Dental Devices and Materials. Various dental devices and materials have been tested for ferromagnetism. While many of them demonstrated deflection forces, only a few of these pose a possible risk to patients undergoing MRI because they are magnetically activated devices.

Heart Valves. Many of the commercially available heart valve prostheses have been tested for ferromagnetism. The majority of these displayed measurable deflection forces; however, the deflection forces were relatively insignificant compared with the force exerted by the beating heart. Therefore patients with these heart valve prostheses may safely undergo MRI.

Intravascular Coils, Filters, and Stents. Less than half of the different intravascular coils, filters, and stents tested were ferromagnetic [152, 159, 162]. These ferromagnetic devices are usually attached firmly into the vessel wall after approximately four to six weeks following introduction [159]. Therefore it is unlikely that any of them would become dislodged by attraction from magnetic forces presently used for MRI. Patients with intravascular coils, filters, or stents in which there is a possibility that the device is not properly positioned or held firmly in place should not undergo MRI.

Ocular Implants. Various ocular implants have been evaluated for ferromagnetism [163]. Of these, the Fatio eyelid spring and retinal tack made from martensitic stainless steel displayed measurable deflection forces. While it is unlikely that the associated deflection forces would cause movement or dislodgment of these implants, it is possible that a patient with one of these implants would be uncomfortable or sustain a minor injury during MRI.

Orthopedic Implants, Materials, and Devices. Most orthopedic implants, materials, and devices tested for ferromagnetism have been demonstrated to be made from nonferromagnetic materials. Therefore patients with these particular orthopedic implants, materials, and devices may be imaged safely by MRI. The Perfix interference screw used for reconstruction of the anterior cruciate ligament, while composed of ferromagnetic material, does not pose a hazard to the patient undergoing MRI because of the significant force that holds it in place in vivo. However, the resulting imaging artifact precludes diagnostic assessment of the knee using MRI.

Otological Implants. The cochlear implants evaluated for ferromagnetism are considered to be contraindicated for MRI. In addition to being attracted by static magnetic fields, these implants are also electronically and/or magnetically activated. Only one of the remaining tested otological implants has associated deflection forces [164]. This implant, the McGee stapedectomy piston prosthesis composed of platinum and ^{17}Cr-^{4}Ni stainless steel was made on a limited basis during the middle of 1987 and was recalled by the manufacturer. Patients with this otological implant were issued warning cards that instruct them to not be examined by MRI.

Pellets, Bullets, Shrapnel, etc. Most of the pellets and bullets previously tested for ferromagnetism are composed of nonferromagnetic materials [150, 152]. Ammunition found to be ferromagnetic typically came from foreign countries and/or was used by the military. Shrapnel usually contains various amounts of steel and therefore presents a potential hazard for MRI. Furthermore, since pellets, bullets, and shrapnel may be contaminated with ferromagnetic materials, these objects represent relative contraindications for MRI. Patients with these foreign bodies should be regarded on an individual basis with respect to whether the object is positioned near a vital neural, vascular, or soft tissue structure. This may be assessed by taking a careful history and using plain film radiography to determine the location of the foreign body.

Penile Implants and Artificial Sphincters. One of the penile implants tested for ferromagnetism displayed significant deflection forces. Although it is unlikely that this implant, the Dacomed Omniphase, would cause serious injury to a patient undergoing MRI, it would undoubtedly be uncomfortable for the patient. Therefore, this implant is regarded as a relative contraindication for MRI. Artificial sphincters that have been tested are made from nonferromagnetic materials. However, at least one artificial sphincter currently undergoing clinical trials has a magnetic component and, therefore, patients with this device should not undergo MRI.

Vascular Access Ports. Of the various vascular access ports tested for ferromagnetism, two showed measurable deflection forces, but the forces were felt to be insignificant relative to the in vivo application of these implants [149]. Therefore, it is considered safe to perform MRI in a patient that may have one of these previously tested vascular access ports. The exception to this is any vascular access port that is "programmable" or electronically activated. Patients with this type of vascular access port should not undergo MRI.

Miscellaneous. Various types of other metallic implants, materials, and foreign bodies have also been tested for ferromagnetism. Of these, the cerebral ventricular shunt tube connector (type unknown) and tissue expander which is magnetically activated exhibited deflection forces that may pose a risk to patients during MRI. An "O-ring" washer used as a vascular marker also showed ferromagnetism, but the deflection force was determined to be minimal relative to the in vivo use of this device.

Each of the contraceptive diaphragms tested for ferromagnetism displayed significant deflection forces. However, we have performed MRI on patients with these devices who did not complain of any sensation related to movement of these objects. Therefore, scanning patients with diaphragms is not believed to be considered to be physically hazardous to patients.

According to the Policies, Guidelines, and Recommendations for MR Imaging Safety and Patient Management information issued by the Society for Magnetic Resonance Imaging Safety Committee [120], patients with electrically, magnetically, or mechanically activated, or electrically conductive devices should be excluded from MRI unless the particular device has been previously shown (i.e., usually by ex vivo testing procedures) to be unaffected by the electromagnetic fields used for clinical MRI and there is no possibility of injuring the patient. During the screening process for MRI, patients with these objects should be identified before their examination and prior to being exposed to the electromagnetic fields used for this imaging technique. There are implants, materials, devices, or other foreign bodies that have yet to be evaluated for MRI compatibility which may be encountered in the clinical setting. Patients that have untested objects should not be allowed to undergo MRI.

■ Screening Patients with Metallic Foreign Bodies

Patients may present to MRI with a history of metallic foreign bodies such as slivers, bullets, shrapnel, or other types of metallic fragments. The relative risk of scanning these patients is dependent upon the ferromagnetic properties of the object, the geometry and dimensions of the object, and the strength of the static and gradient magnetic fields of the MR system. Also important is the strength with which the object is fixed within the tissue and whether or not it is positioned in or adjacent to a potentially hazardous site of the body such as a vital neural, vascular, or soft tissue structure.

A patient that encounters the static magnetic field of an MR system with an intraocular metallic foreign body is at a particular risk for significant eye injury. The single reported case of a patient that experienced a vitreous hemorrhage resulting in blindness, underwent MRI on a 0.35-T scanner and had an occult intraocular metal fragment that was 2.0×3.5 mm in size dislodge during the procedure [165]. This incident emphasizes the importance of adequately screening patients with suspected intraocular metallic foreign bodies prior to MRI.

Research has demonstrated that small intraocular metallic fragments as small as 0.1×0.1×0.1 mm in size are detected using standard plain film radiographs [166]. Although thin slice (i.e., <3 mm) computed tomography has been demonstrated to detect metallic foreign bodies in size down to approximately 0.15 mm, it is unlikely that a metallic fragment of this size would be dislodged during MR imaging, even with a static magnetic field up to 2.0 T [166]. Metallic fragments of various sizes and dimensions ranging from 0.1×0.1×0.1 mm to 3.0×1.0×1.0 mm in size have been examined to determine if they were moved or dislodged from the eyes of laboratory animals during exposure to a 2.0-T MRI system [166]. Only the largest fragment (3.0×1.0×1.0 mm) rotated, but did not cause any discernable damage to the ocular tissue [166]. Therefore, the use of plain film radiography may be an acceptable technique for identifying or excluding an intraocular metallic foreign body that represents a potential hazard to the patient undergoing MRI [120]. Patients with a high suspicion of having an intraocular metallic foreign body (for example, a metal worker exposed to metallic slivers with a history of an eye injury) should have plain film radiographs of the orbits to rule-out the presence of a metallic fragment prior to exposure to the static magnetic field. If a patient with a suspected ferromagnetic intraocular foreign body has no symptoms and plain film series of the orbits does not demonstrate a radiopaque foreign body, the risk of performing MRI is minimal [120].

Using plain film radiography to search for metallic foreign bodies is a sensitive and relatively inexpensive means of identifying patients who are unsuitable for MRI and can also be utilized to screen out patients who may have metal fragments in other potentially hazardous sites of the body [120].

Each MRI site should establish a standardized policy for screening patients with suspected foreign bodies. The policy should include guidelines as to which patients require work-up by radiographic procedures, the specific procedure to be performed (e.g., number and type of views, position of the anatomy), and each case should be considered on an individual basis. These precautions should be taken with regard to patients referred to MRI in any type of MR system regardless of the field strength, magnet type, and the presence or absence of magnetic shielding [120].

■ Performing MRI During Pregnancy

While MRI is not believed to be hazardous to the fetus, only a few investigations have examined the teratogenic potential of this imaging modality. By comparison, literally thousands of studies have been performed to examine the possible hazards of ultrasound during pregnancy, and controversy still exists concerning the safe use of this nonionizing-radiation imaging technique.

Most of the earliest studies conducted to determine possible unwanted bioeffects during pregnancy showed negative results [17, 22, 26, 31, 41, 47, 82]. More recently one study examined the effects of MRI on mice exposed during mid-gestation [22]. No gross embryotoxic effects were observed, however, there was a reduction in crown-rump length [22]. In another study performed by Tyndall and Sulik [74], exposure to the electromagnetic fields used for a simulated clinical MRI examination caused eye malformations in a genetically prone mouse strain. Therefore, it appears that the electromagnetic fields used for MRI have the ability to produce developmental abnormalities.

A variety of mechanisms exist that could produce deleterious bioeffects with respect to the developing fetus and the use of electromagnetic fields during MRI [86, 88, 89, 102, 108, 109, 118]. In addition, it is well-known that cells undergoing division, as in the case of the developing fetus during the first trimester, are highly susceptible to damage from different types of physical agents. Therefore, because of the limited data available at the present time, a cautionary approach is recommended for the use of MRI in pregnant patients.

The current guidelines of the FDA requires labeling of MRI devices to indicate that the safety of MRI when used to image the fetus and the infant "has not been established" [107]. In the United Kingdom the acceptable limits of exposure for clinical MRI recommended by the National Radiological Protection Board in 1983 specify that "it might be prudent to exclude pregnant women during the first three months of pregnancy" [108].

According to the Safety Committee of the Society for Magnetic Resonance Imaging [120] (this information has also been adopted recently by the American College of Radiology), MRI is indicated for use in pregnant women if other nonionizing forms of diagnostic imaging are inadequate or if the examination provides important information that would otherwise require exposure to ionizing radiation (e.g., X-ray, CT). For pregnant patients it is recommended to inform them that to date there has been no indication that the use of clinical MRI during pregnancy has produced deleterious effects. However, as noted by the FDA, the safety of MRI during pregnancy has not been proved [107].

Patients who are pregnant or suspect they are pregnant must be identified prior to undergoing MRI in order to assess the risks versus the benefits of the examination. Since there is a high spontaneous abortion rate in the general population during the first trimester of pregnancy (i.e., >30%), particular care should be exercised with the use of MRI during the first trimester because of associated potential medicolegal implications relative to spontaneous abortions.

■ MRI and Claustrophobia, Anxiety, and Panic Disorders

Claustrophobia and a variety of other psychological reactions including anxiety and panic disorders may be encountered by as many as 5%–10% of patients undergoing MR imaging. These sensations originate from several factors, including the restrictive dimensions of the interior of the scanner, the duration of the examination, the gradient-induced noises, the ambient conditions within the bore of the scanner [167–175]. It should be noted that there has been no prior comparison the incidence of claustrophobia in patients undergoing MR procedures in open-field MR systems versus conventional-design MR systems to substantiate that a more open-configuration improves patient tolerance.

Fortunately, adverse psychological responses to MRI are usually transient. However, there has been a report of two patients with no prior history of claustrophobia who tolerated MRI with great difficulty and had persistent claustrophobia that required long-term psychiatric treatment [168]. Since adverse psychological responses to MRI typically delay or require cancellation of the examination, several techniques have been developed and may be used to avert these problems [120, 167–176]. These include the following:

1. Brief the patient concerning the specific aspects of the MRI examination including the level of gradient-induced noise to expect, the internal dimensions of the scanner, and the length of the examination, etc.
2. Allow an appropriately screened relative or friend to remain with the patient during the procedure.
3. Use headphones with calming music to decrease the repetitive noise created by the gradient coils.
4. Maintain physical or verbal contact with the patient throughout the examination.
5. Place the patient in a prone position with the chin supported by a pillow. In this position, the patient is able to visualize the opening of the bore and thus alleviate the "closed-in" feeling. An alternative method to reduce claustrophobia is to place the subject feet-first instead of head first into the scanner.
6. Use scanner-mounted mirrors, mirror or prism glasses within the scanner allows the patient to see out the scanner.
7. Use a large light at either end of the scanner to decrease the anxiety of being in a long dark enclosure.
8. Use a blindfold on the patient so that he/she is unaware of the close surroundings.
9. Use relaxation techniques such as controlled breathing and mental imagery. Also, several case reports have shown hypnotherapy to be successful in reducing MRI related claustrophobia and anxiety.
10. Use psychological "desensitization" techniques prior to the MRI examination.

Several investigators have recently attempted to compare the effectiveness of some of the above mentioned techniques in reducing MRI induced anxiety and/or claustrophobia [169, 170, 173]. One such study demonstrated that providing detailed information about the MRI procedure in addition to "relaxation exercises" successfully reduced the anxiety level of a group of patients both before and during MRI. A similar anxiety reduction could not be shown in patients provided with only information or "stress reduction" counseling. Relaxation methods have also been shown to significantly decrease anxiety during other medical procedures.

Monitoring Patients During MRI

Because the typical MR system is constructed such that the patient is placed inside a cylindrical structure, routine observations and vital signs monitoring is not a trivial task. Conventional monitoring equipment was not designed to operate in the MRI environment where static, gradient, and RF electromagnetic fields can adversely affect the operation of these devices. Fortunately, MR-safe monitors have been developed and are commonly used in in-patient and out-patient MRI centers [177–186].

Physiological monitoring is required for the safe utilization of MRI in patients who are sedated, anesthetized, comatose, critically ill or unable to communicate with the MR system operator. All of the above categories of patients should be routinely monitored during MRI and, considering the current availability of MRI-safe monitors, there is no reason to exclude these types of patients from MRI. Every physiological parameter that can be obtained under normal circumstances in the intensive care unit or operating room can be monitored during MRI, including heart rate, systemic blood pressure, intracardiac pressure, end-tidal carbon dioxide, oxygen saturation, respiratory rate, skin blood flow, and temperature [178–185]. In addition, there are now MR-safe ventilators for patients who require ventilatory support.

Monitors that contain ferromagnetic components (e.g., transformers, outer casings) can be strongly attracted by middle- and high-field MR systems, posing a serious hazard to patients and possible damage to the MR system. Since the intensity of standard static magnetic field falls off as the third power of the distance from the magnet, simply placing the monitor a suitable distance from the MR system is sufficient to protect the operation of the device and to help prevent it from becoming a potential projectile [182, 185]. If monitoring equipment is not placed in a permanently fixed position, instructions should be given to all appropriate personnel regarding the hazards of moving this equipment too close to the MR system [182, 185].

In addition to being influenced by the static magnetic field, monitors may be adversely affected by electromagnetic interference from the gradient and RF pulses from the MR system [182, 185]. In these instances increasing the length of the patient-monitor interface and positioning the equipment outside the RF-shielded room (e.g., the control room) enables the monitor to operate properly. It is usually necessary to position all monitors with cathode ray tubes at a location in the magnetic fringe field such that the display is not "bent" or distorted.

Certain monitors emit spurious electromagnetic noise that can result in moderate to severe imaging artifacts [182, 185]. These monitors can be modified to work during MRI by adding RF-shielded cables, using fiber-optic transmission of the signals (which is becoming increasingly the method of choice in the MRI environment), or using special outer casing. Also, special filters may be added to the monitor to inhibit electromagnetic noise.

Of further concern is the fact that some monitoring equipment can be potentially harmful to patients if special precautions are not followed [182, 182, 185, 187–189]. A primary source of adverse MR system and physiological monitor interactions has been the interface that is used between the patient and the equipment because this usually requires a conductive cable or other device. The presence of a conductive material in the immediate MR system area is a safety concern because of the potential for monitor-related burns. For example, there has been a report of an unfortunate accident involving an anesthetized patient who sustained a third-degree burn of the finger associated with using a pulse oximeter during MRI [188]. Investigation of this incident revealed that the cable leading from the pulse oximeter to the finger probe may have been looped during MRI and the gradient and/or RF magnetic fields induced sufficient current to exorbitantly heat the finger probe, resulting in the finger burn [188]. This problem may also occur with the use of electrocardiographic lead wires or any other cable that may be looped or form a conductive loop that contact the patient.

Therefore, the following is recommended to prevent potential monitor-related accidents from occurring:

1. Monitoring equipment should only be utilized by trained personal.
2. All cables and lead wires from monitoring devices that come into contact with the patient (e.g., the monitor-patient interface) should be positioned so that no conductive loops are formed.
3. Monitoring devices that do not appear to operate properly during MRI should be immediately removed from the patient and the magnetic environment.

The following is a brief description of some of the techniques of monitoring various physiological parameters:

Monitoring Blood Pressure

Noninvasive blood-pressure monitors typically utilize the oscillometric technique for measuring blood pressure, using a pressure transducer connected to a pressure cuff via a pneumatically filled hose. Certain monitors (e.g., Omega 1400, In-vivo Research Laboratories, Broken Arrow, OK) have adjustable audible and visual alarms and a strip-chart recorder. Occasionally, the cuff inflation tends to disturb lightly sedated patients, especially pediatric patients, which may cause them to move and distort the MR image. For this reason, the noninvasive blood-pressure monitor may not represent the optimal instrument for obtaining vital signs in all patient groups. Direct pressure monitoring of systemic and/or intracardiac pressures, if necessary, can be accomplished using a fiber-optic pressure transducer made entirely of plastic.

Monitoring Respiratory Rate, Oxygenation, and Gas Exchange

Monitoring of respiratory parameters during MRI of sedated or anesthetized patients is particularly important because the medications used for these procedures may produce complications of respiratory depression. Therefore, as a standard of care, a pulse oximeter, capnograph, or capnometer should always be used to monitor patients who are sedated or anesthetized during MRI.

The respiratory monitors utilized successfully on sedated pediatric or adult patients (e.g., the model 515 Respiration Monitor and model 8800 Capnometer, Biochem International, Waukesha, Wisconsin) are relatively inexpensive and can be modified for use during MR imaging by simply lengthening the plastic tubing interface to the patient so that the monitors can be placed at least 8 feet from the unshielded MR imager.

Pulse oximeters are used to record oxygen saturation and heart rate. Commercially available, modified pulse oximeters using hard wire cables have been previously used to monitor sedated and anesthetized patients during the MRI study and the recovery period with moderate success. These pulse oximeters tend to work intermittently during MRI due to interference from the gradient and/or RF electromagnetic fields. In certain instances, patients have been burned, presumably as a result of excessive current being induced in inappropriately looped conductive cables attached to the patient probes of the pulse oximeters [187–189].

Portable fiber-optic pulse oximeters are available for use during MR procedures [190]. Using fiber-optic technology to obtain and transmit physiological signals from patients undergoing MRI has been demonstrated to be a technique that does not have any associated MRI-related electromagnetic interference. It is physically impossible for a patient to be burned using this fiber-optic monitor during MRI because there are no conductive pathways formed by any metallic materials.

Monitoring Cutaneous Blood Flow

Cutaneous blood flow can be monitored during MRI by means of the laser-Doppler velocimetry technique. This noninvasive measurement technique uses laser light that is delivered to and detected from the region of interest by flexible, graded-index fiber-optic light wires. The Doppler-broadening of laser light scattered by moving red blood cells within the tissue is analyzed in real time by an analogue processor that is indicative of instantaneous blood velocity and the effective blood volume and flow. A small circular probe can be attached to any available skin surface of the patient. Areas with a relatively high cutaneous blood flow (such as the hand, finger, foot, toe, or ear) yield the best results.

Hard-copy tracings obtained by laser-Doppler velocimetry can be used to determine the patient's heart rate, respiratory rate and cutaneous blood flow. An audible signal may be activated to permit the operator to hear blood flow changes during monitoring. This technique of continuous physiological monitoring is particularly useful when there is concern about disturbing a sedated patient because it is easily tolerated.

Monitoring Heart Rate

Monitoring the electrocardiogram during MRI is typically required for cardiac imaging, gating to reduce imaging artifacts from the physiological motion of cerebral spinal fluid in the brain and spine, and for determining the patient's heart rate. Artifacts caused by the static, gradient, and RF electromagnetic fields may severely distort the morphology of the electrocardiogram, making determination of cardiac rhythm during MRI extremely difficult and unreliable. Although sophisticated filtering techniques can be used to attenuate the artifacts from the gradient and RF fields, the static magnetic field produces an augmentation of the T-wave, as previously mentioned, and other nonspecific waveform changes that are in direct proportion to the strength of the field, which cannot be easily counterbalanced.

In some instances, static magnetic field-induced augmented T waves have a higher amplitude than the R waves, resulting in false triggering and an inaccurate determination of the beats per minute. Electrocardiogram artifacts can be minimized during MRI by the following: using special filters, using electrocardiogram electrodes with minimal metal, selecting lead wires with minimal metal, twisting or braiding the lead wires, and using special lead placements [184].

The previously mentioned pulse oximeters may also be used accurately to record heart rate during MRI examinations. These devices have probes that may be attached to the finger, toe, or ear lobe of the patient.

References

1. Adzamli IK, Jolesz FA, Blau M (1989) An assessment of blood-brain barrier integrity under MRI conditions: brain uptake of radiolabeled Gd-DTPA and In-DTPA-IgG. J Nucl Med 30:839
2. Barber BJ, Schaefer DJ, Gordon CJ et al (1990) Thermal effects of MR imaging: worst-case studies in sheep. Am J Roentgenol 155:1105–1110
3. Bartels MV, Mann K, Matejcek M et al (1986) Magnetresonanztomographie und Sicherheit: elektroenzephalographische und neuropsychologische Befunde vor und nach MR-Untersuchungen des Gehirns. Fortschr Rontgenstr 145 (4):383–385
4. Besson J, Foreman EI, Eastwood LM et al (1984) Cognitive evaluation following NMR imaging of the brain. J Neurol Neurosurg Psychiatry 47:314–316
5. Bore PJ, Galloway GJ, Styles P et al (1986) Are quenches dangerous? Magn Reson Imaging 3:112–117
6. Bourland JD, Nyenhuis JA, Mouchawar GA et al (1990) Physiologic indicators of high MRI gradient-induced fields. In: Book of abstracts. Society of Magnetic Resonance in Medicine, p 1276
7. Brody AS, Sorette MP, Gooding CA et al (1985) Induced alignment of flowing sickle erythrocytes in a magnetic field. A preliminary report. Invest Radiol 20:560–566
8. Brody AS, Embury SH, Mentzer WC et al (1988) Preservation of sickle cell blood flow patterns during MR imaging. An in vivo study. Am J Roentgenol 151:139–141
9. Brummett RE, Talbot JM, Charuhas P (1988) Potential hearing loss resulting from MR imaging. Radiology 169:539–540
10. Budinger TF, Fischer H, Hentschel D et al (1991) Physiological effects of fast oscillating magnetic field gradients. J Comput Assist Tomogr 15:909–914
11. Carson JJL, Prato FS, Drost DJ et al (1990) Time-varying fields increase cytosolic free Ca2+ in HL-60 cells. Am J Physiol 259:C687–C692
12. Cohen MS, Weisskoff R, Rzedzian R et al (1990) Sensory stimulation by time-varying magnetic fields. Magn Reson Med 14:409–414
13. Cooke P, Morris PG (1981) The effects of NMR exposure on living organisms. II. A genetic study of human lymphocytes. Br J Radiol 54:622–625
14. Doherty JU, Whitman GJR, Robinson MD et al (1985) Changes in cardiac excitability and vulnerability in NMR fields. Invest Radiol 20 (2):129–135
15. Fischer H (1989) Physiological effects of fast oscillating magnetic field gradients. Radiology 173:(P)382
16. Garber HJ, Oldendorf WH, Braun LD et al (1989) MRI gradient fields increase brain mannitol space. Magn Reson Imaging 7:605–610
17. Geard CR, Osmak RS, Hall EJ et al (1984) Magnetic resonance and ionizing radiation: a comparative evaluation in vitro of oncongenic and genotoxic potential. Radiology 152:199–202
18. Gore JC, McDonnell MJ, Pennock JM et al (1982) An assessment of the safety of rapidly changing magnetic fields in the rabbit: implications for NMR imaging. Magn Reson Imaging 1:191–195
19. Gremmel H, Wendhausen H, Wunsch F (1983) Biologische Effekte statischer Magnetfelder bei NMR-Tomographie am Menschen. Wissenschaftliche radiologische Klinik, Christian-Albrechts-University, Kiel
20. Gulch RW, Lutz O (1986) Influence of strong static magnetic fields on heart muscle contraction. Phys Med Biol 31 (7):763–769
21. Hammer BE, Wadon S, Mirer SD et al (1991) In vivo measurement of RF heating in Capuchin monkey brain. In: Book of abstracts. Society of Magnetic Resonance in Medicine, p 1278
22. Heinrichs WL, Fong P, Flannery M et al (1988) Midgestational exposure of pregnant balb/c mice to magnetic resonance imaging. Magn Reson Imaging 6:305–313
23. Hong CZ, Shellock FG (1989) Short-term exposure to a 1.5 Tesla static magnetic field does not effect somatosensory evoked potentials in man. Magn Reson Imaging 8:65–69
24. Innis NK, Ossenkopp KP, Prato FS et al (1986) Behavioral effects of exposure to nuclear magnetic resonance imaging: II. Spatial memory tests. Magn Reson Imaging 4:281–284
25. Jehenson P, Duboc D, Lavergne T et al (1988) Change in human cardiac rhythm by a 2 Tesla static magnetic field. Radiology 166:227–230
26. Kay HH, Herfkens RJ, Kay BK (1988) Effect of magnetic resonance imaging on Xenopus Laevis embryogenesis. Magn Reson Imaging 6:501–506
27. Keltner JR, Roos MS, Brakeman PR et al (1990) Magnetohydrodynamics of blood flow. Magn Reson Med 16:139–149
28. Kido DK, Morris TW, Erickson JL et al (1987) Physiologic changes during high field strength MR imaging. Am J Neuroradiol 8:263–266
29. LaPorte R, Kus L, Wisniewski RA et al (1990) Magnetic resonance imaging (MRI) effects on rat pineal neuroendocrine function. Brain Res 506:294–296
30. McRobbie D, Foster MA (1985) Cardiac response to pulsed magnetic fields with regard to safety in NMR imaging. Phys Med Biol 30:695–702
31. McRobbie D, Foster MA (1985) Pulsed magnetic field exposure during pregnancy and implications for NMR foetal imaging: a study with mice. Magn Reson Imaging 3:231–234
32. Messmer JM, Porter JH, Fatouros P et al (1987) Exposure to magnetic resonance imaging does not produce taste aversion in rats. Physiol Behav 40:259–261
33. Montour JL, Fatouros PP, Prasad UR (1988) Effect of MR imaging on spleen colony formation following gamma radiation. Radiology 168:259–260
34. Muller S, Hotz M (1990) Human brainstem auditory evoked potentials (BAEP) before and after MR examinations. Magn Reson Med 16:476–480
35. Niemann G, Schroth G, Klose U et al (1988) Influence of magnetic resonance imaging on somatosensory potential in man. J Neurol 235:462–465
36. Ngo FQH, Blue JW, Roberts WK (1987) The effects of a static magnetic field on DNA synthesis and survival of mammalian cells irradiated with fast neutrons. Magn Reson Med 5:307–317
37. Osbakken M, Griffith J, Taczanowsky P (1986) A gross morphologic, histologic, hematologic, and blood chemistry study of adult and neonatal mice chronically ex-

posed to high magnetic fields. Magn Reson Med 3:502–517
38. Ossenkopp KP, Kavaliers M, Prato FS et al (1985) Exposure to nuclear magnetic imaging procedure attenuates morphine-induced analgesia in mice. Life Sci 37:1507–1514
39. Ossenkopp KP, Innis NK, Prato FS et al (1986) Behavioral effects of exposure to nuclear magnetic resonance imaging. I. Open-field behavior and passive avoidance learning in rats. Magn Reson Imaging 4:275–280
40. Papatheofanis FJ, Papthefanis BJ (1989) Short-term effect of exposure to intense magnetic fields on hematologic indices of bone metabolism. Invest Radiol 24:221–223
41. Peeling J, Lewis JS, Samoiloff MR et al (1988) Biological effects of magnetic fields on the nemtode Panagrellus redivivus. Magn Reson Imaging 6:655–660
42. Prasad N, Kosnik LT, Taber KH et al (1990) Delayed tumor onset following MR imaging exposure. In: Book of abstracts. Society of Magnetic Resonance in Medicine, p 275
43. Prasad N, Prasad R, Bushong SC et al (1990) Effects of 4.5 T MRI exposure on mouse testes and epididymes. In: Book of abstracts. Society of Magnetic Resonance in Medicine, p 606
44. Prasad N, Bushong SC, Thornby JI et al (1984) Effect of nuclear resonance on chromosomes of mouse bone marrow cells. Magn Reson Imaging 2:37–39
45. Prasad N, Lotzova E, Thornby JI et al (1987) Effects of MR imaging on murine natural killer cell cytotoxicity. Am J Roentgenol 148:415–417
46. Prasad N, Lotzova E, Thornby JI et al (1990) The effect of 2.35-T MR imaging on natural killer cell cytotoxicity with and without interleukin-2. Radiology 175:251–263
47. Prasad N, Wright DA, Ford JJ et al (1990) Safety of 4-T MR imaging: a study of effects of developing frog embryos. Radiology 174:251–253
48. Prasad N, Wright DA, Forster JD (1982) Effect of nuclear magnetic resonance on early stages of amphibian development. Magn Reson Imaging 1:35–38
49. Prato FS, Ossenkopp KP, Kavaliers M et al (1987) Attenuation of morphine-induced analgesia in mice by exposure to magnetic resoance imaging: Seperate effects of the static, radiofrequency and time-varying magnetic fields. Magn Reson Imaging 5:9–14
50. Redington RW, Dumoulin CL, Schenck JL et al (1988) MR imaging and bio-effects in a whole body 4.0 Tesla imaging system. In: Book of abstracts, vol 1. Society of Magnetic Resonance Imaging, p 20
51. Reid A, Smith FW, Hutchison JMS (1982) Nuclear magnetic resonance imaging and its safety implications: follow-up of 181 patients. Br J Radiol 55:784–786
52. Roschmann P (1991) Human auditory system response to pulsed radiofrequency energy in RF coils for magnetic resonance at 2.4 to 170 MHz. Magn Reson Med 21:197–215
53. Sacks E, Worgul BV, Merriam GR et al (1986) The effects of nuclear magnetic resonance imaging on ocular tissues. Arch Ophthalmol 104:890–893
54. Schwartz JL, Crooks LE (1982) NMR imaging produces no observable mutations or cytotoxicity in mammalian cells. Am J Roentgenol 139:583–585
55. Shellock FG, Schaefer DJ, Gordon CJ (1986) Effect of a 1.5 T static magnetic field on body temperature of man. Magn Reson Med 3:644–647
56. Shellock FG, Crues JV (1987) Temperature, heart rate, and blood pressure changes associated with clinical MR imaging at 1.5 T. Radiology 163:259–262
57. Shellock FG, Schaefer DJ, Grundfest W et al (1986) Thermal effects of high-field (1.5 Tesla) magnetic resonance imaging of the spine: clinical experience above a specific absorption rate of 0.4 W/kg. Acta Radiol [Suppl] 369:514–516
58. Shellock FG, Gordon CJ, Schaefer DJ (1986) Thermoregulatory responses to clinical magnetic resonance imaging of the head at 1.5 Tesla: Lack of evidence for direct effects on the hypothalamus. Acta Radiol [Suppl] 369:512–513
59. Shellock FG, Crues JV (1986) Corneal temperature changes associated with high-field MR imaging using a head coil. Radiology 167:809–811
60. Shellock FG, Crues JV (1988) Temperature changes caused by clinical MR imaging of the brain at 1.5 Tesla using a head coil. Am J Neuroradiol 9:287–291
61. Shellock FG, Schaefer DJ, Crues JV (1989) Effect of a 1.5 tesla static magnetic field on body and skin temperatures of man. Magn Reson Med 11:371–375
62. Shellock FG, Schaefer DJ, Crues JV (1989) Alterations in body and skin temperatures caused by MR imaging: is the recommended exposure for radiofrequency radiation too conservative? Br J Radiol 62:904–909
63. Shellock FG, Rothman B, Sarti D (1990) Heating of the scrotum by high-field-strength MR imaging. Am J Roentgenol 154:1229–1232
64. Shivers RR, Kavaliers M, Tesky CJ et al (1987) Magnetic resonance imaging temporarily alters blood-brain barrier permeability in the rat. Neurosci Lett 76:25–31
65. Shuman WP, Haynor DR, Guy AW et al (1988) Superficial and deep-tissue increases in anesthetized dogs during exposure to high specific absorption rates in a 1.5-T MR imager. Radiology 167:551–554
66. Sperber D, Oldenbourg R, Dransfeld K (1984) Magnetic field induced temperature change in mice. Naturwissenschaften 71:100–101
67. Stick VC, Hinkelmann ZK, Eggert P et al (1991) Beeinflussen starke statische Magnetfelder in der NMR-Tomographie die Gewebedurchblutung? (Strong static magnetic fields of NMR: do they affect tissue perfusion?). Fortschr Rontgenstr 154 (3):326–331
68. Stojan L, Sperber D, Dransfeld K (1988) Magnetic-field-induced changes in the human auditory evoked potentials. Naturwissenschaften 75:622–623
69. Sweetland J, Kertesz A, Prato FS et al (1987) The effect of magnetic resonance imaging on human congnition. Magn Reson Imaging 5:129–135
70. Teskey GC, Prato FS, Ossenkopp KP et al (1988) Exposure to time varying magnetic fields associated with magnetic resonance imaging reduces fentanyl-induced analgesia in mice. Bioelectromagnetics 9:167–174
71. Tesky GC, Ossenkopp KP, Prato FS et al (1987) Survivability and long-term stress reactivity levels following repeated exposure to nuclear magnetic resonance imaging procedures in rats. Physiol Chem Phys Med NMR 19:43–49
72. Thomas A, Morris PG (1981) The effects of NMR exposure on living organisms. I. A microbial assay. Br J Radiol 54:615–621
73. Tyndall DA, Sulik KK (1991) Effects of magnetic resonance imaging on eye development in the C57BL/6 J mouse. Teratology 43:263–275
74. Tyndall DA (1990) MRI effects on the tertogenicity of X-irradiation in the C57BL/6 J mouse. Magn Reson Imaging 8:423–433
75. Vogl T, Krimmel K, Fuchs A et al (1988) Influence of magnetic resonance imaging on human body core and intravascular temperature. Med Phys 15:562–566
76. Von Klitzing L (1986) Do static magnetic fields of NMR influence biological signals. Clin Phys Physiol Measurement (Bristol) 7 (2):157–160
77. Von Klitzing L (1989) Static magnetic fields increase the power intensity of EEG of man. Brain Res 483:201–203
78. Von Klitzing L (1991) A new encephalomagnetic effect in human brain generated by static magnetic fields. Brain Res 540:295–296

79. Weiss J, Herrick RC, Taber KH et al (1990) Bio-effects of high magnetic fields: a study using a simple animal model. Magn Reson Imaging 8 (S1):166
80. Willis RJ, Brooks WM (1984) Potential hazards of NMR imaging. No evidence of the possible effects of static and changing magnetic fields on cardiac function of the rat and guinea pig. Magn Reson Imaging 2:89–95
81. Withers HR, Mason KA, Davis CA (1985) MR effect on murine spermatogenesis. Radiology 156:741–742
82. Wolff S, Crooks LE, Brown P et al (1980) Tests for DNA and chromosomal damage induced by nuclear magnetic resonance imaging. Radiology 136:707–710
83. Yamagata H, Kuhara S, Eso Y et al (1991) Evaluation of dB/dt thresholds for nerve stimulation elicited by trapezoidal and sinusoidal gradient fields in echo-planar imaging. In: Book of abstracts. Society of Magnetic Resonance in Medicine, p 1277
84. Vyalov AM (1967) Magnetic fields as a factor in the industrial enviroment. Vestn Akad Med Nauk 8:72–79
85. Vyalov AM (1974) Clinico-hygenic and experimental data on the effect of magnetic fields under industrial conditions. In: Kholodov Y (ed) Influence of magnetic fields on biological objects. Moscow 1971 (translated by the JPRS). Joint Publications Research Service 63 (38):20–35
86. Barnothy MF (1964) Biological effects of magnetic fields, vol 1 and 2. Plenum, New York, p 1969
87. Persson BR, Stahlberg F (1989) Health and safety of clinical NMR examinations. CRC, Boca Raton
88. Tenforde TS (1979) Magnetic field effects on biological systems. Plenum, New York
89. Michaelson SM, Lin JV (1987) Biological effects and health implications of radiofrequency radiation. Plenum, New York
90. Tenforde TS (1986) Thermoregulation in rodents exposed to high-intensity stationary magnetic fields. Bioelectromagnetics 7:341–346
91. Beischer DE, Knepton J (1964) Influence of strong magnetic fields on the electrocardiogram of squirrel monkey (Saimiri sciures). Aerospace Med 35:939–944
92. Tenforde TS, Gaffey CT, Moyer BR et al (1983) Cardiovascular alterations in Macaca monkeys exposed to stationary magnetic fields. Experimental observations and theoretical analysis. Bioelectromagnetics 4:1–9
93. Dimick RM, Hedlund LW, Herfkens RJ et al (1987) Optimizing electrocardiographic electrode placement for cardiac-gated magnetic resonance imaging. Invest Radiol 22:17–22
94. Abdullakhozhaeva MS, Razykov SR (1986) Structural changes in central nervous system under the influence of a permanent magnetic field. Bull Exp Biol Med 102:1585–1587
95. Hong CZ (1987) Static magnetic field influence on human nerve function. Arch Phys Med Rehabil 68:162–164
96. Budinger TF (1981) Nuclear magnetic resonance (NMR) in vivo studies: known thresholds for health effects. J Comput Assist Tomogr 5:800–811
97. Shellock FG, Crues JV (1988) MRI: safety considerations in magnetic resonance imaging. MRI 2:25–30
98. Shellock FG (1989) Biological effects and safety aspects of magnetic resonance imaging. Magn Reson Q 5:243–261
99. Kanal E, Talagala L, Shellock FG (1990) Safety considerations in MR imaging. Radiology 176:593–606
100. Reilly JP (1989) Peripheral nerve stimulation by induced electric currents: exposure to time-varying magnetic fields. Med Biol Eng Comput 27:101–112
101. Bernhardt J (1979) The direct influence of electromagnetic fields on nerve and muscle and muscle cells of man within the frequency range of 1 Hz to 30 MHz. Radiat Environ Phys 16:309–323
102. Adey WR (1981) Tissue interactions with nonionizing electromagnetic fields. Physiol Rev 61:435–514
103. Watson AB, Wright JS, Loughman L (1973) Electrical thresholds for ventricular fibrillation in man. Med J Aust 1:1179–1182
104. Modan B (1988) Exposure to electromagnetic fields and brain malignancy: a newly discovered menance? Am J Indust Med 13:625–627
105. Brown HD, Chattopadhyay SK (1988) Electromagnetic-field exposure and cancer. Cancer Biochem Biophys 9:295–342
106. Pool R (1990) Electromagnetic fields: the biological evidence. Science 249:1378–1381
107. FDA (1988) Magnetic resonance diagnostic device; panel recommendation and report on petitions for MR reclassification. Fed Reg 53:7575–7579
108. NCRP (1986) Report no 86. Biological effects and exposure criteria for radiofrequency electromagnetic fields. National Council on Radiation Protection and Measurements, Bethesda
109. Erwin DN (1988) Mechanisms of biological effects of radiofrequency electromagnetic fields: an overview. Aviat Space Environ Med 59 [11, Suppl]:A21–A31
110. Gordon CJ (1986) Thermal physiology. In: Biological effects of radiofrequency radiaton. EPA-600/8-830-026 A, Washington DC, pp 4/1–4/28
111. Gordon CJ (1987) Normalizing the thermal effects of radiofrequency radiation: body mass versus total body surface area. Bioelectromagnetics 8:111–118
112. Gordon CJ (1988) Effect of radiofrequency radiation exposure on thermoregulation. ISI Atlas Sci Plants Anim 1:245–250
113. Beers J (1989) Biological effects of weak electromagnetic fields from 0 Hz to 200 MHz: a survey of the literature with special emphasis on possible magnetic resonance effects. Magn Reson Imaging 7:309–331
114. Coulter JS, Osbourne SL (1936) Short wave diathermy in heating of human tissues. Arch Phys Ther 17:679–687
115. Bottomley PA, Edelstein WA (1981) Power disposition in whole body NMR imaging. Med Phys 8:510–512
116. Bottomley PA, Redington RW, Edelstein WA et al (1985) Estimating radiofrequency power disposition in body NMR imaging. Magn Reson Med 2:336–349
117. Wickersheim KA, Sun MH (1987) Fluoroptic thermometry. Med Electr, April: 84–91
118. Berman E (1984) Reproductive effects. In: Biological effects of radiofrequency radiation. EPA 600/8-83-026 A
119. Michaelson SM, Lin JC (1987) Biological effects and health implications of radiofrequency radiation. Plenum, New York
120. Shellock FG, Kanal E (1991) Policies, guidelines, and recommendations for MR imaging safety and patient management. J Magn Reson Imaging 1:97–101
121. Hurwitz R, Lane SR, Bell RA et al (1989) Acoustic analysis of gradient-coil noise in MR imaging. Radiology 173:545–548
122. Goldman AM, Grossman WE, Friedlander PC (1989) Reduction of sound levels with antinoise in MR imaging. Radiology 173:549–550
123. McJury M, Stewart RW, Crawford D, Toma E (1997) The use of active noise control ANC to reduce acoustic noise generated during MRI scanning: some initial results. Magn Reson Imaging 15:319–322
124. Hayes DL, Holmes DR, Gray JE (1987) Effect of a 1.5 Tesla nuclear magnetic resonance imaging scanner on implanted permanent pacemakers. J Am Coll Cardiol 10:782–786
125. Gangarosa RE, Minnis JE, Nobbe J et al (1987) Operational safety issues in MRI. Magn Reson Imaging 5:287–292

126. Alagona P, Toole JC, Maniscalco BS et al (1989) Nuclear magnetic resonance imaging in a patient with a DDD pacemaker. Pacing Clin Electrophysiol 12:619
127. Edelman RR, Shellock FG, Ahladis J (1990) Practical MRI for the technologist and imaging specialist. In: Edelman RR, Hesselink J (eds) Clinical magnetic resonance imaging. Saunders, Philadelphia
128. Lauck G, von Smekal A, Wolke S, Seelos KC, Jung W, Manz M, Leuderitz B (1995) Effects of nuclear magnetic resonance imaging on cardiac pacemakers. Pacing Clin Electrophysiol 18:1549–1555
129. Gimbel JR, Johnson D, Levine PA, Wilkoff BL (1996) Safe performance of magnetic resonance imaging on five patients with permanent cardiac pacemakers. Pacing Clin Electrophysiol 19:913–919
130. Hofman MB, de Cock CC, van der Linden JC, van Rossum AC, Visser FC, Sprenger M, Westerhof N (1996) Transesophageal cardiac pacing during magnetic resonance imaging: feasibility and safety considerations. Magn Reson Med 35:413–422
131. ECRI Health Devices Alert (1988) A new MRI complication?
132. Dormer KJ, Richard GJ, Hough JVD et al (1981) The use of rare-earth magnet couplers in cochlear implants. Laryngoscope 91:1812–1820
133. Heller JW, Brackmann DE, Tucci DL, Nyenhuis JA, Chou CK (1996) Evaluation of MRI compatibility of the modified nucleus multichannel auditory brainstem and coclear implants. Am J Otol 17:724–729
134. Youssefzadeh S, Baumgartner W, Dorffner R, Gsteottner W, Trattnig S (1998) MR compatibility of Med EL coclear implants: clinical testing at 1.0 T. J Comput Assist Tomogr 22:346–350
135. Shellock FG (1989) Ex vivo assessment of deflection forces and artifacts associated with high-field MRI of "mini-magnet" dental prostheses. Magn Reson Imaging 7 [Suppl 1]:IT-03
136. Liang MD, Narayanan K, Kanal E (1989) Magnetic ports in tissue expanders: a caution for MRI. Magn Reson Imaging 7:541–542
137. Lund G, Nelson JD, Wirtschafter JD et al (1986) Tatooing of eyelids: magnetic imaging artifacts. Opthamal Surg 17:550–553
138. Sacco DA, Steiger DA, Bellon EM et al (1987) Artifacts caused by cosmetics in MR imaging of the head. Am J Roentgenol 148:1001–1004
139. Jackson JG, Acker JD (1987) Permanent eyeliner and MR imaging. Am J Roentgenol 149:1080
140. Pusey E, Lufkin RB, Brown RKJ et al (1986) Magnetic resonance imaging artifacts: mechanism and clinical significance. Radiographics 6:891–911
141. Chou CK, McDougall JA, Chan KW (1997) RF heating of implanted spinal fusion stimulator during magnetic resonance imaging. IEEE Trans Biomed Eng 44:367–373
142. Buchli R, Boesiger P, Meier D (1988) Heating effects of metallic implants by MRI examinations. Magn Reson Med 7:255–261
143. Davis PL, Crooks L, Arakawa M et al (1981) Potential hazards in NMR imaging: heating effects of changing magnetic fields and RF fields on small metallic implants. Am J Roentgenol 137:857–860
144. Shellock FG, Crues JV (1987) High-field MR imaging of metallic biomedical implants: an in vitro evaluation of deflection forces and temperature changes induced in large prostheses. Radiology 165:150
145. Shellock FG, Crues JV (1988) High-field MR imaging of metallic biomedical implants: an ex vivo evaluation of deflection forces. Am J Roentgenol 151:389–392
146. Dujovny M, Kossovsky N, Kossowsky R et al (1985) Aneurysm clip motion during magnetic resonance imaging: in vivo experimental study with metallurgical factor analysis. Neurosurgery 17:543–548
147. Shellock FG, Schatz CJ, Shelton C et al (1990) Ex vivo evaluation of 9 different ocular and middle-ear implants exposed to a 1.5 Tesla MR scanner. Radiology 177 (P):271
148. Shellock FG, Schatz CJ (1991) High-field strength MRI and otologic implants. Am J Neuroradiol 12:279–281
149. Shellock FG, Meeks T (1991) Ex vivo evaluation of ferromagnetism and artifacts for implantable vascular access ports exposed to a 1.5 T MR scanner. J Magn Reson Imaging 1:243
150. Teitelbaum GP, Yee CA, Van Horn DD et al (1990) Metallic ballistic fragments: MR imaging safety and artifacts. Radiology 175:855–859
151. Shellock FG (1988) MR imaging of metallic implants and materials: a compilation of the literature. Am J Roentgenol 151:811–814
152. Shellock FG, Curtis JS (1991) MR imaging and biomedical implants, materials, and devices: an updated review. Radiology 180:541–550
153. Holtas S, Olsson M, Romner B et al (1988) Comparison of MR imaging and CT in patients with intracranial aneurysm clips. Am J Neuroradiol 9:891–897
154. Huttenbrink KB, Grobe-Nobis W (1987) Experimentelle Untersuchungen und theoretische Betrachtungen uber das Verhalten von Stapes-Metall-Prothesen im Magnetfeld eines Kernspintomographen. (Experiments and theoretical considerations on behaviour of metallic stapedectomy-protheses in nuclear magnetic resonance imaging.). Laryngol Rhinol Otol 66:127–130
155. Becker R, Norfray JF, Teitelbaum GP et al (1988) MR imaging in patients with intracranial aneurysm clips. Am J Neuroradiol 9:885–889
156. Randall PA, Kohman LJ, Scalzetti EM et al (1988) Magnetic resonance imaging of prosthetic cardiac valves in vitro and in vivo. Am J Cardiol 62:973–976
157. Romner B, Olsson M, Ljunggren B et al (1989) Magnetic resonance imaging and aneurysm clips. J Neurosurg 70:426–431
158. Augustiny N, von Schulthess GK, Meier D et al (1987) MR imaging of large nonferromagnetic metallic implants at 1.5 T. J Comput Asisst Tomogr 11:678–683
159. Teitelbaum GP, Bradley WG, Klein BD (1988) MR imaging artifacts ferromagnetism, and magnetic torque of intravascular filters, stents, and coils. Radiology 166:657–664
160. Yuh WTC, Hanigan MT, Nerad JA et al (1991) Extrusion of a magnetic eye implant after MR examination: a potential hazard to the enucleated eye. In: Book of abstracts. American Society of Neuroradiology, p 97
161. Dujovny M, Dujovny N, Fiat D, Gundamraj NR, Misra M, Serdar Alp M, Zhao, YJ (1996) Magnetic field gradients in the MRI suite and their effects on aneurysm clips. Neurol Res 18:483-486
162. Kotsakis A, Tan KH, Jackson G (1997) Is MRI a safe procedure in patients with coronary stents n situ? Int J Clin Pract 51:349
163. Marra S, Leonetti JP, Konior RJ, Raslan W (1995) Effect of magnetic resonance imaging on implantable eyelid weights. Ann Otol Rhinol Laryngol 104:448–452
164. Chou CK, McDougall JA, Can KW (1995) Absence of radiofrequency heating from auditory implants during magnetic resonance imaging. Bioelectromagnetics 16:307–317
165. Kelly WM, Pagle PG, Pearson A et al (1986) Ferromagnetism of intraocular foreign body causes unilateral blindness after MR study. Am J Neuroradiol 7:243–245
166. Williams S, Char DH, Dillon WP et al (1988) Ferrous intraocular foreign bodies and magnetic resonance imaging. Am J Ophthalmol 105:398–401
167. Flaherty JA, Hoskinson K (1989) Emotional distress during magnetic resonance imaging. N Engl J Med 320:467–468

168. Fishbain DA, Goldberg M, Labbe E et al (1988) Long-term claustrophobia following magnetic resonance imaging. Am J Psychiatry 145:1038–1039
169. Quirk ME, Letendre AJ, Ciottone RA et al (1989) Anxiety in patients undergoing MR imaging. Radiology 170:463–466
170. Quirk ME, Letendre AJ, Ciottone RA et al (1989) Evaluation of three psychological interventions to reduce anxiety during MR imaging. Radiology 173:759–762
171. Hricak H, Amparo EG (1984) Body MRI: alleviation of claustrophobia by prone positioning. Radiology 152:819
172. Weinreb JC, Maravilla KR, Peshock R et al (1984) Magnetic resonance imaging: improving patient tolerance and safety. Am J Roentgenol 143:1285–1287
173. Klonoff EA, Janata JW, Kaufman B (1986) The use of systematic desentization to overcome resistance to magnetic resonance imaging (MRI) scanning. J Behav Ther Exp Psychiatry 17:189–192
174. Granet RB, Gelber LJ (1990) Claustrophobia during MR imaging. N J Med 87 (6):479–482
175. Phelps LA (1990) MRI and claustrophobia. Am Fam Phys 42 (4):930
176. McGuinness TP (1984) Hypnosis in the treatment of phobias: a review of the literature. Am J Clin Hyp 26:261–272
177. Karlik SJ, Heatherley T, Pavan F et al (1988) Patient anesthesia and monitoring at a 1.5 T MRI installation. Magn Reson Med 7:210–221
178. Barnett GH, Ropper AH, Johnson KA (1988) Physiological support and monitoring of critically ill patients during magnetic resonance imaging. J Neurosurg 68:244–250
179. Dunn V, Coffman CE, McGowan JE et al (1985) Mechanical ventilation during magnetic resonance imaging. Magn Reson Imaging 3:169–172
180. McArdle CB, Nicholas DA, Richardson CJ et al (1986) Monitoring of the neonate undergoing MR imaging: technical considerations. Radiology 159:223–226
181. Roth JL, Nugent M, Gray JE et al (1985) Patient monitoring during magnetic resonance imaging. Anesthesiology 62:80–83
182. Shellock FG (1986) Monitoring during MRI. An evaluation of the effect of high-field MRI on various patient monitors. Med Electr, Sept: 93–97
183. Shellock FG (1990) Monitoring sedated patients during MRI. Radiology 177:586 (letter)
184. Wendt RE, Rokey R, Vick GW et al (1988) Electrocardiographic gating and monitoring during NMR imaging. Magn Reson Imaging 6:89–95
185. Holshouser BA, Hinshaw DB, Shellock FG (1991) Sedation, anesthesia, and physiologic monitoring during MRI. In: Hasso AN, Stark DD (eds) Catagorical course syllabus, spine and body magnetic resonance imaging. American Roentgen Ray Society
186. Keeler EK, Casey FX, Engels H, Lauder E Pirto CA, Reisker T, Rogers J, Schaefer, DR, Tynes T (1998) Accessory equipment considerations with respect to MRI compatibility. J Magn Reson Imaging 8:12–18
187. Kanal E, Applegate GR (1990) Thermal injuries/incidents associated with MR imaging devices in the US: a compilation and review of the presently available data. In: Book of abstracts. Society for Magnetic Resonance Imaging, p 274
188. Shellock FG, Slimp G (1989) Severe burn of the finger caused by using a pulse oximeter during MRI. Am J Roentgenol 153:1105
189. Kanal E, Shellock FG (1990) Burns associated with clinical MR examinations. Radiology 175:585
190. Shellock FG, Myers SM, Kimble K (1992) Monitoring heart rate and oxygen saturation during MRI with a fiber-optic pulse oximeter. Am J Roentgenol 158:663–664

Diagnostic Procedures and Protocols D

Open-Field Magnetic Resonance Imaging: Diagnostic Procedures and Protocols in the Brain

1

W. W. Orrison Jr.

■ Introduction

Magnetic resonance imaging (MRI) is currently performed with scanners operating at field strengths ranging from 0.02 to 4.0 T [1–5]. Multiple manufacturers now supply open design MRI systems that operate predominately at field strengths below 0.5 T. Issues regarding field strength remain controversial and largely unresolved. This includes diagnostic yield, imaging sequences, manufacturer variation, diagnostic accuracy, adequacy of image quality, cost effectiveness, and safety [6–16]. In spite of these unresolved issues clinical MR units operating at 0.5 T or below may make up as much as 80% of the systems in use in developed countries, and more than 2000 of these lower field strength systems are operational in the United States. At least six manufacturers offer an array of clinical MR systems below 0.6 T, with the sales of open design systems rapidly increasing. Brain imaging on high-field strength magnets in general provides higher resolution, but such systems are more costly to site, operate, and maintain. Open design low-field strength systems tend to demonstrate higher contrast with slightly less resolution; however, costs for siting, operation, and maintenance are significantly lower. In addition, patient tolerance is often superior to that seen in a high-field environment. Technical factors can be critical at both high and low field; however, lower field strength systems tend to be more heavily criticized [10].

■ High-Contrast Versus High-Resolution MRI

As field strength changes in MR, there is a direct effect on relaxation times [17–19]. A shortening of T1 occurs as the field strength decreases, and there is thus an improvement in signal-to-noise per unit time at lower fields. This results in improved lesion contrast [19].

When interpreting brain images at lower field strengths it is important to remember that as the field strength decreases, contrast increases. In general, a high-field-strength scanner provides higher resolution. This implies that if there is a detectable difference in tissue contrast, the higher-field-strength magnet demonstrates smaller regions of difference, and the images are clearer. However, when there is no difference in contrast, regardless of size, the lesion is not apparent. The use of MR contrast agents is based in part on this principle. When lesion contrast is not evident on routine MR and not enhanced by contrast, the lesion goes undetected. Since lower field strength improves contrast on MR, there is the possibility of detecting lesions with low-field MR that go undetected by either high-field MR or contrast-enhanced high-field MR. An example is the report of the longitudinal relaxation rate, 1/T1 values of mobile water protons at lower field strengths for distinguishing between pituitary tumor types [20]. Figure 1 also illustrates this point in a case of herpes simplex encephalitis detected by T2 imaging at low field (0.06 T) but undetected by T2 at 1.5 T. Imaging sequences such as fluid-attenuated inversion recovery (FLAIR) may eliminate this low-field advantage in many cases (Fig. 2).

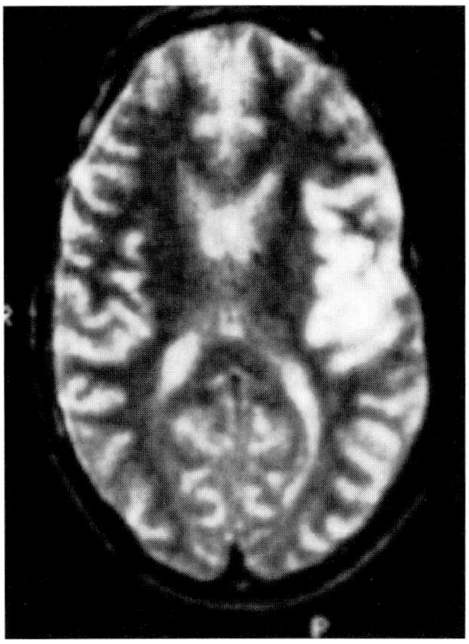

Fig. 1. T2-weighted open-design, low-field MRI demonstrating marked abnormal signal intensity in the left medial temporal lobe. High-field MR interpreted as normal. (Image from a 0.64-T Toshiba open MR system)

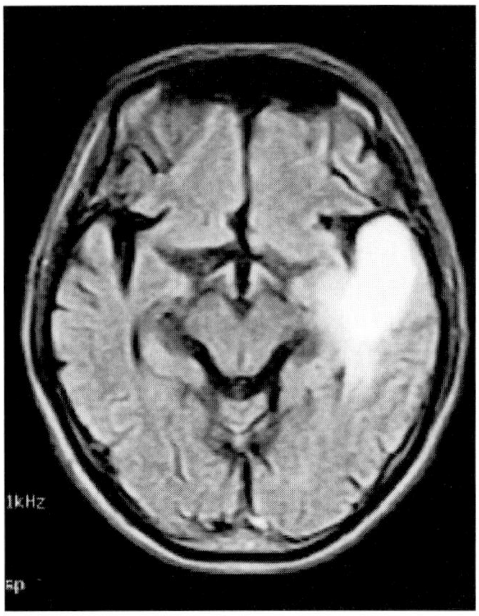

Fig. 2. FLAIR sequence (TR 5500, TE 104, TI 1550) demonstrating "black CSF" and abnormal hyperintensity in the left temporal lobe on this heavily T2-weighted sequence. (Image from a GE 0.2-T open-design magnet)

■ Technical Factors

In brain imaging at lower field strengths the more open designed magnet frequently allows imaging of patients who are unable to tolerate the older "long-bore" design. Although "short-bore" systems are becoming more widely available, in all probability the most open design will continue to be preferred by many patients. The availability of an open magnet often dictates that the patient being scanned is either younger or more difficult. However, as a direct result of this open design these more difficult patients frequently require less sedation. It is common practice in open MRI to reserve sedation for only those patients who are unable to follow instructions, regardless of age. Successful imaging of children as young as 3 years of age has routinely been accomplished on open systems by having the parent or other family member accompany the patient in the scan room. This individual can stand or sit next to the patient, if necessary, and simply holding the patient's hand in some instances is sufficient to al-

Table 1. Brain protocols supplied by manufacturers for T1 sagittal slice orientation

	Fonar	GE	Hitachi	Picker	Siemens	Toshiba	Toshiba
Field strength (T)	0.35 T	0.2 T	0.3 T	0.23 T	0.2 T	0.35 T	0.064 T
Scan time	3:56	6:34	2:52	11:31	4:12	5:22	9:00
Repetition time	600	483	550	30	588	500	68
Echo time TE1/TE2	30	26	25	10	15	20	24
Number of averages	2	5	2	1	3	2	1
Field of view	240	19×19	240	360	16×22	20×20	110
Number of slices	11	7	11	120	19	8	32
Slice thickness (mm)	5	3.0	5	1.5	5	3.0	4.5
Flip angle (degrees)	90	90	90	35	90	90	45
Matrix hor/ver	192×256	256×160	192×192	180×256	134×256	160×256	256×256

Table 2. Brain protocols supplied by manufacturers for T2 axial slice orientation

	Fonar	GE	Hitachi	Picker	Siemens	Toshiba	Toshiba
Field strength (T)	0.35 T	0.2 T	0.3 T	0.23 T	0.2 T	0.35 T	0.064 T
Scan time (min)	8:54	12:28	8:06	9:48	7:22	9:41	17:00
Repetition time	2700	3700	4100	3630	4284	3000	2000
Echo time TE1/TE2	115	96	130	120	106	20	105
Number of averages	1	4	84	1	3	1	2
Field of view	240	24×24	240	300	19×22	20×20	110
Number of slices	17	22	16	23	19	12	14
Slice thickness (mm)	5	5	5	5	5	3	10
Flip angle (degrees)	90	90	90	100	90	90	90
Matrix hor/ver	192×256	256×192	224×224	162×256	170×256	192×256	256×256

Table 3. Brain protocols supplied by manufacturers for FLAIR axial slice orientation

	GE	Hitachi	Picker	Siemens	Toshiba
Field strength (T)	0.2 T	0.3 T	0.23 T	0.2 T	0.35 T
Scan time	10:06	6:24	10:42	7:19	5:46
Repetition time	5500	8000	3961	6000	8000
Echo time TE1/TE2	112	117	120	93	120
Inversion time	1550	1800	1600	1600	1900
Number of averages	2	87	1	2	2
Field of view	24×24	240	300	19×22	22×22
Number of slices	9	14	20	9	22
Slice thickness (mm)	8	5	7	5	6
Flip angle (degrees)	90	90	90	90	90
Matrix hor/ver	256×128	192×192	162×256	168×256	224×256

low for satisfactory completion of the scan. It is also possible to keep younger children quiet in the magnet for extended periods of time by having a parent or sibling actually lie next to the child in the scanner. This can also serve as an effective adjunct to sedation for children who are reluctant to cooperate even when having received a full dose of sedative.

In general, imaging of the brain involves the use of T1-, T2-, and intermediate-weighted sequences. Image quality can be significantly enhanced for the T1 weighted sequences by using a gradient echo technique rather than a spin echo sequence. As with all gradient echo sequences, motion can be a significant degrading factor in image quality, and if patient motion is severe, a spin echo sequence can be substituted. At field strengths in the range of 0.06 T a typical gradient echo sequence can be substituted. At field strengths in the range of 0.06 T a typical gradient echo sequence would include a TR of 68, TE of 24, and FA of 60 or a similar configuration for adequate image quality. At 0.23 T excellent image quality can be obtained on an open MR system using TR of 30, TE of 10, and FA of 35. A detailed summary of manufacturer supplied brain protocols successfully used in open systems of varying field strengths is included in Tables 1–3.

As with high-field imaging, standard T2 and proton density (intermediate) weighted sequences are usually obtained on lower field strength imaging systems. The value of these techniques in imaging of the brain is well established, and for a rapid screen T2-weighted sequences may be suffi-

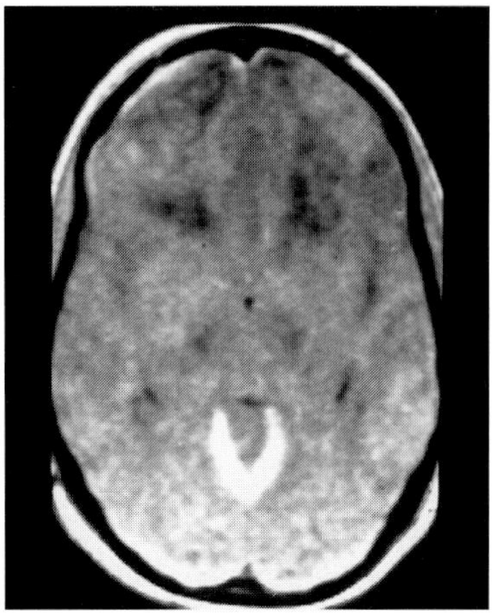

Fig. 3. T1 (TR 68, TE 24, FA 60) open-design, low-field MRI examination demonstrating acute SAH as markedly high signal intensity. (Image obtained on a 0.64-T Toshiba open MR system)

cient to exclude significant pathology. However, an additional advantage of lower field strength systems is the ability to detect changes that may go undetected at higher field (see Fig. 1, above). Another example is in the area of acute subarachnoid hemorrhage (SAH) where T1-, T2-, and proton density weighted imaging may be negative at high field but obvious on T1 weighted low-field images (Fig. 3). Therefore in general it is advantageous to perform at least both T1- and T2-weighted sequences on all patients referred for a brain evaluation.

Fluid-Attenuated Inversion Recovery

The advent of fluid-attenuated inversion recovery (FLAIR) imaging has drastically altered the evaluation of the brain by MR, and has given the brain imager yet another advantage in the diagnosis of cerebral pathology. FLAIR sequences produce heavily T2-weighted and cerebrospinal fluid (CSF) nulled images of the brain on MR. This novel method of imaging was first described by the group from Hammersmith Hospital in the United Kingdom and demonstrates dramatic changes on MRI that may otherwise go undetected [1–3, 8, 21]. By reducing the signal from CSF and enhancing the T2 weighting FLAIR sequences provide a unique opportunity to evaluate brain pathology (see Fig. 2). Clinical applications of FLAIR have been demonstrated in disease processes including SAH, cerebral infarction, brain trauma, cerebral neoplasms, inflammatory conditions, and most notably demyelinating diseases [1, 5–7, 21].

The routine use of FLAIR is recommended for all brain evaluations regardless of field strength, but, again, lower field strength scanners may prove to be advantageous in this regard. Higher field strength systems tend to demonstrate significant and often severe artifacts on FLAIR sequences. The artifacts that result from CSF or vascular flow and pulsation on high-field FLAIR images are less of a problem at lower field, and in some cases at low field can be virtually eliminated (Fig. 4).

One of the most significant limitations of FLAIR imaging has been the presence of signifi-

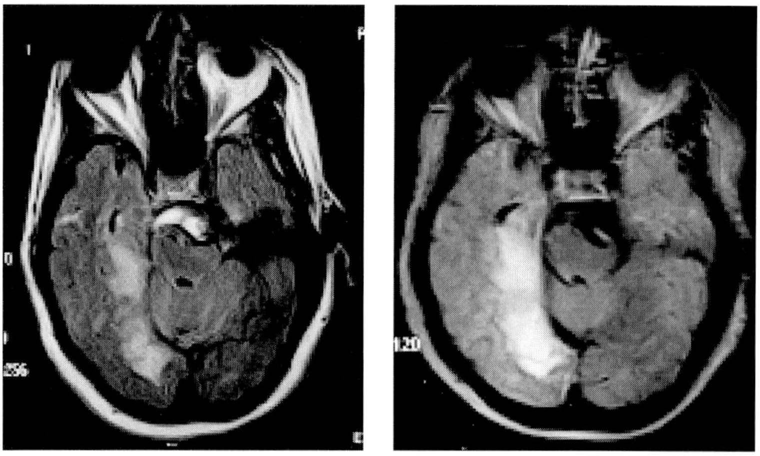

a b

Fig. 4. a A 1.5-T FLAIR image (TR 8243, TE 112, T1 1600) demonstrating a right posterior cerebral artery infarction. Note the artifact in the prepontine cistern identified as high signal. (Image from a 0.23-T Picker open MR system) **b** A 0.23-T FLAIR image (TR 4752, TE 120, TI 1600) demonstrating the right posterior artery infarction seen in **a**, but without the prepontine flow artifact that is prominent on high-field MR. (Image from a 0.23-T Picker open MR system) cant artifacts that are particularly related to CSF motion. These are often encountered in the region of the lateral ventricles, foramen of Monroe, third ventricle, cerebral aqueduct, and fourth ventricle. These artifacts at high-field can be particularly problematic when attempting to evaluate cerebral pathology adjacent to regions of the brain that are contiguous with or adjacent to pulsatile CSF. One of the advantages of open MRI scanning at lower field strengths is a notable absence of these artifacts (see Figs. 4, 13).

■ Contrast Agents

Contrast agents improve the diagnostic power of MR in several ways. Both the conspicuity of abnormalities and better demarcation of their borders are achieved through the use of MR contrast agents. The viable areas of neoplasms may be distinguished from surrounding edema in some cases and contrast also helps to date abnormalities, specifically with regards to cerebral infarctions.

The ideal contrast agent must be both effective and safe. The main objective of contrast agents in imaging is to enhance image contrast to render normal and pathological anatomy more conspicuous. Great advances have been made toward both of these ends, and while some drawbacks exist, research and development of new and improved contrast agents persists. Generally there is little difference between the use of contrast agents in children and in adults, the main difference being one of dose, based on weight and age. Children also tend to have a lower incidence of adverse reaction than adults, whether mild or severe, to all contrast agents [22].

Contrast agents are administered to patients in liquid form and function within the bloodstream or CSF. Accordingly the inherent properties of density, viscosity, and osmolality effect their safety and efficacy [23].

The United States Food and Drug Administration has approved three MRI contrast agents for intravenous administration: Magnevist (gadopentetate dimeglumine injection, Berlex Laboratories), Omniscan (gadodiamide injection, Nycomed), and ProHance (gadoteridol injection, Bracco Diagnostics). Since the element gadolinium is the base of all of these contrast agents, they all have similar mechanisms of action, biodistribution, and half-lives [24–27]. While these agents appear to have remarkably similar effectiveness and safety profiles, some differences do exist.

There are osmolality differences between Magnevist (1960 mmol/kg of water) [28], Omniscan (789 mmol/kg water), and ProHance (630 mmol/kg water). The significance of this osmolality difference, however, is proportionally decreased by the administered volume of these agents being typically quite small.

Gadolinium is not normally present in a mammalian system except in trace amounts and has no known natural functions. It is highly toxic in its ionic form to humans, even at low doses. The contrast agents used for MR enhancement in the United States are gadolinium chelates that localize in the extracellular fluid compartment to be then rapidly excreted by the kidney. As the gadolinium ion is toxic, it must be complexed with ligands.

For all of these agents, the adverse reaction rate seems to be less than 4% [25, 29–42]. The adverse reactions that are most commonly experienced seem to be nausea, emesis, hives, headache, and local injection site reactions, such as irritation or a burning or cool sensation. The incidence of the anaphylactoid reactions that have been reported with all three of these FDA-approved intravenous MR contrast agents is so exceedingly rare that it is difficult to attempt to place any significance on these rates. At worst, the rate of this extreme sort of reaction from any of these agents is probably in the 1:100,000 range, and this may be as high as 1:450,000.

The use of Magnevist has been associated with transient elevations in serum bilirubin (3%–4% of patients) that seems to spontaneously reverse within 24–48 h [31, 43]. The use of ProHance has not resulted in reports of such alterations in blood chemistry. All MRI contrast agents have been associated with delayed reactions of hypertension, vasovagal responses, and syncope. There are no known contraindications for Magnevist, Omniscan, or ProHance.

The administration of MRI contrast agents during pregnancy and lactation has not been determined to be without risk. To date no clinical trials have been reported on pregnant women. The studies performed on animals, however, using doses much higher than those employed clinically have produced a number of severe adverse effects on the fetus. Gadopentetate dimeglumine does cross the placenta and has been found in the fetal bladder [44]. The rate of clearance of MRI contrast agents from the amniotic fluid cycle has not been assessed. Until more data become available, routine administration of any of the MRI contrast agents in pregnant patients should not occur, unless the potential benefit justifies the risk to the fetus. It is also recommended that mothers refrain from breast feeding, while continuing to express milk, for 24 h following gadopentetate administration.

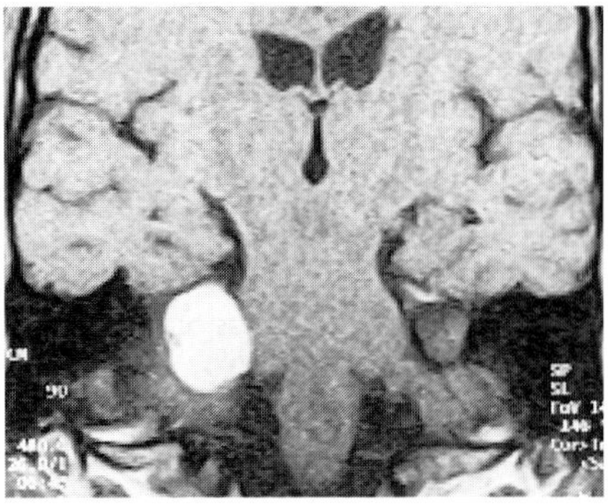

Fig. 5. Postcontrast MR (TR 480, TE 26) demonstrating enhancing right-sided acoustic neuroma from a Siemens 0.2-T open MR system. (Mark Leszczynski, RT, Memorial Open MRI, Houston, Texas, used with permission)

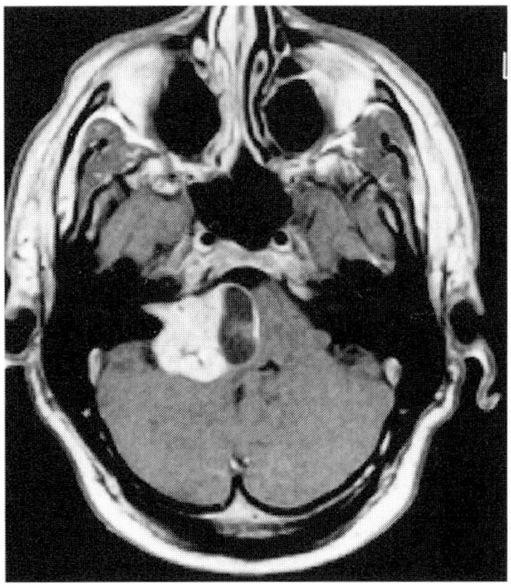

Fig. 6. Postcontrast T1 image (TR 650, TE 25) of an extra-axial acoustic neuroma. (Image from a 0.3-T Hitachi open MR system)

Our clinical experience with gadolinium imaging on low-field open-MRI has resulted in the use of a T1-weighted gradient echo technique with a bolus of one half of a 0.1 mmol/kg dose of gadolinium DTPA, with drip infusion of the remaining one-half dose diluted in 50 cc sterile water [45]. Due to the longer scan times required at lower fields, the drip infusion technique provides optimum levels of gadopentetate dimeglumine at the actual times of image acquisition. Some low-field centers report using approximately 0.15–0.2 mmol/kg single injections with similarly improved results. The use of open low-field or 1.5-T bore-type MR appears comparable, in our experience, for cranial central nervous system disease with or without contrast (Figs. 5, 6, 9, 25).

In general, the indications for the use of contrast in the brain are similar for high- and low-field strength systems. The advantage of the open-design magnets in this regard is the ease of access to the patient for contrast administration and management. It is possible to perform rapid scan sequences on most open design systems, and the role of dynamic sequences in addition to those described in the subsequent section on pituitary imaging remains to be fully established. It is conceivable that dynamic perfusion studies with MR contrast will be an important part of the management of patients with cerebral vascular disease in the future.

■ Safety

Recent reports and at least one survey of MR facilities show potential areas of significant concern regarding safety, with a number of accidents and death associated with MR having been reported [46–50].

Numerous studies have been performed to investigate the potential bioeffects of MRI. The majority of these studies support the widely held view that no significant biological health risks are associated with the use of this modality. The effects on humans and biological systems of strong static magnetic fields are not well understood.

Some of the literature does include data that appear to be contradictory; however, no evidence has demonstrated conclusively any irreversible or hazardous biological effects related to humans being exposed to acute, short-term static magnetic fields of strengths up to 2.0 T [22].

Certain devices must be precluded from entering the magnet room, for reasons of them being mechanically attracted by the field of the magnet or having their function altered by the presence of the fields. The FDA requires labeling of MR systems to indicate that the device is contraindicated for patients who have implants such as internal cardiac pacemakers, implantable cardiac defibrillators, cochlear implants, neurostimulators, bone-growth stimulators, implantable electronic drug infusion pumps, and similar devices, since electromagnetic fields produced by the MR system may seriously interfere with the operation of these devices [51].

Our three 1.5-T sites have had at least four documented incidences of ferromagnetic objects unintentionally entering the magnetic field and being drawn into the magnet. In one of these instances there was minimal injury when during equipment repair, a repairman and his equipment were drawn into the magnet. In a second instance, a significant injury could have occurred if a patient had been present in the magnet when a metallic writing pen was pulled from a radiologist's pocket as he entered the magnet room. There have been two instances of minor burns related to metallic objects touching the patient during the scan. We have experienced none of these adverse effects in 10 years of open design magnet use at lower field strengths.

Concern for injury from internal or external metallic objects is minimal or nonexistent at very low-field strengths. MR facilities report accidents primarily involving static ferromagnetic objects that became projectiles when subjected to the pull of the magnetic field. Additional injuries have been encountered from MR accessories causing burns [46–50]. A potential injury includes the effect of high magnetic fields that are in general considered safe, but this is unproven. There is a more immediate danger of injury from damage to devices such as implanted pacemakers [47]. An additional problem is that MR accidents are probably grossly underreported [46–50]. Measurements of magnetic forces and torques at 0.064 T support the added safety for patients from both internal and external metal objects when being scanned in open design low-field systems [52].

At higher field strengths several safety concerns exist for scanning patients who have certain ferromagnetic implants, materials, or foreign bodies. Primarily this is because of the possibility of movement or dislodgment of these objects [53–55]. The possibility exists also of current induction, excessive heating, and the misinterpretation as an abnormality of an artifact produced by such an object [53, 55–59]. Several considerations must be taken into account before allowing a patient who has a ferromagnetic object to be scanned, including (a) the strength of the magnetic field to which the patient is exposed, (b) the degree of ferromagnetism manifest by an object, (c) the mass and geometry of the object and its location and orientation in a patient, and (d) the length of time the object has been in place.

For patients who present to the MRI with a history of metallic foreign bodies such as shrapnel, bullets, slivers, or other types of metallic fragments the risk depends on several factors. A patient encountering the static magnetic field of an MR system with an intraocular metallic foreign body, for example, is at significant risk for a serious eye injury. One patient was blinded at the completion of his MR examination on the way out of the MR imager [60]. A patient undergoing an MR examination at one scanner has absolutely no assurance that it is necessarily safe to undergo another MR scan at the same or another location. It has been established that the use of plain film radiography may be an acceptable technique for identifying or excluding an intraocular metallic foreign body that represents a hazard [61].

The hazard of open-design 0.064-T MR regarding intraocular ferromagnetic metal fragments has been evaluated using both in vitro and in vivo animal experiments [62]. An important observation during these experiments was the fact that all motion was increased by increasing the speed at which fragments entered or exited the magnetic field. Regardless of field strength, the forces acting on metallic fragments, and the subsequent risk to patients, can be effectively reduced by decreasing the speed of entry into and the exit from a magnetic field. In other words, regardless of field strength, simply moving the patient in and out of the scan field slowly significantly reduces patient risk.

At least two dozen patients with cardiac pacemakers have been placed in MRI systems, either intentionally or inadvertently. The documentation is such that at least five of these individuals have died, although it should be stressed that the cause of death in these patients is unknown. A study demonstrating total pacemaker inhibition [63] and pacemaker malfunction in another [64] has serious safety implications for studying patients who have pacemakers being imaged. It is commonly understood that scanning any patient who has a cardiac pacemaker is contraindicated.

No standardized testing criteria exist by which MR compatibility claims may be assessed [65, 66]. Not even the term "MR compatible" is defined. No standardization exists that ensures that in such devices as implanted intracranial aneurysm clips, for example, that clips produced from one run are identical in ferromagnetic properties to those of another. This explains why some researchers find some clips "MR compatible" and others find the same clip types respond to the presence of a strong magnetic field. At this point several physicians have decided not to scan any patient with an intracranial aneurysm clip in place until firm guidelines are established [22]. If MR scanning is deemed imperative, the lower field open design magnet may offer less risk than the traditional 1.5-T bore-type systems.

The sensations of claustrophobia and a variety of other unpleasant psychological reactions including anxiety and panic are encountered by as many as 5%–10% of patients during or precipitating MRI. The originating factors include the narrow dimensions of the interior of the bore-type of scanner; the length of the examination; the banging, gradient-induced noises; the encompassing and dark conditions within the traditional bore of the scanner, and other factors [67–75]. Offering an open design magnet is probably the most effective solution to these problems.

■ Cranial Imaging

MR in Brain Disorders

Virtually every type of brain pathology is responded to clinically through the utilization of MR. Since treatment may be dramatically altered, the value of a normal MR scan is not to be underestimated [76]. The decrease in clinic visits, patient concern, and physicians' and other health care professionals' time are relevant in terms of financial and psychological relief [77]. It could be said that the normal brain MR might be one of the most cost-effective studies in all medicine. Considering this is one of the most expensive areas of the health care system, it is certainly warranted to try to exit the patient from this costly system, as well as relieve them of the high stakes that accompany brain disorders [76]. Neoplasms, infections, cerebrovascular disease, head trauma, intracranial hemorrhage, and white matter disease are several disease categories for which the use of MR has proved essential [77].

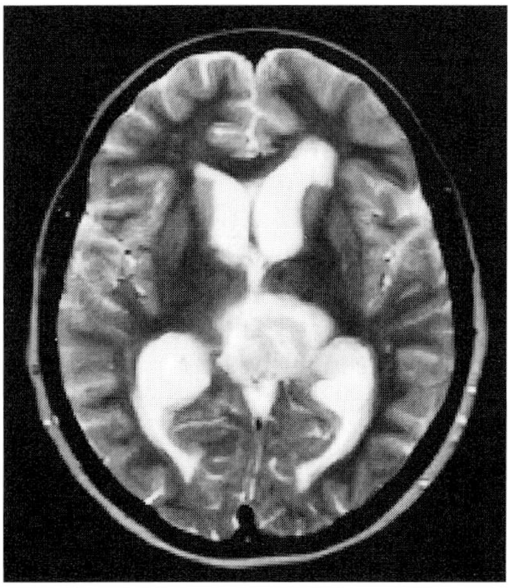

Fig. 7. T2-weighted image (TR 3900, TE 120) of a high-grade glioma. (Image from a 0.3-T Hitachi open MR system)

Neoplasms

Obviously much more attention is given to the abnormal than the normal brain MRI. New primary brain tumors are identified in approximately 40,000 patients in the United States each year, which may result in paralysis, dementia, seizures, and death [77]. Mass effect, edema, hemorrhage, and contrast enhancement are the recognizable characteristics of a neoplasm on MR. Because of the nature of the brain, the classifications of benign or malignant pathology may not apply, as the most "benign" of tumors can be devastating if located in a critical part of the brain [76]. Until recently the location of an intracranial neoplasm was more telling than the cell type of the neoplasm. Even if considered histologically "benign," many intracranial neoplasms are thought to "behave" in a malignant manner.

The availability of functional brain imaging [77] has changed the traditional approach to intracranial masses including neoplasms. Malignant neoplasms once thought to be unresectable because of their close anatomic relationship to vital areas of brain function are now being successfully resected without resulting loss of function. This is due to the location not being as closely related to "vital" brain regions as would be anticipated from

Fig. 8. T1 (TR 68, TE 24, FA 60) open-design, low-field MRI demonstrating ring enhancing mass from metastatic disease following administration of gadolinium. (Image from a 0.64-T Toshiba open MR system)

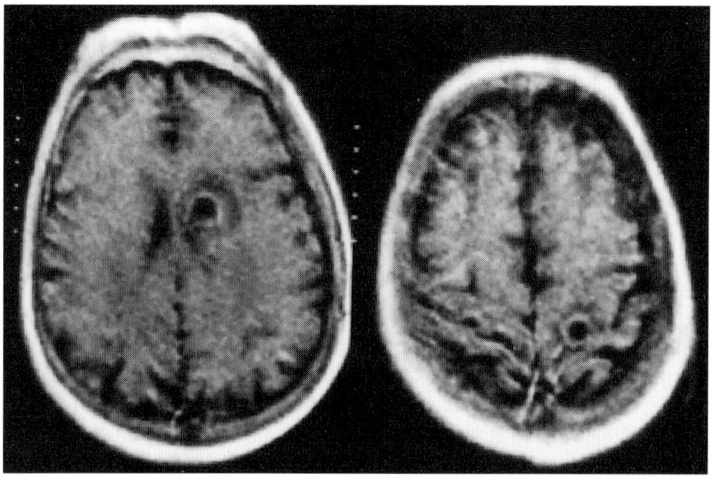

traditional predictions. The number of neoplasms that can be effectively treated is increasing, even though many continue to be refractory to treatment. Although most functional magnetic resonance imaging (fMRI) is currently limited to high-field bore types of systems, fMRI has been performed successfully on lower field strength magnets. The role of fMRI on open design low-field systems remains to be defined.

The two most important criteria for evaluation of images of intracranial neoplasms are age of the patient and location of the mass [77, 78]. On MR brain tumors are often described as being intra-axial, within the brain substance, or extra-axial, outside the brain substance. Benign tumors are frequently extra-axial and easier to resect surgically (Fig. 6). Most often intra-axial, malignant tumors frequently extend far into the brain beyond the appearance on MR (Fig. 7). Surgical cure is difficult, recurrence common, and these tumors include metastatic cancer from other organ systems [76].

Most commonly arising from primary neoplasms of the lung and breast, metastatic cancer represents approximately 25% of all brain tumors (Fig. 8). Metastatic brain tumors may also arise from the gastrointestinal tract, the genitourinary tract, and melanoma [76].

Infections

Infection of the brain is becoming one of the more common indications for brain imaging and may be the result of extension of infectious conditions in the sinuses, ear, orbit, or superficial soft tissues. The bloodstream can carry the infection from various parts of the body. Many of these conditions respond rapidly to treatment which make these some of the most urgent and important scans performed. Early treatment of brain infection may mean the difference between the patient recovering, being severely incapacitated, or dying [76] (Fig. 9).

Often congenital central nervous system (CNS) infections are caused by what is referred to as the TORCH agents: toxoplasmosis, rubella, cytomegalovirus, and herpes simplex virus. Other important causes of congenital CNS infections are human immunodeficiency virus (HIV) and syphilis [79].

The most common form of CNS infection is meningitis [80]. This condition can be divided into three general categories: acute pyogenic meningitis (most often bacterial infections), lymphocytic meningitis (usually viral), and chronic meningitis (examples are tuberculosis and coccidioidomycosis).

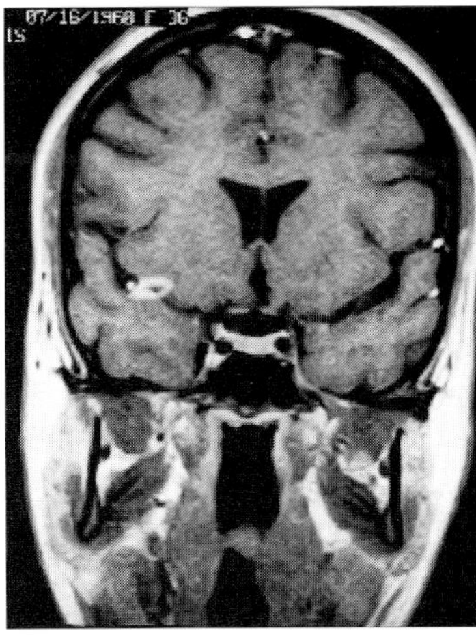

Fig. 9. Postcontrast enhanced MR (TR 500, TE 25) demonstrating a ring enhancing inflammatory lesion. (Image from a 0.3-T Hitachi open MR system)

In the evaluation of patients with suspected meningitis, MRI is superior to computed tomography (CT) [22]. Precontrast T1-weighted images may demonstrate obliterated cisterns that enhance strongly following contrast administration. In severe cases extension of enhancing subarachnoid exudate deep into the sulci can be seen.

Meningitis is conspicuous on postcontrast T1-weighted images; however, unenhanced MR images often do not detect active meningeal inflammation [82, 83]. In chronic meningitis contrast-enhanced T1-weighted MR scans reveal the characteristic basal meningeal inflammatory pattern seen on contrast-enhanced CT studies [84].

The earliest stage of purulent brain infection is cerebritis [80]. This diffuse infection often leads to abscess formation with characteristic neuroimaging features [85]. The organisms most frequently isolated from cerebral abscesses are streptococci, including both aerobic and anaerobic, and staphylococci. Gram-negative organisms, however, are an increasing cause of cerebral abscess [86].

In MR the findings in brain abscess vary with time. An ill-defined subcortical hyperintense zone can be noted on T2-weighted images during the initial, early cerebritis stage. In postcontrast T1-weighted studies poorly delineated enhancing areas within the isointense to mildly hypointense edematous region may be disclosed.

The central necrotic area is typically hyperintense to brain on proton-density and T2-weighted sequences during the late cerebritis stage. On T1-weighted images the thick, somewhat irregularly marginated rim appears isointense to mildly hyperintense and isointense to relatively hypointense

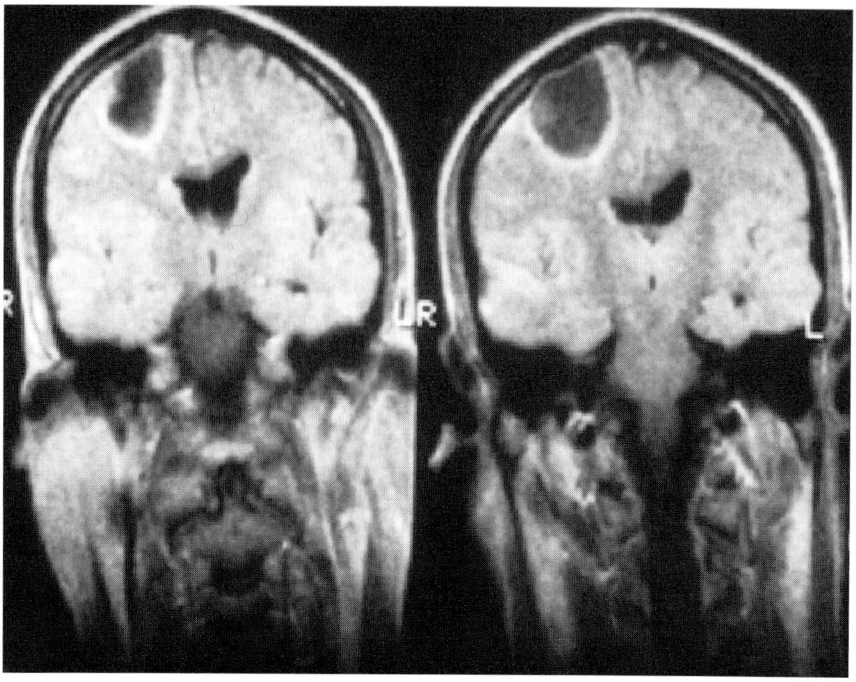

Fig. 10. T1 (TR 68, TE 24, FA 60) open-design, low-field MRI demonstrating rim enhancement in a cerebral abscess following gadolinium administration. (Image from a 0.64-T Toshiba open MR system)

on proton density and T2-weighted scans. In nearly all cases peripheral edema is present. Following contrast administration the rim enhances intensely (Fig. 10). Satellite lesions are commonly present [87]. The collagenous abscess capsule is visible on unenhanced scans, during the early and late capsule stages, as a comparatively thin-walled, well-delineated isointense to slightly hyperintense ring that becomes hypointense on T2-weighted sequences.

While encephalitis is usually viral, it may be caused by a broad spectrum of agents. In the United States and Europe this diffuse, nonfocal brain parenchymal inflammatory disease is most commonly caused by herpes simplex encephalitis.

The typical early findings of MR include gyral edema on T1-weighted images and high signal intensity in the temporal lobe or cingulate gyrus on T2-weighted scans. Often the signal abnormalities extend into the insular cortex and spare the putamen. In the early stages enhancement following contrast administration is unusual [88]. While petechial hemorrhages occur, they are uncommonly identified early in the disease process. As previously demonstrated, open low-field MR may be advantageous in the early diagnosis of this and other progressive brain disorders (see Fig. 1).

Fungi are single-celled organisms that are very different from bacteria in size, structural complexity, chemical composition, and their pathological effects on the central nervous system [89]. Imaging findings vary depending on the specific fungus involved. Gelatinous-appearing pseudocysts are produced by cryptococcus, and these extend along enlarged perivascular spaces, particularly in the basal ganglia. Imaging of aspergillosis usually shows that of multifocal hemorrhagic mycetomas or penetrating or large vessel cerebral infarcts, since this is an angioinvasive fungus. In CNS coccidioidomycosis, what is usually seen is meningeal inflammation with infectious purulent and caseous granulomas. Communicating hydrocephalus is common, and the basal meninges may appear notably thickened [90].

CNS infections can be caused by several different parasites and include toxoplasmosis, cysticercosis, schistosomiasis, sparganosis, amebiases, and echinococcosis. Imaging findings are related to the stage of the infection at presentation [92]. On imaging studies obtained during the vesicular stage of parenchymal cysticercosis, the larva appears as a round CSF-like cyst with a mural nodule that represents its scolex (head). Edema and cyst wall enhancement occur on imaging studies during the colloidal vesicular stage. In the granular nodular stage, the residual cyst is typically isointense compared to brain on unenhanced T1-weighted images and isointense to hypointense on T2-weighted sequences. By the final, nodular calcified stage, the granulomatous lesion has contracted to a fraction of its initial size and is completely mineralized [91].

Imaging findings of miscellaneous parasitic infections vary with the disease stage, although multiple conglomerate, ring-enhancing lesions with striking peripheral edema are typical [92]. In sparganosis, imaging findings are not distinguishable from other granulomas or neoplastic masses [93]. In echinococcosis, also known as hydatid disease, the imaging findings are striking. What is typical is a single, thin-walled spherical CSF-density cyst in the parietal area [92]. Rarely multilocular or multiple lesions occur.

Vascular Disease

The third leading cause of death in the United States is cerebrovascular disease, most of which affects individuals over the age of 55, and is related to atherosclerotic disease. Patients presenting for MR with cerebrovascular disorders commonly suffer from one of three conditions: (a) a transient ischemic attack (TIA), a neurological deficit that clears in less than 24 h, (b) a reversible ischemic neurological deficit (RIND), in which the neurological deficit lasts longer than 24 h but clears, or (c) cerebrovascular accident (CVA), or completed stroke, in which the patient does not recover all lost neurological function. A "stroke in progress" is a fourth condition for which MR (and particularly MRA) may be used. This medical emergency is now often treated in a manner similar to a heart attack. Every second counts in this circumstance. It has been possible to entirely reverse strokes that would have otherwise left the patient paralyzed [76].

With standard spin-echo MRI arterial patency may be difficult to assess. Vessel occlusion with intraluminal thrombus is usually present when intraluminal signal that is isointense with brain on long TR/short TE or long TR/long TE is observed [94]. In-flow phenomena, however, as well as slow or in-plane flow in tortuous, ectatic vessels can mimic intraluminal thrombi. The presence of a normal "flow void" does not exclude significant extracranial carotid stenosis [94, 95].

Diminished blood flow to all parts (global) or selected areas (regional or focal) of the brain is referred to as cerebral ischemia [96]. Stroke is a dynamic process that changes over time, involving the location and degree of cerebral ischemia and resulting infarction. The parameters of flow decrement, location, duration, and tissue volume involved [96] are predicated by ischemic manifestations. Progressing in stages, a stroke moves from ischemia to actual infarction [97].

The lay term "stroke" encompasses a heterogeneous group of widely differing cerebrovascular disorders. Four major types include cerebral infarction, primary intracerebral hemorrhage (ICH), SAH, and venous occlusions. In cerebral ischemia the imaging findings vary significantly over time. More often acute infarcts are identified and localized on MR compared to CT scans (see Fig. 4) [98]. Open low-field imaging may prove particularly helpful in the management of these patients who often require extensive life support assistance. In addition, areas of ischemia can often be detected within minutes of the acute event. On standard spin-echo MR scans obtained within 24 h of the ictus, 80% of acute infarcts are visible [99]. On MR the earliest findings are vascular flow-related abnormalities, including absence of normal flow void and slow flow with intravascular arterial enhancement [100]. Within minutes of symptom onset, these signs are detectable [101, 102]. In nearly three-quarters of acute cortical infarcts, intravascular enhancement is seen [101].

Early on, T1-weighted images also manifest morphological changes, particularly brain swelling. Such anatomic changes may precede the development of increased signal on proton density or T2-weighted sequences. While usually not observed before 8 h on high-field, T2 hyperintensity does occur (Fig. 11). These changes may be detected within the first hour on lower field strength open-design MR systems where tissue contrast is greater. In about one-third of cases abnormal meningeal enhancement is seen adjacent to cortical infarcts that are aged 1–3 days [101]. In 10%–20% of patients standard high-field MRI sequences fail to detect acute stroke [103].

As mentioned above, because cerebral infarction is a dynamic process, its imaging manifesta-

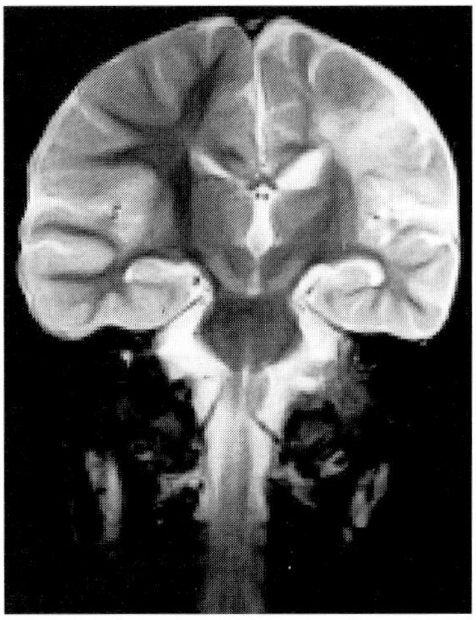

Fig. 11. T2 image (TR 4000, TE 48) in cerebral infarction. Note the cortical and subcortical increased signal intensity of the left hemisphere. (Images from a 0.2-T Siemens MR system. Margareta Arens, MD, St. Barbara Klinik, Hessen, Germany, used with permission)

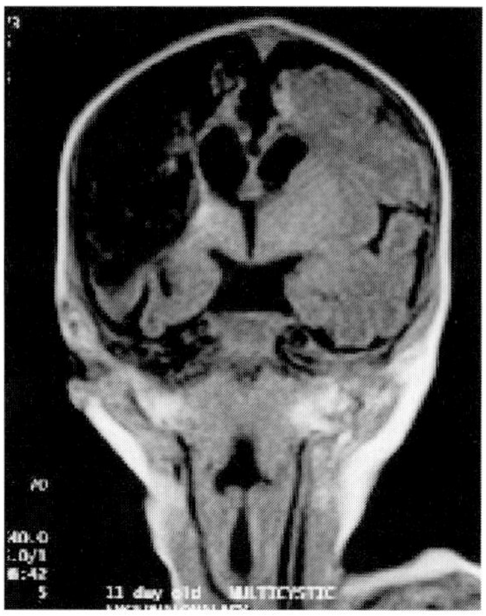

Fig. 12. A T1-weighted image (TR 540, TE 15) of encephalomalacia from a Siemens 0.2-T MR system. (Margareta Arens, MD, St. Barbara Klinik, Hessen, Germany, used with permission)

tions continue to evolve with time. Within 2–4 days after ictus the two earliest signs of acute infarction of intravascular and meningeal enhancement begin to diminish [101]. The parenchymal contrast enhancement that ensues can persist for weeks. Becoming more prominent, edema appears hypointense to cortex on T1-weighted images and hyperintense on T2-weighted images. Mass effect increases and then gradually diminishes.

A noticeable decrease in signal intensity is sometimes observed on T2-weighted images during the second post-ictal week. The initially high-signal changes may largely regress or even disappear. It is likely that this "fogging" effect is due to a reduction in edema and leakage of proteins from cell lysis [104, 105].

The end result of the destructive process of prolonged ischemia is chronic infarction. The pathological hallmarks of stroke residua are volume loss and gliosis, both reflected in gross specimens of chronic infarcts. On MR focal well-delineated low-attenuation or encephalomalacic areas are seen in the affected vascular distribution. The loss of cerebral tissue volume is reflected in the prominence of the adjacent sulci and the enlargement of the ipsilateral ventricle (Fig. 12). After 8–10 weeks the enhancement disappears. Rarely dystrophic calcification may occur in the infarcted brain [106].

Since relaxation times are prolonged in both, the MR differentiation of subacute from chronic (<2 weeks) infarction on standard spin-echo sequences may be difficult because relaxation times are prolonged in both [107]. Mass effect and contrast enhancement are absent in old infarcts (>8–10 weeks). Ipsilateral brain stem atrophy and hyperintensity on T2 or FLAIR imaging may result from wallerian degeneration of axons and their myelin sheaths [108] (Fig. 13). Gyriform signal changes can sometimes be identified on T1-weighted images if cortical hemorrhage or secondary calcification has occurred. These are either hypo- or hyperintense depending on the age of the hemorrhage. Old infarcts reveal ribbon-like very hypointense foci on T2-weighted images [109].

Lacunar infarcts, which account for 15%–25% of all strokes [110], are seen as rounded or slitlike lesions on MR that are hypointense to brain on

a 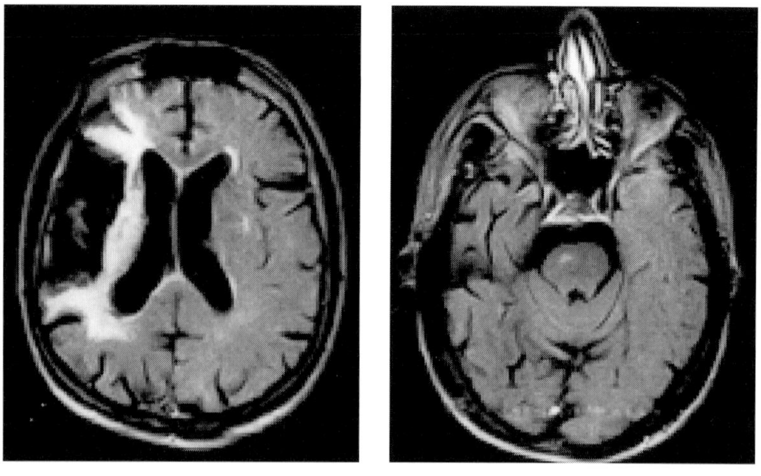 b

Fig. 13. a FLAIR image (TR 4750, TE 120, TI 1600) demonstrating a right middle cerebral artery infarction. (Image from 0.23-T Picker open MR system.) **b** FLAIR image (TR 4750, TE 120, TI 1600) demonstrating wallerian degeneration associated with the right middle cerebral artery infarction in **a**. Note the abnormal increased signal intensity in the right pons and the absence of artifacts (compare to Fig. 4a). (Image from a 0.23 T Picker open MR system)

T1-weighted images. On T2-weighted sequences well-delineated hyperintense areas are identified. Following contrast administration, some late acute or early subacute lacunar infarcts may enhance [110].

Hypoxic-ischemic encephalopathy (HIE) results from global rather than focal brain injury (see Fig. 12). Common causes of HIE are severe prolonged hypotension, cardiac arrest with successful resuscitation, profound neonatal asphyxia, and carbon monoxide inhalation. Most frequently the sites of brain involvement are the basal ganglia and parasagittal areas. Border zone area hyperintensities are revealed on T2-weighted images. Striking enhancement can occur after contrast administration.

Differentiating between ischemia and a neoplasm can at times be difficult. Often imaging findings that suggest stroke includes a full thickness lesion that affects gray and white matter and follows a typical vascular distribution. The cortex is affected and the underlying white matter spared in a stroke, while tumors tend to involve the white matter and spare the cortex. A stroke tends to be wedge-shaped or serpentine, whereas a tumor is usually round, lobulated, or infiltrating.

MR may also be of benefit in the evaluation of other vascular lesions such as arteriovenous malformations, aneurysms, vasculitis, and direct vessel injury (Fig. 14).

Head Trauma

With two million cases in the United States each year, traumatic brain injury is one of the most common types of insult in the United States. MR and particularly open design MR is frequently becoming utilized for this injury [76]. MR can better identify several types of lesions associated with head trauma than CT, including contusions, shearing injury of the white matter, subdural hematomas, and anoxic injury [111] (Fig. 15).

The reasons emergency patients with head injury were in the past evaluated by CT were both logistical and clinical. Siting requirements at one time dictated that MR scanners be located a considerable distance from emergency rooms. Also, it was difficult and sometimes impossible to manage these acutely injured patients effectively in most MR scanners. However, it is now possible to locate an open-field magnet near an emergency department providing the opportunity to compare patients who undergo examination by the respective modalities [111].

While previous studies of MRI indicated that this modality was more sensitive than CT in detecting many types of traumatic lesions [112–124], blinded studies support the claim that a positive MR is more predictive of actual trauma than a positive CT for all forms of traumatic injury, excluding fracture [111]. The appropriate acute surgical management in cases of head trauma continues for the most part to rely on CT as the diagnostic modality of choice [125–129]. CT appears to be satisfactory as the initial diagnostic test in the comatose or dramatically neurologi-

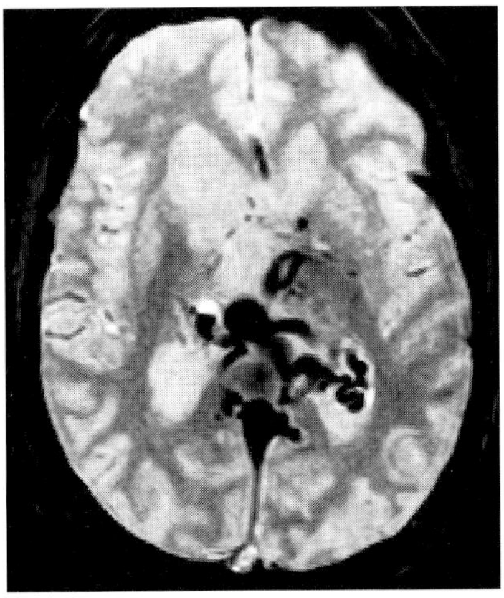

Fig. 14. Gradient echo MR (TR 610, TE 35, FA 30) demonstrating a large arteriovenous malformation. Note the probable area of focal hemorrhage seen as marked hyperintensity. (Imaged from a 0.3-T Hitachi open MR system)

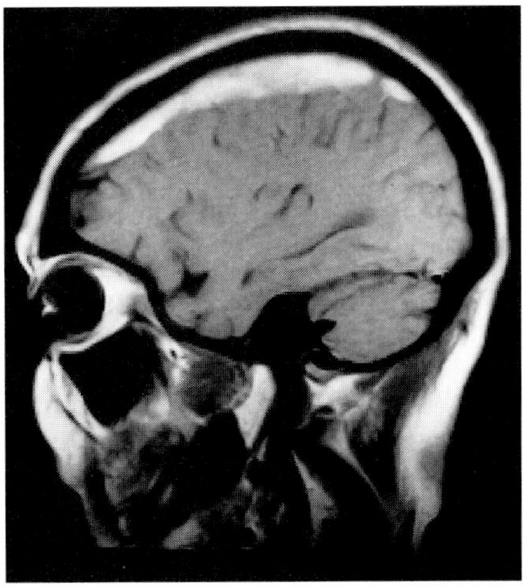

Fig. 15. T1-weighted MR (TR 650, TE 25) demonstrating a subdural hematoma. (Image from a 0.3-T Hitachi open MR system)

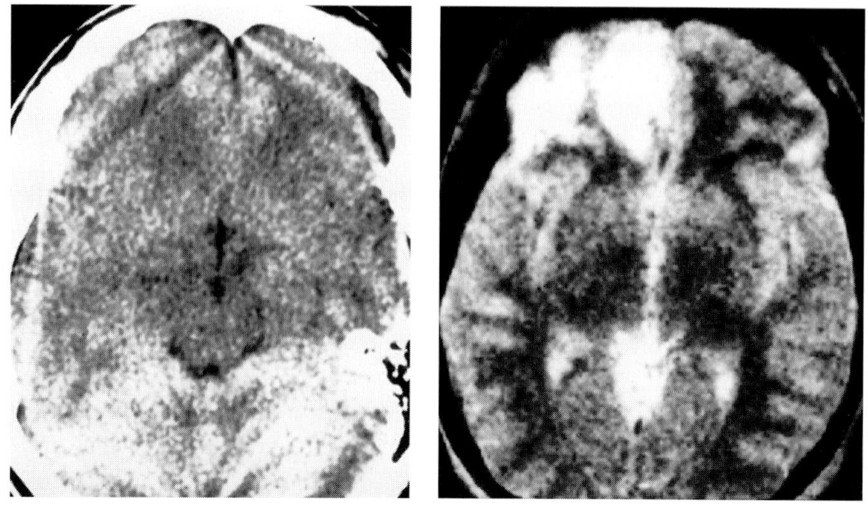

Fig. 16. **a** CT demonstrating no significant abnormality. (Image from a 0.3-T Hitachi open MR system.). **b** T2-weighted (TR 2000, TE 105) open-design MRI demonstrating extensive cerebral contusions performed on the same day as **a**. (Image from a Toshiba 0.64-T open design MR system)

cally impaired head-injured patient due to current widespread availability, speed, and accessibility. It must be recognized that the inability of CT to detect multiple types of cerebral injury has been substantiated by pathological confirmation [115, 130–132]. Acute brain injury can be more accurately assessed with MR, improving quantitative and qualitative analysis of the extent of acute brain injury. It is no longer adequate to use a normal CT scan as evidence that patients with head injury do not suffer severe neuropsychological or delayed neurological impairments as a result of undetected cerebral lesions (Fig. 16).

In the United States over half of the significant head injuries occur as a result of automobile accidents [133]. A sensitive and objective tool is necessary not only to sort out the relevance of persistent complaints when litigation is in process or pending; more importantly, alteration in medical treatment of these patients may be indicated by lesions that are undetected by CT. Patients with significant cerebral lesions may warrant closer observation, more aggressive and earlier rehabilitation efforts, and a more gradual or prolonged convalescent period, possibly even fluid restriction [111].

In determining the value of an open-field scanner in the emergency setting, what becomes apparent is a need for a systematic approach. These patients should receive initial CT scans as soon as possible, followed by MR within the first 24 h. When MR is performed and CT scans are not available, our protocol calls for an axial T1-weighted scan. This significantly improves the detection of SAH and ICH at lower field strengths [134–136] (see Fig. 3). To accommodate the large number of cranial MR referrals from this protocol it has been necessary to establish a limited MR examination. This limited examination consists of axial proton density and T2-weighted images and is performed only when a CT scan is available from the preceding 24 h. This is charged as a combination study, and represents a 50% reduction in cost of the two examinations performed separately.

Provided a CT scan has been performed, our study indicates that MRI performed within 24 h of the initial head trauma should be adequate. It has also been demonstrated conclusively that a negative CT scan is not sufficient to exclude large contusions, shearing injury, and extra-axial fluid collection [111]. These disorders may require less acute neurosurgical or medical intervention.

The additional information provided by an MR scanner in the emergency room may alter patient care significantly. The open design system allows the management of acutely injured patients. While CT and MR are complementary in the evaluation of head trauma, MR has been demonstrated to be significantly more sensitive for a broad range of common posttraumatic brain insults [111].

Hemorrhage

The appearance of hemorrhage may be the most difficult area to understand in all of MR brain imaging. The several published studies on the appearance of blood on MR attest that there is as much disagreement as there is agreement on this topic. To a large extent this is due to the fact that field strength has been ignored when hemorrhage on MR is considered. A common pattern in the appearance of intraparenchymal hemorrhage is identifiable when the field strength of the scanner is included [136].

T1- and T2-weighted images show hyperintensity in the hyperacute stage of hemorrhage (bleeding that is less than 24 h in age). As the field strength decreases, T1 is much more hyperintense, with T2 rapidly losing intensity as the field strength increases. Hyperacute blood is therefore white on T1 at low-field strength and white on T2 at both high and low-field strengths, but not for long at higher field strengths (see Fig. 3) [76].

Aging blood becomes acute (1 day to 1 week) and loses intensity on both T1 and T2 sequences at all field strengths. At higher field strengths it becomes darker more rapidly on T1- and particularly on T2-weighted sequences. This is attributed to a combination of clot retraction and deoxyhemoglobin formation as well as red blood cell settling and packing (Fig. 17) [76].

Blood continues to age and becomes subacute (2 weeks–1 month) as it goes through several phases. Intracellular methemoglobin begins to form, and T1-weighted sequences show the blood as white (increased signal intensity or hyperintensity), while the T2 sequences show decreased signal continually (Fig. 18). Then the methemoglobin becomes extracellular as the red blood cells lyse, and blood becomes hyperintense (white) on T2 sequences also [76].

Blood is generally referred to as chronic when it becomes more than 1 month old. When it is chronic, it remains hyperintense on both T1- and T2- weighted sequences until replaced by CSF. Then it is usually hyperintense (white) on T2 and hypointense (black) on T1. Figure 19 summarizes the changes that blood goes through on MR, and illustrates the effect of field strength on the appearance of blood over time. For the most part, blood exhibits the exact same changes at all field strengths, with a more rapid time course at lower field strengths. This can be summarized on T1 and T2 sequences in the following manner and visualized in Fig. 19.

On T1, blood begins as hyperintense (especially on low field) where this increased signal persists much longer than at high field) and decreases rapidly to hypointensity. During this same time T2 sequences show acute blood also going from hyper- to hypointense but decreasing to a much lower intensity on T2 (black blood) as compared to the signal decrease on T1. This process

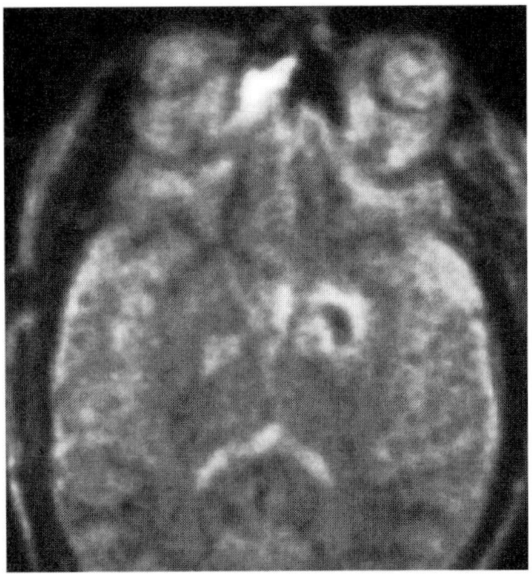

Fig. 17. T2 MRI (TR 2000, TE 105) demonstrating decreased signal intensity in a hemorrhagic focus. (Image from a Toshiba 0.64-T open-design MR system)

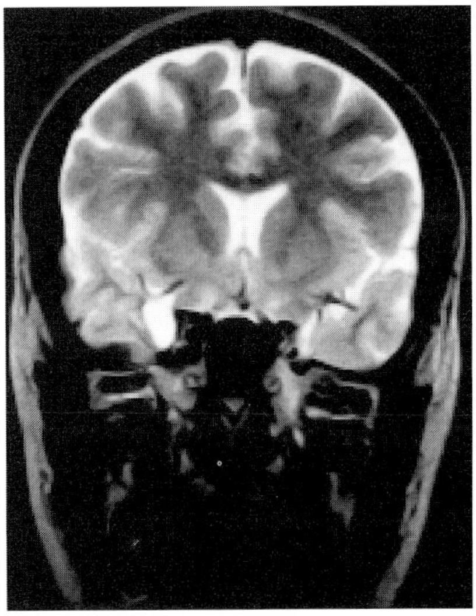

Fig. 18. High signal intensity of methemoglobin on T2 sequence (TR 3900, TE 117) resulting from an aneurysm. (Image from a 0.3 T Hitachi open MR system)

of signal loss represents well oxygenated intact red blood cells (hyperintense on T1 and T2) going through a process of oxygen loss, red cell dehydration, and clot formation with clot retraction (hypointense on T1 and T2). At this stage the deoxyhemoglobin in the retracted clot filled with dehydrated cells appears of low signal on T1 and black on T2. As methemoglobin begins to form in the intact red blood cells, T1 signal increases until the lesion begins to appear hyperintense (white) while on T2 the lesion remains hypointense (black). With lysis of the red blood cells, free methemoglobin forms, and this is hyperintense on both T1 and T2. The lesion is now there-

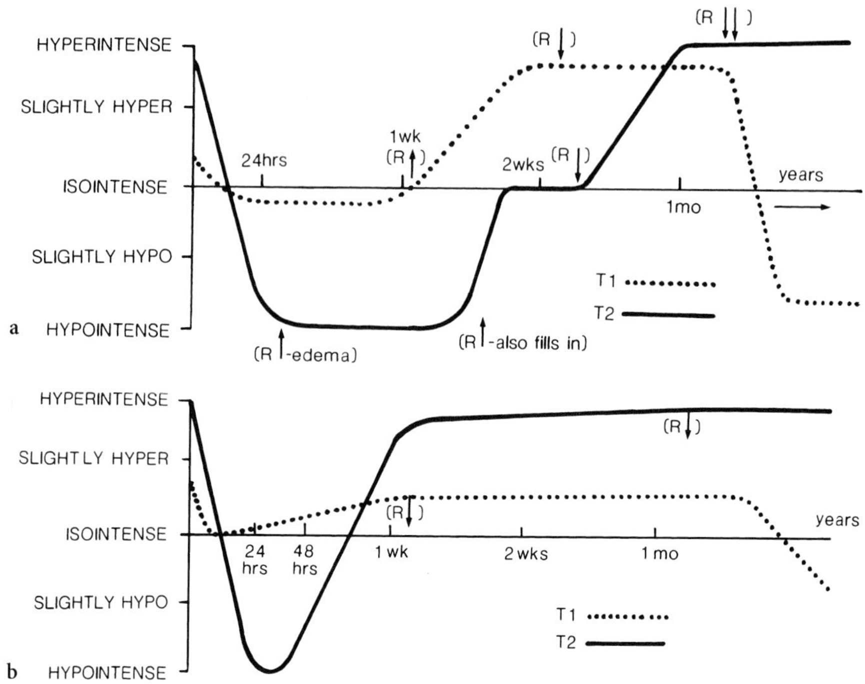

Fig. 19. **a** Graph indicating the temporal pattern of hemorrhage at high field (*R*, rim of lesion). **b** Graph indicating the temporal pattern of hemorrhage as seen on low-field open-design systems (*R*, rim of lesion)

fore white on both T1 and T2. A hemosiderin ring forms around both T1 and T2 but is far more evident on T2 as the blood ages. Finally, if replaced by CSF, the lesion is hypointense on T1 but remains hyperintense on T2.

In conclusion, definite temporal patterns for the evolution of hemorrhage exist. The variability that is so marked and observed in hemorrhages can be explained by several factors including time, biochemical change, and structural alterations in the evolving hematoma [136]. The patterns identified above can aid in the approach, identification, and final diagnosis of an intracranial hemorrhage [136]. In time the heterogeneity in the appearance of hemorrhage may provide insight into the pathophysiological changes occurring in the brain.

White Matter Disease

MR is the most effective imaging technique with regards to white matter disease. White matter disease may be classified as either demyelinating or dysmyelinating. The term dysmyelinating disease is used to describe a group of conditions in which there is a lack of normal myelin (white matter) formulation in the brain. Conditions such as metachromatic leukodystrophy, Krabbe's disease (globoid cell leukodystrophy), Canavan's disease (spongiform leukodystrophy), Alexander's disease (fibrinoid leukodystrophy), and adrenal leukodystrophy are examples of dysmyelinating disease. All of these disorders have in common a lack or delay in the formation of normal white matter that results in severe neurological abnormalities and/or early death [138].

In contrast to the dysmyelinating diseases, where no normal myelin forms, demyelinating conditions are diseases in which there is a loss of normally formed myelin. These are commonly referred to as primary or secondary. Primary demyelinating diseases are those that destroy the myelin sheath, tend to spare other parts of the nervous system such as nerve cells and supporting structures, and demonstrate a relative lack of wallerian degeneration [139–141]. Secondary refers to conditions that may result in a loss of myelin, and this category includes ischemia, anoxia, infection, toxic agents, and diseases of unknown etiology (Fig. 20). The term "white matter disease" could include most diseases of the central nervous system, when it is used in reference to secondary demyelinating processes [139–145].

Multiple sclerosis (MS) is the most common condition that results in the loss of normally formed myelin [138, 146] (Fig. 21). While the cause of MS remains unknown, it is believed to involve autoimmune-mediated demyelination in

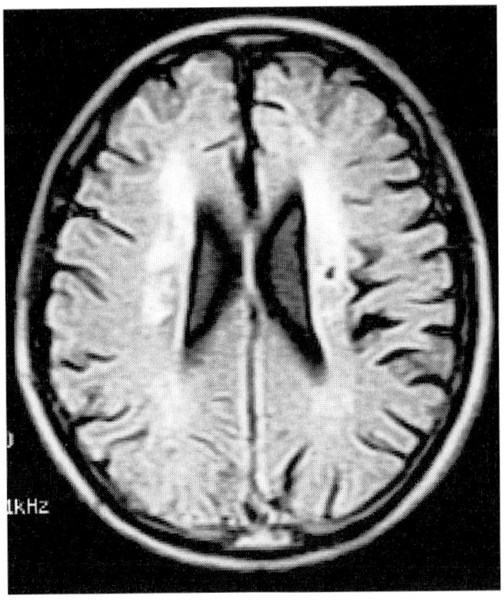

Fig. 20. FLAIR image (TR 5500, TE 112, TI 1550) demonstrating periventricular and subcortical white matter disease on a GE 0.2-T open MRI system

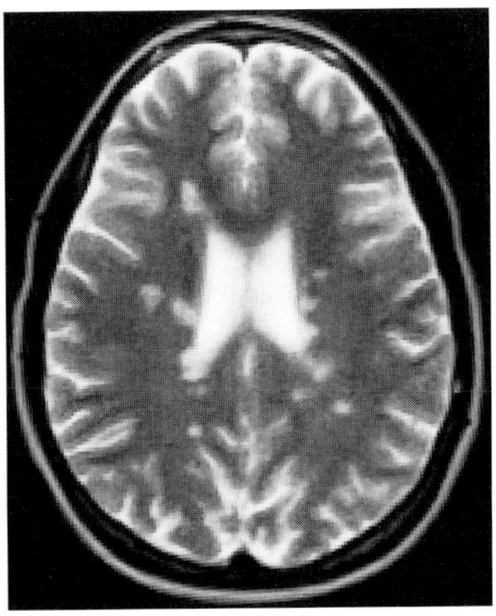

Fig. 21. Axial T2-weighted MR (TR 5605, TE 117) of MS plaques from a 0.2-T Siemens open MR system. (Donald Schnapf, DO, York Imaging Center, Pennsylvania, used with permission)

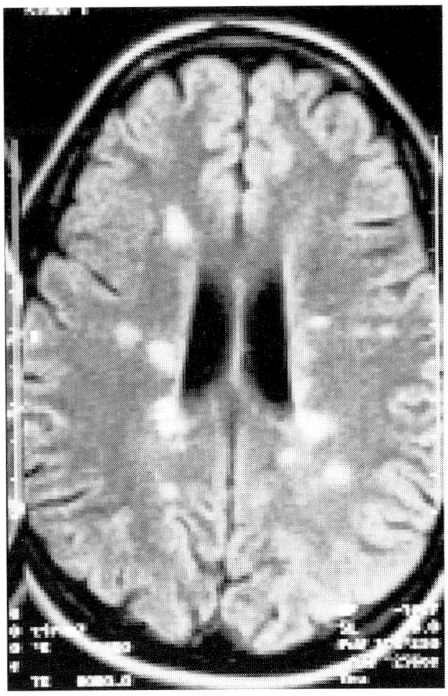

Fig. 22. A FLAIR image (TR 6000, TE 93) demonstrating "Dawson's fingers" from a 0.2-T Siemens scanner. (Donald Schnapf, DO, York Imaging Center, Pennsylvania, used with permission)

genetically susceptible individuals [146–150]. The role of inheritance is not understood, even though an increased incidence of subclinical demyelination has been demonstrated in asymptomatic first-order relatives of MS patients [148]. Patients with this disease present with highly variable forms of clinical presentation; indeed, it is the broad variety of neurological symptoms that occur at different times that often lead to a suspicion of MS.

A prospective 2-year study demonstrated the sensitivity of MRI in detecting MS to be nearly 85% and exceeding all other tests, including CT [151]. On standard MR scans most foci that are identified are clinically silent [152, 153]. Most often MS "plaques" are iso- to hypointense on T1-weighted scans and hyperintense compared to brain on T2-weighted scans (Fig. 4). In order to establish the MR diagnosis of MS most require the presence of three or more discrete lesions that are 5 mm or greater in size, as well as lesions that occur in a characteristic location and have a compatible clinical history [154, 155]. It is typical to find oblong lesions at the callososeptal interface. Also characteristic is pervenular extension into the deep white matter, the so-called Dawson's finger [155] (Fig. 22).

The MS lesions often appear as round or ovoid areas with a "beveled" (lesion within a lesion) appearance on T1- and proton density weighted studies. In severe cases confluent periventricular lesions are common (Fig. 23). In about 10% of long-standing severe MS cases, abnormal basal ganglia hypointensity is seen. Following contrast administration enhancement represents blood-brain barrier disruption. Enhancement is seen during the active dysmyelinating stage as highly variable and typically transient [138]. Solid as well as ringlike enhancement patterns are evident [156]. While most MS plaques do not enhance following contrast administration [154], enhanced T1-weighted scans can detect additional lesions that are not apparent on T2 weighted imaging

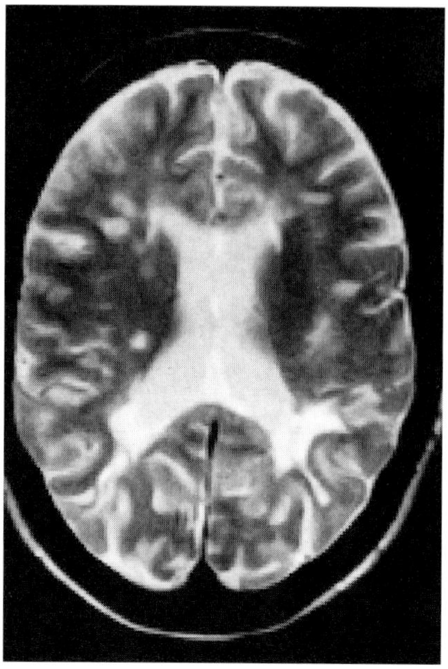

Fig. 23. A T2 MR (TR 2880, TE 90) demonstrating all features of MS including confluent periventricular lesions. (Image obtained from a 0.3-T Hitachi open MR system)

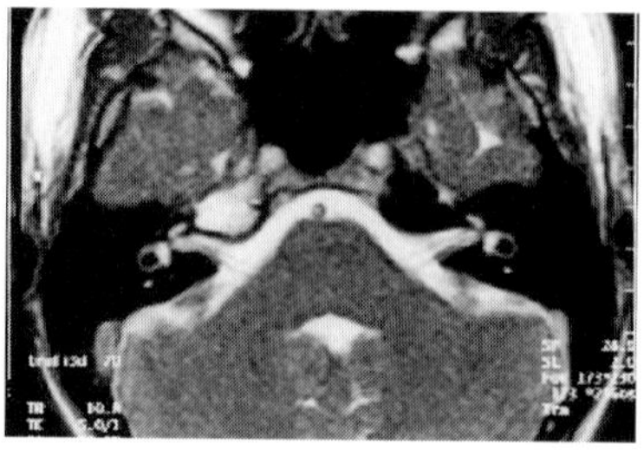

Fig. 24. Fast spin echo sequence demonstrating seventh and eighth nerves on a 0.2 T Siemens open MR system. (Michael Deimling, PhD, Siemens, Erlangen, Germany, used with permission)

[152]. Certain solitary or very atypical MS lesions may be indistinguishable from abscess or neoplasm [157, 158].

Optic neuritis particularly and other cranial neuropathies are common in patients with MS. On T2-weighted imaging lesions in the brainstem tracts and nuclei are seen, whereas contrast-enhanced T1-weighted studies may delineate enhancement in the nerves themselves. What proves useful in separating optic nerve enhancement from high-signal orbital fat are fat-saturation and short-inversion recovery scans [159]. The use of black CSF techniques or FLAIR results in white lesions against a black CSF signal that makes missing the lesions nearly impossible (see Figs. 2, 13, 20, 22).

Imaging of internal auditory canal and pituitary structures were in the past limited to high-field systems. However, imaging of these regions is now readily accomplished using open-design low-field scanners (see Figs. 5, 6, 24).

■ Pituitary Imaging

Improved tissue contrast and multiplanar capability make MR the preferred imaging method for evaluating patients with suspected sellar and parasellar abnormalities. In patients with symptoms or signs of pituitary dysfunction or visual field deficits MR is the primary imaging modality, while coronal CT remains the diagnostic imaging method of choice in patients in whom an MR study is contraindicated. The following protocols have been successfully employed at field strengths from 0.6 to 1.5 T for the evaluation of the pituitary. Routine dynamic scanning has been performed regardless of field strength with scans being initiated after IV injection of a bolus of 0.1 mmol/kg gadolinium DTPA. A CT dynamic protocol has also been included here for the rare patient in whom MR is contraindicated.

Protocol: Pituitary High-Field MR (Siemens)

1. Sagittal localizer.
2. T1 coronal dynamic (begin when Gd bolus is started): TR 1200 TE 1 matrix 128×256, FOV 300, thickness 3 mm, ACQ 1, slices 5 (×8), time 29 s ×8.
3. T1 coronal routine: TR 300 TE 15 matrix 192×256, FOV 300, thickness 3 mm, ACQ 4, slices 10 (4 min).
4. Routine T1 sagittal: TR 700, TE 15, matrix 256×256, FOV 240, thickness 5 mm, ACQ 2, slices 23 (6 min).
5. Proton density and T2 axial: TR 2500, TE 22/90 matrix 192×256, FOV 240, thickness 5 mm, ACQ 1, slices 20 (8 min).

Protocol: Pituitary High-Field MR (GE)

1. Sagittal localizer.
2. T1 coronal dynamic (begin when Gd bolus is started): TR 32, TE 6, FA 20 (SPGR), matrix 256×128, FOV 240, thickness 3 mm, ACQ 2 (2 slice locations), single-slice technique, time-25 s (per slice) ×8 (sequence time 1 min; scan time 5 min).
3. T1-coronal routine: TR 600, TE 12, matrix 256×128, FOV 160, thickness 3 mm, ACQ 4, slices 14 (5 min).
4. Routine T1 sagittal: TR 600, TE 12 matrix 256×128, FOV 160, thickness 3 mm, ACQ 4, slices 14 (5 min).

5. Proton density and T2 axial: TR 2800, TE 30/100, matrix 256×192, FOV 200, thickness 5 mm, ACQ 0.075, slices 20 (7 min).

Protocol: Pituitary Open Low-Field MR (Toshiba)
1. Center the pituitary gland by scout view or fluoro-mode.
2. Three-axis locator (scout view).
3. TR 150, TE 30, matrix 256×256, FOV 125, thickness 10 mm, ACQ 1, slices-1 (×8) time 38 s (×8).
4. T1 coronal routine: TR 110, TE 15, FA 60, matrix 256×256, FOV 110, thickness 2.5 mm, ACQ 2, slices 16 (9 min, 56 s).
5. Reconstruct coronal, sagittal, and axial planes at 1.25 mm, film at 4× magnification.

Protocol: Pituitary Open Low-field MR (Picker)
1. Center the pituitary gland by scout view or fluoro-mode.
2. T1 coronal dynamic TR 250, TE 15, FA 35, matrix 25/256, FOV 300, thickness 3 mm, ACQ 1, slices 1×5, time 1:04 (×5).
3. Reconstruct sagittal and axial planes.

Protocol: Coronal Sellar CT
1. Position patient supine with head at maximum extension with shoulder elevation.
2. Scout view.
3. Gantry tilt 140° posterior or true coronal plane.
4. Program dynamic technique (8–13 slices as required for pituitary fossa).
5. Bolus with 40 g iodinated contrast.
6. Begin scanning with thinnest slices as rapidly as possible through the pituitary fossa.
7. Following dynamic scan, repeat high-resolution coronal CT.
8. Photograph at 2× magnification.
9. Reconstruct sagittal and axial images.
10. Measure gland height at stalk and at maximum size.

A wide variety of pathological processes have been described in the sellar and parasellar region [160–163].

The abnormal finding that is most striking on both dynamic and routine neuroimaging of the pituitary gland is a focal defect in the gland following contrast administration. The diagnosis is frequently that of a pituitary adenoma, when this finding is combined with other abnormalities of the gland (Fig. 25) [164]. A pituitary adenoma, clinically categorized as functioning or nonfunctioning, may be defined as a benign neoplasm of the anterior pituitary gland (adenohypophysis). Radiologically an adenoma is described as a microadenoma or macroadenoma based on size. A microadenoma is less than 10 mm in diameter and a macroadenoma is greater than 10 mm in diameter. More often the microadenomas are functioning and typically secrete prolactin, growth hormone, or ACTH. Macroadenomas, less often functioning, are more likely to present with neurological signs and symptoms from mass effect on the optic chiasm or cranial nerves (Fig. 26) [164–166]. Prior to contrast enhancement macroadenomas can be expected to demonstrate isointensity or hyperintensity relative to cerebral gray matter. Signal inhomogeneity may present as a result of tumor necrosis, cyst formation, or hemorrhage. Minimal to moderate enhancement is typical following the administration of gadolinium on MR. The objective of an MR examination is primarily to evaluate possible suprasellar or parasellar extension, even though these lesions are readily identifiable without contrast in many instances. It is possible to best evaluate compression of the optic chiasm, invasion of the cavernous sinuses, or extension into the sphenoid sinus following administration of intravenous contrast by MR. The possibility of an aneurysm should be indicated by the presence of a large flow void on MR, and MR angiography can be performed at the same setting.

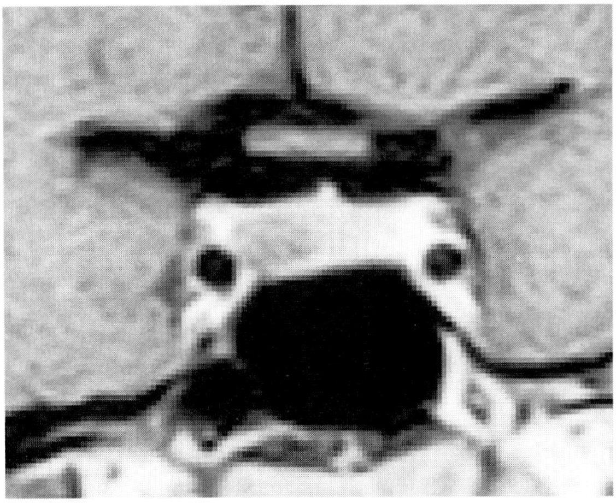

Fig. 25. A T1 postcontrast MR (TR 472, TE 26) demonstrating a pituitary microadenoma identified as a focal area of decreased signal within the enhancing pituitary gland. (Image from a 0.2-T Siemens open MR system. Mark Leszczynski, RT, Memorial Open MRI, Houston, Texas, used with permission)

Findings most commonly encountered in the evaluation of microadenomas, which may be common to both microadenomas and macroadenomas, include: (a) focal defect in the gland follow-

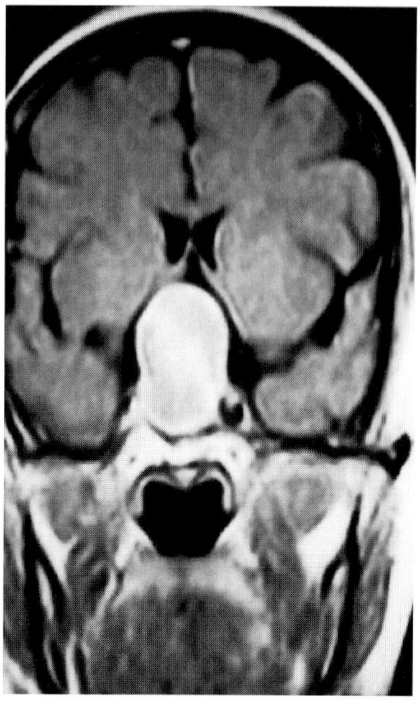

Fig. 26. T1-weighted MR (TR 68, TE 24, FA 30) postgadolinium contrast enhancement demonstrating a pituitary macroadenoma. (Image from on a 0.64-T Toshiba open design MR system)

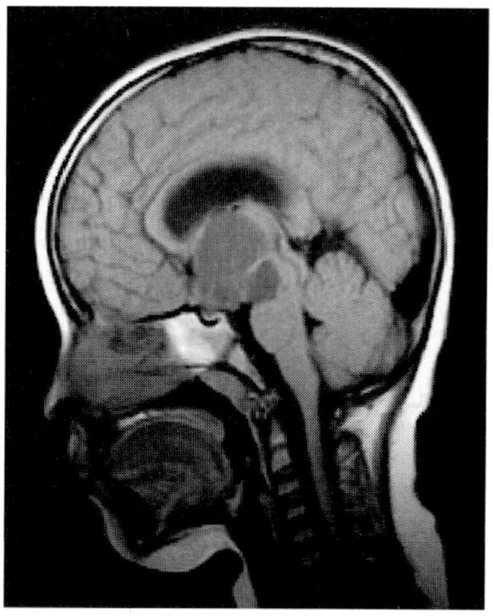

Fig. 27. T1-weighted MR (TR 600, TE 30) demonstrating a large suprasellar cystic mass. (Image from a 0.35-T Fonar MR system)

ing contrast enhancement (particularly evident on dynamic images), (b) upward convexity of the superior margin of the pituitary gland, (c) asymmetric gland enlargement, (d) increased gland height, (e) stalk deviation, and (f) focal erosion of the floor of the sella (often difficult to appreciate on MR). When more of the findings are present, there is a greater likelihood of pituitary adenoma. However, as stated above, the strongest indicator of pituitary microadenoma is a focal region of hypointensity following contrast administration [164, 165, 167–169].

A precursor of pituitary adenoma may be represented by pituitary hyperplasia. Pituitary hyperplasia or hypertrophy may be the result of normal hormonal influences occurring during early development, puberty, and pregnancy [170, 171]. Abnormal extrapituitary influences may also result in pituitary hyperplasia, occurring as a result of bronchial carcinomas, islet cell tumors, and carcinoid tumors, for example [172]. Following contrast enhancement pituitary hyperplasia demonstrates a uniformly enlarged and enhancing gland without evidence of a focal defect. In a uniformly enlarged pituitary gland, dynamic images are particularly valuable in excluding a focal defect.

The location of craniopharyngiomas may be both intrasellar and suprasellar [161, 167, 173]. Craniopharyngiomas arise from squamous epithelial clefts of Rathke's pouch and are slowly growing benign neoplasms. These tumors present primarily in children or young adults, but may also be seen in middle or later age groups. These neoplasms contain both cystic and solid components with the cystic areas containing cholesterol or blood. The signal intensity of the cystic component is variable on MR but may also be hyperintense as a result of cholesterol or blood. Cystic regions are typically hypodense on CT. Craniopharyngiomas are most often heterogeneous, and this is not related to location [161, 167, 173] (Fig. 27).

In addition to adenomas and craniopharyngiomas, tumors such as meningiomas, metastatic disease, gliomas, lymphomas, pinealomas, choristomas, dermoids, epidermoids, teratomas, and lipomas also occur in this location.

A sella that is partially or completely filled with cerebrospinal fluid is referred to as an "empty sella." Frequently the gland is small and positioned posteriorly and inferiorly against the sellar floor. An empty sella is rarely accompanied by endocrine dysfunction or an associated pituitary adenoma.

■ Diagnostic Yield and Reader Experience

Diagnostic efficacy is considered of primary importance in the evaluation of any imaging modality. This remains a concern regardless of other issues that may be involved, including risk and cost. Therefore imaging systems that may offer a significant reduction in cost and risk would generally be considered of little value unless at least an acceptable level of diagnostic efficacy had been demonstrated. Well-controlled and blinded studies have shown similar diagnostic accuracy for low, middle-, and high-field MR systems [174].

The development of MRI has been paralleled with controversy regarding optimum field strength since the first clinical applications of MR in 1982 [175, 176]. After more than 15 years of continued research and clinical use this issue remains unresolved [175–178]. In a study comparing the diagnostic efficacy of MRI at 0.064 T with CT and with MRI at 1.5 T in cranial central nervous system disease, statistical measurements of sensitivity, specificity, and reader confidence were addressed [179].

The results from this study indicate that the difference in diagnostic capability of MR imagers at field strengths of 0.064 and 1.5 T is small for most central nervous system diseases and between 0% and 10% in most cases. Many additional factors must be considered when evaluating diagnostic accuracy for clinical care, including the radiologist's experience, the patient population, availability of the clinical history, and effective use of the MR imager, which includes thoroughness of the examination, appropriate use of pulse sequences, and use of MRI contrast material. Instead of establishing the superiority of one imaging system, technique, or field strength, research generally demonstrates that each system provides diagnostically valuable images, and that it is critical to know how to use each system to its best advantage [175, 176, 180–188].

It is important to include consideration not only of the quality of the images but the clinical history of the patient and the capability of the radiologist when assessing diagnostic accuracy. In the above study an incomplete or inadequate history accounted for as much as 100% loss in sensitivity in the category of abscess or infection. We found as much as 15% loss of diagnostic sensitivity as a result of variations in reader capability, diligence, and attention. Therefore issues such as history and reader variability accounted for far more than scanner type in missed diagnoses. Radiologists and physicians in a competitive environment are aware that quality of interpretation, availability of comparative studies, direct and complete clinical history, and radiological training have measureless influence on individual patient care. Issues of quality assurance have been partly deflected by the predominant focus on type of imager and field strength with those issues that actually make the most clinical difference avoided. In other words, both the literature and common experience confirm that no amount of scanner improvements can account for inherent deficiencies in the physician reading the scan.

While inherent scanner limitations do exist, there appear to be little in the way of diagnostic differences between high- and low-field MR images. The specificity of low-field MRI and even CT may be substantially superior to that with high-field MRI in some cases [179].

The literature indicates that bore-type high-field and open-design low-field MR imagers are diagnostically equivalent for detection of central nervous system disease [189]. Many additional factors must be considered when evaluating this conclusion, such as the experience of the radiologist, the type of patient being evaluated, the availability of appropriate history, maximum utilization of the MR scanner, length of the study, and patient safety. Literature studies have generally found that most imaging systems provide diagnostically valuable information at varying field strengths and for a broad range of diseases [1–5, 12, 136, 189–195].

It is not surprising that differences in reader interpretation and the effect of information such as appropriate clinical history are more significant than the diagnostic imaging modality utilized. However, time, cost-effectiveness, and safety are additional factors that should be considered in MR applications.

Even the most technologically advanced and sophisticated imaging technology has serious limitations. We must continue to recognize a patient's uniqueness and the distinctiveness of each individual's condition. Each person's brain is capable of markedly different physiological and functional responses to the presence of pathology; this may significantly influence treatment outcomes and options. Open design MR systems provide yet another tool to assist in the care of our wonderfully complex patients.

■ References

1. Lotz H, Ekelund L, Hietala SO, Wickman G (1988) Low-field (0.02) MR imaging of the whole body. J Comput Assist Tomogr 12 (6):1006–1013
2. Seppon RE, Sipponen JT, Sivula A (1985) Low-field (0.02) nuclear magnetic resonance imaging of the brain. J Comput Assist Tomogr 9:237–241
3. Sipponen JT, Sepponen RE, Tantu JL, Sivula A (1985) Intracranial hematomas studied by MR imaging at 0.17 and 0.02 T. J Comput Assist Tomogr 9:698–704
4. Kormano M, Raininko R, Katevuo K (1987) Magnetic resonance imaging of intracranial neoplasms at 0.02 T. Acta Radiol 28:369–374
5. Barfuss H, Fisher H, Hentschel D et al (1988) Whole-body MR imaging and spectroscopy with a 4-T system. Radiology 169:811–816
6. Mitchell MD (1996) Efficacy studies of low-field-strength MR imaging: feast or famine. Radiology 200 (1):284

7. Drejer J, Thomsen HS, Tanttu J (1995) Low-field imaging of the spine: a comparative study of a traditional and a new, completely balanced gradient-echo sequence. Acta Radiol 36:505–509
8. Fagerlund M, Björnebrink, Elelund L, Toolanen G (1992) Ultra low field MR imaging of cervical spine involvement in rheumatoid arthritis. Acta Radiol 33 (2):89–92
9. Hittmair K, Turetschek K, Gomiscek G, Stiglbauer R, Schurawitzki H (1996) Field strength dependence of MRI contrast enhancement: phantom measurements and application to dynamic breast imaging. Br J Radiol 69 (819):215–220
10. Friedman DP, Rosetti GF, Flanders AE, Piccoli C, Rao VM, Mitchell DG et al (1995) MR imaging: quality assessment method and ratings at 33 centers. Radiology 196 (1):219–226
11. Ignelzi RJ (1993) The potential role of low field MR with open design in assessing ligamentous injury in acute cervical trauma. Surg Neurol 39:519–529
12. Kent LD, Larson EB (1988) Magnetic resonance imaging of the brain and spine. Ann Intern Med 108:402–424
13. Cooper LS, Chalmers TC, McCally M, Berrier J, Sacks HS (1988) The poor quality of early evaluations of magnetic resonance imaging. JAMA 259:3277–3280
14. Margulis AR (1988) About articles of judgment. Radiology 169:576–577
15. Freiherr G, Stephenson GM (1990) Indifference to safety heightens MR risks. Diagn Imaging 12 (6):79–83
16. New PFJ, Rosen BR, Brady TJ et al (1983) Potential hazards and artifacts of ferromagnetic and nonferromagnetic surgical and dental materials and devices in nuclear magnetic resonance imaging. Radiology 147:139–148
17. Koenig SH, Brown RD, Adams D, Emerson D, Harrison CG (1984) Magnetic field dependence on 1/T1 in tissue. Invest Radiol 19:76–81
18. Rinck PA, Fischer HW, Elst LV, Van Haverbeke Y, Muller RN (1988) Field cycling relaxometry: medical applications. Radiology 168:843–849
19. Kaufman L, Arakawa M, Hale J, Rothschild P, Carlson J, Hake K, Kramer D, Lu W, Van Heteren J (1989) Accessible magnetic resonance imaging. Magn Reson Q 5:283–297
20. Duffy KR, Spiller M, Lansen TA, Rifkinson-Mann S, Valsamis MP, Koenig SH, Kasoff SS, Brown RD, Tenner M (1992) Very low magnetic field strengths differentiate secreting from non-secreting pituitary adenomas. Proceedings of the 1992 meeting of the American Association of Neurological Surgeons, pp 334–335
21. Tsuchiya K, Mizutani Y, Hachiya J (1996) Preliminary evaluation of fluid-attenuated inversion-recovery MR in the diagnosis of intracranial tumors. AJNR Am J Neuroradiol 17:1081–1086
22. Kanal E, Shellock FG (1998) Magnetic resonance: bioeffects and safety. In: Orrison WW Jr (ed) Neuroimaging. Saunders, Philadelphia (in press)
23. Sell J. Contrast agents in neuroradiology. In: Orrison WW Jr (ed) Neuroimaging. Saunders, Philadelphia (in press)
24. Oksendal A, Hals P (1993) Biodistribution and toxicity of MR imaging contrast media. J Magn Reson Imaging 3:157–165
25. Harpur E, Worah D, Hals P, Holtz E, Furuhama K, Nomura H (1993) Preclinical safety assessment and pharmacokinetics of gadodiamide injection, a new magnetic resonance imaging contrast agent. Invest Radiol 28:S280–S343
26. Tweedle M, Eaton S, Eckelman W et al (1988) Comparative chemical structure and pharmacokinitics of MRI contrast agents. Investigative Radiology 23 [Suppl 1]:S236–S239
27. Tweedle M (1992) Physiochemical properties of gadoteridol and other magnetic resonance contrast agents. Invest Radiol 27 [Suppl 1]:S2–S6
28. Watson A, Rocklage S, Carvlin M (1991) Contrast media. In: Stark D, Bradley W (eds) Magnetic resonance imaging. Mosby, St Louis
29. McLachlan S, Lucas M, DeSimone D et al (1992) Worldwide safety experience with gadoteriodol injection (ProHance). In: Book of abstracts. Society of Magnetic Resonance in Medicine, p 1426
30. LaFlore J. Goldstein H, Rogan R, Keelan T, Ewell A (1989) A prospective evaluation of adverse experiences following the administration of Magnevist (gadopentetate dimeglumine) injection. In: Book of abstracts. Society of Magnetic Resonance in Medicine, p 1067
31. Niendorf H, Dinger J, Haustein J, Cornelius I, Alhassan A, Claub W (1991) Tolerance data of Gd-DTPA: a review. Eur J Radiol 13:15–20
32. Takebayashi S, Sugiyama M, Nagase M, Matsubara S (1990) Severe adverse reaction to IV gadopentetate dimeglumine. Am J Roentgenol 14:912–913
33. Shellock FG, Hahn P, Mink JH, Itskovich E (1993) Adverse reaction to intravenous gadoteridol. Radiology 189:1–2
34. Salonen O (1990) Case of anaphylaxis and four cases of allergic reaction following Gd-DTPA administration. J Comput Assist Tomogr 14:912–913
35. Tishler S, Hoffman JC (1990) Anaphylactoid reactions to IV gadopentetate dimeglumine. Am J Neuroradiol 11:1167
36. Tardy B, Guy C, Barral G. Page Y, Ollagnier M, Bertrand C (1992) Anaphylactic shock induced by intravenous gadopentetate dimeglumine. Lancet 339:494
37. Omohundro J, Elderbrook M, Ringer T (1992) Laryngospasm after administration of gadopentetate dimeglumine. J Magn Reson Imaging 1:729–730
38. Chan C, Bosanko C, Wang A (1989) Pruritis and paraesthesia after IV adminstration of Gd-DTPA. Am J Neuroradiol 10:S53
39. McAlister V, Kissane J (1990) The effect of Gd-dimeglumine on subcutaneous tissues: a study with rats. Am J Neuroradiol 11:325–327
40. Cohan R, Elder RA, z et al (1991) Extravascular toxicity of two magnetic resonance contrast agents: preliminary experience in the rat. Invest Radiol 26:224–226
41. Kanal E, Applegate G, Gillen C (1990) Review of adverse reactions, including anaphylaxis, in 5260 cases receiving Gadolinium-DTPA by bolus injection. Radiology 177 (P):159
42. Harbury O (1991) Generalized seizure after IV gadopentetate dimeglumine. Am J Neuroradiol 12:666
43. Harpur E, Worah D, Halls P, Holtz E, Furuhama K, Nomura H (1993) Preclinical safety assessment and pharmacokinetics of gadodiamide injection, a new magnetic resonance imaging contrast agent. Invest Radiol 28:S280
44. Elster AD (1994) Questions and answers in magnetic resonance imaging. Mosby Year Book, St Louis
45. Hadford DJ, Orrison WW Jr, Stimac GK, Kelsey CA (1989) Ultra low-field gd-DTPA-enhanced MR imaging: dosage and administration. Radiology 173 (P):255
46. Freiherr G, Stephenson GM (1990) Indifference to safety heightens MR risks. Diagn Imaging 12 (6):79–83
47. Bieze J (1992) Careful patient screening crucial to MRI safety. Diagn Imaging 57/58:63
48. FDA receives reports of burns caused by MRI scanning units (1992) Radiol Today 9:1
49. Klucznik RP, Carrier DA, Pyka R, Haid RW (1993) Placement of a ferromagnetic intracerebral aneurysm clip in a magnetic field with a fatal outcome. Radiology 187:855–856
50. Kelley W, Paglen PG, Pearson JA, San Diego AG, Soloman MA (1986) Ferromagnetism of intraocular foreign body causes unilateral blindness after MR study. AJNR 7:234–245

51. FDA Magnetic resonance diagnostic device (1988) Panel recommendation and report on petitions for MR reclassification. Fed Reg 53:7575–7579
52. Sheldon P, Kaufman L, Carlson J (1991) Forces and torques produced by a 640-Gauss permanent magnet on ferromagnetic objects. J Neuroimaging 1:184–190
53. Shellock FG, Crues JV (1988) MRI: safety considerations in magnetic resonance imaging. MRI 2:25–30
54. Shellock FG (1989) Biological effects and safety aspects of magnetic resonance imaging. Magn Reson Q 5:243–261
55. Kanal E, Talagala L, Shellock FG (1990) Safety considerations in MR imaging. Radiology 176:593–606
56. Lund G, Nelson JD, Wirtschafter JD et al (1986) Tatooing of eyelids: magnetic imaging artifacts. Opthamic Surg 17:550–553
57. Sacco DA, Steiger DA, Bellon EM et al (1987) Artifacts caused by cosmetics in MR imaging of the head. Am J Roentgenol 148:1001–1004
58. Jackson JG, Acker JD (1987) Permanent eyeliner and MR imaging. Am J Roentgenol 149:1080
59. Pusey E, Lufkin RB, Brown RKJ et al (1986) Magnetic resonance imaging artifacts: mechanism and clinical significance. Radiographics 6:891–911
60. Kelly WM, Pagle PG, Pearson A et al (1986) Ferromagnetism of intraocular foreign body causes unilateral blindness after MR study. Am J Neuroradiol 7:243–245
61. Shellock FG, Kanal E (1991) Policies, guidelines, and recommendations for MR imaging safety and patient management. J Magn Reson Imaging 1:97–101
62. Kelsey CA, King JN, Keck GM, Chiu MT et al (1991) Ocular hazard of metallic fragments during MR imaging at 0.064 T. Radiology 180:282–283
63. Hayes DL, Holmes DR, Gray JE (1987) Effect of a 1.5 tesla nuclear magnetic resonance imaging scanner on implanted permanent pacemakers. J Am Coll Cardiol 10:782–786
64. Erlebacher JA, Cahill PT, Pannizzo F, Knowles JR (1986) Effect of magnetic resonance imaging on DDD pacemakers. Am J Cardiol 57:437–440
65. Kanal E, Shellock F (1993) MR imaging of patients with intracranial aneurysm clips. Radiology 187:612–614
66. Kanal E, Shellock F (1994) The value of published data regarding MR compatibility of metallic implants and devices. Am J Neuroradiol 15:1394–1396
67. Flaherty JA, Hoskinson K (1989) Emotional distress during magnetic resonance imaging. N Engl J Med 320:467–468
68. Fishbain DA, Goldberg M, Labbe E et al (1988) Long-term claustrophobia following magnetic resonance imaging. Am J Psychiatry 145:1038–1039
69. Quirk ME, Letendre AJ, Ciottone RA et al (1989) Anxiety in patients undergoing MR imaging. Radiology 170:463–466
70. Quirk ME, Letendre AJ, Ciottone RA et al (1989) Evaluation of three psychological interventions to reduce anxiety during MR imaging. Radiology 173:759–762
71. Hricak H, Amparo EG (1984) Body MRI: alleviation of claustrophobia by prone positioning. Radiology 152:819
72. Weinreb JC, Maravilla KR, Peshock R et al (1984) Magnetic resonance imaging: improving patient tolerance and safety. Am J Roentgenol 143:1285–1287
73. Klonoff EA, Janata JW, Kaufman B (1986) The use of systematic desensitization to overcome resistance to magnetic resonance imaging (MRI) scanning. J Behav Ther Exp Psychiatry 17:189–192
74. Granet RB, Belber LJ (1990) Claustrophobia during MR imaging. N J Med 87 (6):479–482
75. Phelps LA (1990) MRI and claustrophobia. Am Fam Physician 42 (4):930
76. Woodward P, Orrison WW Jr (1997) MRI optimization: a hands-on approach. McGraw Hill, New York
77. Orrison WW Jr, Sanders JA (1995) Clinical brain imaging: computerized axial tomography and magnetic resonance imaging. In: Orrison WW, Jr, Lewine JD, Sanders JA, Hartshorne MF (eds) Functional brain imaging. Mosby Year Book, St Louis, pp 97–144
78. Haughton VM, Rimm AA, Sobocinski KA et al (1986) A blinded clinical comparison of MR imaging and CT in neuroradiology. Radiology 160:751–755
79. Osborn AG (1994) Infections of the brain and its linings. In: Osborn AG (ed) Diagnostic neuroradiology, Mosby-Year Book, Inc., St. Louis, MO, pp 673–712
80. Barkovich AJ (1990) Infections of the nervous system. In: Barkovich AJ (ed) Pediatric neuroimaging. Raven, New York, pp 293–325
81. Chang KH, Han MH, Roh JK et al (1990) Gd-DTPA-enhanced MR imaging of the brain in patients with meningitis: comparison with CT. AJNR 11:69–76
82. Chang KH, Han M-H, Roh J-K et al (1991) Gd-DTPA enhanced MR imaging in intracranial tuberculosis. Neuroradiology 238:340–344
83. Matthews VP, Kuharik MA, Edwards MK et al (1988) Gd-DTPA enhanced MR imaging of experimental meningitis: evaluation and comparison with CT. AJNR 9:1045–1050
84. Offenbacher H, Fazekas F, Schmidt R et al (1991) MRI in tuberculosis meningoencephalitis: report of four cases and review of the neuroimaging literature. J Neurol 238:340–344
85. Zimmerman RD, Weingarten K (1991) Neuroimaging of cerebral abscesses. Neuroimaging Clin North Am 1:1–16
86. Okagaki H (1989) Fundamentals of neuropathology, 2nd edn. Igaku-Shoin, New York
87. Haimes AB, Zimmerman RD, Morgello S et al (1989) MR imaging of brain abscesses. AJNR 10:279–291
88. Barloon TJ, Yuh WTC, Knepper LE et al (1990) Cerebral ventriculitis: MR findings J Comput Assist Tomogr 14:272–275
89. Bazan C III, Rinaldi MG, Rauch RR, Jinkins JR (1991) Fungal infections of the brain. Neuroimaging Clin North Am 1:57–88
90. Bowen BC, Post MJD (1991) Intracranial infection. In: Atlas SW (ed) Magnetic resonance imaging of the brain and spine. Raven, New York, pp 501–538
91. Zee C-S, Segall HD, Boswell W et al (1988) MR imaging of neurocysticercosis. J Comput Assist Tomogr 12:927–934
92. Chang KH, Cho SY, Hesselink JR et al (1991) Parasitic diseases of the central nervous system. Neuroimaging Clin North Am 1:159–178
93. Tsai M-D, Chang C-N, Ho Y-S et al (1993) Cerebral sparganosis diagnosed and treated with stereotactic techniques. J Neurosurg 78:129–132
94. Lane JI, Flanders AE, Doan HT, Bell RD (1991) Assessment of carotid artery patency in routine spin-echo MR imaging of the brain. AJNR 12:819–826
95. Osborn AG (1994) Stroke. In: Osborn AG (ed) Diagnostic neuroradiology. Mosby-Year Book, Inc., St. Louis, MO, pp 330–338
96. terPenning B (1992) Pathophysiology of stroke. Neuroimaging Clin North Am 2:389–408
97. Bryan RN (1990) Imaging of acute stroke. Radiology 177:615–616
98. Shuaib A, Lee D, Pelz D et al (1992) The impact of magnetic resonance imaging on the management of acute ischemic stroke. Neurology 42:816–818
99. Bryan RN, Levy LM, Whitlow WD et al (1991) Diagnosis of acute cerebral infarction: comparison of CT and MR imaging, AJNR 12:611–620
100. Mueller DP, Yuh WTC, Fisher DJ et al (1993) Arterial enhancement in acute cerebral ischemia: clinical and angiographic correlation. AJNR 14:661–668

101. Elster AD, Moody DM (1990) Early cerebral infarction: gadopentetate dimeglumine enhancement. Radiology 177:627–632
102. Yuh WTC, Crain MR, Loes DJ et al (1991) MR imaging of cerebral ischemia: findings in the first 24 hours. AJNR 12:621–629
103. Alberts MJ, Faulstich ME, Gray L (1992) Stroke with negative brain magnetic resonance imaging. Stroke 23:663–667
104. Elster AD (1992) Enhancement patterns in cerebral infarction. MRI 30–33
105. Asato R, Okumaura R, Konishi J (1991) "Fogging effect" in MR of cerebral infarct. J Comput Assist Tomogr 15:160–162
106. Parisi J, Place C, Nag S (1988) Calcification in a recent cerebral infarct: radiologic and pathologic correlation. Can J Neurol Sci 15:192–195
107. Lundblom N, Katevuo K, Kumo M et al (1992) T1 in subacute and chronic brain infarctions: time-dependent development. Invest Radiol 27:673–680
108. Kuhn MJ, Mikulis DJ, Ayoub DM et al (1989) Wallerian degeneration after cerebral infarction: evaluation with sequential MR imaging. Radiology 172:170–182
109. Boyko OB, Burger PC, Shelburne JD, Ingram P (1992) Non-heme mechanisms for T1 shortening: pathologic, CT, and MR elucidation. AJNR 13:1439–1445
110. Regli L, Regli F, Maeder P, Bogousslavski J (1993) Magnetic resonance imaging with gadolinium contrast in small deep (lacunar) cerebral infarcts. Arch Neurol 50:175–180
111. Orrison WW Jr, Gentry LR, Stimac GK, Tarrel RM, Espinosa MC, Cobb LC (1994) Blinded comparison of cranial CT and MR in closed head injury evaluation. AJNR Am J Neuroradiol 15:351–356
112. Zimmerman RA, Bilaniuk LT, Hackney DB, Goldberg HI, Grossman RI (1986) Head injury: early results comparing CT and high-field MR. AJNR Am J Neuroradiol 7:757–764
113. Gentry LR, Godersky JC, Thompson BH (1989) Traumatic brain stem injury: MR imaging. Radiology 171:177–187
114. Gentry LR, Godersky JC, Thompson BH (1988) MR imaging of head trauma: review of the distribution and radiopathologic features of traumatic lesions. AJNR Am J Neuroradial 9:101–110
115. Gentry LR, Godersky JC, Thompson B, Dunn VD (1988) Prospective comparative study of intermediate-field MR and CT in the evaluation of closed head trauma. AJNR Am J Neuroradiol 9:91–100
116. Han JS, Kaufman B, Alfidi RJ et al (1984) Head trauma evaluated by magnetic resonance and computed tomography: a comparison. Radiology 150:71–77
117. Hesselink JR, Dowd CF, Healy ME, Hajek P, Baker LL, Luerssen TG (1988) MR imaging of brain contusions: a comparative study with CT. AJNR Am J Neuroradiol 9:269–278
118. Gentry LR, Thompson B, Godersky JC (1988) Trauma to the corpus callosum: MR features. AJNR Am J Neuroradiol 9:1129–1138
119. Moon KL Jr, Brant-Zawadzki M, Pitts LH, Mills CM (1984) Nuclear magnetic resonance imaging of CT-isodense subdural hematomas. AJNR Am J Neuroradiol 5:319–322
120. Levin HS, Handel SF, Goldman AM, Eisenberg HM, Guinto FC (1985) Magnetic resonance imaging after "diffuse" nonmissile head injury. Arch Neurol 42:963–968
121. Langfitt TW, Obrist WD, Alavi A et al (1986) Computerized tomography, magnetic resonance imaging, and positron emission tomography in the study of brain trauma: preliminary observations. J Neurosurg 64:760–767
122. Gandy SE, Snow RB, Zimmerman RD, Deck MDF (1984) Cranial nuclear magnetic resonance imaging in head trauma. Ann Neurol 16:254–257
123. Snow RB, Zimmerman RD, Gandy SE, Deck MDF (1986) Comparison of magnetic resonance imaging and computed tomography in the evaluation of head injury. Neurosurgery 18:45–52
124. Jenkins A, Teasdale G, Hadley MDM, MacPherson P, Rowan JO (1986) Brain lesions detected by magnetic resonance imaging in mild and severe head injuries. Lancet 2:445–446
125. French BN, Dublin AB (1977) The value of computerized tomography in the management of 1000 consecutive head injuries. Surg Neurol 7:171–183
126. Zimmerman RD, Danziger A (1982) Extracerebral trauma. Radiol Clin North Am 20:105–121
127. Moseley IF, Zilkha E (1976) The role of computerized axial tomography (EMI-scanning) in the diagnosis and management of cranio-cerebral trauma. J Neuroradiol 3:277–296
128. Bricolo AP, Pasut LM (1984) Extradural hematoma: toward zero mortality. Neurosurgery 14:8–12
129. Seelig JM, Becker DP, Miller JD, Greenberg RP, Ward JD, Choi SC (1981) Traumatic acute subdural hematoma: major mortality reduction in comatose patients treated within four hours. N Engl J Med 304:1511–1518
130. Adams JF, Genneralli TA, Graham DI (1982) Brain damage in non-missile head injury observations in man and subhuman primates. In: Smith WT, Cavanagh JB (eds) Recent advances in neuropathology, vol 2. Churchill Livingstone, Edinburgh, pp 165–190
131. Adams JH, Graham DI, Scott G, Parker LS, Doyle D (1980) Brain damage in fatal non-missile head injury. J Clin Pathol 33:1132–1145
132. Cooper PR, Maravilla K, Kirkpatrick J et al (1979) Traumatically induced brain stem hemorrhage and the computerized tomographic scan: clinical pathological, and experimental observations. Neurosurgery 4:115–124
133. Baker SP (1989) Injury science comes of age (editorial). JAMA 262:2284–2285
134. Yoon HC, Lufkin RB, Vinuela F, Bentson J, Martin N, Wilson G (1988) MR of acute subarachnoid hemorrhage. AJNR Am J Neuroradiol 9:404–405
135. Janousek A (1991) Head injuries: three years experience with ultra-low-field MRI. Neuroradiology 33 [Suppl]:616–617
136. Chaney RK, Taber KH, Orrison WW, Hayman LA (1992) Magnetic resonance imaging of intracerebral hemorrhage at different field strengths. Neuroimaging Clin North Am 2:25–51
137. Atlas SW, Grossman RI, Gomori JM et al (1987) Hemorrhagic intracranial malignant neoplasms: spin-echo MR imaging. Radiology 164:71–77
138. Osborn AG (1994) Acquired metabolic, white matter, and degenerative diseases of the brain. In: Osborn AG (ed) Diagnostic neuroradiology. Mosby-Year Book, Inc., St. Louis, MO, pp 748–778
139. Escourolle R, Poirier J (1973) Pathology of the central nervous system; demyelinating diseases. Manual of basic neuropathology. Saunders, Philadelphia, pp 128–135
140. Merritt HH, Moses HL, Moses L (1979) A textbook of neurology; diseases of the myelin sheath, 6th edn. Lea and Febiger, Philadelphia, pp 767–824
141. Adams RD, Victor M (1981) Principles of neurology; multiple sclerosis and allied demyelinative diseases. McGraw-Hill, New York, pp 647–663
142. Mendes JH, Kinsbourne M, Batzdorf U, Gabriel RS, Weil ML (1974) Textbook of child neurology; heredodegenerative diseases. Lea and Febiger, Philadelphia, pp 101–113

143. Holland BA (1987) Diseases of white matter. Magnetic resonance imaging of the central nervous system. Raven, New York, pp 259–278
144. Barkovich AJ (1987) Pediatric neuroimaging; metabolic and destructive brain disorders. Raven, New York, pp 259–278
145. Leestma JE (1988) Forensic neuropathology. Raven, New York, pp 137–156
146. Edwards MK, Bonnin JM (1991) White matter diseases. In: Atlas SW (ed) Magnetic resonance imaging of the brain and spine. Raven, New York, pp 467–500
147. Merrill JE, Graves MC, Mulder DG (1992) Autoimmune disease and the nervous system: biochemical, molecular, and clinical update. West J Med 156:639–646
148. Tienari PJ, Salonen O, Wikstrom J et al (1992) Familial multiple sclerosis: MRI findings in clinically affected and unaffected siblings. J Neurol Neurosurg Psychiatr 55:883–886
149. Niebler G, Harris T, Davis T, Raos K (1992) Fulminant multiple sclerosis. AJNR 13:1547–1551
150. Kepes JJ (1993) Large focal tumor-like demyelinating lesions of the brain: intermediate entity between multiple sclerosis and acute disseminated encephalomyelitis. A study of 31 patients. Ann Neurol 33:18–27
151. Lee KH, Hashimoto SA, Hooge JP et al (1991) Magnetic resonance imaging of the head in the diagnosis of multiple sclerosis: a prospective 2-year follow-up with comparison of clinical evaluation, evoked potentials, oligoclonal banding, and CT. Neurology 41:657–660
152. Barkhof F, Scheltens P, Frequin STFM et al (1992) Relapsing-remitting multiple sclerosis: sequential enhanced MR imaging vs. clinical findings in determining disease activity. AJR 159:1041–1047
153. Capra R, Marciano N, Vignolo LA et al (1992) Gadolinium-pentetic acid magnetic resonance imaging in patients with relapsing remitting multiple sclerosis. Arch Neurol 49:687–689
154. Runge VM (1992) MRI of multiple sclerosis in the brain. MRI 2–10
155. Yetkin FZ, Haughton VM (1992) Common and uncommon manifestations of MS on MRI. MRI 13–18
156. Powell T, Sussman JG, Davies-Jones GAB (1992) MR imaging in acute multiple sclerosis: ring-like appearance in plaques suggesting the presence of paramagnetic free radicals. AJNR 13:1544–1546
157. Giang DW, Poduri KR, Eskin TA et al (1992) Multiple sclerosis masquerading as a mass lesion. Neuroradiology 34:150–154
158. Zagzag D, Miller DC, Kleinman GM et al (1993) Demyelinating disease versus tumor in surgical neuropathology. Am J Surg Pathol 17:537–545
159. Miller DH, MacManus DG, Bartlett PA et al (1993) Detection of optic nerve lesions in optic neuritis using frequency-selective fat-saturation sequences. Neuroradiology 35:156–158
160. Osborn AG (1990) MRI of the sellar/juxtasellar region. I. Intrasellar and suprasellar masses. MRI 19–30
161. Osborn AG (1991) Handbook of neuroradiology. Mosby Year Book, St Louis, pp 331–343
162. Naidich TP, Pinto RS, Kushner MJ, Lin JP, Kricheff II, Leeds NE, Chase NE (1976) Evaluation of sellar and parasellar masses by computed tomography. Radiology 120:91–99
163. Zimmerman RA (1990) Imaging of the intrasellar, suprasellar, and parasellar tumors. Semin Roentgenol 25:174–197
164. Sakamoto Y, Takahashi M, Korogi Y, Bussaka H, Ushio Y (1991) Normal and abnormal pituitary glands: gadopentetate dimeglumine-enhanced MR imaging. Radiology 178:441–445
165. Patel SC, Sanders WP (1990) MRI of the pituitary gland: adenomas. MRI 12–20
166. Tindall GT, Barrow DL (1986) Pathology of the pituitary gland. Disorders of the pituitary. Mosby, St Louis, pp 203–229
167. Johnson DE, Woodruff WW, Allen IS, Cera PJ, Funkhouser GR, Coleman LL (1991) MR imaging of the sellar and juxtasellar regions. Radiographics 11:727–758
168. Bonneville JF, Cattin F, Moussa-Bacha K, Portha C et al (1983) Dynamic computed tomography of the pituitary gland: the "Tuft sign." Radiology 149:145–148
169. Orrison WW Jr, Watridge CB, Gabatin AR, Pretorius HT, Floyd JP III et al (1983) Dynamic computed tomographic scanning of the pituitary gland. Radiology 149 (P):262
170. Tien RD, Kucharczyk J, Bessette J, Middleton M (1992) MR imaging of the pituitary gland in infants and children: changes in size, shape, and MR signal with growth and development. AJR 158:1151–1154
171. Elster AD, Chen MY, Williams DW, Key LL (1990) Pituitary gland: MR imaging of physiologic hypertrophy in adolescence. Radiology 174:681–685
172. Tindall GT, Barrow DL (1986) Acromegaly. Disorders of the pituitary. Mosby, St Louis, pp 203–229
173. Pusey E, Kortman KE, Flannigan BD, Tsuruda J, Bradley WG (1987) MR characterization. AJNR 8:439–444
174. Bradley WG Jr, Waluch V, Yadley RA, Wycoff RR (1984) Comparison of CT and MR in 400 patients with suspected disease of the brain and cervical spinal cord. Radiology 152:695–702
175. Chen CN, Sank VJ, Cohen SM, Hoult DI (1986) The field dependence of NMR imaging. I. Laboratory assessment of signal-to-noise ration and power deposition. Magn Reson Med 3:722–729
176. Loult DI, Chen CN, Sank VJ (1986) The field dependence on NMR imaging. II. Arguments concerning an optimal field strength. Magn Reson Med 3:730–746
177. A special issue on MRI (1988) Health Technol 2:20–23
178. Kaufman L, Crooks LE (1987) Field strength issues in MRI. Adm Radiol 6:17–19
179. Orrison WW Jr, Stimac GK, Stevens EA, LaMasters DL et al (1991) Comparison of CT, low-field-strength MR imaging and high-field-strength MR imaging. Work in progress. Radiology 181:121–127
180. Kent LD, Larson EB (1988) Magnetic resonance imaging of the brain and spine. Ann Intern Med 108:402–424
181. Gentry LR, Godersky JC, Thompson B, Dunn VD (1988) Prospective comparative study of intermediate-field MR and CT in the evaluation of closed head trauma. AJR 150:673–682
182. Hirsch WL Jr, Hryshko FG, Sekhar LN et al (1988) Comparison of MR imaging, CT, and angiography in the evaluation of the enlarged cavernous sinus. AJNR 9:907–915
183. Bradley WG Jr, Waluch V, Yadley RA, Wycoff RR (1984) Comparison of CT and MR in 400 patients with suspected disease of the brain and cervical spinal cord. Radiology 152:695–702
184. Brant-Zawadzki M, Davis PL, Crooks LE et al (1983) NMR demonstration of cerebral abnormalities: comparison with CT. AJNR 4:117–124
185. Han JS, Kaufman B, Alfidi RJ et al (1995) Head trauma evaluated by magnetic resonance and computed tomography: a comparison. Radiology 150:71–77
186. Hesselink JR, Dowd CF, Healy ME, Hajek P, Baker LL, Luerssen TG (1988) MR imaging of brain contusions: a comparative study with CT. AJNR 9:269–278
187. Jacobs L, Kinkel WR, Polachini I, Kinkel RP (1986) Correlations of nuclear magnetic resonance imaging, computerized tomography, and clinical profiles in multiple sclerosis. Neurology 36:27–34
188. Haughton VM, Rimm AA, Sobocinski KA et al (1986) A blinded clinical comparison of MR imaging and CT in neuroradiology. Radiology 160:751–755

189. Norman D (1987) Vascular disease: hemorrhage. In: Brant-Zawadski M, Norman D et al (eds) Magnetic resonance imaging of the central nervous system. Raven, New York, pp 209–220
190. Beers GJ, Raque GH, Wagner GG, Shields CB, Nichols GR II, Johnson JR, Meyer JE (1988) MR imaging in acute cervical spine trauma. J Comput Assist Tomogr 12 (5):755–761
191. Kerslake RW, Jaspan T, Worthington BS (1991) Magnetic resonance imaging of spine trauma. Br J Radiol 64:386–402
192. Kulkarni MV, McArdle CB, Kopanicky D, Miner M, Cotler HB, Lee KF, Harris JH (1987) Acute spinal cord injury: MR imaging at 1.5 T. Radiology 164:837–843
193. Mirvis SE, Geisler FH, Jelinek JJ, Joslyn JN, Gellad F (1988) Acute cervical spine trauma: evaluation with 1.5 T MR imaging. Radiology 166:807–816
194. Tarr RW, Drolshagen LF, Kerner TC, Allen JH, Partain CL, James AE Jr (1987) MR imaging of recent spinal trauma. J Comput Assist Tomogr 11 (3):412–417
195. Seeger LL (1989) The shoulder. In: Bassett LW, Gold RH, Seeger LL (eds) MRI atlas of the musculoskeletal system. Deutscher Ärzte Verlag, Cologne, pp 95–128

Magnetic Resonance Imaging of the Head and Neck

2

A. Borges · P. Villablanca · Y. Anzai · J. Curran
K. Blackwell · R. B. Lufkin

■ Introduction

Magnetic resonance (MR) has revolutionized head and neck imaging and has replaced computed tomography (CT) as the imaging study of choice for many lesions of the extracranial head and neck. MR easily surpasses CT in its ability to differentiate subtle differences in soft tissue boundaries in the head and neck. The beam-hardening artifacts on CT images from dental amalgam and dense cortical bone of the mandible, skull base, shoulders, and other areas are also not a problem with MR imaging. Multiplanar imaging capabilities and lack of ionizing radiation make MR the most suitable imaging technique for many diseases of the head and neck. Although CT is still essential for nonneoplastic diseases in the paranasal sinuses, inflammatory or congenital diseases in the temporal bone, and abscess search for the neck, MR is the study of choice for most head and neck tumors [1–3]. Now open MR scanners make MR even more accessible to patients with suspected pathology of the head and neck.

Head and neck cancers are often more accessible by visual inspection or palpation compared to those in the brain, chest, and abdomen. The key role of any imaging modality in most head and neck cancers is to identify deep infiltration of tumors [1–3]. Mucosal changes are for the most part best evaluated by direct inspection during physical examination. MR is a powerful tool for determination of extension of disease and relationship to the major vascular structures, which helps therapeutic planning. Blood flow and vascularity determinations can be performed with a combination of gadolinium and/or MR angiography eliminating the need for many invasive diagnostic angiographic procedures [4].

Understanding anatomy helps tremendously narrow the differential diagnosis of disease in the head and neck. Probably nowhere else in the body do anatomical boundaries provide more important clues to the etiology of a disease process. Even when the exact nature of the offending process cannot be determined, disruptions of facial planes and muscle interfaces help to define surgery or radiation therapy management of the patient.

■ Technique

Radiofrequency Coils

Surface coils greatly increase the signal to noise ratio and allow higher spatial resolution of most examinations of the area [5, 6]. Specially designed anterior neck or solenoid neck coils are now used in routine clinical practice. The use of the appropriate coil is an essential factor in head and neck MR imaging, especially in the larynx, temporal bone, and orbit. Although acceptable images of the sinuses, nasopharynx, and oropharynx may be obtained with the standard head coil, a dedicated neck coil is still necessary for staging of cervical nodal disease.

Dual phased array surface coils provide extremely high-resolution with higher signal to noise ratio compared to standard surface coils. Each phased array coil has its own preamplifier, receiver channel, and digitizer, allowing collection of data and generation of images individually and subsequent combination into a composite image [7]. This is especially valuable in MR imaging of the temporal bone. Appropriate coil selection is essential in order to obtain high quality images to improve diagnostic accuracy.

MR Pulse Sequences

High signal fat on T1-weighted images permits anatomical details to be well delineated that are often not seen on CT. T1- and T2-weighted SE images sufficiently provide excellent fat/tumor and muscle/tumor contrast, respectively. Gadolinium contrast agents are valuable in certain head and neck applications such as perineural spread or leptomeningeal invasion, depiction of tumor necrosis, cyst, and abscess. There is much less use of gadolinium in the head and neck than in the CNS. To some extent this probably reflects the fact that, unlike the brain, in the extracranial head and neck, T2-weighted tissue changes often correspond to regions of gadolinium enhancement changes. Because of abundant high signal fat, gadolinium enhancement can sometimes obscure the delineation of tumor margin. Fat suppression technique [8–10] has been investigated throughout the head and neck and is now used most consistently in the orbit.

Fast spin echo (FSE) has almost completely replaced conventional T2-weighted spin echo imaging [11, 12]. In FSE acquisition multiple refocused echoes are generated during a single TR (usually 8–16 echo trains), resulting in short scan time and better signal to noise ratio. This technique is especially useful with lower field open systems. With FSE technique image quality is improved by reducing motion artifact as well as susceptibility artifact from the air in the sinuses or airway. Contrast is manipulated through the reordering of phase encoding views so that the views with the lowest spatial frequency are obtained in the echoes nearest the desired effective echo time [13]. The drawbacks of FSE include fewer slices obtained for the same TR. A notable difference compared to routine SE in the head and neck is higher signal from fat, which is presumably due to echoes generated at the relatively short effective echo times, which still has T1-weighted contrast. In addition to some gadolinium studies, fat suppression has been applied to T2 FSE to mini-

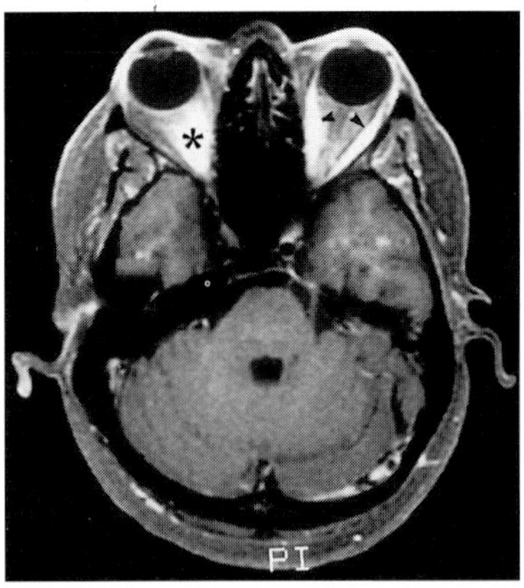

Fig. 1. Noncontrast fat suppression T1 weighted image through the orbit shows typical fat suppression failure in the inferior aspect of orbital fat (*asterisk*), immediately cranial to the maxillary sinus air. This artifact is due to focal magnetic field inhomogeneity and should not be misinterpreted as pathological

mize this effect. Fat suppression failure or undesired water suppression remains a potential problem for interpretation of those sequences [14] (Fig. 1). Careful attention should be paid not to misinterpret this artifact as a pathology.

The standard MR sequence of the head and neck should at least include T1-weighted spin echo axial and coronal images and T2-weighted imaging. Sagittal images are valuable for evaluation of the status of the preepiglottic space, base of the tongue, mastoid portion of the facial nerve, and other midline pathology. Gadolinium enhancement is useful when intracranial extension, perineural spread, or questions about necrosis or cyst are present. Fat suppression gadolinium enhanced technique is useful for the detection of perineural extension of tumor or orbital pathologies.

■ Temporal Bone

MR is the imaging modality of choice for patients presenting with sensorineural hearing loss (SNHL) [15, 16]. High-resolution technique is critically important in the imaging of the temporal bone and submillimeter pixel resolution is practically mandatory (Fig. 2). These images allow clear demonstration of labyrinthine structures [17–19]. MR imaging is indicated for patients with suspected retrocochlear sensorineural hearing loss to search for a tumor in the cerebellopontine angle and/or the internal auditory canal.

Acoustic schwannoma arising from the vestibulocochlear nerve is the most common neoplasm of the cerebellopontine angle cistern. Although 85% of acoustic tumors arise from the vestibular nerve, sensorineural hearing loss is the most common initial manifestation because a large tumor compresses the cochlear nerve. MR is the best imaging modality to detect intracanalicular acoustic tumor because of its ability to demonstrate the nerve structure itself (Fig. 3). The acoustic tumor is easily seen as an enhancing extra-axial mass extending into the internal acoustic canal. Gadolinium-enhanced images provide clear delineation of tumor extent and improve detection of the intracanalicular acoustic tumor.

High-resolution T2 FSE images with dual-phased array coils have caused some investigators to consider whether gadolinium is necessary for diagnosis [20, 21]. There are few cases in which high-resolution T2 FSE might miss a tumor that could be detected as a small area of enhancement only in a postgadolinium enhanced image. Several investigators reported that such small areas of enhancement of the nerve without a mass can be seen in inflammatory conditions such as neuritis or labyrinthitis and do not require surgery [22–24]. Such patients with a small area of enhancement with stable symptoms are now often treated conservatively with imaging follow-up rather than immediate surgery for what might be an inflammatory (nonsurgical) condition.

Meningioma is the second common cerebellopontine angle tumor, arising from the dural surface of the cerebellopontine angle and internal acoustic canal. Meningiomas usually present as a mass with wide dural attachments and are eccentric to the porus, whereas acoustic tumors

a

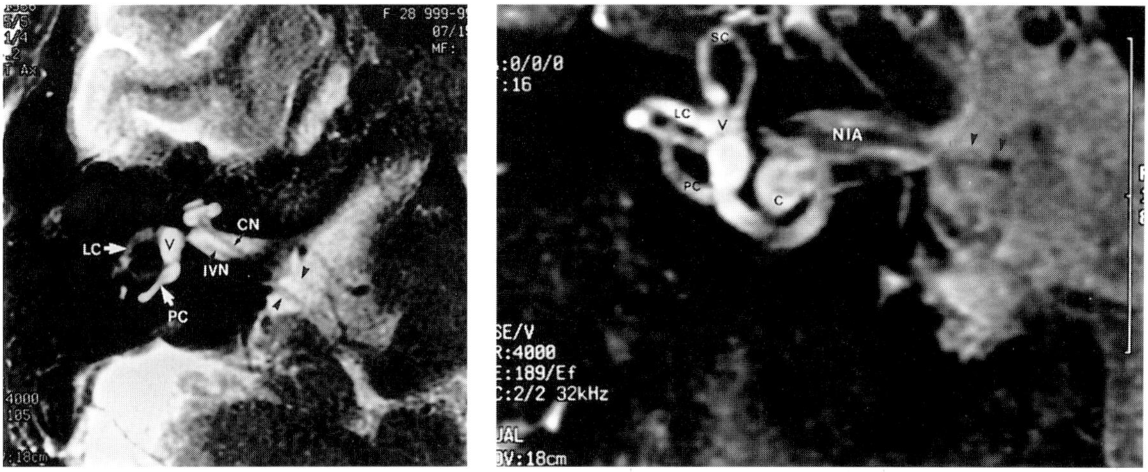

b

Fig. 2a,b. High-resolution T2-weighted FSE image of the temporal bone. Three-dimensional reconstructed axial (**a**) and coronal (**b**) images of the inner ear structures with maximum intensity projection method. Note the superb delineation of the 7th and 8th nerve complex. *CN*, Cochlear nerve; *IVN*, inferior vestibular nerve; *V*, vestibule; *PC*, posterior semicircular canal; *LC*, lateral semicircular canal; *SC*, superior semicircular canal; *C*, cochlea

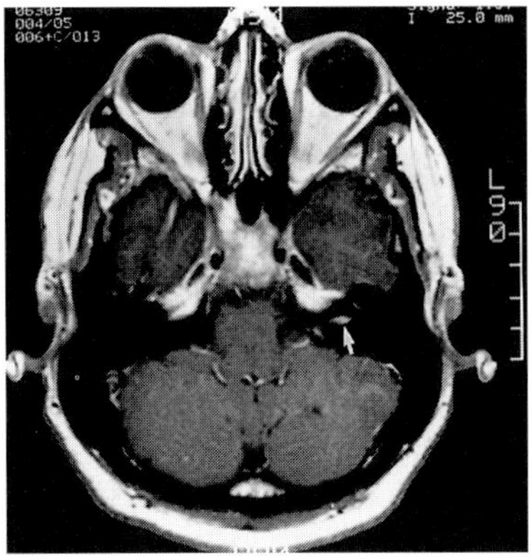

Fig. 3. Gadolinium-enhanced T1-weighted axial image shows a small focus of enhancement within the internal auditory canal, representing an intracanalicular acoustic neurinoma

usually are a more spherical mass centered on the porus with acute bone-tumor angles. Meningiomas are isointense to the cerebral cortex on both T1- and T2-weighted images in the majority of cases. Hyperostosis and dural thickening are often associated with meningioma. Following gadolinium administration, meningioma characteristically shows homogenous enhancement of tumor and adjacent dura.

Epidermoid (congenital cholesteatomas) originates from embryonic ectodermal inclusion located anywhere in the temporal bone or in the adjacent extradural, epidural or intracranial spaces. Common locations of epidermoid in the temporal bone are the middle ear, external ear, petrous apex, and mastoid antrum. The congenital cholesteatomas in the middle ear appear as a well defined soft tissue mass with a normal tympanic membrane. The petrous apex cholesteatoma, on the other hand, represents an expansive mass associated with destructive bony changes of the petrous trabeculae. This should be differentiated from other lesions arising from the petrous apex, such as cholesterol granuloma, mucoceles, histiocytosis X, neuromas, carotid aneurysms, primary bone, and cartilaginous lesions. The epidermoid contains keratin debris and solid cholesterol. The majority of congenital cholesteatomas show low or intermediate signal on T1- and high signal on T2-weighted images. Signal intensity of the lesion differentiates it from cholesterol granulomas that have high signal on both T1 and T2 images [25]. The absence of gadolinium enhancement of the epidermoid also helps differentiate it from acoustic tumor or meningioma.

Glomus jugulare tumor is usually centered at the jugular foramen and associated with cortical bone destruction. MR shows an enhancing mass on postgadolinium T1-weighted images and heterogeneous signal intensity on T2-weighted images. The typical MR appearance of glomus tumor is the so called "salt and pepper appearance," which reflects the vascular nature of the tumor. High signal foci represent subacute hemorrhage or slowly flowing blood and low signal serpentine areas represent the flow void of tumor vessels (Fig. 4). This appearance may be seen in other hypervascular masses and is not specific for a glomus tumor. The absence of these signs does not necessarily exclude a diagnosis of glomus tumor.

CT remains the imaging study of choice at present time for inflammatory disease and conditions resulting in conductive hearing loss. Important information about the status of the ossicles and

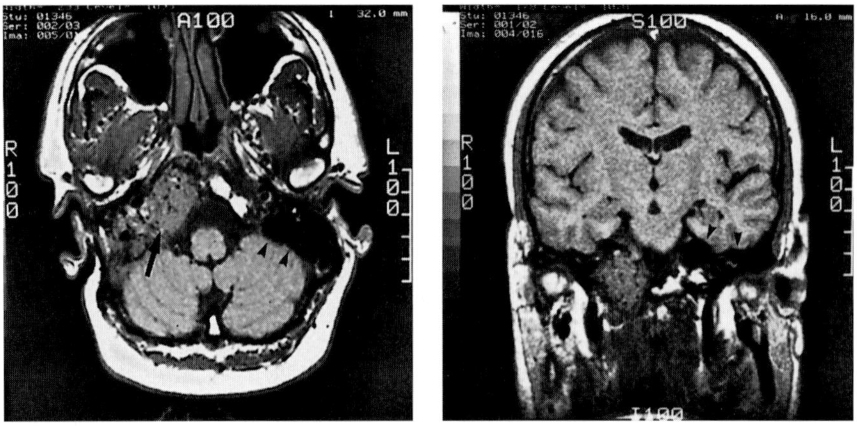

a b

Fig. 4a,b. T1-weighted axial image shows a large heterogeneous mass centered in the right jugular foramen (*arrow*). Multiple foci of low intensity most likely represent flow void from tumor vessels. Axial and coronal images demonstrate high signal bone marrow in the skull base replaced by the tumor, consistent with bone destruction. Surgery and pathology revealed glomus jugulare tumor bony covering of the facial nerve canal is still best obtained with CT. CT can also best visualize tumors and metabolic diseases affecting the middle ear and mastoid air cells. For the remainder of lesions of the temporal bone, CT and MR will continue to play complementary roles in the imaging work-up. Depending on the location and particular pathology, each of the imaging modalities contribute information.

■ Salivary Glands

The preferred method of imaging the salivary glands has evolved with new development in imaging technology and clinical needs. While sialography is still used to evaluate some inflammatory or autoimmune diseases of the salivary glands, CT can be used for sialolithiasis or infectious disease such as abscess. CT of the salivary glands may be obscured by beam hardening artifact from the skull base and dental amalgam. MR has replaced CT for the imaging evaluation of the majority of masses in the major salivary glands. Although inflammatory lesions or calculus are most common in the submandibular gland, approximately 80% of major salivary gland tumors occur in the parotid gland. Therefore MR is most frequently used for evaluation of parotid masses.

The main roles of MR imaging in the parotid gland tumor are: (a) differentiation between benign and malignant tumors, (b) differentiation between extrinsic parapharyngeal space masses and intrinsic parotid masses, and (c) definition of the relationship of the facial nerve to the parotid tumor. Is the tumor superficial, deep or combined? Does the tumor extend into the temporal bone, which necessitates partial temporal bone resection?

Parotid parenchyma appears high signal on T1-weighted image due to its relatively high fat content. Therefore T1-weighted images delineate parotid tumor very well, since the majority of parotid tumors appear low signal (Fig. 5). T1-weighted axial images should be obtained first to find a lesion. This sequence is supplemented with coronal or sagittal views when there is a question of temporal bone involvement. By finding parapharyngeal fat between deep lobe of the parotid gland and a tumor, the differentiation of an intraparotid gland mass from extraparotid parapharyngeal mass is possible.

Although high grade malignant tumor has been reported to be low signal on T2-weighted images [26], practically speaking benign and malignant tumors are not reliably differentiated

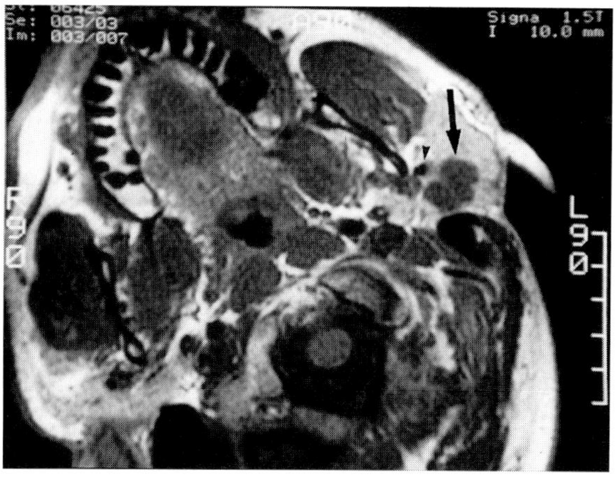

Fig. 5. Pleomorphic adenoma of the left parotid gland. T1-weighted axial image shows low intensity somewhat lobulated mass (*arrow*) within the left parotid gland The tumor is located in the superficial lobe of the parotid gland. The vetro mandibular vein is normal (*arrowhead*)

based on signal characteristics. MR can only rarely suggest the histology of tumors such as a Warthin tumor in multilobulated bilateral cystic masses seen in an elderly male. Fine-needle aspiration is a simple, minimally invasive method to define the cytology of the tumor and has been widely applied in large clinical series [27–29].

The real advantage of MR in imaging of the parotid space is its ability to more accurately determine the relationship of the tumor to the facial nerve [30]. The superficial and deep lobes of the parotid gland are not actual anatomical structures but are rather conceptual areas based on the plane defined by the course of the facial nerve. Malignant tumors in close relation to the facial nerve may require excision of part of that structure and subsequent microsurgical repair. Perineural extension is a well-known phenomenon for adenoid cystic carcinoma although this can be seen in other pathologies, such as mucoepidermoid carcinoma or squamous cell carcinoma. Gadolinium administration is useful for evaluation of abnormal enhancement of the facial nerve. Access to larger deeper lesions may require division and reflection of the ramus of the mandible. Information about deep invasion is easily obtained with MR imaging.

Multiple and often bilateral lymphoepithelial cysts are one of the head and neck manifestations of HIV infection [31], along with lymphoid tissue hyperplasia and lymph adenopathy.

Multifocal tumors can be seen in recurrent pleomorphic adenoma (Fig. 6), if initial excision was merely enucleation or partial resection. Pleomorphic adenoma can recur even 15–20 years

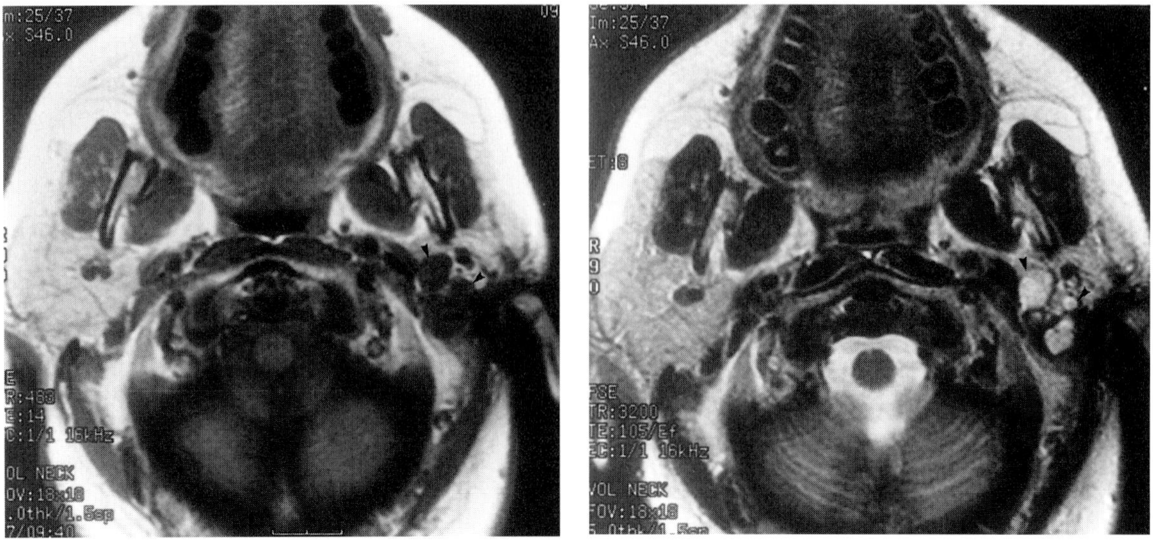

a b

Fig. 6 a, b. Recurrent pleomorphic adenoma. The patient had a pleomorphic adenoma of the left parotid gland resected 8 years previously presented with submucosal mass in the left oropharynx. T2-weighted FSE image clearly demonstrates multiple foci of high signal masses within the prestyloid parapharyngeal space as well as left parotid bed

after initial surgery and could potentially become malignant (so-called carcinoma ex pleomorphic adenoma). Oncocytomas may also be multiple and bilateral.

Lymph node metastases can be seen in the parotid gland, usually within the superficial lobe. The common primary sites which metastasize to the intraparotid lymph nodes are skin cancer in the face, the external auditory canal, or the scalp. Primary parotid lymphoma is very rare but usually shows diffuse swelling with infiltrative mass.

Paranasal Sinuses

While the mainstay for imaging inflammatory paranasal sinus disease or fibro-osseous disease will continue to be CT, MR may be substituted for the evaluation of advanced neoplastic lesions. Although cortical bone and air do not return a signal on MR, cortical bone can be visualized as a dark line (signal void) between the layers of high signal soft tissue and mucosa covering the sinus wall. Erosions of the bony walls can be demonstrated on MR as the absence of signal void normally present in cortical bone (Fig. 7). MR provides superior delineation of sinus tumor extension over contrast-enhanced CT scan and is the clear study of choice in advanced disease [32, 33]. Tumor extension to the pterygoid muscle, the retromolar trigone, the buccal or lingual alveolar ridges is readily visualized on MR. Special attention should be paid to search for perineural extension or leptomeningeal spread when a sinus tumor extends to the pterygopalatine fossa. MR allows differentiation of tumor from most secondary obstructed sinus secretion on T2-weighted images.

MR signal characteristics of sinus secretion varies depending on its protein concentration and free water proton content [34]. Most fluid in the sinuses appears hypointense on T1- and hyperintense on T2-weighted images. As protein concentration increases, sinus secretions become hyperintense on T1- and T2-weighted images. Further increasing protein concentration (over 25%–28%) with almost no free water results in extremely dark signal on both T1- and T2-weighted images (signal void). Fungus infection (mycetoma) also causes this signal void on both T1- and T2-weighted images, simulating well-pneumatized normal sinuses [35, 36]. This is due to the presence of paramagnetic substances such as manganese, iron, and calcium as well as desiccated debris within mycetoma, which do not contain free water. The fungus infection can often be demonstrated as an area of slightly increased density on CT.

Although MR has limited value for the evaluation of simple sinusitis, there is potential role of MR for evaluation of the intracranial complications from severe sinusitis. These include meningitis, encephalitis, brain abscess, subdural empyema, and thrombophlebitis. Frontal sinus mucocele or pyocele is potentially life threatening. Once the posterior wall of frontal sinus is disrupted due to increased pressure, meningitis, encephalitis or

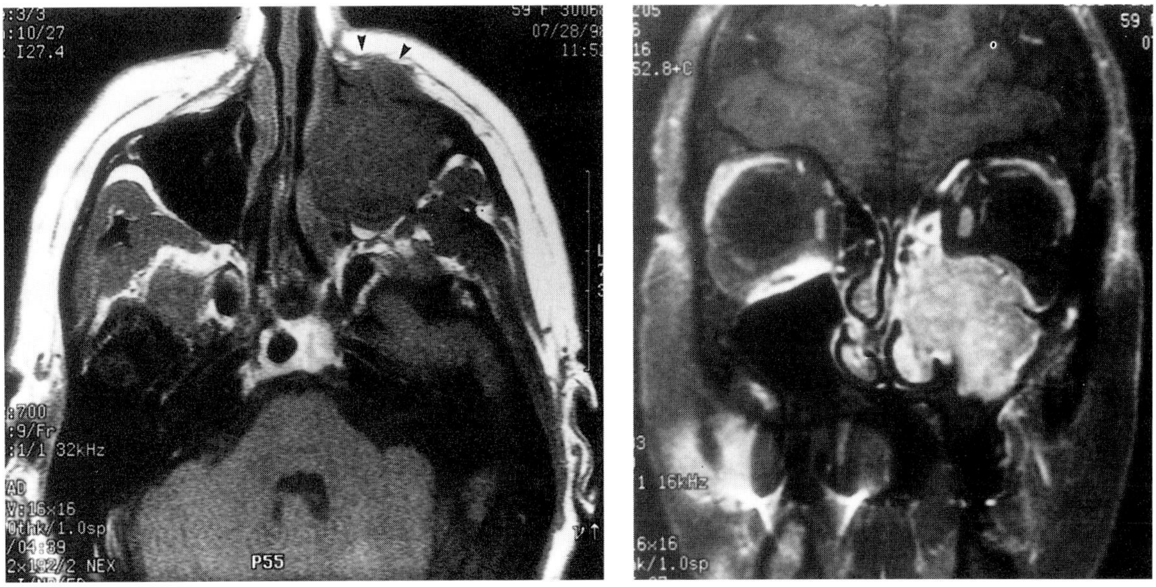

a b

Fig. 7 a, b. Left maxillary sinus adenocarcinoma. There is a large lobulated tumor (*arrowhead*) arising from the left maxillary sinus involving the left infratemporal fossa as well as the nasal cavity

brain abscess can be easily formed in the frontal lobe. Gadolinium-enhanced MR imaging is useful for early detection of these complications. Mucormycosis, commonly seen in diabetic patients, and some invasive forms of aspergillosis often appear as an aggressive mass in association with skull base destruction.

■ Nasopharynx and Parapharyngeal Space

The nasopharynx, the most cranial part of the upper aerodigestive tract, is located above the hard palate and underneath the clivus. The configuration of the nasopharynx is dominated by a very tough fascial membrane called the pharyngobasilar fascia. This tough fascia represents a continuation of the pharyngeal constrictor muscles and extends from the base of the skull down to the level of hard palate. Its function is to maintain the airway as an open channel for breathing during normal activities and during chewing. Only malignant tumors and very aggressive infectious processes such as mucormycosis cause disruption of the pharyngobasilar fascia (Fig. 8) [37–39]. The lateral nasopharyngeal wall consists of the torus tubarius with the eustachian tube opening anteriorly, and fossa of Rosenmuller in the posterolateral position. Two small muscles attach the skull base to the mucosal space in nasopharynx: the tensor and levator veli palatini muscles. These are seen on MR T1-weighted images as thin areas of low signal immediately lateral to the mucosal surface of the nasopharynx. Lateral to the tensor veli palatini muscle is the parapharyngeal space which is mainly filled with fat. The retropharyngeal space is separated from nasopharyngeal mucosal space by the pharyngobasilar fascia. The retropharyngeal space only contains several lymph nodes (retropharyngeal nodes) and fat. The lateral retropharyngeal nodes, so-called Rouvierre nodes, lie medial to the internal carotid artery and anterolateral to the prevertebral muscles. The retropharyngeal nodes are nearly impossible to assess by physical examination and not easily removable by surgery yet have important prognostic significance in the cancer patient.

The tensor veli palatini muscle is enveloped in a fascial plane of its own which divides the parapharyngeal space into two compartments [40]. The tensor veli palatini muscle fascia passes posterior to the styloid process and divides the space into a lateral compartment which is called the prestyloid space and a medial compartment called the poststyloid space. Pathologies originating from each compartment are different. It is therefore important to clearly identify the anatomical boundaries of this compartment. The majority of prestyloid space masses are salivary gland tumors and most poststyloid masses are of neurovascular origin, such as neuronal tumors, paraganglioma, and occasionally extracranial aneurysm [41] (Fig. 9). Metastatic tumor and lymphoma can be seen in both compartments. The medial pterygoid

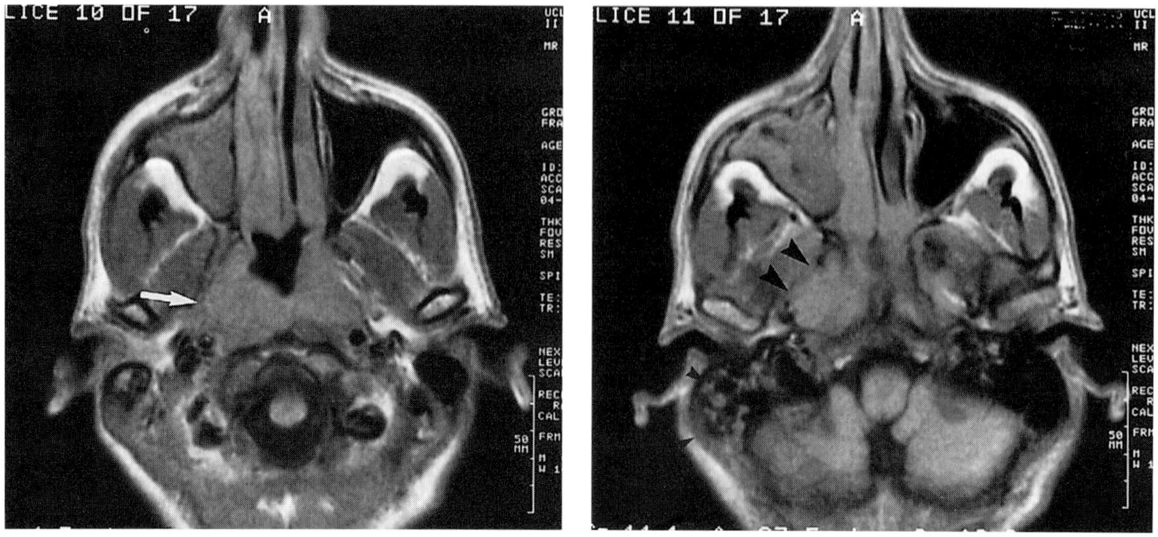

a b

Fig. 8 a, b. Nasopharyngeal carcinoma. T1-weighted axial image shows a bulky mass occupying the nasopharynx extending into the right parapharyngeal space (*arrow*). The image slightly higher than (**a**) shows destruction of the pharyngobasilar fascia (*arrowhead*), indicating an aggressive process. Note the unilateral fluid within the right and the mastoid air cells

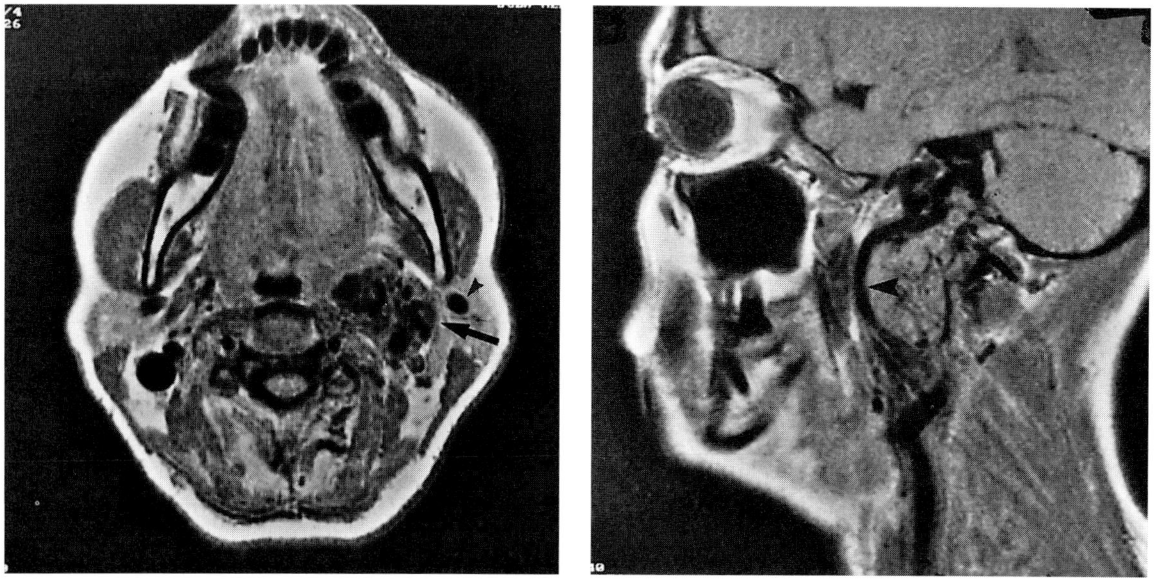

a b

Fig. 9 a, b. Glomus vagale tumor. A middle age male with a history of metastatic cancer presented with a mass on the left. T1-weighted (**a**) axial (**b**) sagittal images show a mass in the left poststyloid parapharyngeal space with anterior displacement of the vessels

muscle fascia separates the infratemporal fossa from the prestyloid parapharyngeal space. These two fascial planes generally fuse at their skull base attachment, which is immediately medial to the foramen ovale. The mandibular branch of the trigeminal nerve is within the infratemporal fossa, not in the parapharyngeal space.

The deep nasopharynx remains one of the blind areas of clinical examination. Its proximity to the skull base makes cancers in this region particularly devastating. The most common complaints of patients presenting with nasopharyngeal tumors are nasal obstruction, cranial nerve palsy, unilateral serous otitis media, and cervical lymph node metastases. Most malignancies of the nasopharynx are squamous cell carcinoma. Other nasopharyngeal tumors, such as lymphoma and plasmacytoma, tend to be bulkier and infiltrate

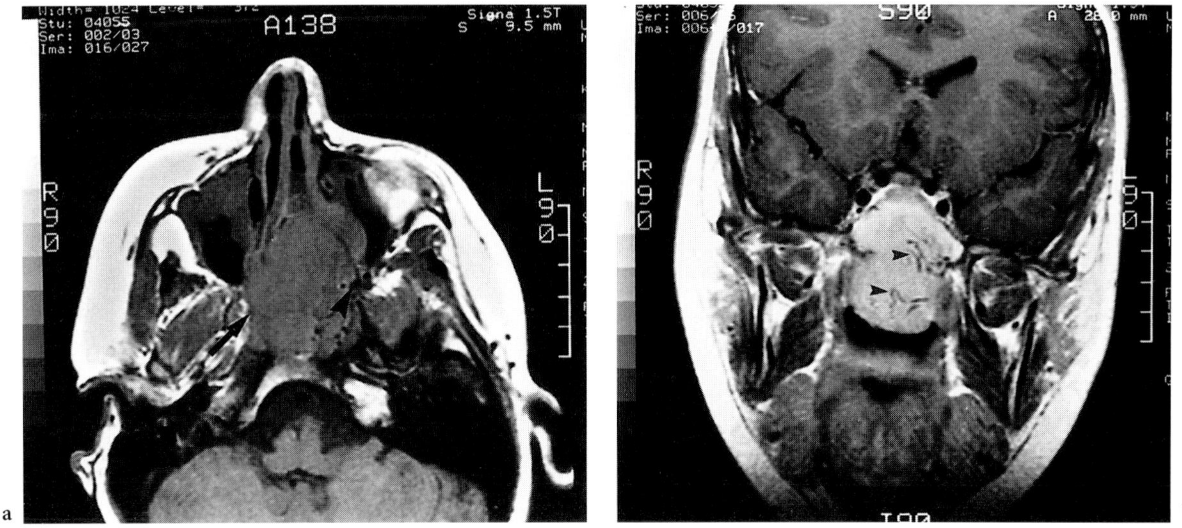

Fig. 10 a, b. A 13-year-old boy presented with nasal obstruction and recurrent epistaxis. Noncontrast T1 (**a**) and post-gadolinium coronal images (**b**) demonstrate a bulky mass within the posterior choana to the nasopharynx (*arrow*). The tumor involves the left pterygopalatine fossa (*arrowhead*) and fills the entire sphenoid sinus. Flow voids are present (**b**, *arrowheads*). Surgery and pathology revealed juvenile angiofibroma

more widely than squamous carcinoma [42]. In children, rhabdomyosarcomas are also encountered in the nasopharynx. A nasopharyngeal mass with pterygopalatine fossa invasion in a teenage male is strongly suggestive of juvenile angiofibroma (Fig. 10).

If a patient has symptoms of cranial nerve involvement, gadolinium should be administered and the skull base, jugular foramen, and the cavernous sinus should be thoroughly searched. In particular, direct coronal and sagittal MR scans are valuable to assess craniocaudal extension of tumor or skull base involvement, which help radiation therapy planning. Abnormalities of the skull base are detected by replacement of the normal high signal bone marrow with low signal neoplasm or enhancement within the marrow cavity. Nasopharyngeal tumors have a tendency to infiltrate beneath the mucosa and extend over wide areas with little superficial evidence of their presence. This is especially true in recurrent disease following therapy where the mucosa can return to a relatively normal appearance but where deep infiltration persists. MR is particularly well suited to compliment the clinical examination in this situation.

■ Oropharynx and Oral Cavity

Continuous with the nasopharynx, the oropharynx is bordered by the hard palate superiorly and the vallecula inferiorly, including the palatine tonsil, tonsillar fossae, the base of tongue, and the posterior pharyngeal wall from the level of soft palate to the tip of the epiglottis. The oral cavity is subclassified into several categories; the alveolus and gingiva, the hard palate, the retromolar trigone, the buccal mucosa, the anterior tongue, and the floor of mouth. Physical examination and visual inspection of these lesions reveal mucosal color changes, induration, or ulceration. MR images may not show significant abnormalities, if tumor spread is limited to the mucosal surface. On the other hand, deeply infiltrating tumor with limited mucosal change may be underestimated by physical examination alone. The main purposes of MR is to evaluate the extent of deep infiltration of the primary tumor and nodal disease [43–45]. Occasionally an infiltrating tumor may have spread to the nasopharynx or the supraglottic larynx, which might change the management of the patients.

T2-weighted images clearly delineate tumor margin, as all tongue musculature appears low signal on T2 as opposed to higher signal tumor (Fig. 11). Several anatomic regions need to be evaluated in order to plan surgical management. These are the neurovascular bundles, midline fibrous septum, mandible, base of tongue, and glossopalatinus sulcus. At least one hypoglossal nerve and one lingual artery must be retained in order to perform hemiglossectomy. A total glossectomy is a much more involved procedure, requiring myocutaneous flap reconstruction. Following total glossectomy, swallowing and speech

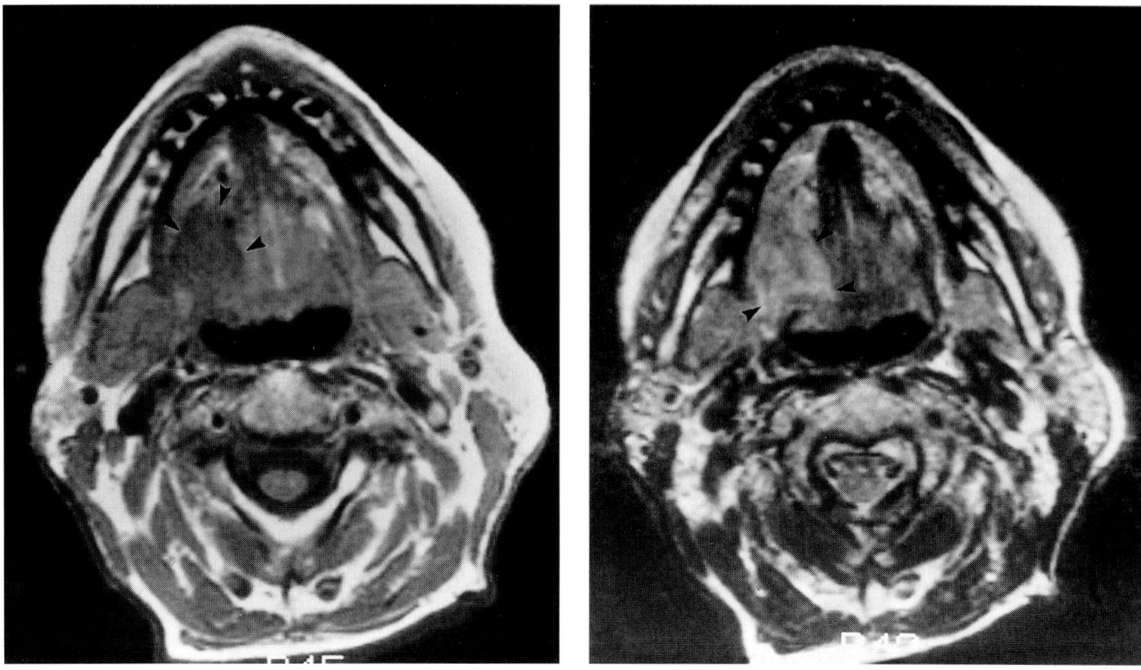

a b

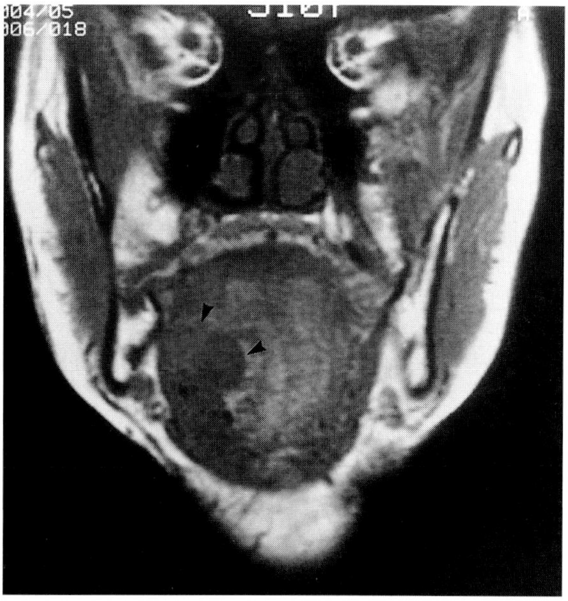

c

Fig. 11. Images show a large tumor infiltrating the right side of the tongue, extending into the base of tongue, not crossing the midline (*arrowhead*). **a** T1 weighted axial view. **b** T2 weighted axial view. **c** T1 weighted coronal view

function is significantly impaired. The lingual artery is easily visible between the genioglossus muscle and the interdigitation of the styloglossus and hyoglossus muscles [43]. Disruption of the diaphragm of the floor of the mouth, (the mylohyoid muscle) clearly indicates a far advanced tumor. Involvement of mandible is an important factor, which usually necessitates composite resection of that structure. Careful inspection of marrow signal within the mandible is essential, since the area of involvement may be more extensive than clinically suspected. Adenoid cystic carcinomas frequently extend along perineural lymphatics. Gadolinium-enhanced MR images are helpful in this situation to demonstrate the enhancement of the involved nerve [44]. The intimate association of the lateral portion of the tongue with the glossopalatinus muscle and glossopharyngeal sulcus means that these tumors have ready access to the tonsillar beds by direct extension. Frequently it is impossible to state whether the tumor originated in the tongue, the glossopharyngeal sulcus, or the tonsillar bed.

Carcinomas of the base of tongue (posterior to the foramen cecum) are particularly troublesome. Because of their inaccessibility they are usually not discovered until a late stage. Three-quarters of the tumors are reported to have metastases at the time of initial examination. Nodal metastases are frequently bilateral because of the bilateral drainage of the posterior third of the tongue. Tumors of the base of the tongue have a propensity to spread laterally into the glossopharyngeal sulcus and the tonsillar bed and posteriorly into the vallecula and preepiglottic space. Since minor asymmetry of the mucosal surface of the base of tongue is relatively common, an MR finding suggestive of early base of tongue tumor is the disruption of the intrinsic muscle layer, which is best seen on sagittal T1-weighted image [46].

The remaining anterior lesions of the buccal space, retromolar trigone, alveolar ridge, and lips are readily accessible by visual inspection or palpation and imaging studies seldom play a role in the diagnosis of these tumors. Posterior pharyngeal wall tumors are quite rare. They infiltrate locally and extend to the retropharyngeal lymphatics and jugular nodes. The primary tumors are easily seen by clinical examination, but at times their extensions may be obscure. Their nodal spreads constitute the principal indication for radiological investigation.

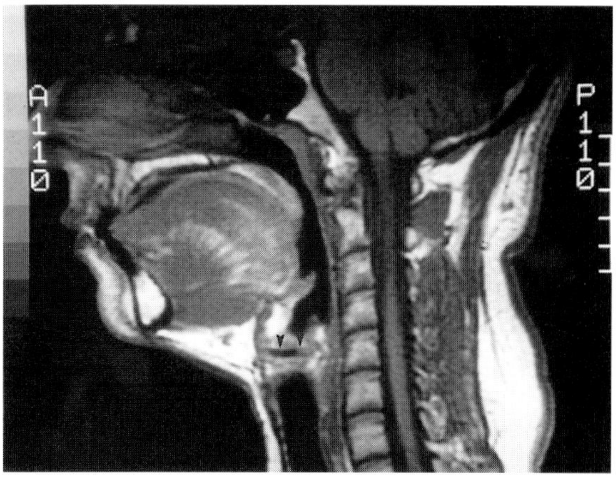

Fig. 12. Normal paramidline sagittal image is used as a landmark for MR imaging of the larynx. Epiglottis, preepiglottic fat, base of the tongue are clearly seen on sagittal image. Axial and coronal images should be obtained parallel and perpendicular to the true vocal cord, based on the sagittal image. The laryngeal ventricle is visible as a signal void (*arrowhead*)

■ Larynx and Hypopharynx

Understanding the laryngeal skeleton is a key to being comfortable with laryngeal anatomy. Three major (hyaline) cartilages (thyroid cartilage, cricoid cartilage, and arytenoid cartilage) and hyoid bone make up the framework of the larynx. The epiglottis, made of elastic cartilage, which does not normally calcify, maintains its flexibility to protect the airway from aspiration. The small triangular shaped arytenoid cartilage has three processes, the vocal process attached to the vocal cord, the muscular process attached to intrinsic laryngeal muscles, and the superior process attached to the aryepiglottic fold. When the top of the cricoid lamina and the arytenoid cartilage are seen in the same axial view, that indicates the level of the true vocal cord. If no cricoid cartilage but only the superior process of the arytenoid is seen, that is the level of the false cord. The subglottic level starts roughly 1 cm below the middle portion of the laryngeal ventricle.

The intrinsic musculature of the larynx (thyroarytenoid muscle and vocalis muscle) appear as low signal areas as opposed to bright signal false cord which is rich in fatty glandular tissue. Laryngeal ventricle may be seen as a slit of air on coronal images. Involvement of the intrinsic muscles or the adjacent bright signal areolar tissue planes indicate deep infiltration and spreading tumor. The space lying anterior to the epiglottis, the preepiglottic space, consists of loose fatty, areolar tissue to allow the epiglottis to invert during swallowing. The fatty plane between the thyroid cartilage and false cord is called the paralaryngeal space, which freely communicates with the preepiglottic space (Fig. 12). Tumor invasion to the preepiglottic or paralaryngeal spaces is clearly demonstrated by replacement of the normal high signal fat [8, 47, 48].

The hypopharynx is grossly divided into three anatomical areas; the pyriform sinuses, the retrocricoid region and the posterior pharyngeal wall (which is continuous with the oropharyngeal posterior wall). The aryepiglottic fold separates the laryngeal airway from the pyriform sinuses. The mucosa covered lumen behind the cricoid cartilage is the retrocricoid region. It is important to remember that the apex of the pyriform sinuses corresponds to the level of the true vocal cords. The pyriform sinus and retrocricoid hypopharynx are so intimately associated with the larynx that resection of tumors in these regions often necessitates surgery of the larynx. The hypopharynx becomes the cervical esophagus at the inferior border of the cricoid cartilage.

Laryngeal Cancer

Cancer of the larynx is usually described in terms of the levels involved, i.e., supraglottic (Fig. 13), glottic (Fig. 14), subglottic, and transglottic disease. The treatment depends on the levels and location of involvement. The loss of natural voice function resulting from a total laryngectomy can be devastating to many individuals. Less radical laryngeal resections that allow the preservation of natural speech and the protective sphincter mechanism of the larynx have been developed for certain smaller laryngeal tumors. Specifically, all techniques require an intact cricoid cartilage and at least one mobile arytenoid upon which to construct a functional voice box.

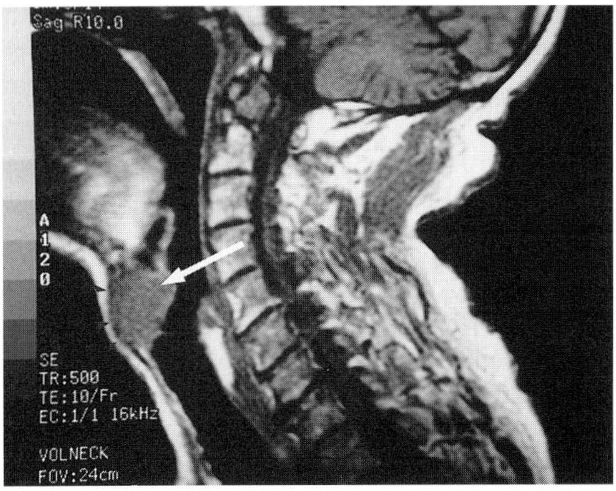

Fig. 13. Anterior supraglottic cancer invading the preepiglottic space. There is complete obliteration of high signal preepiglottic fat by the low signal tumor (*arrow*), resulting in anterior bulging of the thyrohoid membrane (*arrow*)

Key MR findings which affect management of larynx cancer patients are; (a) craniocaudal extension crossing the laryngeal ventricle, (b) cartilage invasion; (c) superior extension to the base of tongue, (d) subglottic extension, (e) extension across the midline (to the contralateral vocal cord), and (f) extralaryngeal spread [48]. The appropriate treatment decision depends on these factors.

The vertical spread of tumors should be carefully documented, especially whether the supraglottic cancer crosses the laryngeal ventricle. If this extension is present, the classical supraglottic laryngectomy is usually not performed, since the incision is made directly through the laryngeal ventricle (Fig. 13). Coronal and sagittal MR images with T1-weighted pulsing sequences readily demonstrate craniocaudal extent of disease.

The growth patterns of supraglottic cancer are divided into two forms: (a) anterior supraglottis, predominantly affecting the epiglottis, (b) posterolateral supraglottis, involving the aryepiglottic fold and arytenoid. Anterior supraglottic cancer often spreads to the preepiglottic space. The presence of preepiglottic space invasion alone does not preclude supraglottic laryngectomy. However, massive infiltration of the preepiglottic space abutting the thyrohyoid membrane can easily lead to extralaryngeal spread through penetration in the region of the neurovascular bundle (superior laryngeal artery, vein and nerve; Fig. 13). If the supraglottic tumor involves the tongue base, a partial glossectomy is necessary. Extensive extralaryngeal spread may ultimately render the tumor unresectable.

a

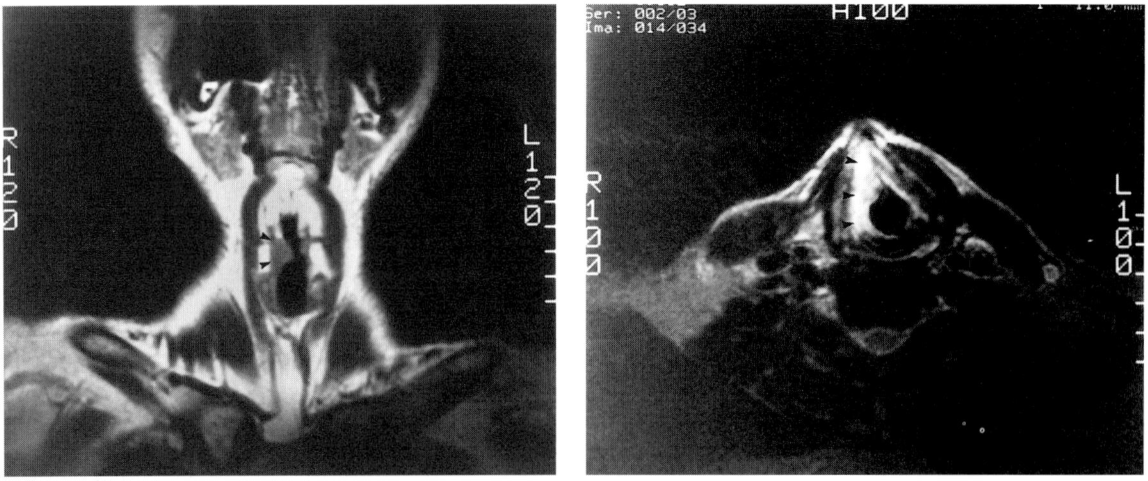

b

Fig. 14. Glottic cancer. **a** Coronal T1W image shows a soft tissue mass involving the true vocal cord (*arrowheads*). The supraglottic and subglottic larynx are clear. **b** T2 weighted axial image shows that the increased signal of the mass (*arrowheads*) extends from the anterior commissure posteriorly but does not involve the contralateral cord

The lateral wall of the aryepiglottic fold is technically the medial wall of the pyriform sinus. This is an area of overlap between the larynx and hypopharynx, and it may not always be possible to tell from which region a tumor arises based on MR images. Marginal cancer tends to spread along the aryepiglottic fold into the arytenoid. Tumor involving the interarytenoid region regardless of tumor size requires total laryngectomy, since at least one arytenoid needs to remain intact in order to save the larynx. In advanced cases tumor extends into the true vocal cord or the cricoarytenoid cartilage, resulting in cord fixation. Therefore special attention should be paid to the signal intensity and soft tissues within the cricoarytenoid joint, cricothyroid joint, and interarytenoid region. Cartilage invasion and extralaryngeal spread are rare for a pure marginal supraglottic cancer.

Imaging of thyroid cartilage invasion is a controversial topic. Initial studies have reported that MR is the best method to detect the cartilage invasion from the laryngeal cancer. Consensus at this time is that MR has a higher sensitivity of detecting cartilage destruction but lower specificity than CT. MR tends to produce more false-positive results than CT due to fibrosis or nonspecific inflammation [49, 50]. Findings indicating thyroid cartilage invasion are signal reduction in the dark signal rim of cortex or within the fatty marrow. When cartilage invasion is present, cure with radiation therapy alone is often not possible.

Hypopharyngeal Cancer

Pyriform sinus cancers behave more aggressively than endolaryngeal lesions and comprise 10%–20% of "laryngeal" cancers. They are actually cancers of the hypopharynx. Pyriform sinus cancers arising from the medial wall extend laterally into the paralaryngeal space and medially into the vocalis muscle, resembling marginal supraglottic lesions [51]. However, those from the lateral wall of the pyriform sinus extend outside the larynx via the cricothyroid joint, destroying the thyroid cartilage (Fig. 15). The primary tumor and cervical lymph nodes may form bulky masses in the neck. The important landmarks for conservative surgery of pyriform sinus cancers are similar to those used for supraglottic laryngectomy. Lesions high in the pyriform sinus can be treated with supraglottic laryngectomy, with the incision made through the laryngeal ventricle. A lesion reaching the apex of the pyriform sinus (which corresponds to the level of true vocal cord), needs total laryngectomy. Therefore, caudal extension is the most important finding to be determined. The anterior aspect of the retrocricoid hypopharynx is the mucosal covering of the posterior surface of the cricoid (Fig. 16). Total laryngectomy is usually required for retrocricoid cancers.

■ Unknown Primary

The patient presenting with a solitary, metastatic cervical lymph node presents one of the most interesting challenges in head and neck can-

a

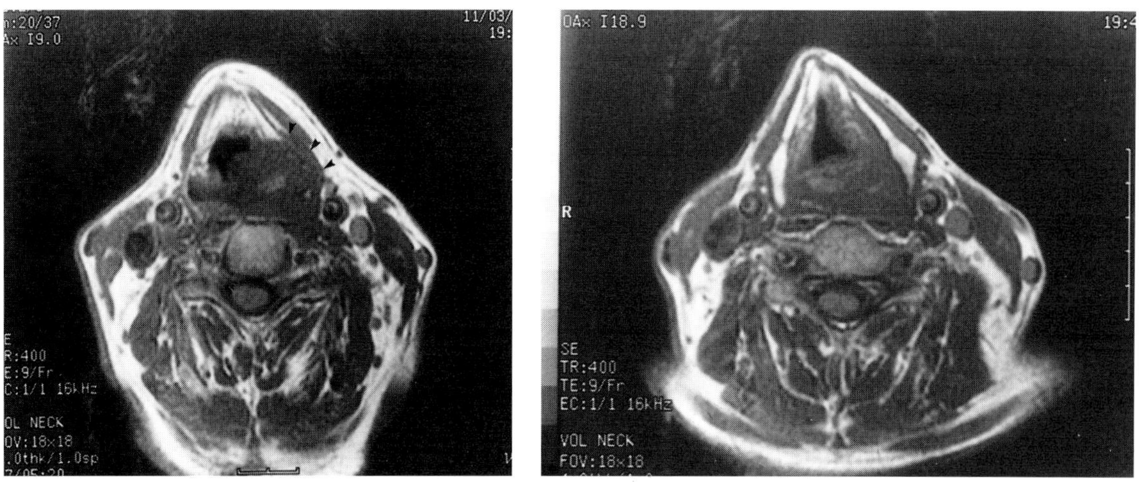

b

Fig. 15. Piriform sinus cancer. **a** Axial T1W image at the level of the high supraglottis shows a posterior piriform sinus mass on the left. The high signal marrow in the adjacent ossified thyroid cartilage has been replaced by tumor (*arrowheads*). **b** T1 weighted axial image more inferiorly shows the pyriform sinus mass which widens the cricothyroid joint

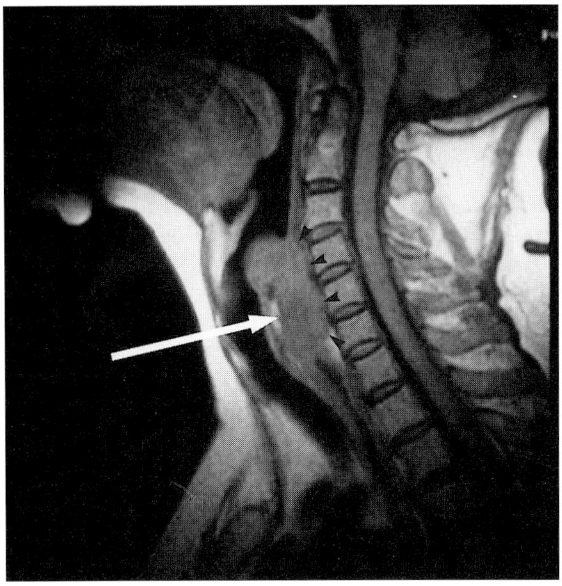

Fig. 16. Retrocricoid hypopharyngeal cancer. There is a mass (*arrowhead*) located behind the cricoid cartilage (*arrow*), extending into the cervical esophagus (below the lower margin of the cricoid cartilage)

cers. This is the so-called unknown primary situation, where the metastasis is clinically evident but the location of the primary tumor is unknown. Sound surgical principles dictate that the primary tumor should be managed at the same setting as the metastasis.

Three common blind areas in the head and neck during endoscopic examination are the nasopharynx, pyriform sinus, and base of tongue. Careful inspection in those three areas on MR is essential. The level of lymph node enlargement may to some extent suggest the primary site. MR allows detection of clinically occult primary sites in selected cases. In some cases the primary tumor disappears or is found, leaving only the lymph node metastasis. Patients whose primary site presents after the completion of a full dose of radiation therapy and/or radical neck dissection have a worse prognosis than those in whom a primary tumor is never found. Attempts should be made to search for the primary site so that boost radiation therapy can be added and unnecessary irradiation can be minimized.

Lymph Node Metastases

The presence of nodal metastases has a strong influence on prognosis of any head and neck cancer. The diagnosis of nodal metastases has been based on morphological features, such as size, internal architecture, and marginal appearance of nodes. Signal characteristics of MR on T1- and T2-weighted images for both benign and malignant nodes unfortunately overlap [52]. Criteria used for MR diagnosis of cervical nodal metastases are essentially the same as those established in the CT era [53–56]. Gadolinium-enhanced MR imaging does not appear to improve the accuracy of detection of metastatic lymph nodes [57].

Recently a new intravenous reticuloendothelial MR contrast agent called AMI 227 (Advanced Magnetics, Cambridge, Mass.), an ultrasmall superparamagnetic iron oxide, has been tested in a few clinical trials. The small iron particles (size of 17–21 nm) are taken up by elements of the reticuloendothelial system, including liver, spleen, and lymph nodes [58]. Normal functioning nodes reduce their signal following intravenous administration of iron oxide. On the other hand, metastatic nodes replaced by cancer cells which do not possess normal phagocytotic activity, remain high signal on postcontrast images. Iron oxide enhanced MR imaging has been reported to be more accurate for detection of nodal metastases than size criteria in head and neck cancer patients [59]. Safety issues as well as efficacy of this agent in postoperative or postradiation patients remain to be investigated in a large clinical trials.

Conclusion

Experience over the last 15 years indicates that magnetic resonance is now the imaging modality of choice to evaluate the majority of head and neck tumors. Spatial resolution has been dramatically improved compared to prototype MR imaging. A number of pulse sequences have been developed in the clinical use of head and neck MR. Gadolinium agents are essential when the skull base or intracranial extension is a major question. Development of new iron-based MR contrast agents may potentially improve detection of cervical nodal metastases.

References

1. Mancuso AA. Hanafee WN (1985) Computed tomography and magnetic resonance imaging of the head and neck, 2nd edn. Williams and Wilkins, Baltimore, pp 428–497
2. Mancuso AA, Hanafee W (1983) Elusive head and neck carcinomas beneath intact mucosa. Laryngoscope 93:133–139
3. Lufkin R, Hanafee W (1989) MR atlas of head and neck anatomy. Raven, New York

4. Ross JS (1995) Magnetic resonance angiography of the head and neck. A teaching file, 1st edn. Mosby, St Louis, pp 264–292
5. Lufkin RB, Hanafee W (1985) Application of surface coils to NMR anatomy of the larynx. AJNR 6:492–497
6. Lufkin RB, Votruba J, Reicher M, Bassett L, Smith DS, Hanafee WN (1986) Solenoid surface coils in magnetic resonance imaging. AJR 146:409–412
7. Hayes CE, Hattes N, Roemer PB (1991) Volume imaging with MR phased arrays. Magn Reson Med 18:309–319
8. Axel L, Dougherty L (1985) Chemical shift selective magnetic resonance imaging of multiple line spectra by selective saturation. J Magn Reson 66:189–194
9. Keller PJ, Hunter WW, Schmalbrock P (1987) Multiselection fat-water imaging with chemical shift selective presaturation. Radiology 164:539–541
10. Barkos JA, Dillon WP, Crew WM (1991) Orbit, skull base, and pharynx: contrast enhanced fat suppression MR imaging. Radiology 179:191–198
11. Zoarski GH, Mackey K, Anzai Y, Hanafee WN, Melki PS, Mulkern R, Jolsez FA, Lufkin RB (1993) Head and neck: initial clinical experience with fast spin echo MR imaging. Radiology 188:323–327
12. Lewin JS, Curtin HD, Ross JS, Weissman JL, Obuchowski NA, Tkach JA (1994) Fast spin-echo imaging of the neck: comparison with conventional spin-echo, utility of fat suppression, and evaluation of tissue contrast characteristics. AJNR 15 (7):1351–1357
13. Mulkern RV, Wong STS, Winalski C, Joesez FA (1990) Contrast manipulation and assessment of 2D and 3D RARE sequences. Magn Reson Imaging 8:557–566
14. Anzai Y, Lufkin R, Jabour BA, Hanafee W (1992) Fat suppression failure artifacts simulating pathology on frequency selective fat suppression MR imaging in the head and neck. AJNR 13:879–884
15. Swartz JD, Harnsberger HR (1992) Imaging of the temporal bone, 2nd edn. Thieme, New York, pp 1–20
16. Hasso AN, Smith DS (1989) The cerebellopontine angle. Semin Ultrasound CT MR 10 (3):280–301
17. Brogen M, Charkeres DW, Schudbrock P (1991) High resolution 3DFT MR imaging of the endolymphatic duct and soft tissue of the otic capsule. AJNR 12:1–11
18. Tanioka H, Shirakawa T, Machida T, Sasaki Y (1991) Three dimensional reconstructed MR imaging of the inner ear. Radiology 178:141–144
19. Brogan M, Chakeras DW (1990) Gd-DTPA-Enhanced MR Imaging of Cochlear Schwannoma. AJNR11:407–408
20. Allen RW, Harnsberger HR, Davis WL, King BD, Parkin JL, Apfelbaum RI (1993) MR imaging and the diagnosis of acoustic schwannoma: is contrast enhancement necessary? Radiology 189 (p):141
21. Remely KB, Stillman AE, Loes D (1993) High resolution fast SE MR imaging of the internal auditory canal: is T1 weighted contrast enhanced imaging still necessary? Radiology 189 (p):141
22. Seltzer S, Mark AS (1991) Contrast enhancement of the labyrinth on MR scans in patients with sudden hearing loss and vertigo: evidence of labyrinthine disease. AJNR 12:13–16
23. Mark AS, Seltzer S, Harnsberger HR (1993) Sensorineural hearing loss: more than meets the eye? AJNR 14 (1):37–45
24. Han MH, Jabour, BA, Andrews JC, Canalis RF, Chen FH, Anzai Y et al (1991) Nonneoplastic enhancing lesions mimicking intracanalicular acoustic neuroma on Gadolinium-enhanced MR images. Radiology 179:795–796
25. Greenberg JJ, Oot RF, Wismer GL, Davis KR, Goodman ML, Weber AE et al (1988) Cholesterol granuloma of the petrous apex: MR and CT evaluation. AJNR 9:1205–1214
26. Som PM, Biller HF (1989) High-grade malignancies of the parotid gland: identification with MR imaging. Radiology 173 (3):823–826
27. Teresi LM, Lufkin RB, Wortham DG, Abemayor E, Hanafee WN (1987) Parotid masses: MR imaging. Radiology 163:405–409
28. Casselman J, Mancuso AA (1987) Major salivary gland masses: comparison of MR imaging and CT. Radiology 165:183–189
29. Batsakis JG (1979) Tumors of the head and neck: clinical and pathological considerations, 2nd edn. Williams and Wilkins, Baltimore, p 194
30. Teresi L, Lufkin R, Kolin E, Hanafee W et al (1987) MRI of the intraparotid facial nerve. AJNR 8 (2):253–259
31. Shugar JM, Som PM, Jacobson AL, Ryan JR, Bernard PJ, Dickman SH (1988) Multicentric parotid cysts and cervical adenopathy in AIDS patients. A newly recognized entity: CT and MR manifestations. Laryngoscope 98 (7):772–775
32. Moore J, Potchen M, Waldenmaier N, Sierra A, Potchen EJ (1986) High-field magnetic resonance imaging of paranasal sinus inflammatory disease. Laryngoscope 96 (3):267–271
33. Som PM, Shapiro MD, Biller HF, Sasaki C, Lawson W (1988) Sinonasal tumors and inflammatory tissues: differentiation with MR imaging. Radiology 167 (3):803–808
34. Som PM, Dillon WP, Fullerton GD, Zimmerman RA, Rajagopalan B, Marom Z (1989) Chronically obstructed sinonasal secretions: observations on T1 and T2 shortening. Radiology 172 (2):515–520
35. Som PM, Dillon WP, Curtin HD, Fullerton GD, Lidov M (1990) Hypointense paranasal sinus foci: differential diagnosis with MR imaging and relation to CT findings. Radiology 176:777–781
36. Zinreich SJ, Kennedy DW, Malat J, Curtin HD, Epstein JI, Huff LC, Kumar AJ, Johns ME, Rosenbaum AE (1988) Fungal sinusitis: diagnosis with CT and MR imaging. Radiology 169 (2):439–444
37. Dillon WP, Mills CM, Kjos B et al (1984) Magnetic resonance imaging of the nasopharynx. Radiology 152:731–737
38. Teresi LM, Lufkin RB, Vinuela F et al (1987) MR imaging of the nasopharynx and floor of the middle cranial fossa. Part I. Normal anatomy. Radiology 164:811–816
39. Teresi LM, Lufkin RB, Vinuela F et al (1987) MR imaging of the nasopharynx and floor of the middle cranial fossa. Part II. Malignant tumors. Radiology 164:817–821
40. Curtin HD (1987) Separation of the masticator space from the parapharyngeal space. Radiology 163:195–204
41. Som PM, Sacher M, Stollman AL, Biller HF, Lawson W (1988) Common tumors of the parapharyngeal space: refined imaging diagnosis. Radiology 169 (1):81–85
42. Som PM (1992) Head and neck imaging, 2nd edn. Mosby, St Louis
43. Lufkin RB, Wortham DG, Dietrich RB, Hoover LA, Larsson SG, Kangarloo H, Hanafee WN (1986) Tongue and oropharynx: findings on MR imaging. Radiology 161 (1):69–75
44. Vogl T, Bruning R, Grevers G, Mees K, Bauer M, Lissner J (1988) MR imaging of the oropharynx and tongue: comparison of plain and Gd-DTPA studies. J Comput Assist Tomogr 12 (3):427–433
45. Lufkin RB, Larsson SG, Hanafee W (1983) NMR anatomy of the larynx and tongue base. Radiology 148:173–175
46. Gromet M, Homer MJ, Carter BL (1982) Lymphoid hyperplasia at the base of the tongue. Radiology 144:825–828
47. Lufkin RB, Hanafee WN, Wortham D, Hoover L (1986) Larynx and hypopharynx: MR imaging with surface coils. Radiology 158:747–754
48. Curtin HD (1989) Imaging of the larynx: current concepts. Radiology 173 (1):1–11
49. Becker M, Zbaren P, Laeng H, Stoupis C, Porcellini B, Vock P (1995) Neoplastic invasion of the laryngeal car-

tilage: comparison of MR imaging and CT with histopathologic correlation. Radiology 194:661–669
50. Curtin HD (1995) Importance of imaging demonstration of neoplastic invasion of laryngeal cartilage (editorial; comment). Radiology 194 (3):643–644
51. Larsson SV, Mancuso A, Hoover L, Hanafee W (1981) Differentiation of pyriform sinus cancer from supraglottic laryngeal cancer by computed tomography. Radiology 141:427–432
52. Dooms GC, Hricak H, Moseley MD, Bottles K, Fisher M, Higgins CB (1985) Characterization of lymphadenopathy by magnetic resonance relaxation times: preliminary results. Radiology 155:691–697
53. Mancuso AA, Maceri D, Rice D, Hanafee W (1981) CT of cervical lymph node cancer. AJR 136:381–385
54. Mancuso AA, Harnsberger HR, Muraki AS et al (1983) Computed tomography of cervical and retropharyngeal lymph nodes: normal anatomy. Radiology 148:709–714
55. Som PM (1992) Detection of metastasis in cervical lymph nodes: CT and MR criteria and differential diagnosis. AJR 158 (5):961–969
56. Som PM (1987) Lymph nodes of the neck. Radiology 165 (3):593–600
57. Yousem DM, Som PM, Hackney DB, Schwaibold F, Hendrix RA (1992) Central nodal necrosis and extracapsular neoplastic spread in cervical lymph nodes: MR imaging versus CT. Radiology 182 (3):753–759
58. Anzai Y, McLachlan S, Moris M, Saxton R, Lufkin RB (1994) Dextran covered superparamagnetic iron oxide: the first human use of a new MR contrast agent for assessing lymph nodes in the head and neck. AJNR 15:87–94
59. Anzai Y, Blackwell K, Hirschowitz S, Rogers J, Sato Y, Yuh WTC, Runge V, Lufkin RB (1994) Initial clinical experience with Dextran-coated superparamagnetic iron oxide for detection of lymph node metastases in patients with head and neck cancer. Radiology 192:709–715

Low-Field Dedicated Extremity Magnetic Resonance Imaging

3

E. Dion · C.G. Peterfy · S. Anderson · H.K. Genant

Introduction

In the current climate of cost containment, there is increased need for radiologists to identify more cost-effective approaches to the imaging of common musculoskeletal disorders and to justify their special role in healthcare delivery. This is particularly true in the area of magnetic resonance imaging (MRI), where some of the basis for cost escalation has recently been directed. These conditions have created a greater awareness among radiologists of the potential benefits of low field strength MRI and innovative magnet designs, such as open and interventional magnets and, most recently, dedicated extremity scanners.

Dedicated extremity MRI (E-MRI), which became commercially available in the United States in 1993, represents a radical departure from the traditional whole-body magnet design that has dominated clinical MRI thus far. To image an extremity with a conventional whole-body magnet, the entire body must be placed within the bore of the magnet. With E-MRI, however, only the extremity is inserted into the bore, while the rest of the body remains outside (Fig. 1). This unique design offers a number of practical and economic advantages, including lower cost, facilitated siting, improved patient comfort, and reduced patient risk. Currently there are two E-MRI systems approved for use in the United States: the Artoscan (Esaote, Genoa, Italy; distributed in the United States by Lunar, Madison, WI), which uses a 0.2 T permanent magnet with a small circumferential bore, and the Magna-SL (MagnaLab, New York, NY), a 0.3 T open system. However, many more systems are expected to enter the marketplace in the near future.

This chapter reviews the strengths and weaknesses of low-field E-MRI, and points to ways that this technology can actually expand the envelope of MRI in the face of cost containment to incorporate new clinical indications and underserved markets that thus far have not benefited greatly from MRI.

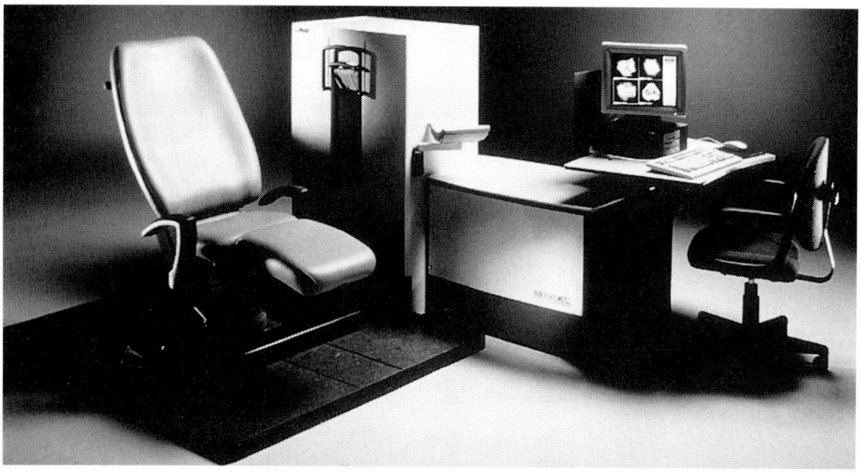

Fig. 1. Dedicated E-MRI. Example of a circumferential small-bore 0.2-T extremity MRI system. (From Artoscan, Lunar Corporation, Madison, WI; with permission)

■ Reduced Cost and Space Requirements

High cost has been a principal impediment to the use of MRI in a number of important clinical applications, such as the evaluation of acute extremity trauma and osteomyelitis, and the use of MRI as a screening tool for diseases, such as osteoarthritis, which may develop morphological changes long before clinical symptoms emerge. In addition to substantially lower purchase price (less than 20% the cost of whole-body scanners) and maintenance costs (20%–30% that of whole-body MRI), E-MRI scanners are considerably less expensive to site. Because of their small footprint and low fringe field, E-MRI can be housed in as little as 100 ft^2 of space. Moreover, E-MRI scanners are relatively light weight (as little as 800 kg) and therefore do not require any structural reinforcement of the examination room. These features enable E-MRI to operate in an environment not previously accessible to MRI. Notable examples include the emergency department and, even more intriguingly, the physician's office. Office-based MRI is particularly cogent to the growing movement towards deinstitutionalization of healthcare [1].

The implications of this are far reaching. Lowering the technical cost of MRI allows a greater proportion of the total reimbursement to reflect image interpretation: the true deliverable of this diagnostic examination. Such a margin is desirable under any circumstance, but can be particularly advantageous in a capitated environment. However, in addition to making MRI utilization for established musculoskeletal indications more cost effective, E-MRI can potentially capture markets previously dominated by low-cost radiographic imaging. Large-volume markets, such as acute extremity trauma and arthritis, offer particularly intriguing opportunities for this technology.

This blade, however, has two sides. As MRI becomes less expensive and more accessible to mainstream medicine, there will be greater competition for the technology from outside Radiology. Consistent with this, the majority of E-MRI systems in the United States have been purchased by orthopedic surgeons, not radiologists.

■ Patient Comfort and Safety

About 5% of patients cannot complete a whole-body MRI examination due to claustrophobia. A larger proportion of patients find the experience unpleasant, sometimes requiring sedation to cope. This is particularly true of children who often require heavy sedation or anesthesia. Open magnets are less claustrophobic, but E-MRI completely eliminates the problem by allowing all but the patient's extremity to remain outside the scanner. Additionally, patients enjoy direct contact with the technician, who is seated in the same room with them during the examination.

Keeping the body of the patient out of the main magnetic field also reduces the risk of biohazards associated with metal. The fringe field of the Artoscan is 4 ft from the center of the bore (i.e., where the patient is seated during the examination) is only 1 G (Fig. 2). The ambient magnetic field in some subway systems may be ten times this value. While the FDA has not yet lifted the existing restrictions to imaging subjects with aneurysm clips, metal fragments in the eyes, pacemakers or other contraindications to conventional MRI, the risk of E-MRI to those patients in

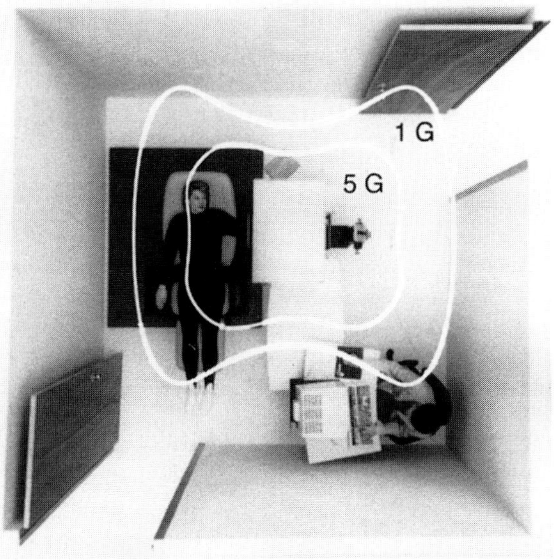

Fig. 2. Dedicated E-MRI. The fringe field of the Artoscan (Lunar) E-MRI scanner. The 1-G line is only 4 ft from the center of the bore of the magnet. Accordingly, E-MRI is safer to operate. A low fringe field along with the small size and low weight of the system make siting convenient and inexpensive. (From Lunar Corporation, Madison, Wis., with permission)

whom these potential contraindications are not detected during the pre-scan screening is clearly reduced. Moreover, metallic objects, such as oxygen tanks, wheelchairs, intravenous poles, computers, etc. can be brought close to the magnet without special consideration.

■ Technical and Diagnostic Performance

Anatomical Coverage/Patient Positioning

One limitation of E-MRI is that only the distal two thirds of an extremity can be evaluated. This excludes the shoulder and hip, which presently account for a significant proportion of the musculoskeletal volume.

There are also restrictions in the maximum field of view available. For example the Artoscan provides 11 cm of effective field of view (FOV). This does not pose a significant problem for evaluating most intra-articular abnormalities. However, in some cases (e.g., large soft-tissue masses, malignant bone tumors with potential satellite lesions, extensive infection) multiple scans with repositioning may be necessary to gain adequate coverage. In a series of 2437 consecutive examinations, however, Passariello reported that only 2% could not be successfully completed [2].

An additional consideration in patient positioning is the distribution of magic-angle phenomenon. This phenomenon reflects the angular anisotropy of T2 relaxation in hydrated collagen-containing structures. Under normal circumstances, collagen constrains the mobility of water protons and promotes dipole-dipole interactions and therefore T2 relaxation. As a result, collagen-containing tissues, such as tendons, ligaments and menisci, show such rapid T2 relaxation (<1 ms) that even the shortest TE attainable with conventional MRI are too long to capture any signal from these structures. Accordingly, tendons, ligaments and menisci typically appear signal-less on all pulse sequences. However, because of the highly regular structure of collagen, water protons constrained within collagen fibers tumble at different rates in different directions. When the internuclear vector between these water protons is oriented at 55° relative to the static magnetic field (B_0), one component of T2 relaxation is nulled and the aggregate T2 time increases considerably. As a result of this, signal can be seen on short-TE images in segments of tendons or ligaments in which the collagen fibers are oriented at 55° to B_0. In order to avoid misinterpretation, foci of intratendinous signal should be verified on long-TE images. However, in some cases, e.g., meniscal tear, this is not possible, and reorientation of the limb relative to B_0 may be necessary [3]. Knowledge of the arrangement of collagen within the articular structures of interest and of the orientation of B_0 is therefore useful for determining the optimal limb positioning for a particular clinical application.

In most superconducting magnets B_0 is aligned parallel to the long axis of the bore. In the Artoscan, however, B_0 runs horizontally across the short axis of the magnet bore. This alters the distribution of magic-angle effects on images acquired with the Artoscan. For example, magic-angle phenomenon often arises in the extensor carpi ulnaris tendon as it curves across the distal tip of the ulna when the hand is imaged in the usual position, with the thumb turned upwards. As this tendon is occasionally the site of clinically occult rupture in rheumatoid arthritis, short-TE images in these patients can be misleading, and should either be verified with heavily T2-weighted images or acquired with the hand in supination or pronation.

Image Quality

In any discussion of diagnostic utility it is important to acknowledge the fundamental differ-

Table 1. Preliminary experience with E-MRI of the knee

		Meniscal tear		ACL tear	
	n	*n*	Sens./spec.	*n*	Sens./spec.
Barile et al. [15]	157	134	100/73	84	100/97
Kersting-Sommerhoff et al. [16]	210	163	92/87	106	90/100
Masciocchi et al. [17]	233	186	95/97	106	97/99

ence between intermediate measures of "image quality" and more clinically meaningful measures of "diagnostic power." Difficulties in coming to grips with this distinction has been a major stumbling block in the long-standing and sometimes acrimonious debate over which field strength is optimal for MRI. Arguments in support of high field strength MRI often focus on technical parameters that scale with field strength (e.g., SNR) or on subjective qualities tied to image esthetics. Of the small handful of studies that have formally compared the diagnostic power of high-field MRI with that of low-field MRI, most have failed to find any significant difference [4–8].

Despite the fact that E-MRI has been available in the United States since 1993, very little formal assessment of the diagnostic power of this modality has reached the literature. The preliminary evidence, however, is encouraging and appears to have parody with conventional MRI (Table 1). Several studies in the knee, for example, have demonstrated high sensitivity and specificity of E-MRI for both meniscal tear and cruciate ligament tear. Kersting-Sommerhoff found discrepancies between high and low field MRI in only 8% of 20 patients studied prospectively.

■ Clinical Applications

Certainly E-MRI shows promise as a low-cost alternative to conventional MRI for evaluating cruciate ligament tears, meniscal pathology, and other established indications. However, even more intriguing are the implications of this modality to conditions that could benefit from MRI without placing significant demands on spatial resolution, imaging speed, T2* effects or spectral separation, but which for practical and economic reasons have thus far been dominated by radiography, scintigraphy, or even clinical examination. Such conditions include acute fracture, osteomyelitis, arthritis, possible neoplasia, as well as a host of nonspecific complaints that are responsible for bringing many patients repeatedly to their physicians office, but for which the expense and inconvenience of conventional MRI is felt not to be justified. The following discussion explores each of these potential niche applications of E-MRI.

Acute Fracture

Fractures of the extremities (Figs. 3, 4), particularly those involving the scaphoid, talus or the tibial plateau, are often occult on initial radiographs despite costly special views. In order to avoid the sometimes serious consequences of missing these fractures (e.g., nonunion, malunion, osteonecrosis), clinically suspected cases are often unnecessarily immobilized and subjected to serial reevaluations. This results in increased costs and greater patient morbidity. Moreover, with the growing popularity of rollerblading, skateboarding and snowboarding the incidence of these injuries is on the rise.

MR imaging is currently the most sensitive technique for detecting nondisplaced fractures, but in many cases, cost is prohibitive. Low cost and high diagnostic accuracy make E-MRI well suited to service this large population. Because of its small size and easy siting, an E-MRI system could easily be placed in or very close to a busy Emergency Room. Not only could E-MRI identify fractures that would otherwise have been missed with conventional radiography, it could rule out fractures in the much larger proportion of patients who had clinically suspected fractures and would therefore have received unnecessary immobilization and follow-up examinations.

In a recent examination of 45 consecutive patients with upper extremity trauma and negative initial radiographs, E-MRI identified 25 fractures in 20 patients (49%), including 4 scaphoid fractures that subsequently became evident on follow-up radiography [9]. Twenty-three (51%) of the 45 cases showed no evidence of fracture. E-MRI showed a diagnostic accuracy for fracture of 100%. As expected, fractures were most conspicuous on STIR images. However, T1-weighted 3D gradient echo, which could be acquired in as little as 4 min, was equally accurate (100%). In each case, a fracture line could be delineated on the E-MR image.

Heller et al. [10] recently completed a cost-effectiveness study of MRI in suspected scaphoid fracture using decision-tree analysis and three-way sensitivity testing. Based on probabilities derived from a 10-year meta-analysis of the literature on scaphoid fracture, and cost values derived from 1995 Medicare reimbursement rates, MRI

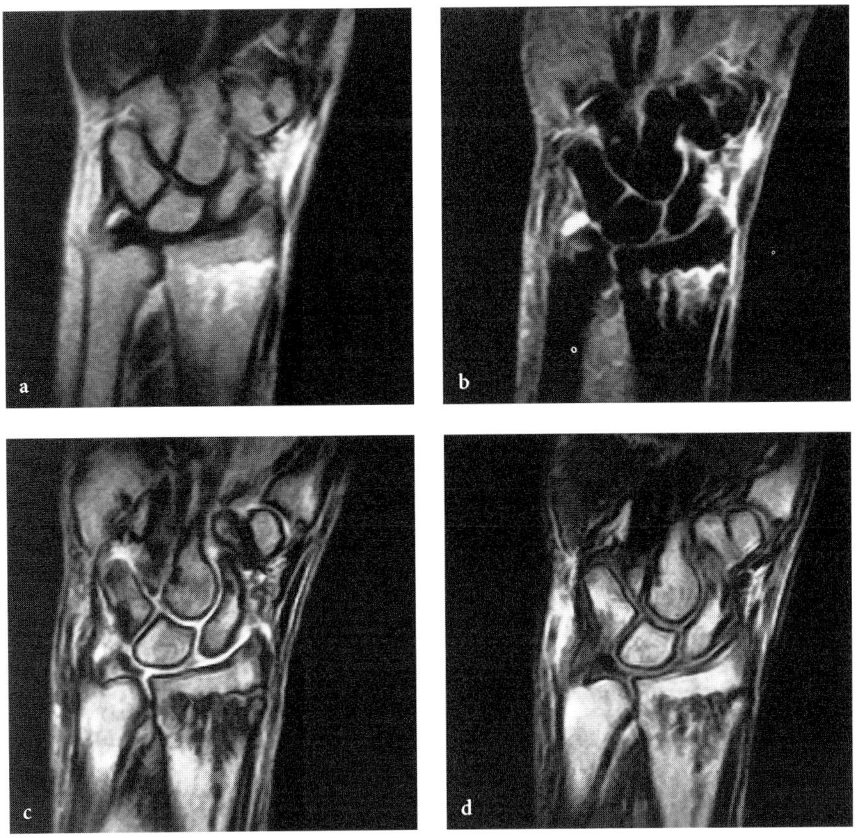

Fig 3 a–d. Radiographic occult fracture of the radius. The fracture line and bone marrow edema are both clearly visible on spin echo T2 (**a**), STIR sequence (**b**), gradient recalled echo 50/18/α: 15° (**c**), gradient recalled echo 50/16/α: 60° (**d**)

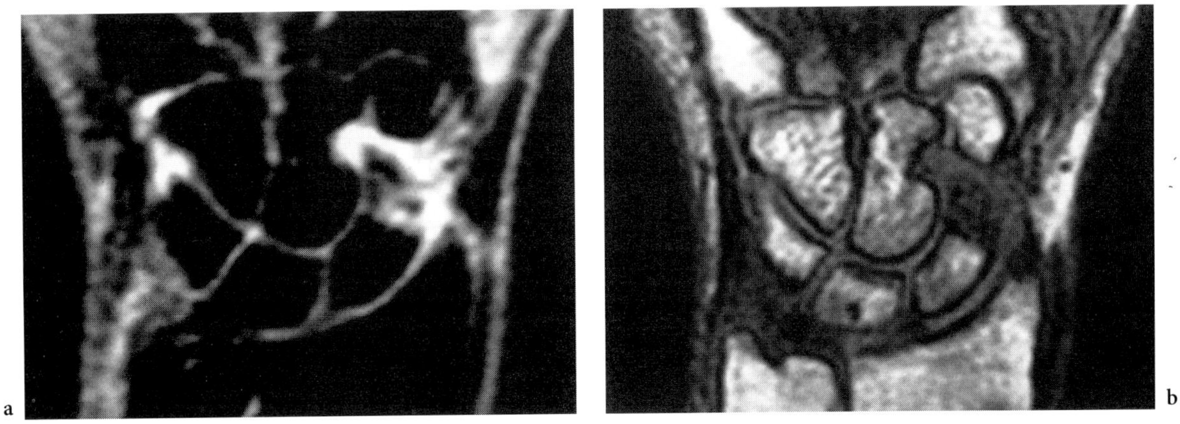

Fig. 4 a, b. Persistent pain after trauma of the wrist. X-rays of the wrist were considered as normal. **a** STIR image, used as a screening sequence in trauma patients, demonstrated fluid and fracture of the scaphoid. **b** T1-weighted spin echo image confirms the fracture line and a bone marrow edema in the distal portion of the scaphoid

was found to be more cost effective than immobilization with follow-up clinical examination and radiography, as long as the cost of MRI was kept below \$ 240. Parity with serial radiography and clinical examination was reached if the prevalence of scaphoid fracture rose above 46% (the true probability based on the meta-analysis was only 20%), the sensitivity of radiography rose above 86% (the true probability was only 40%), or the cost of clinical evaluation and immobilization dropped below \$ 86 (the Medicare reimbursement was \$ 144). Correspondingly, as the prevalence of scaphoid fracture decreased and that of associated injuries increased, the threshold cost for MRI increased. If one also factors in intangible benefits to the patient, such as alleviation of anxiety associated with uncertainty about the diagnosis of a condition with potentially serious downstream implications, and freedom from unnecessary immobilization and repeat visits to the physician and imaging center, the actual value of MRI increases further.

Similar methods could be used to help establish guidelines for managing other types of injuries, such as suspected tibial plateau fracture or fracture of the ankle.

Ligament Injuries

In addition to fracture, extremity trauma is often associated with injury to ligamentous structures. E-MRI is capable of visualizing most important ligaments directly and can establish their integrity during the same imaging examination used to assess the fractures.

Ligamentous injuries are particularly common in the ankle. Usually these involve the anterior talofibular ligament of the lateral collateral complex, and are relatively easy to evaluate clinically. Occasionally, however, other ligaments, such as the spring ligament, the talocalcaneal ligament in the sinus tarsi or the distal tibiofibular syndesmosis, are injured. These ligaments are more difficult to evaluate clinically and may therefore benefit more from E-MRI. Similarly triangular fibrocartilage and scapholunate ligament tears in the wrist, ulnar collateral ligament injury in the elbow, or cruciate or collateral ligament tear in the knee can be easily evaluated with E-MRI. E-MRI may also be useful for differentiating nondisplaced tears of the ulnar collateral ligament of the thumb from Stenner lesions that require open reduction and internal fixation [11].

Patients with Orthopedic Hardware

One intriguing application of E-MRI, and low-field systems in general, is imaging patients with metallic hardware in or near a joint. Artifacts created by metal usually limit opportunities to monitor with MRI patients who have undergone internal fixation or arthroplasty. Evaluation of postoperative complaints in these patients must thus rely on clinical evaluation or conventional radiography. The severity of metallic artifacts, however, depends on a number of technical factors, and can be reduced significantly when appropriate measures are taken. For example, metallic artifacts are most severe on gradient-echo images and minimal on fast spin-echo images. Metallic artifacts also scale with magnetic field strength and are therefore less severe on low-field images. Metallic artifacts are further reduced when the long axis of the hardware is aligned with B_0 and the direction of phase encoding. Knowledge of the relationship between the anatomy in question and the relative orientation of the metal hardware, B_0 and phase encoding are therefore useful for planning an imaging protocol for a patient with orthopedic hardware. As stated above, the orientation of B_0 in E-MRI is transverse to the long axis of the magnet bore. Consequently screws in a buttress plate on the lateral tibial plateau of the knee, for example, are oriented transverse to the long axis of the knee and therefore cause minimal artifacts (Figs. 5, 6), while the buttress plate itself, which is perpendicular to B_0, produces larger artifacts. These considerations should be kept in mind when imaging a patient with hardware.

Bone Marrow Abnormalities

A variety of conditions have associated findings in the bone marrow. As was discussed above for acute bone trauma, for most of these conditions MRI is currently felt to be the most sensitive method of detection. Since marrow abnormalities typically cover large areas of bone, high spatial resolution is not a necessity for adequate imaging. Accordingly, E-MRI can play a useful role in evaluating these conditions to the extent that they involve accessible regions of the anatomy.

Osteomyelitis is thus an important potential application for E-MRI. While radiography depends on trabecular and to a lesser extent cortical bone destruction to demonstrate osteomyelitis and is therefore notoriously insensitive, MRI is exquisitely sensitive because of its ability to detect even small elevations in marrow water content. E-MRI thus offers a cost-effective and reliable way to exclude osteomyelitis in high risk patients, such as diabetics (Fig. 7) and patients receiving immunosuppressive therapy. E-MRI may also be useful for monitoring antibiotic therapy and potentially for directing tissue-sparing surgery in these patients.

E-MRI can also differentiate avascular necrosis from stress fracture in patients receiving systemic steroids. While avascular necrosis typically shows a wavy margin of reactive or regenerative tissue delimiting a devitalized vascular territory, linear signal abnormalities in bone are suggestive of stress fracture.

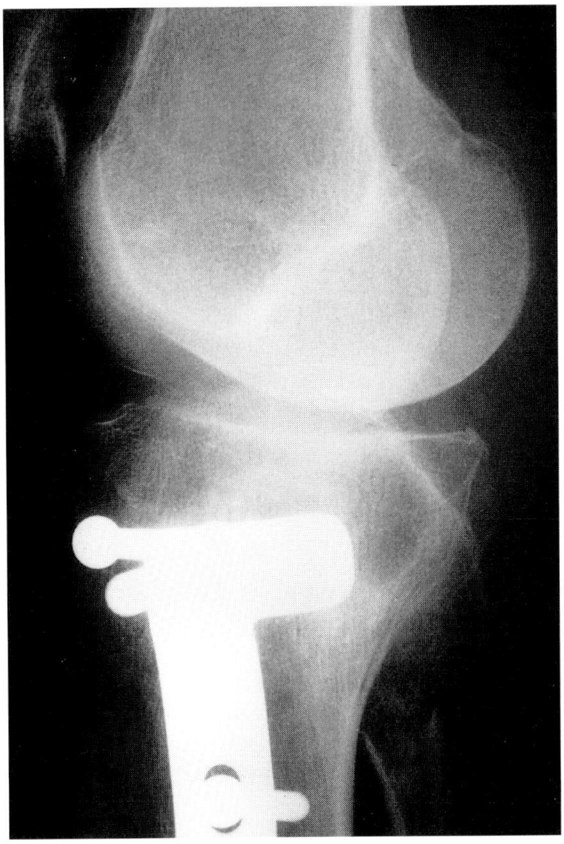
a

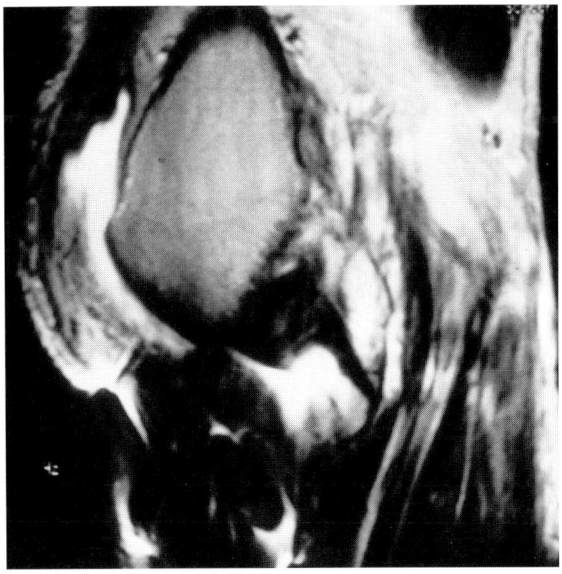
b

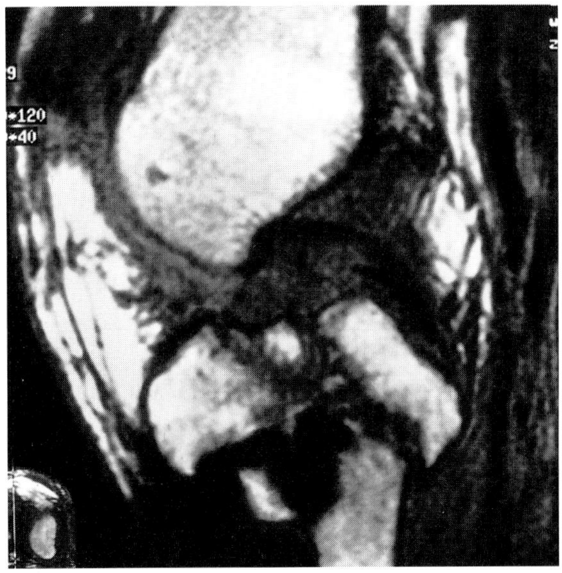

c

Fig 5a–c. Reduced metallic artifacts with 0.2-T extremity MRI. **a** Lateral radiograph of the knee shows metallic fixation hardware for remote tibial plateau fracture, but no other abnormalities to explain persistent pain in this patient several months after surgery. **b** Sagittal T2-weighed fast spin echo image of the same knee acquired at 1.5 T (Signa, General Electric) is distorted by metallic artifacts and offers no convincing explanation for the patient's pain. **c** Sagittal T1-weighted 3D gradient recalled echo image acquired at 0.2 T (Artoscan, Esaote/Lunar) shows markedly fewer metallic artifacts from the fixation hardware and reveals a large unfixed fracture fragment of tibial plateau at the insertion of the posterior cruciate ligament

Arthritis

Patients with arthritis represent a large population for whom imaging has had relatively little to offer thus far. Conventional whole-body MRI has already been shown to be twice as sensitive as radiography for detecting osseous erosions in patients with rheumatoid arthritis [12, 19] (Fig. 8) and 89% accurate in diagnosing early rheumatoid arthritis in patients who lack radiographic changes [13] (Fig. 9). In patients with established rheumatoid arthritis, MRI can detect clinically occult tendinitis and tendon rupture, and thus direct preemptive tenosynovectomy [12]. Moreover, MRI is uniquely capable of quantifying synovitis and its response to therapy [12], and measuring small quantities of cartilage loss over time [15, 16]. A principal obstacle to the acceptance of MRI for these purposes has been concern over cost and accessibility. E-MRI thus offers a way of bringing MRI to this underserved population in a cost-effective manner.

■ Conclusion

In summary, E-MRI represents an intriguing technological advance which offers a number of practical and economic advantages over conventional whole-body MRI. These include lower cost, more convenient and inexpensive siting, greater patient comfort and safety, and lower vulnerabil-

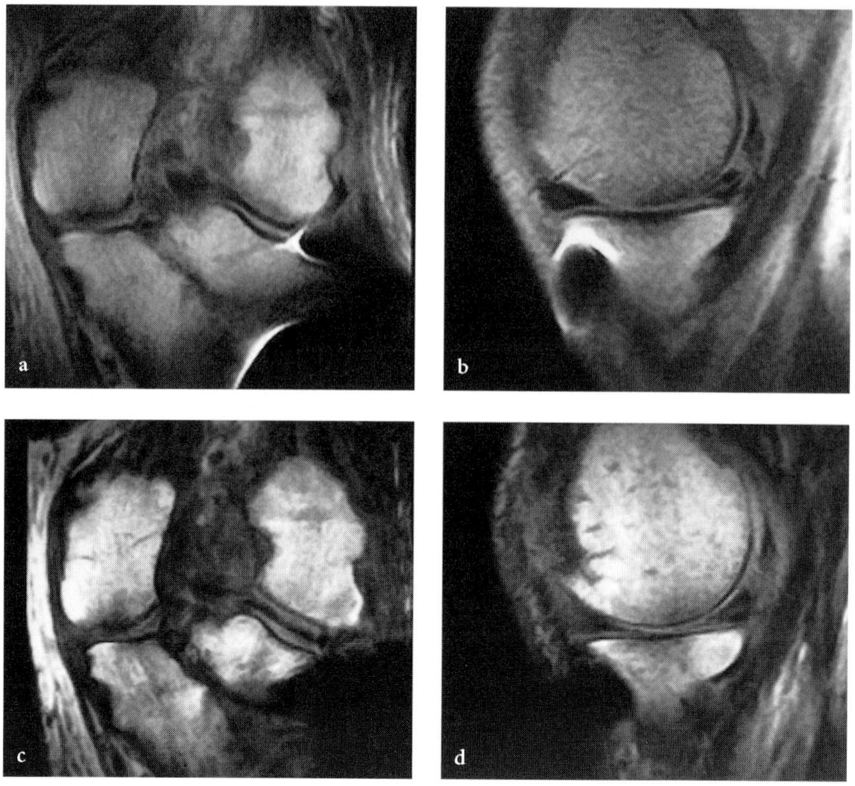

Fig 6a–d. Tibial plateau fracture treated by internal screw fixation. Several months after surgery, the patient complained of knee pain. No displacement was seen on the X-ray and on E-MRI coronal images (**a, c**). A meniscal posterior horn tear is visible on sagittal images gradient recalled echo (**b**) and T1-weighted spin echo (**d**)

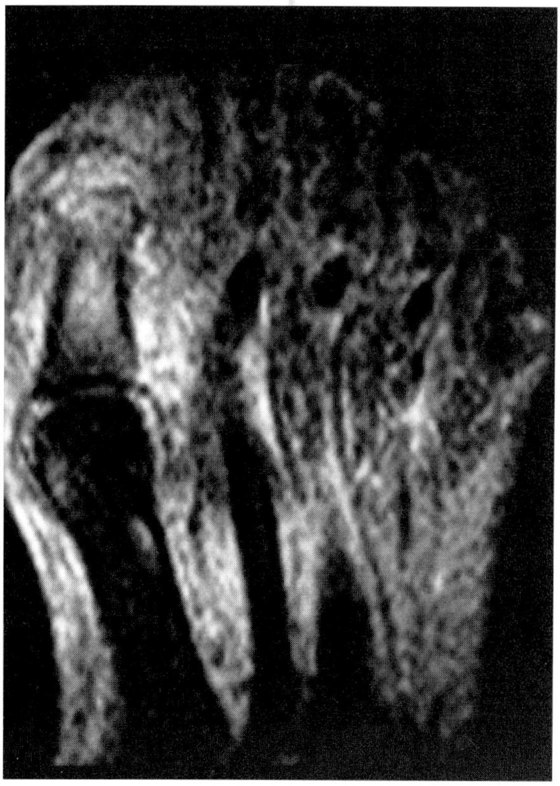

a

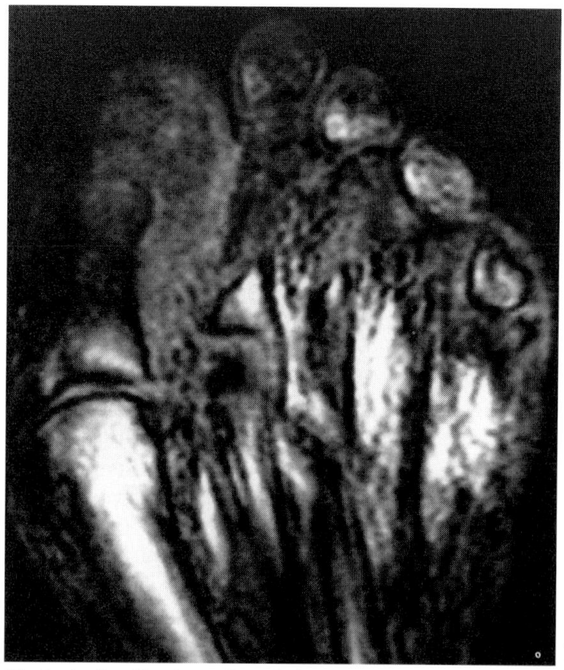

b

Fig 7a, b. Insulin-dependent diabetic patient with persistent pain 3 months after resection of the distal phalanx. Bone marrow edema and adjacent cellulitis are visible on STIR (**a**) and T1-weighted spin echo image (**b**) consistent with osteomyelitis of the proximal phalanx

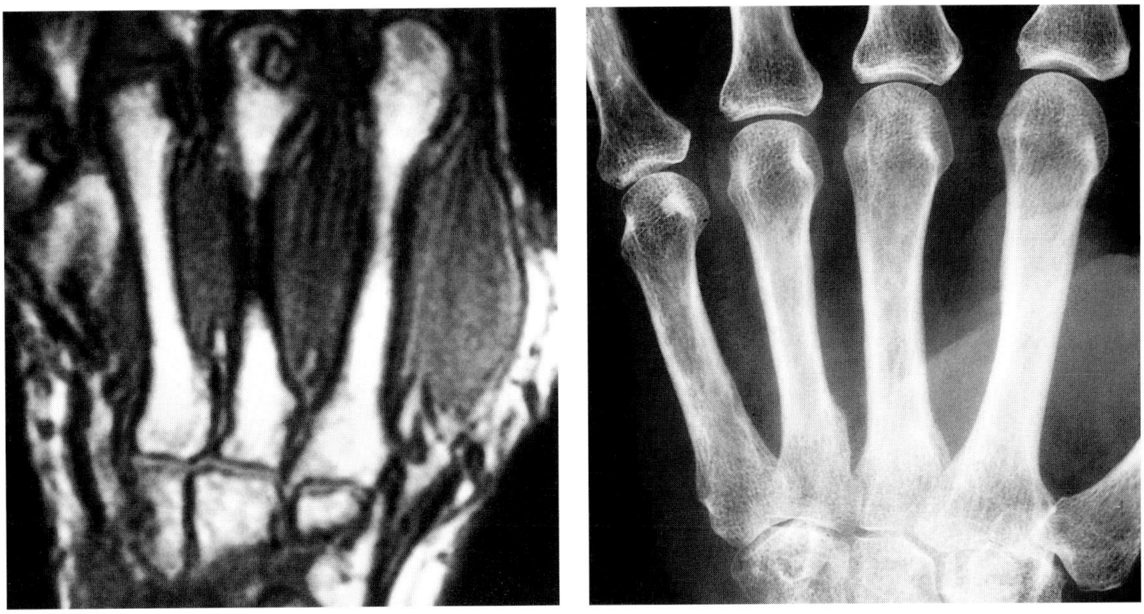

a b

Fig. 8. **a** Coronal spin echo T1-weighted image of the hand of a rheumatoid patient showing a large erosion of the 3rd and some signal changes in the 2nd metacarpal head. **b** The X-rays of the same hand were considered normal

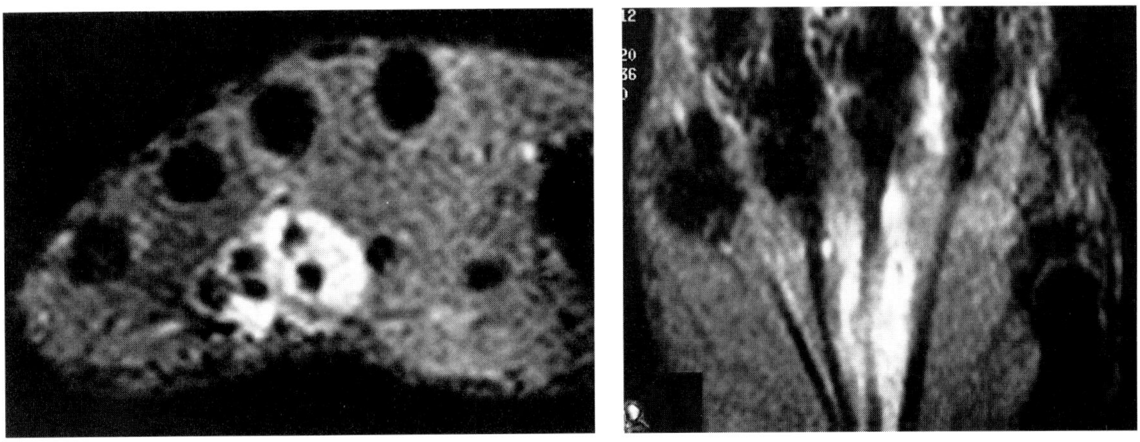

a b

Fig 9. Axial (**a**) and coronal (**b**) STIR images. Tenosynovitis of the flexor tendons in the right hand

ity to magnetic susceptibility artifacts. Limitations include inaccessibility of the shoulder or hip, practical restrictions in bore size and field of view, and controversies surrounding the tradeoffs associated with low field strength imaging.

Not only can E-MRI facilitate imaging in children and claustrophobic patients, and bring greater cost-effectiveness to the evaluation of musculoskeletal conditions, such as meniscal tears, for which the role of MRI is already well established, it may ultimately expand the envelope of MRI to include new clinical populations that have thus far been dominated by radiography and scintigraphy. These include patients with acute extremity trauma, suspected osteomyelitis, arthritis, or periarticular metallic hardware, as well as patients with vague and nonspecific joint complaints, for whom the perceived cost and inconvenience of conventional MRI is considered to be excessive.

Also at issue is the potential impact of this technology on the franchise on MRI that Radiology has enjoyed thus far. As MRI becomes less expensive and more portable, it also becomes increasingly accessible to those outside Radiology who would covet this unique tool. Radiology must not, however, abrogate the stewardship of this modality to others less capable of maximizing its potential or directing its development. It is important therefore that radiologists become more familiar with E-MRI, and take a more active hand in defining its appropriate applications and establishing high standards for its use.

Acknowledgements. Portions of this chapter were adapted from [20]. Work with the Artoscan was supported by grants from Esaote (Genoa, Italy) and Lunar (Madison, WI).

References

1. Bell RA (1996) Economics of MRI technology. J Magn Reson Imaging 6:10–25
2. Passiarello R, Masciocchi C, Barile A, Mastantuono M, De Bac S, Satragno L (1995) Niche MR unit shows promise in extremities. Diagn Imaging Eur 17–20
3. Peterfy CG, Janzen DL, Tirman PFJ, van Dijke CF, Pollack M, Genant HK (1994) Magic-angle phenomenon: a cause of increased signal in the normal lateral meniscus on short-TE MR images of the knee. AJR 163:149–154
4. Jack CR, Berquist TH, Miller GM et al (1990) Field strength in neuro-MR imaging: a comparison of 0.5 T and 1.5 T. J Comput Assist Tomogr 14:505–513
5. Steinberg HV, Alarcon JJ, Bernardino ME (1990) Focal hepatic lesions: comparative MR imaging at 0.5 and 1.5 T. Radiology 174:153–156
6. Orrison WW, Stimac GK, Stevens EA et al (1991) Comparison of CT, low-field-strength MR imaging, and high-field-strength MR imaging. Work in progress. Radiology 181:121–127
7. Barnett MJ (1993) MR diagnosis of internal derangements of the knee: effect of field strength on efficacy. AJR 161:115–118
8. Rutt BK, Lee DE (1996) The impact of field strength on image quality in MRI. J Magn Reson Imaging 6:57–62
9. Häckl F, Peterfy CG, Gindele A et al (1996) Excluding radiographically occult fractures with low-cost dedicated extremity MR imaging. 96th annual meeting of the American Roentgen Ray Society, San Diego, May 1996
10. Heller et al (1997) Cost effectivness of dedicated extremity MRI. International Society for Magnetic Resonance in Medicine, Vancouver
11. Spaeth HJ, Abrams RA, Bock GW, Trudell D, Hodler J, Botte MJ, Petersen M, Resnick D (1993) Gamekeeper thumb: differentiation of nondisplaced and displaced tears of the ulnar collateral ligament with MR imaging. Work in progress. Radiology 188 (2):553–556
12. Palmer WE, Rosenthal DI, Shoenberg OI et al (1995) Quantification of inflammation in the wrist with gadolinium-enhanced MR imaging and PET with 2-[F-18]-fluoro-2-deoxy-D-glucose. Radiology 196:645–655
13. Sugimoto H, Takeda A, Masuyama J, Furuse M (1996) Early-stage rheumatoid arthritis: diagnostic accuracy of MR imaging. Radiology 198:185–192
14. Rubens DJ, Blebea JS, Totterman SMS, Hooper MM (1993) Rheumatoid arthritis: evaluation of wrist extensor tendons with clinical examination versus MR imaging – a preliminary report. Radiology 187:831–838
15. Peterfy CG, van Dijke CF, Janzen DL et al (1994) Quantification of articular cartilage in the knee by pulsed saturation transfer and fat-suppressed MRI: optimization and validation. Radiology 192:485–491
16. Peterfy CG, van Dijke CF, Lu Y et al (1995) Quantification of articular cartilage in the metacarpophalangeal joints of the hand: accuracy and precision of 3D MR imaging. AJR 165:371–375
17. Barile A, Masciocchi C, Mastantuono M, Passariello R, Satragno L (1995) The use of a "dedicated" MRI system in the evaluation of knee joint diseases. Clin MRI 5:79–82
18. Kersting-Sommerhoff B, Hof N, Lenz M, Reinisch M, Riel KA, Gerhardt P (1996) MRI of the knee using a 0.2 T dedicated system: diagnostic accuracy, cost-effectiveness and clinical acceptance. First International Symposium on Musculoskeletal Magnetic Resonance Imaging, San Francisco, January
19. Masciocchi C, Barile A, Navarra F et al (1994) Clinical experience of osteoarticular MRI using a dedicted system. MAGMA 2:545–550
20. Peterfy CG, Roberts T, Genant HK (1997) Dedicated extremity MRI. Radiol Clin North Am 35:1–20

General Pediatric Applications for Open-Field Magnetic Resonance Imaging

4

T. R. Hall · M. I. Boechat · S. J. Westra

■ Introduction

Since its introduction in the past decade magnetic resonance imaging (MRI) has evolved as an important tool in the evaluation of pediatric diseases. While its role in pediatric neuroimaging is important, we would like to emphasize the uses of open MR in body imaging. The lack of ionizing radiation and multiplanar imaging capability with excellent tissue contrast differentiation plus the development of rapid scanning techniques and improved instrumentation, have made MR especially attractive for use in children [8, 12, 38, 60]. High cost and limited availability are constraints faced when using MR in all patients. Furthermore, the need for sedation is another important issue to consider in this age group. In general, ultrasonography (US) and plain films remain as the initial and sole imaging modalities for many pediatric conditions. MR competes with computed tomography (CT) mainly in the evaluation of the extent and resectability of masses [13, 23]. Open MR is particularly valuable in the pediatric patient because of increased accessibility.

■ Patient Preparation, Sedation, and Monitoring

The long acquisition times for most MR examinations usually require deep sedation for pedia-

Table 1. Sedation protocol

Sedation protocol by age	
0–3 months	NPO 3 h prior to exam Chloral hydrate 50 mg/kg p.o. If not asleep in 20–30 min, repeat half original dose
3–6 months	NPO 4 h prior to examination Chloral hydrate 75 mg/kg p.o. If not asleep in 20–30 min, repeat half original dose
6 months–1 year	NPO 4 h prior to examination Chloral hydrate 100 mg/kg p.o. If not asleep in 20–30 min, repeat half original dose
1 year plus (if nursing staff available)	NPO 4 h prior to exam Nembutal (pentobarbital) i.v. Dose titrated by radiologist until child adequately sedated If awakes during procedure, may be resedated by radiologist
1 year plus (other circumstances)	
1–2 years	As per regime for 6 months–1 year, using chloral hydrate
2 years plus	NPO 4 h prior to examination Pentothal (thiopental sodium) 25 mg/kg per rectum If not asleep in 15 min, repeat half original dose
Use of intravenous	Nembutal (pentobarbital) in children
Loading dose	3.0 mg/kg i.v. (Loading dose may be varied downward in the range 2.0–3.0 mg/kg) First 1.0 mg/kg should be given slowly over 2 min Wait at least 2 min to assess effect
Incremental dose	0.5–1.0 mg/kg i.v. (Lower dose for children who are drowsy but not quite sufficiently sedated) Wait 23 min to assess effect of each increment
Saline flush	Required after each dose to ensure no drug remains in i.v. line (5 + cc in case of central line)
Contraindications	Liver failure Poor renal function Sensitivity to barbiturates or other sedatives Porphyria
Maximum dose	6 mg/kg or 150 mg total
Monitoring	Nurse to monitor sleeping patient continuously until awake MD to administer sedation and available while patient asleep Pulse oximeter while patient being sedated and throughout study Apnea monitor while patient in magnet if pulse oximeter inoperable
Versed may be used (i.v.) for the reversal of a paradoxical reaction in its early stage	
Loading dose	0.1 mg/kg
Incremental dose	0.1 mg/kg not to exceed four times the total loading dose
Saline flush	Required after each to dose to ensure that no drug remains in i.v. line
Contraindications	Known hypersensitivity to benzodiazepines (valium and derivatives), glaucoma
For adverse reaction	Flumazenil 0.005 mg/kg i.v. administered over 45 s; can be repeated in 60-s intervals until desired response is achieved.

tric patients. It is generally worth the effort to spend a few minutes with the child and the parents and explain how the scanner works and what to expect once scanning is in progress. A booklet that is written in lay language is helpful adjunct to support personnel who can answer questions for the parents. Reassurance is very important. with most open geometry MR systems the parents and child may remain "in contact" throughout the examination.

The hospital's anesthesia quality assurance committee reviews all sedation protocols. Our current protocol is summarized in Table 1. The protocol is updated periodically whenever alternative drugs become available for clinical use. Both the American Academy of Pediatrics (AAP) and American Society of Anesthesiologist (ASA) recommend continuous monitoring with pulse oximetry and periodic vital signs during induction of deep sedation, during performance of the scan, and in the recovery period. The sedation protocol should also define discharge criteria and provide for a 24-h follow-up phone call for documentation of delayed or prolonged side effects is considered prudent.

Although our success rate with intravenous sedation (96.7%) and all other agents combined (93.9%) is excellent, some cases require a deeper level of sedation. General anesthesia is scheduled for these patients with a pediatric anesthesiologist in charge of medication administration, airway management, and patient monitoring.

At the completion of the scanning procedure the child is transported to a recovery room in close proximity to the MR suite. Monitoring is continued until the patient is alert enough to take clear liquids by mouth. All patients receive written instructions at discharge. The instructions include information about the recovery period, and about possible delayed side effects of the medication, such as vomiting, irritability, or prolonged sedative effect. They are also provided with a physician contact number, which is through the page operator.

Once the child is sedated, and is ready for scanning, attention is given to patient positioning, immobilization, scanning pulse sequences and imaging planes, and coil selection. Surface coils are particularly useful for children. They improve signal-to-noise ratios and spatial resolution. Coils are selected according to patient size and the body part for evaluation [51]. Creative use of the surface coils improves the quality of the studies and is mandatory in the evaluation of small structures.

■ Pulse Sequences

The basic evaluation of most organ systems involves the use of spin-echo technique, usually in two orthogonal planes (axial/coronal, axial/sagittal), obtaining T1- and T2-weighted images.

Recent advances in MRI techniques have made available an impressive array of imaging choices to the radiologist. The MR signal intensity is a synthesis of the hydrogen concentration and the T1 and T2 relaxation values of the tissues. Depending on the imaging method used – spin echo, inversion recovery, short inversion recovery (STIR), complex rephasing incorporated surface probe (CRISP) – the pulse sequences intervals, echo-delay times, and magnetic field strength-image contrast will greatly vary. Although some basic principles apply to all imaging units, each center must develop its own parameters for optimal imaging of each patient. Studies should be carefully tailored to the type of pathology evaluated, in order to avoid the use of excessive scanner time and redundant sequences.

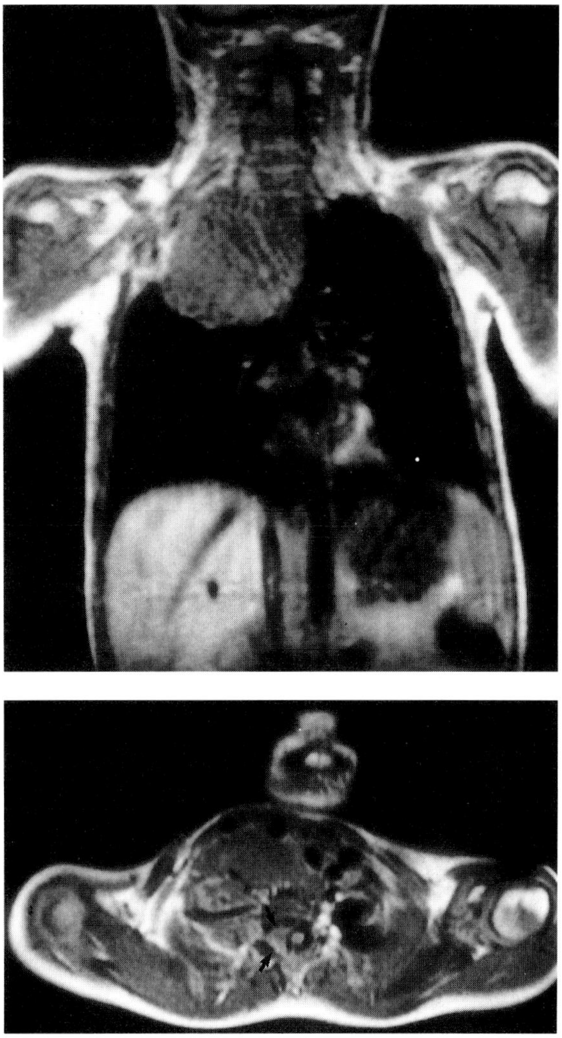

a

b

Fig. 1 a, b. Chest. Neuroblastoma in 5-year-old boy, presenting with Horner syndrome. Coronal (**a**) and axial (**b**) T1-weighted SE images demonstrate a large right apical chest mass. Epidural extension through spinal foramen (**b**, *arrows*) is indicative of posterior mediastinal origin of mass, from superior sympathetic chain ganglion

■ Chest/Cardiovascular Imaging

CT is still the primary imaging modality for the chest when evaluating parenchymal lesions, because of its short scanning time and superior spatial resolution. However, MRI is very useful in the evaluation of the mediastinum, depicting a variety of lesions such as lymphoma, neuroblastoma, cystic hygroma, and other masses [4, 48, 62]. Imaging is usually done in two planes, using at least T1- and T2-weighted sequences (Figs. 1–3).

Imaging of the heart and great vessels with MRI and magnetic resonance angiography (MRA) has improved significantly in the past decade, due mainly to the development of faster pulse sequences, cardiac and respiratory triggering of image acquisition, and cine MRA. Not only can detailed anatomic images of complex cardiovascular anomalies be obtained with either cardiac-gated conventional spin-echo ("black blood") or gradient echo ("white blood") sequences but also physiological information can be acquired (ventricular volumes, ejection fractions, gradients across valves or stenoses and flow quantification [2, 41, 50]. Cardiac MRI in many centers replaces conventional angiocardiography in children in whom echocardiography fails to completely characterize the lesion (Fig. 4). MRI is most useful in the visualization of echocardiographically "blind spots," such as aortic coarctation (Fig. 5 a), vascular rings and slings, branch pulmonary arteries (Fig. 5 b), pulmonary veins, and in general in older children and young adults with congenital heart lesions, in whom no good acoustic window exists to asses cardiac anatomy and function [5, 28].

The choice from a wide array of imaging sequences and planes must be tailored to the clinical question to be answered, and close cooperation with pediatric cardiologists is required. Despite the recent development of some faster scan techniques, sedation is generally required in young and uncooperative children, as most studies take up to one hour to perform. The influence of respiratory motion artifacts is still significant enough to preclude imaging of peripheral airways

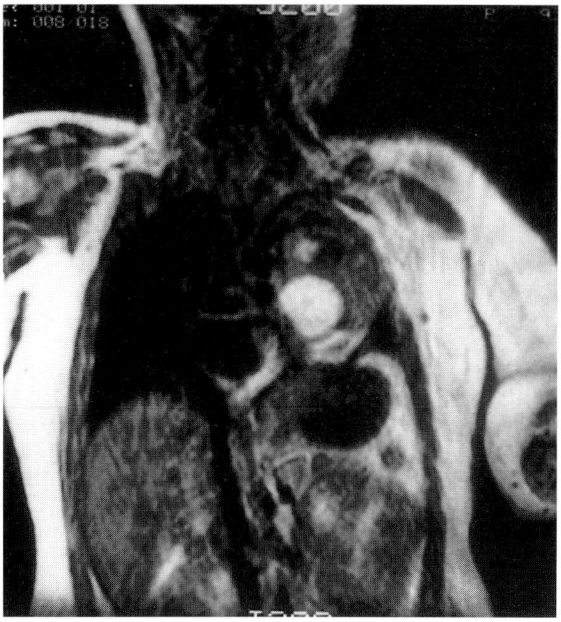

a

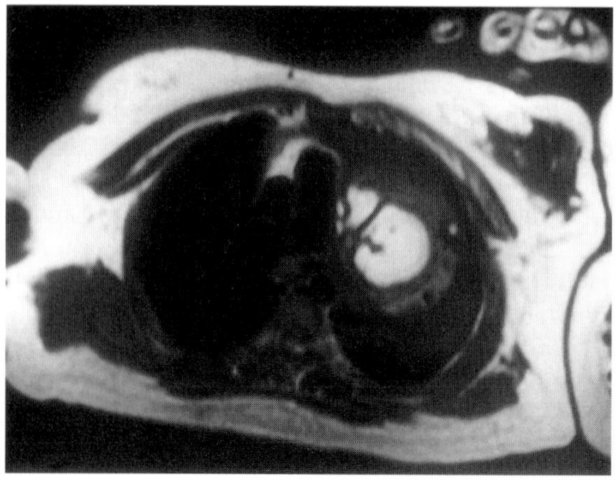

b

Fig. 2 a, b. Mediastinum. Teratoma in 5-year-old girl. Coronal (**a**) and axial (**b**) T1-weighted SE images demonstrate a well-demarcated mass with homogeneous soft-tissue and septated fatty components in the anterior mediastinum. Note compression of left pulmonary artery

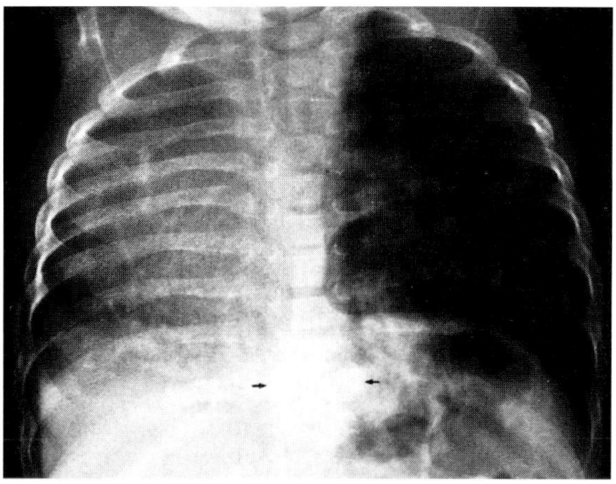

a

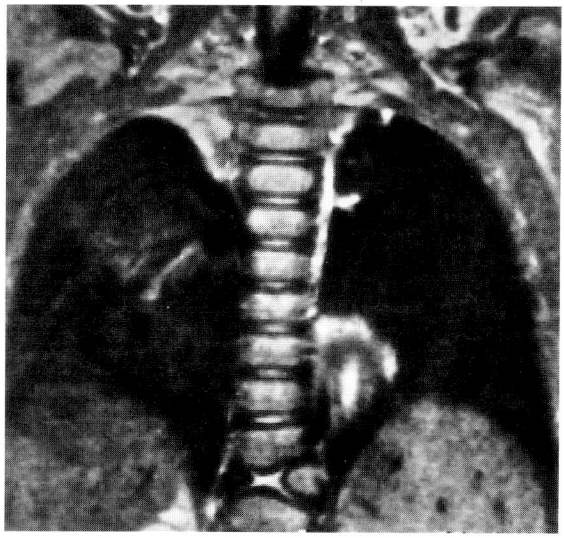

b

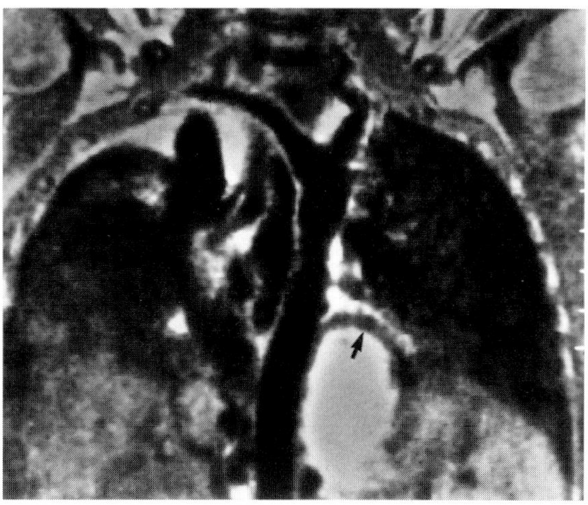

c

Fig. 3 a–c. Chest. Pulmonary sequestration. **a** AP chest radiograph in 6-month-old girl with right lung hypoplasia and recurrent pulmonary infections. **b**, **c** Coronal T2-weighted images demonstrate sequestration as a high-intensity round mass in the left cardiophrenic angle, with systemic arterial supply (*arrow*). Note also butterfly vertebra in lower thoracic spine on **a** (*small arrows*) and **c**

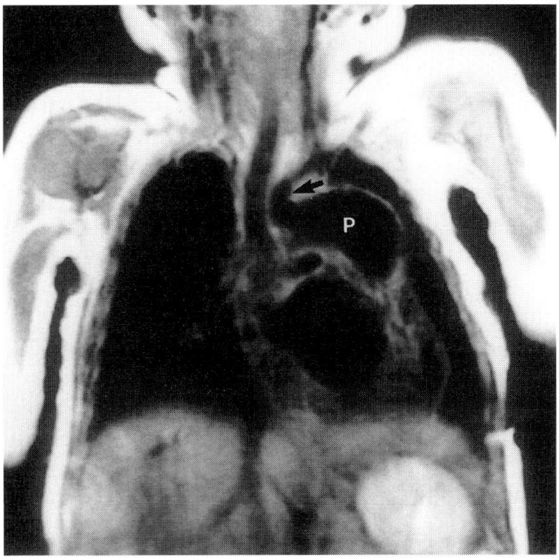

Fig. 4. Cardiovascular. Pseudoaneurysm of pulmonary artery after left modified Blalock-Taussig shunt placement in 3-year-old girl. Coronal cardiac-gated T1-weighted SE image demonstrates relationship between pseudoaneurysm (*P*) and shunt anastomosis (*arrow*)

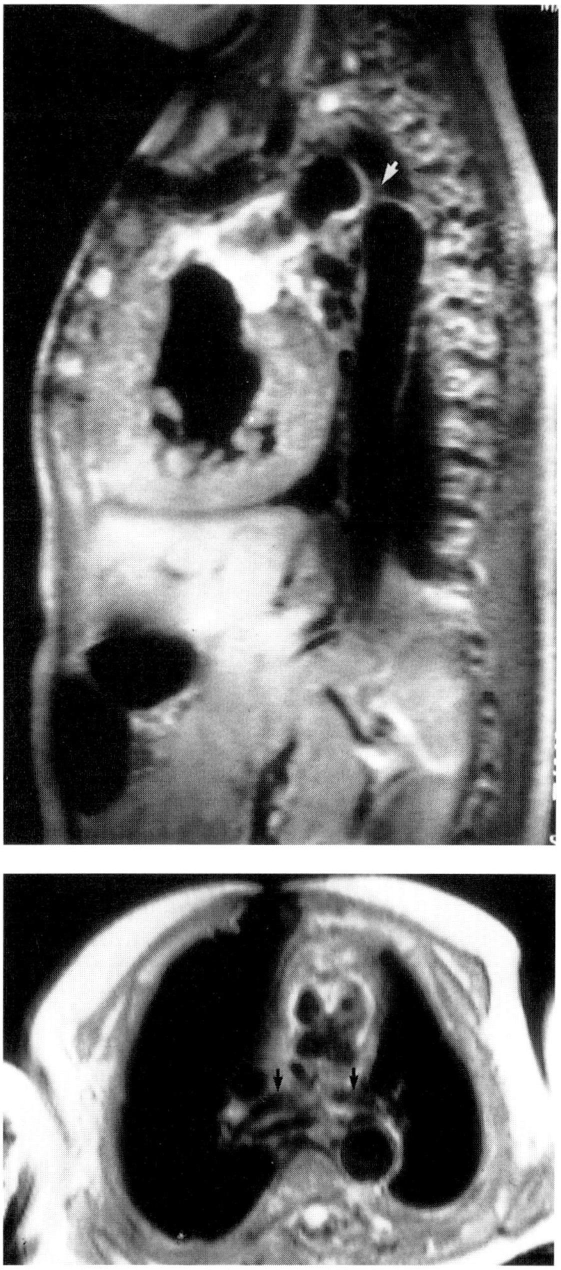

a

b

Fig. 5 a, b. Cardiovascular. **a** Severe aortic coarctation (*arrow*) sagittal-oblique cardiac-gated T1-weighted spin echo image. Note hyperdense material in wall of neoascending aorta) in 5-month-old boy who underwent Norwood repair for hypoplastic left heart syndrome. There is marked myocardial hypertrophy. **b** Both branch pulmonary arteries are hypoplastic (*arrows*; axial T1-weighted image), precluding the placement of a Glenn shunt (SVC to right pulmonary artery)

and vessels, but the development of faster echoplanar sequences with respiratory triggering may resolve this problem. The presence of metallic clips and stents in close proximity to anatomic details to be visualized makes MRI less suitable to image postoperative patients.

The development of MRA pulse sequences has also found wide applications in pediatric peripheral vascular imaging [18]. One of the most frequent indications for vascular studies is the search for a suitable venous access site for central line placement in patients with multiple line complications, who are dependent on total parenteral nutrition. Using 2D time-of-flight MRA with appropriately placed saturation pulses, the entire central venous system can be imaged in a relatively short period of time, without the need for intravenous contrast administration (Fig. 6). Another useful application of MRA is for noninvasive imaging of patients with portal hypertension, who are being considered for portosystemic shunt placement or liver transplantation.

In oncological imaging MRA is used to assess vascular compression by tumor, tumor extension into the renal veins/inferior vena cava (Fig. 7), and patency of the portal vein in patients with liver tumors to determine resectability and surgical approach [23].

In general, color Doppler US is equally useful and often complementary to MRA, but the former is more operator dependent. MRA provides a more global image of vascular anatomy and involvement in disease processes than does color Doppler ultrasound, and is therefore preferred as a preoperative procedure, frequently obviating the need for conventional angiography.

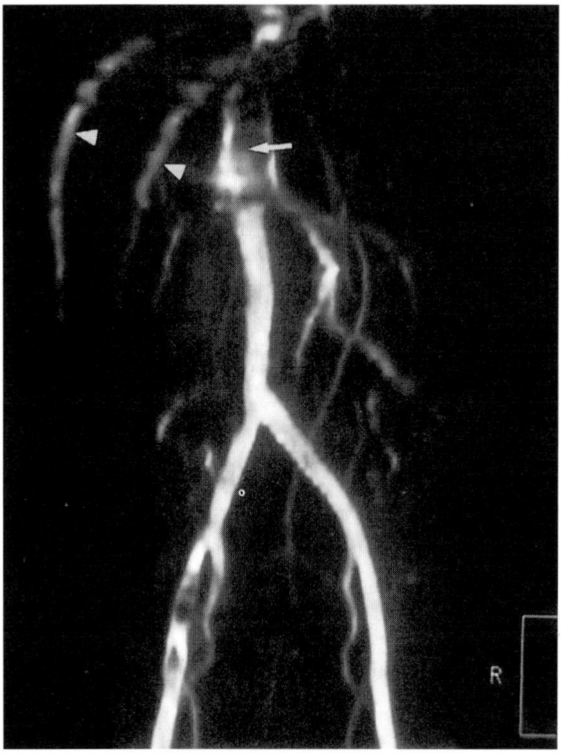

Fig. 6. Cardiovascular. Thrombotic occlusion (*arrow*) of hepatic portion of inferior vena cava in 11-year-old postoperative patient with hypercoagulable state, shown on AP maximum intensity projection image of 2D time-of-flight MR venogram data. Hepatic veins (*arrowheads*) are patent. (Courtesy of Michael Gyepes, MD, Long Beach Memorial Hospital, Calif.)

Abdominal Imaging

Respiratory motion and bowel peristalsis are limiting factors in the evaluation of intra-peritoneal abnormalities. At the time of this writing, there are no satisfactory contrast agents available for bowel opacification, and it may be difficult to distinguish between lymphadenopathy and overlying bowel [3]. MRI plays a significant role in the evaluation of liver and retroperitoneal organs in children. Its most important role is in the evaluation of abdominal neoplasms, an area where CT was until recently the gold standard [13].

When a child presents with an abdominal mass, the initial examination is a plain radiography of the abdomen, followed by US. If US shows a solid lesion that the physician suspects may be a neoplasm, CT or MRI is used to define the origin extent and resectability of the lesion. MRI is also an ideal modality for follow-up study of these patients.

Liver

As previously mentioned, the most commonly used imaging modality in the study of the liver is US. MR, however, has a well defined role in the evaluation of children with liver masses, as it gives precise information about the extent and resectability of lesions, assisting surgeons in surgical planning [14, 15, 74]. Benign and malignant masses are equally well depicted by MR, and

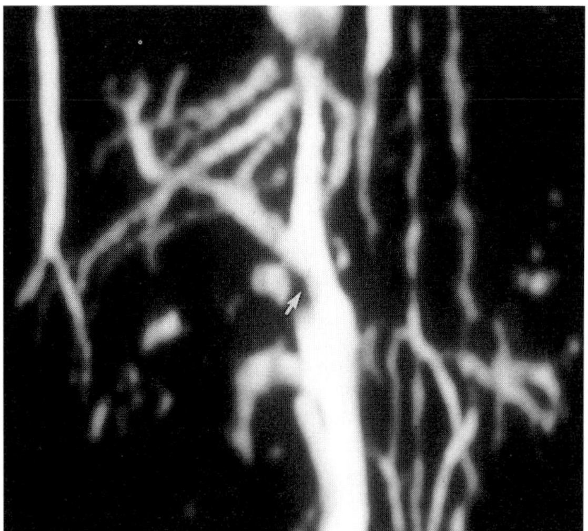

Fig. 7. Cardiovascular. Large right Wilms' tumor in 8-year-old boy. Tumor extension from right renal vein into IVC is well demonstrated on coronal maximum intensity projection image from 2D time-of-flight MRA sequence

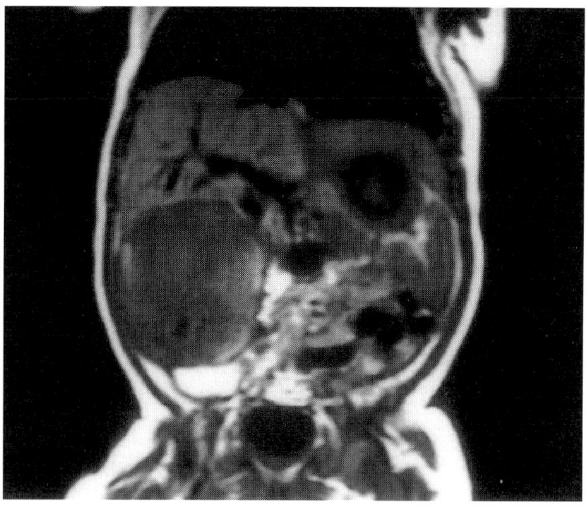

Fig. 8. Liver. Mesenchymal hamartoma originating from inferior right liver in 3-month-old boy presenting with an abdominal mass. Coronal T1-weighted SE image demonstrates sharp delineation between right liver lobe and mass, and relationship to portal vein and gallbladder. During surgery this benign tumor could easily be separated from the liver

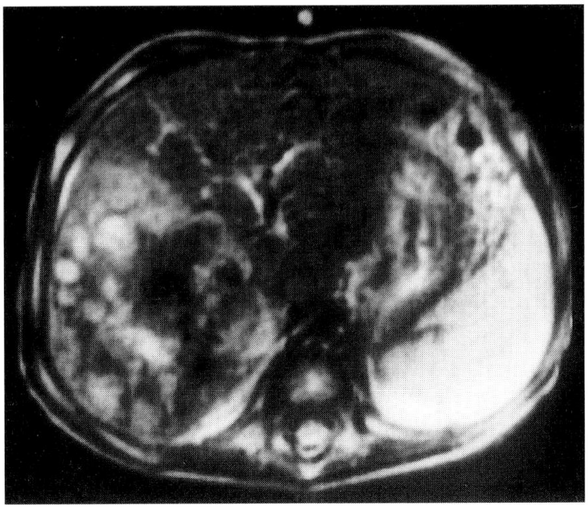

Fig. 9. Liver. Hepatoblastoma in 4-year-old boy, axial T2-weighted image. There is an ill-defined inhomogeneous mass which was confined to the right liver lobe and did not involve the portal vein (not shown). Extended right lobe resection could be performed and was curative

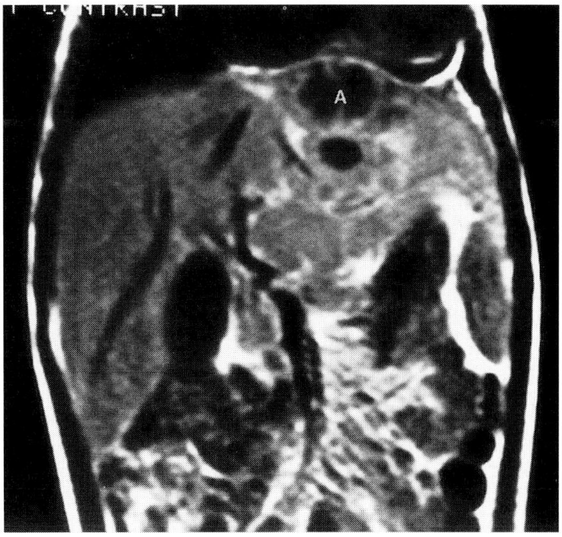

Fig. 10. Liver. Amebic abscess in 3-year-old boy; coronal T1-weighted image shows close proximity of abscess (*A*) in left liver lobe to the heart, indicating risk of intrapericardial rupture. This finding constitutes an urgent indication for percutaneous drainage of the abscess. (Reprinted with permission)

although the imaging findings sometimes allow the radiologist to predict the type of lesion, it should be remembered that neither MR nor CT can provide histological diagnosis (Figs. 8–10).

Axial T1- and T2-weighted sequences are initially used in evaluating the liver and biliary tract. On these images the organ parenchyma is well visualized, and structures such as the portal vein, the origin of celiac axis, and the superior mesenteric artery are clearly seen. The axial plane is also used for evaluation of the common bile duct. Heavily T2-weighted images are especially helpful in the evaluation of liver hemangiomas, as these vascular lesions have increased signal with prolongation of TE/TR [21, 64]. This finding, however, does not occur when there is significant fibrosis within the hemangioma, and the differential diagnosis with other childhood tumors can be difficult. In all cases of hepatic tumors it is important to obtain the patient's history and laboratory findings, and to determine a correlation between them with the imaging information. Hemangiomas are more common in the first year of life, hepatoblastomas have elevated levels of α_1-fetoprotein, and hepatocellular carcinoma is usually associated with chronic liver diseases, such as hepatitis, and tyrosemia.

The MR characteristics of liver tumors are: isointensity or low signal intensity on T1-weighted images, with areas of high signal representing hemorrhage and areas of low signal intensity corresponding to calcifications or necrosis; on T2-weighted sequences, tumors have high signal intensity. Tumor thrombus within the portal vein or inferior vena cava have a similar appearance. MR is also utilized in the postoperative follow up of children with liver tumors, depicting the presence of recurrence and metastatic spread [15].

Generalized liver disease, such as cirrhosis and hemochromatosis, is also imaged well by MRI. Cirrhotic liver appears small, with nonhomogeneous signal intensity, while hemochromatosis has a markedly lower signal intensity because of the deposition of iron and prolongation of T1 relaxation time [39, 65]. More useful than the ability of MR to demonstrate generalized liver disease, is the depiction of vascular anatomy with exquisite detail, without contrast administration. As mentioned above, MRA is very useful in the evaluation of children before and after liver transplantation.

■ Pancreas, Spleen, Mesentery

Although the pancreas, spleen and mesentery can be evaluated by MR, the method is seldom used in children, since it does not offer specific advantages over US or CT, and usually requires sedation of the patient.

■ Kidneys

T1-weighted coronal images are the best to demonstrate the overall appearance of the kidneys, their accurate dimensions, and relationship to adjacent organs. The cortex has higher signal intensity than the medulla, with clear corticomedullary differentiation on T1-weighted images, especially when inversion recovery is used. The renal artery and vein, the ureter, and the pelvicalyceal system all have low signal intensity. Renal pyramids are relatively more prominent in neonates and young children; they become similar to those seen in adult kidneys by about 12 years of age. Signal intensity from adipose tissue (short T1 and long T2 relaxation times) is not visible in the renal hili of young children. It progressively increases with age, when fat starts to accumulate in the region and is clearly visible by puberty [25].

Congenital and acquired anomalies of the urinary tract are usually diagnosed by means of US or CT urogram. The role of MR in the evaluation of children with urinary tract infection is being investigated; the use of inversion recovery sequences with gadolinium is promising [56]. Another area of present research is the evaluation of glomerular function using dynamic MR scanning [30].

Imaging of renal tumors requires either CT or MR; an important limitation of the latter is the long imaging time, that does not allow the depiction of lung metastasis. Therefore in most centers CT is the imaging modality of choice, although MR can exquisitely depict a Wilms tumor, its extension to adjacent organs and inferior vena cava [23, 49].

Wilms tumor is the most common solid intra-abdominal neoplasm in children. MR shows an expansive lesion, with low signal on T1- and high signal on T2-weighted sequences. Areas of hemorrhage are seen as regions of high signal on T1-weighted images. MR is also helpful to differentiate between classic Wilms tumor and Wilms tumor arising from nephroblastomatosis. In the latter group of patients there are multicentric or diffuse tumors and tumor-like lesions; the contralateral kidney should be carefully examined because of the known increased incidence of bilateral lesions. MRI can also be used for the evaluation of liver metastasis, tumor response to chemotherapy, and postsurgical follow-up studies.

Other common renal neoplasms in children include forms of leukemia and lymphoma. Renal infiltration by lymphoma causes focal or generalized enlargement of the kidneys with low signal intensity and loss of corticomedullary differentiation in the involved portion. Involvement of the bone marrow in these patients can also be demonstrated by areas of lower signal intensity on T1-weighted images, a very useful sign in differentiating leukemia and lymphoma from Wilms tumor.

■ Adrenal Glands

With MRI, one can accurately evaluate normal and abnormal adrenal glands especially when T1-weighted coronal images are used. In neonates and young children, the adrenal gland is relatively large and may have convex borders, while in older children, it has straight or slightly concave borders. The signal intensity of the adrenal glands is slightly less than that of the renal cortex, similar to the overall signal intensity of the kidneys, and substantially less than that of perinephric fat. When the kidneys are absent or abnormally located, such as in those patients with renal agenesis or ectopia, the ipsilateral adrenal gland appears flat and plate-like (discoid adrenal gland), and may mimic a kidney.

The most significant role of MRI in the evaluation of adrenal diseases in children is in the assessment of adrenal neoplasms, particularly neuroblastoma [27, 76].

Neuroblastoma is the second most common solid neoplasm in childhood, and it occurs along the sympathetic chain in the nasopharynx, chest, abdomen and pelvis, or the origin may be unknown. The most common location is in the abdomen, in the region of the adrenal glands.

Coronal T1-weighted images should be acquired initially to separate adrenal from paravertebral or renal neoplasm. By clearly visualizing the spine and the spinal cord, it is possible to evaluate intraspinal extension of a lesion confidently and obviate the need for invasive procedures, such as conventional or CT myelography [26] (Fig. 11). Neuroblastoma has a tendency to spread quite early to the retroperitoneal area, encasing and displacing arteries and veins. Demonstration of vascular anatomy is of paramount importance for evaluation of tumor resectability. The aorta and the inferior vena cava are best seen on coronal T1-weighted images, whereas the superior mesenteric artery and the celiac axis are better visualized on the axial plane (Fig. 12). Differentiation between adrenal hemorrhage and hemorrhagic neuroblastoma in newborns is not always possible based on MRI findings alone, and whether to resect the lesion or monitor it with ultrasound until resolution is based primarily on clinical grounds [17, 29, 76] (Fig. 13).

Fig. 11 a, b. Neuroblastoma. Coronal (**a**) and axial (**b**) T1-weighted images in 9-month-old girl, demonstrating paraspinal neuroblastoma (*N*), with ingrowth into spinal canal leading to obliteration of epidural fat (**b**, *arrows*)

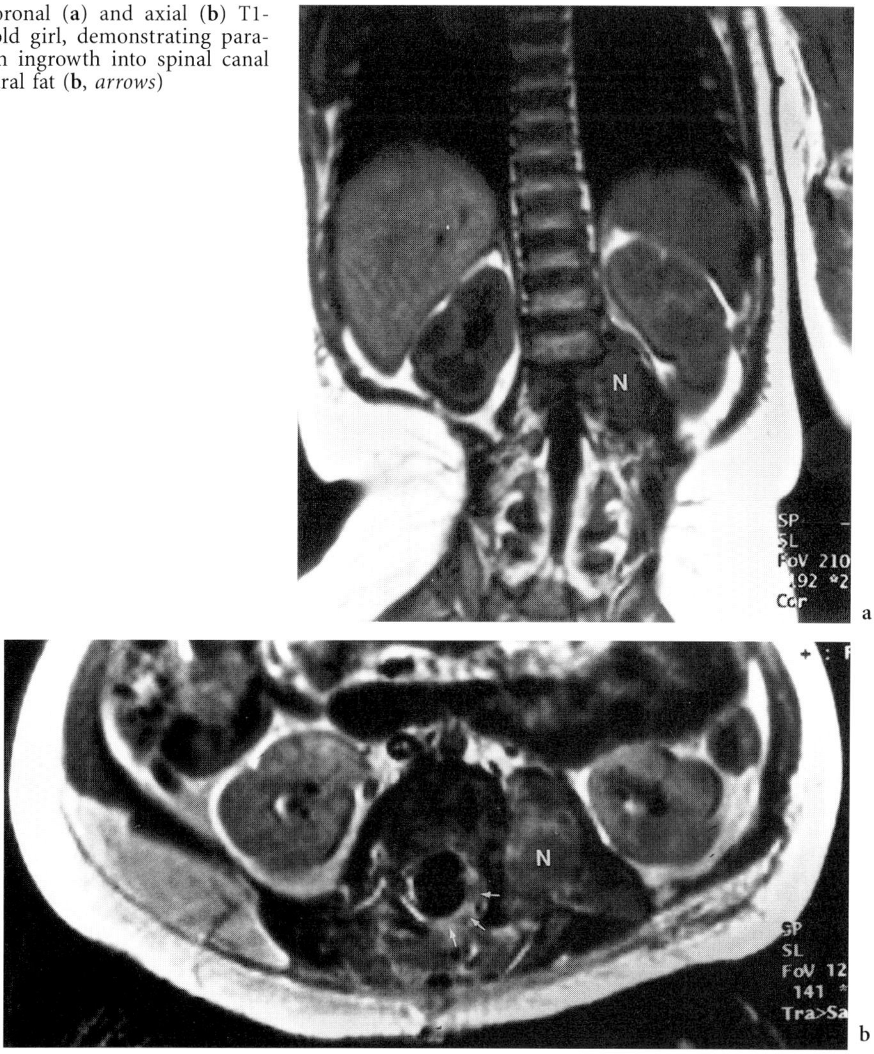

Fig. 12. Adrenal gland. Stage 3 neuroblastoma. Axial T1-weighted spin echo image demonstrates large left retroperitoneal mass (*M*), displacing the aorta (*a*) anteriorly and extending across the midline to the inferior vena cava (*i*)

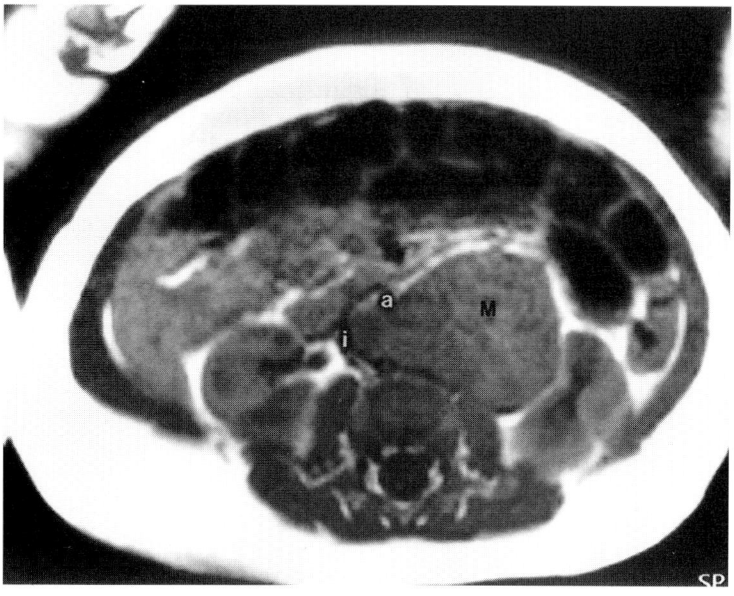

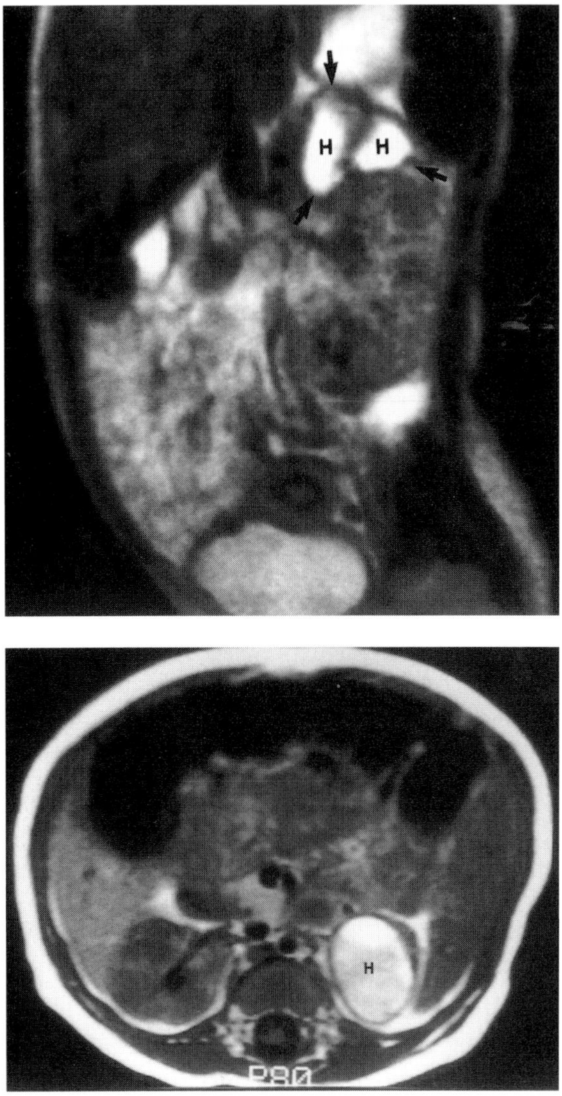

a

b

Fig. 13 a, b. Adrenal gland. Left adrenal hemorrhage associated with renal vein thrombosis in 1-week-old girl. Coronal-oblique T1-weighted image shows left renal enlargement with loss of corticomedullary differentiation, secondary to left renal vein thrombosis. This also caused hemorrhagic infarction (*H*) of the left adrenal gland, which was enlarged but has retained its normal triangular shape (*arrows*). In contrast, adrenal shape is lost in hemorrhagic neuroblastoma in different infant, axial T1-weighted SE image (*B*), in whom hemorrhage (*H*) is seen in the adrenal medulla with preservation and stretching of the cortex

Tumor metastasis to bone, bone marrow, and dura can also be evaluated with MRI (Fig. 14). MRI appears to be more sensitive in detecting marrow and bone metastasis than radionuclide bone scans, although a nuclear medicine bone scan is better for screening. MRI is also more accurate than CT in evaluation of dural metastasis. Spine and long bones are best evaluated in the coronal plane and the brain dura in the sagittal

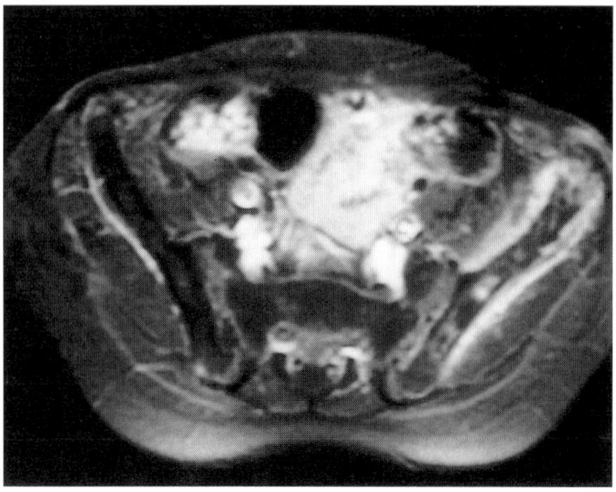

Fig. 14. Stage 4 neuroblastoma metastases to left iliac wing. Axial T1-weighted SE image with fat suppression after gadolinium enhancement shows inhomogeneity of the marrow signal and diffuse periosteal enhancement of the left iliac wing (compare with the normal right side)

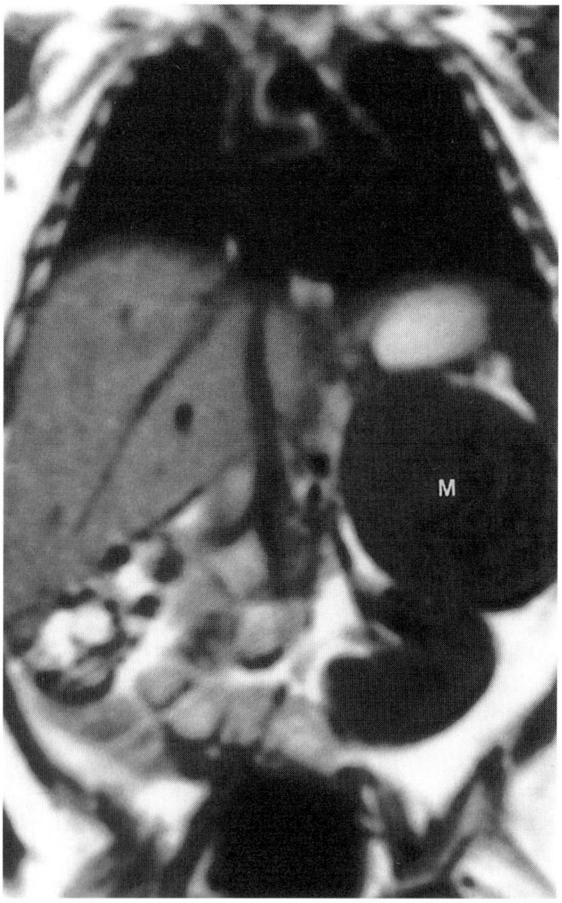

Fig. 15. Adrenal. Adrenal cortical carcinoma in infant with Cushing syndrome. Coronal T1-weighted image demonstrate large left adrenal mass (*M*), with characteristic displacement of left kidney. Despite the regular outline of the mass, malignancy was found in the resection specimen. (Courtesy of Michael Gyepes, MD, Long Beach Memorial Hospital, Calif.)

plane. Again, MRI is the ideal imaging modality after chemotherapy and surgery.

Other adrenal tumors such as pheochromocytoma, ganglioneuroma, adrenal cortical adenoma and carcinoma are much rarer than neuroblastoma in children. MRI demonstrates an adrenal mass with nonspecific signal characteristics, and is used primarily to determine resectability [75] (Fig. 15). In the coronal plane, MRI may specifically demonstrate the extension of adrenal carcinoma into the renal vein, the inferior vena cava, and the right atrium.

In children, as opposed to adults, functional status of adrenal cortical tumors cannot be predicted based on signal characteristics, but the majority of these present clinically with a well-defined endocrine syndrome.

■ Pelvis

The most common indications for pelvic MRI in children are the evaluation of congenital abnormalities of the female pelvis and the study of pelvic soft tissue masses [9, 61]. MR is particularly important in the staging of pelvic malignancies, allowing determination of the site of origin, extent and characteristics of masses [10]. Other indications include evaluation of imperforate anus and undescended testis [58, 69].

Congenital Anomalies

The knowledge of normal embryological development is fundamental to the understanding of abnormalities found in the genitourinary tract. In the absence of antimüllerian hormone secretion by a fetal testis, the müllerian ducts meet in the midline by 8 weeks gestation and subsequently differentiate into the uterus, cervix, fallopian tubes, and proximal two-thirds of the vagina. The urogenital sinus forms the distal one-third of the vagina [1].

Anomalies of müllerian duct development can cause serious complications of sexual function, pregnancy, and labor and are frequently associated with anomalies of the urinary tract, such as absent or ectopic kidneys [33, 34].

The diagnosis and management of disorders of gonadal function or development require complex laboratory and clinical evaluation. It is often necessary to define the pelvic anatomy before a definite diagnosis can be made, or therapeutic action undertaken. This is particularly important in the neonatal period to avoid incorrect gender assignment. A broad spectrum of anomalies of sexual differentiation may exist at birth, including male and female pseudohermaphroditism, gonadal dysgenesis, and true hermaphroditism. The main role of imaging in these cases is to document the presence or absence of a uterus and identification of the gonads. This is usually done by US and sometimes genitography. MR should be used in patients with suspected congenital anomalies for whom the results of either ultrasound or radiographic studies are inconclusive and a precise diagnosis is required for treatment [11, 31, 43].

There are many types of congenital uterine anomalies, the most common is bicornuate uterus. These anomalies can be identified by MR imaging, using T2-weighted sagittal images, supplemented by axial T1- and T2-weighted images, perpendicular to the long axis of uterine body and cervix [19, 53].

Congenital anomalies of the vagina include complete or partial agenesis, stenosis, septation and the presence of an imperforate membrane. Hydrohematometrocolpos refers to the accumulation of fluid and menstrual products in the vagina and uterus. The obstruction results in the accumulation of secretions in the vagina (hydrocolpos) or within the vagina and uterus (hydrometrocolpos), and subsequent appearance of a palpable abdominal or pelvic mass (Fig. 16). It can be secondary to an intact hymen, a vaginal membrane, or vaginal atresia. MR has an important role depicting the level of obstruction and uterine anatomy. The use of very thin contiguous slices in the evaluation of the vagina assists the diagnosis of uterine/vaginal agenesis with normal ovaries seen in Mayer-Rokitansky-Kuster-Hauser syndrome and in the diagnosis of duplicated vagina [31, 68].

Congenital Anorectal Anomalies

Children with imperforate anus need precise pre- and postoperative evaluation. Before surgery it is necessary to establish the level of the anorectal malformation in relation to the levator muscle sling (low, intermediate or high lesion), to decide on the surgical approach and assess the likelihood of attaining rectal continence [58]. Detection of associated renal and spinal malformations is also important.

Plain films do not allow accurate assessment of this pathology. The capability of MR to depict the muscles and their relationship with adjacent structures makes it the ideal method to study the pelvic structures in children with imperforate anus.

After surgery children may develop incontinence due to sphincter or musculature problems,

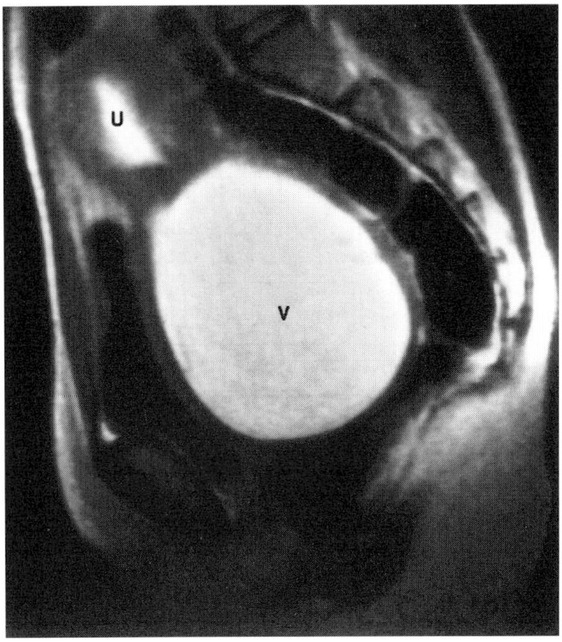

Fig. 16. Pelvis. Midsagittal T1-weighted scan shows high signal intensity mass between bladder and rectum, consistent with hydrometrocolpos. *U*, Uterus; *V*, vagina. (Reprinted with permission)

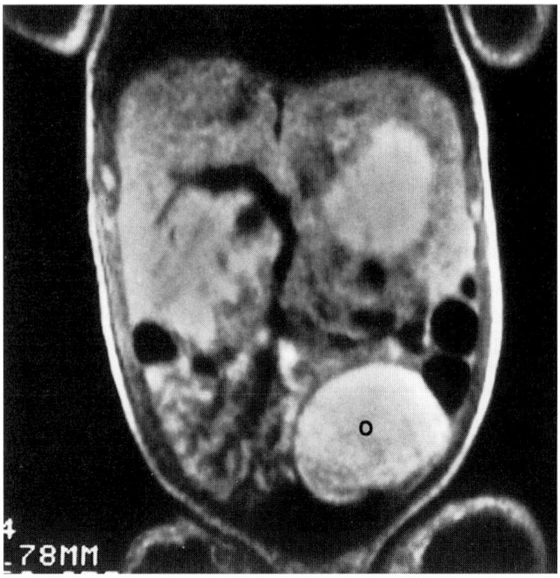

Fig. 17. Pelvis. Newborn girl with palpable mass in left lower abdomen, with high signal intensity on coronal T1-weighted scan, due to hemorrhagic ovarian cyst (*O*). (Reprinted with permission)

such as misplaced neorectum, inadvertently pulled-through mesenteric fat and diverticulation of the rectal lumen. All these abnormalities can be shown by MR [58, 71].

Cloacal Malformations and Extrophy Syndromes

Cloacal malformations involve a combination of abnormalities of the urinary, genital and intestinal tracts, with a common outflow structure, the cloaca. It is seen in phenotypic females and has a good prognosis, with surgical repair and good functional outcome now possible [40].

The extrophy syndromes reflect maldevelopment of the cloacal membrane and defective sub-umbilical abdominal wall development. Extrophy of the bladder is the most common anomaly, accounting for two-thirds of the patients with this condition. Epispadias is the mildest form, whole extrophy of the cloaca is the most severe [77].

Imaging evaluation of this group of patients involves use of multiple catheters, contrast injection under fluoroscopy and US examination of the pelvis, abdomen and spine. MR plays a role in the delineation of the urogenital septum and cloacal membrane, and the relationship between the pelvic structures. It is also used in the assessment of associated spinal abnormalities [47].

Ovarian Lesions

In the neonatal period, genital masses are usually due to hematocolpos/hematometrocolpos or to ovarian cysts (Fig. 17). In older children almost all masses originate from the ovaries, either due to benign cysts of to germ cell tumors [16]. These lesions may be asymptomatic or cause acute pain, if they undergo torsion or rupture. Once again, US is the screening examination performed and directs clinical or surgical management. If the results of the US examination are unclear, MR maybe useful not only in pre-operative evaluation, but also in the staging of tumors.

■ Musculoskeletal System and Bone Marrow

Although there are many similarities in the appearance of the joints in children and adults, some important differences should be noted [20, 46, 67]. The growth plate produces a zone of low signal intensity and is wider in younger children. A line of low signal intensity may be identified at the site of the former growth plate in adolescents, even after radiographic evidence of closure. The ossified portion of the epiphysis contains marrow, thus having a higher signal intensity than the surrounding cartilaginous portion.

Imaging of the musculoskeletal system is done using spin echo, gradient echo and short T1 inversion recovery (STIR) pulse sequences; postgadolinium scans with fat suppression or STIR may be useful to assess soft tissue tumors and to differentiate viable tumor from marrow edema in patients undergoing chemotherapy [73]. Gradient echo scans are mainly used to assess joint cartilage, especially for determining cartilaginous integrity in osteochondritis dissecans. Images in the coronal and sagittal planes are useful in the evaluation of extremities and spine, while imaging in the axial plane is indicated for pelvis and shoulder. When the spin echo technique is used, the MR signal intensity obtained may be high (marrow), low (bone cortex), or intermediate (cartilage and muscle) as a result of added signals from lipid and water protons.

MRI is the modality of choice for evaluation of the bone marrow in children. As the MR signal intensity of the bone marrow is related to the ratio of fat to other cells (in healthy children this ratio is around 50%), the signal is strong and uniform, particularly in the metaphysis and diaphysis. Results are not reliable when one is comparing signal intensity differences of the marrow between two patients or between two examinations on the same patient. Comparison with the signal intensity of an adjacent structure, such as muscle, provides more accurate information. The marrow in a healthy pediatric subject has a uniform signal approximately three times more intense than that of adjacent muscle.

Marrow hyperplasia is characterized by low signal intensity because of decreased marrow fat; it is seen in the bones of patients with sickle cell anemia, hemophilia, and aplastic anemia (Fig. 18). Anemic patients may show normal signal in the epiphysis and abnormal signal in the metaphysis and diaphysis, because most of the hematopoiesis occurs in these areas. Untreated aplastic anemia may show normal signal intensity because of overabundant fat. In the recovery phase, when there is marrow hypercellularity, the signal intensity decreases.

Primary bone tumors, such as osteosarcoma and Ewing sarcoma, are one of the most common indications for imaging of the musculoskeletal system by MRI. Soft tissue and marrow involvement are very well demonstrated, and coronal images provide good assessment of tumor extent, allowing preoperative planning. T1-weighted images of children with osteosarcoma show a lesion with mixed signal intensity, the areas of low signal intensity representing mineralized tumor osteoid. On a T2-weighted sequence the lesion shows high signal intensity; this sequence also demonstrates soft tissue involvement and is usually obtained in the axial plane (Fig. 19). Tumor re-

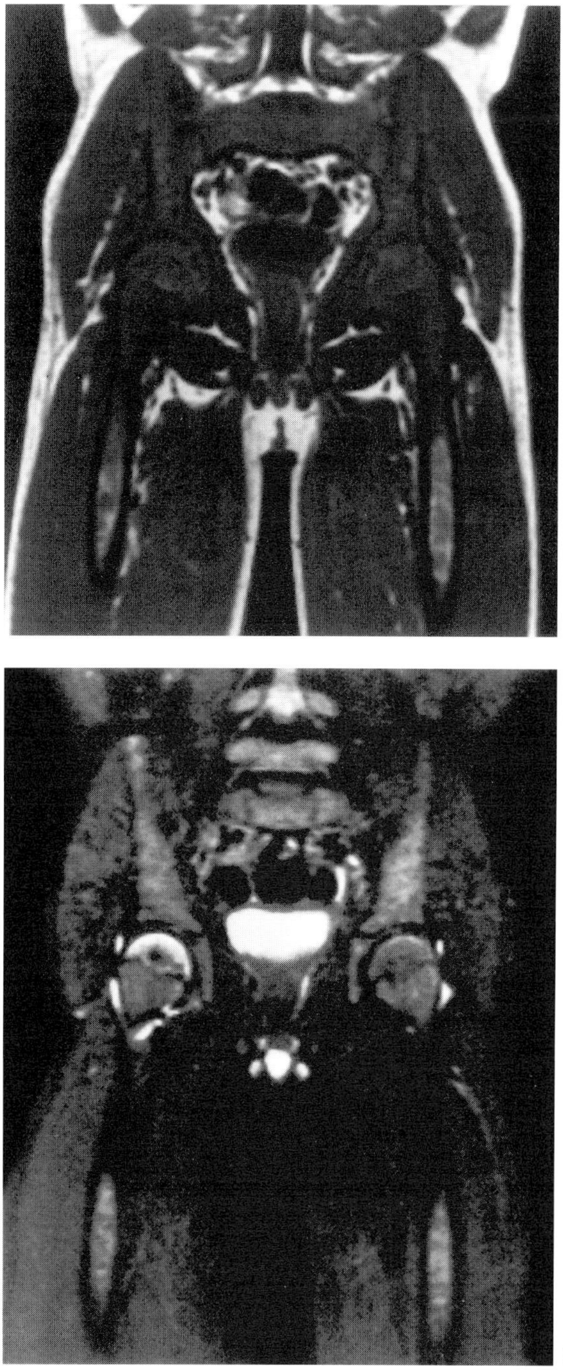

a

b

Fig. 18a,b. Musculoskeletal. Eleven-year-old boy with sickle cell anemia, who presented with acute right hip pain. **a** Coronal T1-weighted scan shows abnormal low signal intensity in both proximal femurs and pelvis due to replacement of fatty marrow by red marrow. Both femoral heads appear identical with abnormal low signal. **b** Only coronal STIR sequence identifies edema in right femoral head, due to aseptic necrosis

sponse to chemotherapy may be monitored sequential using gadolinium-enhanced sequences with fat suppression [72]. Ewing' sarcoma pro-

Fig. 19 a–c. Musculoskeletal. Osteosarcoma in a 7-year-old boy. **a** Coronal image (SE 500/30) is useful to demonstrate the extent of medullary invasion, as areas of decreased signal intensity (*arrowhead*) in contrast with the bright signal of fat in the nondiseased marrow. **b** Axial image. This T1-weighted sequence showed periosteal rupture (*arrowhead*) and the soft-tissue component of this tumor. **c** The T2-weighted image of the axial study again depicts marrow invasion, periosteal disruption, and a soft-tissue component

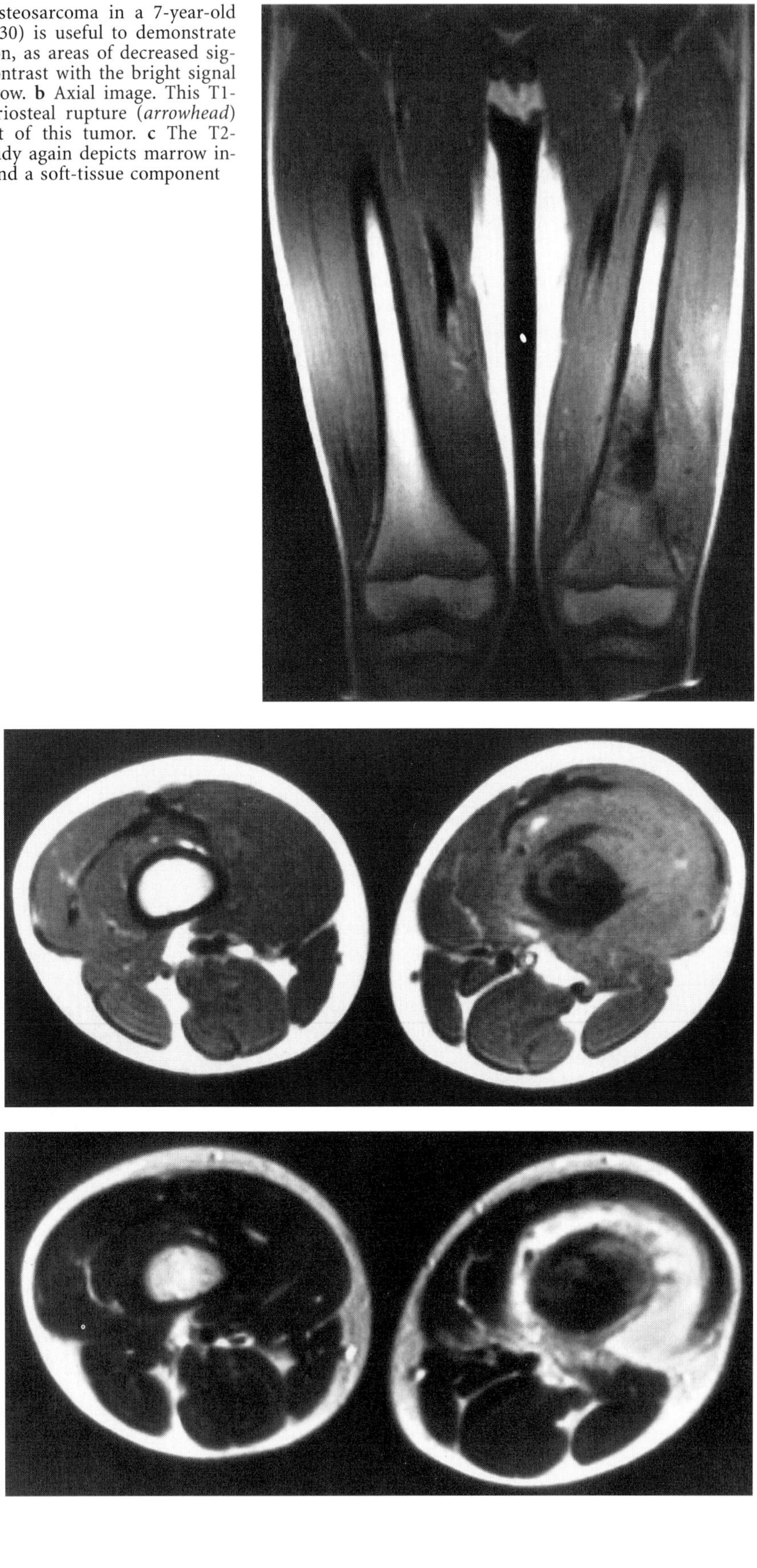

a

b

c

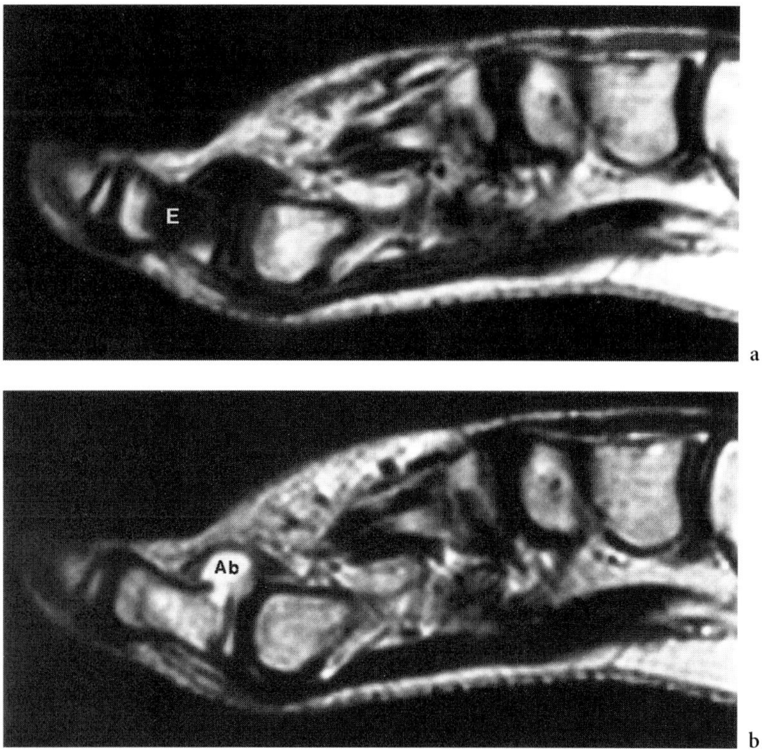

Fig. 20 a, b. Musculoskeletal. Osteomyelitis in proximal phalanx of big toe after minor trauma. **a** T1-weighted image shows bone marrow edema (*E*). **b** T2-weighted image better depicts effusion in metatarsophalangeal joint and subperiosteal abscess (Ab)

duces similar MR images as osteosarcoma, in different locations and age groups.

Metastatic bone disease may also be detected by MRI, although screening these patients with radionuclide bone scan is more desirable. Specific sites of high suspicion may then be selected for evaluation, because total body imaging by MRI is not technically feasible at this time.

Primary soft tissue neoplasms are also well imaged by MRI, depicting tumor size and extent, and depicting involvement of adjacent anatomic compartments, individual muscles, neurovascular structures, and joints. Soft tissue lesions commonly evaluated by MRI include hemangiomas and lymphangiomas (which have low signal on T1 and high signal on T2), lipomas (high signal on T1 and T2), posttraumatic conditions such as scars and myositis (low signal on T1 and T2), and hematomas (acute and chronic hematomas have low signal on T1; subacute hematoma has high signal on T1) [66].

Osteomyelitis may also be detected by MRI and fat-suppressed contrast-enhanced MRI appears to be more sensitive and specific than radionuclide bone scintigraphy [24, 54] (Fig. 20). MR images may be useful when the bone scan and plain films are equivocal or show a normal appearance, but as a screening or localizing test, scintigraphy is preferable.

Aseptic necrosis is well imaged by MRI [45, 70] (Fig. 18). This modality also provides useful information concerning femoral head coverage and incongruity. Therefore it may be employed when evaluating patients with congenital hip dislocation, slipped capital femoral epiphysis, and septic arthritis [55, 57]. Finally, MRI has been shown to be useful in the diagnosis of tarsal, especially fibrous, coalition [75].

References

1. Arey LB (1974) The genital system. In: Developmental anatomy: a textbook and laboratory manual of embryology. Saunders, Philadelphia, p 315
2. Bank ER (1993) Magnetic resonance of congenital cardiovascular disease: Update. Radiol Clin North Am 31:553–572
3. Bissett GS III (1989) Evaluation of potential practical oral contrast agents for pediatric magnetic resonance imaging: Preliminary observations. Pediatr Radiol 20:61–66
4. Bissett GS III (1989) Pediatric thoracic applications of magnetic resonance imaging. J Thorac Imaging 4 (2):51–57
5. Bisset GS III, Kirks DR, Strife JL (1987) Vascular rings: magnetic resonance imaging. AJR 149:251–256
6. Bloomfield EL (1993) Propocol for sedation of pediatric patients. Radiology 186:580–581
7. Bloomfield EL, Masaryk TJ, Caplin A et al (1993) Intravenous sedation for MR imaging of the brain and spine in children: Pentobarbital versus propofol. Radiology 186:93–97

8. Boechat MI (1990) Magnetic resonance imaging of abdominal and pelvic masses in children. Top Magn Reson Imaging 3 (1):25–41
9. Boechat MI (1992) Magnetic resonance imaging of the pediatric pelvis. Radiol Clin North Am 30:807–816
10. Boechat MI (1996) Magnetic resonance imaging of the pediatric pelvis. Radiol Clin North Am (in press)
11. Boechat MI, Kangarloo H (1988) MR imaging in Drash syndrome. J Comput Assist Tomogr 12 (3):405–408
12. Boechat MI, Kangarloo H (1989) MR imaging of the abdomen in children. AJR 152:1245–1250
13. Boechat MI, Kangarloo H (1988) MRI usurping CT's role in pediatric abdomen. Diagn Imaging 10 (2):114–119
14. Boechat Ml, Kangarloo H, Gilsanz V (1988) Hepatic masses in children. Semin Roentgenol 23:185–193
15. Boechat Ml, Kangarloo H, Ortega J et al (1988) Primary liver tumors in children: comparative study between MRI and CT. Radiology 169:727–732
16. Breen JL, Bonamo JF, Maxson WS (1981) Genital tract tumors in children. Pediatr Clin North Am 28:355–367
17. Brill PW, Jagannath A, Winchester P et al (1989) Adrenal hemorrhage and renal vein thrombosis in the newborn: MR imaging. Radiology 170:95–98
18. Burrows PE (1990) Magnetic resonance imaging of the aorta in children. Semin US CT MR 11:221–223
19. Carrington BM, Hricak M, Nuruddin R et al (1990) Mullerian duct anomalies: MR imaging evaluation. Radiology 176:715–720
20. Chung T, Jaramillo D (1995) Normal maturing distal tibia and fibula: Changes with age at MR imaging. Radiology 194:227–232
21. Chung T, Hoffer FA, Burrows PE et al (1996) MR imaging of hepatic hemangiomas of infancy and changes seen with interfreon alpha-2a treatment. Pediatr Radiol 26:341–348
22. Cohen MD (1990) Pediatric sedation. Radiology 175:611–612
23. Cohen MD, Bugaieski EM, Haliloglu M et al (1996) Visual presentation of the staging of pediatric solid tumors. Radiographics 16:523–545
24. Dangman BC, Hoffer FA, Rand FF et al (1992) Osteomyelitis in children: gadolinium-enhanced MR imaging. Radiology 182:743–747
25. Dietrich RB, Kangarloo H (1986) Kidneys in infants and children: evaluation with MR. Radiology 159:215–221
26. Dietrich RB, Kangarloo H (1986) Retroperitoneal mass with intradural extension: value of magnetic resonance imaging in neuroblastoma. AJR 146:251–254
27. Dietrich RB, Kangarloo H, Lenarsky KY et al (1987) Neuroblastoma: the role of magnetic resonance imaging. AJR 148:937–942
28. Fletcher BD, Cohn RC (1989) Tracheal compression and the innominate artery: MR evaluation in infants. Radiology 170:103–107
29. Forman HP, Leonidas JC, Berdon WE et al (1990) Congenital neuroblastoma: evaluation with multimodality imaging. Radiology 175:365–368
30. Fukuda Y, Watanabe H, Tomita T et al (1996) Evaluation of glomerular function in individual kidneys using dynamic magnetic resonance imaging. Pediatr Radiol 26:324–328
31. Gambino J, Caldwell B, Dietrich R, Walot I, Kangarloo H (1992) Congenital disorders of sexual differentiation: MR Findings. AJR 158:363–367
32. Gersovich EO, McGahan JP, Buonocore MH et al (1990) Rediscovery of infant feeding formula with magnetic resonance imaging. Pediatr Radiol 20:147–151
33. Gilsanz V, Cleveland RH (1982) Duplication of the müllerian ducts and genitourinary malformations: part I. The value of excretory urography. Radiology 144:793–796
34. Gilsanz V, Cleveland RH, Reid BS (1982) Duplication of the müllerian ducts and genitourinary malformations: part II. Analysis of malformations. Radiology 144:797–801
35. Glasier CM, Stark JE, Brown R et al (1995) Rectal thiopental sodium for sedation of pediatric patients undergoing MR and other imaging studies. AJNR 16:111–114
36. Greenberg SB, Faerber EN, Aspinall C et al (1993) High-dose chloral hydrate sedation for children undergoing MR imaging: safety and efficacy in relation to age. AJR 161:639–641
37. Greenberg SB, Faerber EN, Radke JL et al (1994) Sedation of difficult-to-sedate children undergoing MR imaging: value of thioridazine as an adjunct to chloral hydrate. AJR 163:165–168
38. Harris TM, Cohen MD (1989) Abdominal magnetic resonance imaging. Pediatr Radiol 20:10–19
39. Hayes Am, Jaramillo D, Levy HL et al (1992) Neonatal hemochromatosis: diagnosis with MR imaging. AJR 159:623–625
40. Hendren WH (1986) Repair of cloacal anomalies: current techniques. J Pediatr Surg 21:1159–1176
41. Ho VB, Kinney JB, Sahn DJ (1996) Contributions of newer MR imaging strategies for congenital heart disease. Radiographics 16:43–60
42. Holshouser BA, Hinshaw DB Jr, Shellock FG (1993) Sedation, anesthesia, and physiologic monitoring during MR imaging: evaluation of procedures and equipment. J Magn Reson Imaging 3:553–558
43. Hricak H, Kim B (1993) Contrast-enhanced MR imaging of the female pelvis. J Magn Reson Imaging 3:297–306
44. Hubbard AM, Markowitz RI, Kimmel B et al (1992) Sedation for pediatric patients undergoing CT and MRI. J Comput Assist Tomogr 16:3–6
45. Jaramillo D, Kasser JR, Villegas-Medina OL et al (1995) Cartilaginous abnormalities and growth disturbances in Legg-Calve-Perthes disease: evaluation with MR imaging. Radiology 197:767–773
46. Jaramillo D, Laor T, Lulkern RV (1994) Comparison between fast spin-echo and conventional spin-echo imaging of normal and abnormal musculoskeletal structures in children and young adults. Invest Radiol 29:803–811
47. Jaramillo D, Lebowitz RL, Hendren WH (1990) Cloacal malformation: radiologic findings and imaging recommendations. Radiology 177:441–448
48. Kangarloo H (1988) Chest MRI in children. Radiol Clin North Am 26:263–275
49. Kangarloo H, Dietrich RB, Ehrlich RM et al (1986) Magnetic resonance imaging of Wilms' tumor. Urology 28:203–207
50. Kastler B, Livolsi A, Germain P et al (1990) Magnetic resonance imaging in congenital heart disease of newborns: preliminary results in 23 patients. Eur J Radiol 10:109–117
51. Lufkin MR, Votruba J, Reicher M et al (1986) Solenoid surface coils in magnetic resonance imaging. AJR 146:409–412
52. Manuli MA, Davies L (1993) Rectal methohexital for sedation of children during imaging procedures. AJR 160:577–580
53. Mintz MC, Thickman DI, Gussman D, Kressel HY (1987) MR evaluation of uterine anomalies. AJR 287–290
54. Morrison WB, Schweitzer ME, Bock GW et al (1993) Diagnosis of osteomyelitis: utility of fat-suppressed contrast-enhanced MR imaging. Radiology 189:251–257
55. Nuss R, Kilcoyne RG, Geraghty S et al (1994) Utility of magnetic resonance imaging for management of hemophilic arthropathy in children. Radiology 192:294–295
56. Pennington DJ, Lonergan G, Haws RM et al (1996) Renal MR imaging with the fast inversion-recovery sequence: enhancement patterns and potential pitfalls. The Society of Pediatric Radiology book of abstracts, Boston, MA, P108:98

57. Ranner G, Ebner F, Fotter R et al (1989) Magnetic resonance imaging in children with acute hip pain. Pediatr Radiol 20:67–71
58. Sato Y, Pringle KC, Bergman RA et al (1988) Congenital anorectal anomalies MR imaging. Radiology 168:157–162
59. Shellock FG (1990) Monitoring sedated pediatric patients during MR imaging. Radiology 177:586–587
60. Siegel MJ (1995) MR imaging of the pediatric abdomen. MRI Clin North Am 3:161–182
61. Siegel MJ (1991) Magnetic resonance imaging of the pediatric pelvis. Semin US CT MR 12:475–505
62. Siegel MJ, Glazer HS, Weiner JI et al (1989) Normal and abnormal thymus in childhood: MR imaging. Radiology 172:367–371
63. Slovis TL, Parks C, Reneau D et al (1993) Pediatric sedation: short-term effects. Pediatr Radiol 23:345–348
64. Stanley P, Geer GD, Miller J et al (1989) Infantile hepatic hemangiomas: clinical features, radiological investigations and treatment in twenty patients. Cancer 64 (4):936–949
65. Stark DD, Moseley ME, Bacon BR et al (1985) Magnetic resonance imaging and spectroscopy of hepatic iron overload. Radiology 154:137–142
66. Stöver B, Laubernberger J, Niemeyer C et al (1995) Hemangiomatosis in children: Value of MRI during therapy. Pediatr Radiol 25:123–126
67. Sugimoto H, Ohsawa T (1994) Ulnar collateral ligament in the growing elbow: MR imaging of normal development and throwing injuries. Radiology 192:417–422
68. Togashi K, Nishimura K, Itoh K et al (1987) Vaginal agenesis: classification by MR imaging. Radiology 162:675–677
69. Troughton AH, Waring J, Longstaff A et al (1990) The role of magnetic resonance imaging in the investigation of undescended testes. Clin Radiol 41:178–181
70. Uno A, Hattori T, Noritake K et al (1995) Legg-Calve-Perthes Disease in the evolutionary period: comparison of magnetic resonance imaging with bone scintigraphy. J Pediatr Orthop 15:362–367
71. Vade A, Reyes H, Wilbur A et al (1989) The anorectal sphyncter after rectal pull-through surgery for anorectal anomalies: MR evaluation. Pediatr Radiol 19:179–183
72. Van der Woude HJ, Bloem JL, Schipper J et al (1994) Changes in tumor perfusion induced by chemotherapy in bone sarcomas: Color Doppler flow imaging compared with contrast-enhanced MR imaging and three-phase bone scintigraphy. Radiology 191:421–431
73. Weinberger E, Shaw DWW, White KS et al (1995) Non-traumatic pediatric musculoskeletal MR imaging: Comparison of conventional and fast-spin-echo short inversion time inversion-recovery technique. Radiology 194:721–726
74. Weinreb JC, Cohen JM, Armstrong E et al (1986) Imaging the pediatric liver. MRI and CT. AJR 147:785–790
75. Wechsler RJ, Schweitzer ME, Deely DM et al (1994) Tarsal coalition: depiction and characterization with CT and MR imaging. Radiology 193:447–452
76. Westra SJ, Zaninovic AC, Hall TR et al (1994) Imaging of the adrenal gland in children. Radiographics 14:1323–1340
77. Wood BP (1990) Cloacal malformations and exstrophy syndromes. Radiology 177:326–327

Interventional Procedures E

Interventional Magnetic Resonance Imaging of the Brain

1

V. Tronnier · A. A. F. DeSalles · Y. Anzai · G. J. Rubino
K. L. Black · R. B. Lufkin

Introduction

Through the technological and clinical advances of the past decade, magnetic resonance imaging (MRI) has become one of the most powerful noninvasive diagnostic tools in the evaluation of the brain. The superior soft-tissue contrast, the oblique and multiplanar imaging capability, and the absence of ionizing radiation have made MRI the imaging modality of choice for most diagnostic applications of the brain. These advantages also make MRI an ideal guide for invasive and interventional procedures in the brain. The high sensitivity of MRI to flow enables the delineation of blood vessels without the use of contrast agents. The absence of beam-hardening artifacts from bone and metal devices allows complex instrumentation approaches to anatomic regions that may be difficult or impossible to reach under conventional computed tomography (CT) guidance. Over a decade of experience with MRI-guided stereotaxis has proven MRI to be an effective and reliable means to visualize and localize neurosurgical targets and a valuable aid in optimizing surgical approaches [1–4].

Recently MRI has been applied to treatment monitoring procedures in the brain such as interstitial therapy and even open surgery [5]. New developments in MRI techniques and MR-compatible instrumentation and the availability of open magnet designs are revolutionizing the role of MRI in guiding and monitoring interventional procedures.

MR-Guided Stereotaxis

From the middle 1980s on, MRI stereotaxis has been successfully employed in neurosurgery to guide biopsies, tumor resection, deep EEG electrode placement, functional target development and resection, and other interventional procedures [6–14]. The noninvasive visualization and localization provided by MRI greatly reduce the surgical invasion necessary to access the target and significantly lower patient morbidity. Several stereotactic systems with localizer frames designed for MRI localization are commercially available: the BRW and CRW (Radionics, Burlington, Mass., USA), Leksell (Elekta Instruments, Atlanta, Ga., USA), Laitinen (Sandström Trade & Technology, Welland, Ont., Canada), and others.

Since MRI is more prone to geometric distortion than CT, the accuracy of MRI stereotaxis must be evaluated. The maximum localization error reported in the literature ranges from 1 to 5 mm [15–18]. The variation in the maximum error may be accounted for partly by the use of different stereotactic systems and different reference imaging modalities (CT, ventriculography, etc.) to which MRI is compared. The spatial accuracy of MRI depends on the linearity and calibration of magnetic field gradients and on magnetic susceptibility artifacts which manifest as spatial distortions. Meticulous quality control should decrease errors in magnetic field linearity and calibration. MRI sequences should use high bandwidth signal acquisition to reduce spatial distortion due to susceptibility effects. Several researchers have proposed practical correction algorithms to further improve the spatial accuracy of MRI [19, 20].

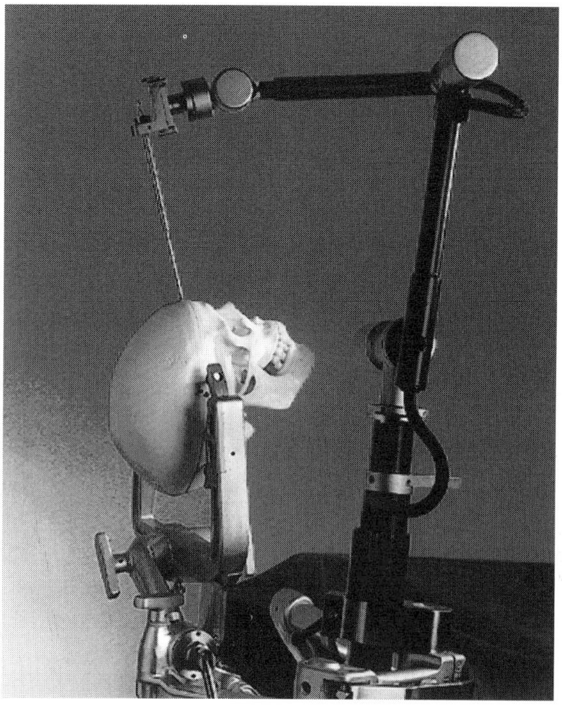

Fig. 1. The Operating Arm System (Radionics Software Applications) provides intraoperative navigation on a previously acquired 3D MR data set

Although accurate and reliable, conventional stereotactic systems require the fixation of a frame to the patient's skull. Recent developments in frameless stereotactic systems will improve patient comfort, localization efficiency, and surgical access in open procedures [21–23]. Projects are underway to develop MR-compatible navigational systems which use arm-based 3-D digitizer or light emitting diode (LED) based optical digitizers registered to the coordinate system of the interventional MR scanner for interactive scan plane control and near real-time MRI monitoring of the interventional procedure (Fig. 1).

■ MR-Guided Biopsy

One of the earliest applications of intracranial interventional MR was to obtain biopsy specimens for tissue diagnosis. As with biopsies elsewhere in the body, the approach utilized for accessing an intracranial lesion is chosen to limit the risk of injury to surrounding vital structures. Either fine needle aspirates or core biopsies can be obtained by utilizing various gauge MR-compatible needles. Also, either frame based or frameless stereotaxis may be used to guide the approach depending on the location and size of the target lesion. Also, either frame based or frameless stereotaxis may be used to guide the approach depending on the location and size of the target lesion. The primary goal of an intervention within the MR scanner, however, will be a frameless procedure with on-line imaging control of the needle trajectory. The point of entry is determined either with an optical tracking device, a gadolinium-filled wand, or simply the surgeon's finger. Fast image sequences (e.g., FISP 2D) allow a near real-time image while advancing the biopsy needle to the desired target. An obvious advantage compared to intraoperative CT is the possibility to take specimens from different tumor areas best displayed by MRI under direct visual control (Fig. 2).

■ MR-Guided Electrode Placement

Another application of interventional MR is to assist in the placement and in postplacement evaluation of intracerebral depth electrodes [37–43]. Intracerebral depth electrodes are used to localize the seizure focus in those patients who are refractory to medical therapy. Prior to the development of this technique such electrodes were placed by inferring their position relative to previously ac-

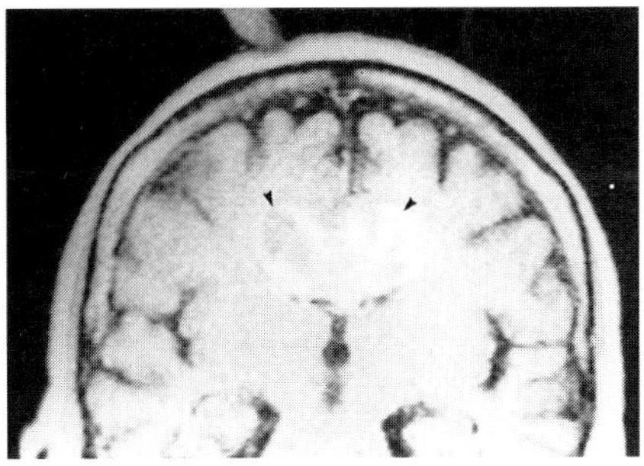

a

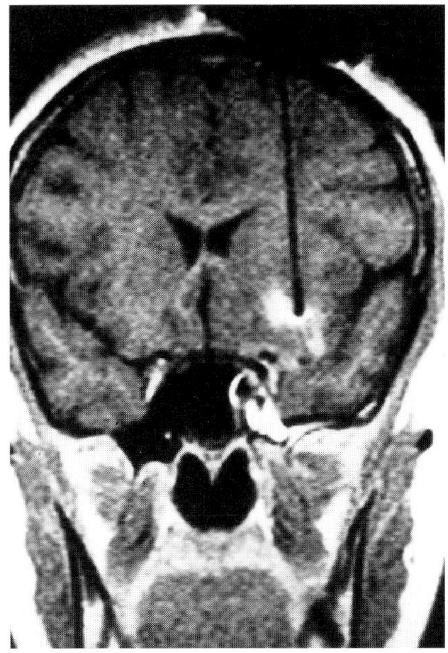

b

Fig. 2. MR-guided biopsy of glioma. **a** Direct localization for approach. Note physicians finger. **b** MR-compatible needle within the glioma in another patient

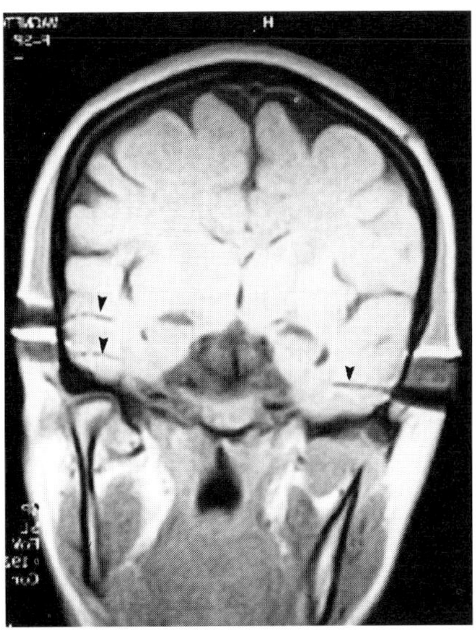

Fig. 3. Deep EEG electrode implantation for patients with medically refractory partial complex seizures who are being considered for possible temporal lobectomy. Coronal MRI obtained with MR-compatible electrodes (*arrow heads*) shows the position in the hippocampal region as well as surrounding soft tissues

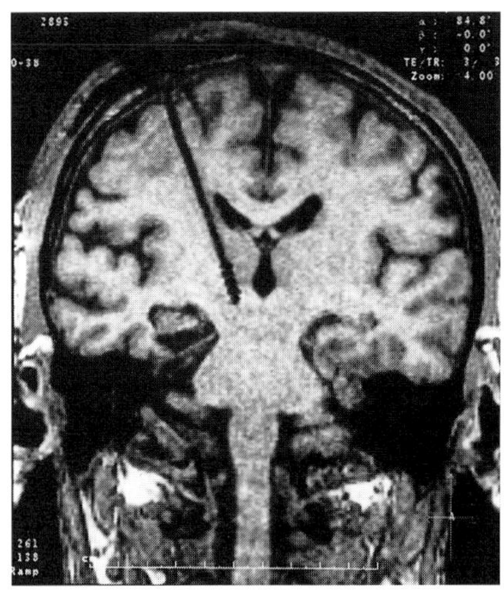

Fig. 4. Intraoperative documentation of an implanted depth electrode for treatment of chronic pain

quired imaging studies. Postplacement examination of electrode placement could not be accurately performed due to the extensive beam-hardening artifact produced by the stainless steel composition of the electrodes during CT. Previously MRI was not feasible because of the ferromagnetic properties of stainless steel and concern for heat and torque production that could result in local brain injury. With the manufacture of different metal compositions such as platinum alloys utilized in electrode production, MRI guidance can be employed during electrode placement to confirm position without risk of brain injury.

Sufficient anatomic detail is obtained to adequately evaluate electrode placement and to avoid possible procedural complications (Fig. 3). This should result in improved anatomic-physiological correlation and surgical outcome for these patients. This should result in improved anatomic-physiological correlation and surgical outcome for these patients. Intraoperative documentation of chronic implanted depth electrode placement for treatment of chronic pain or movement disorders is another reason to establish a correlation between anatomical relationships and intraoperative neurophysiological target determination (Fig. 4).

■ MR-Guided Closed Minimally Invasive Therapeutic Procedures

In the effort to reduce patient morbidity, hospitalization length, and recovery time associated with conventional craniotomy, several researchers are pioneering new, minimally invasive therapeutic techniques which may achieve results comparable to surgical resection or serve as effective palliative measures. In these minimally invasive procedures, it is particularly appealing to employ MRI beyond mere stereotactic localization and begin to use MRI to directly monitor treatment administration. The sensitivity of MRI to temperature change and other acute tissue effects (e.g., edema) enables the physician to interactively adjust treatment parameters to maximize the destruction of pathological tissue and minimize undesirable injury to normal tissue.

Cryoablation

Freezing has been explored as a minimally invasive technique for tissue ablation in the brain. Postoperative MRI of patients who underwent cryothalamotomy demonstrated excellent depiction of the lesions created [24] (Fig. 5). Intraoperative MRI guidance and monitoring of the cryoablation procedure awaits the development of practical MR-compatible freezing devices.

Interstitial Laser Ablation

Traditionally the use of lasers in neurosurgery has been limited to applications in which direct visualization was possible. Now MRI guidance allows stereotactic placement of an interstitial laser probe into a deep tumor through a small burr hole in the skull. Laser energy travels through the optic fiber directly into the tumor and produces heat-induced protein denaturation and coagulation necrosis. However, since the penetration and absorption of laser energy are complex functions of tissue characteristics, it is difficult to predict a priori the extent of tissue damage as a function of dose. Therefore a monitoring technique is required to follow the destructive process in tissue as laser energy is applied. Although CT can show laser-induced tissue changes, these are relatively late findings. Early tissue reaction to laser is missed by CT due to its low soft-tissue contrast [25]. Fortunately, many researchers have demonstrated the ability of MRI to detect acute tissue changes secondary to the application of laser energy [26–30].

Animal studies have characterized the acute and chronic tissue effects of Nd:YAG laser and established the correlation between histopathological findings and their MRI appearance [26, 28, 31]. It has been shown that T2-weighted images are particularly sensitive to tissue changes and can clearly demonstrate concentric rings of central cavitation, coagulation necrosis, and edema around the point of laser application. Higuchi et al. detected similar patterns in T2-weighted images 5 min after laser irradiation in the live rabbit brain.

Since the primary tissue effect of Nd:YAG laser irradiation is thermal damage [32, 33], the thermal sensitivity of MRI can also be exploited to monitor the progress of the laser therapy. The dependence of T1, diffusion coefficient, water proton chemical shift, and other MR parameters on temperature is well known, and these have been utilized for noninvasive thermal mapping during the application of laser and other thermal ablation techniques [34–39]. Knowledge of the temperature distribution in the treatment area allows the surgeon to confirm unambiguously the destruction of the target while avoiding irreversible thermal damage to vital structures.

Interstitial laser therapy is particularly well suited for intraoperative MRI guidance because the laser-delivering optic fiber is intrinsically MR-compatible, and because the application of laser energy does not interfere with MR signal acquisition. Initial clinical experience with MRI-guided interstitial laser therapy has yielded promising results in the treatment of brain tumors [40]. This procedure can be executed under local anesthesia which allows the neurological status of the patient

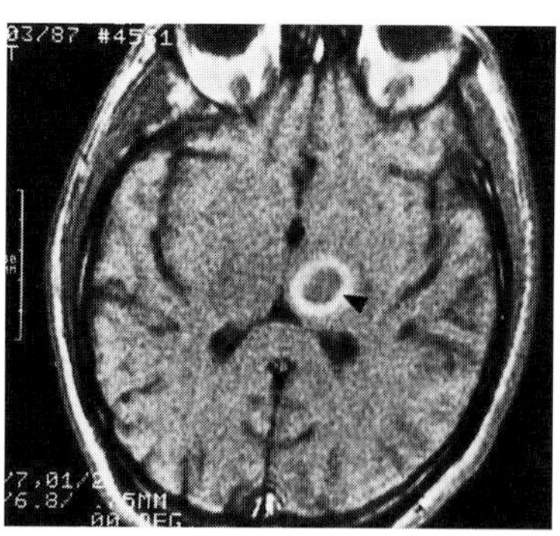

Fig. 5. T1-weighted image obtained several days after stereotactic cryothalamotomy shows the lesion well-circumscribed by a hyperintense ring (*arrowhead*)

to be monitored continuously. MRI guidance enables the physician to minimize damage to normal brain tissue while the absence of systemic toxicity permits repetition of the procedure as necessary.

Radiofrequency Thermal Ablation

Radiofrequency (RF) thermal ablation is a technique of tissue destruction by resistive heating using RF (approx. 500 kHz) electrical current. A probe with a conductive tip is inserted into the target, and RF current is then delivered from the tip to cause focal heating, resulting in protein denaturation and coagulation necrosis. Over three decades of extensive neurosurgical experience with RF has established the efficacy and safety of this ablation technique [41–51]. RF ablation has been used primarily for functional neurosurgical procedures including thalamotomy and pallidotomy for parkinsonism and other movement disorders, leucotomy for intractable pain, and rhizotomy for trigeminal neuralgia. Postoperative MRI has demonstrated excellent depiction of lesion details in patients who underwent RF thalamotomy [43, 52, 53].

Our group has recently completed an initial study of MRI-guided RF ablation of primary and metastatic brain tumors [5, 54]. The procedure used MRI-guided stereotaxis to place an RF probe (Radionics, Burlington, MA) into the tumor through a 2-mm twist-drill hole in the skull (Fig. 6). RF power was then applied to achieve an intratumoral temperature of 80 °C for 1 min. Depending on the shape and size of the tumor the probe position was adjusted, and additional doses were administered. The entire procedure was performed under light sedation and local anesthesia which allowed the surgeon to monitor the neurological status of the patient throughout.

Pretreatment T1- and T2-weighted MR images provided clear depiction of tumor morphology and anatomical relationships with surrounding vital structures and proved critical in planning the best trajectory for the RF probe. MR angiography with 2D time-of-flight sequences also proved use-

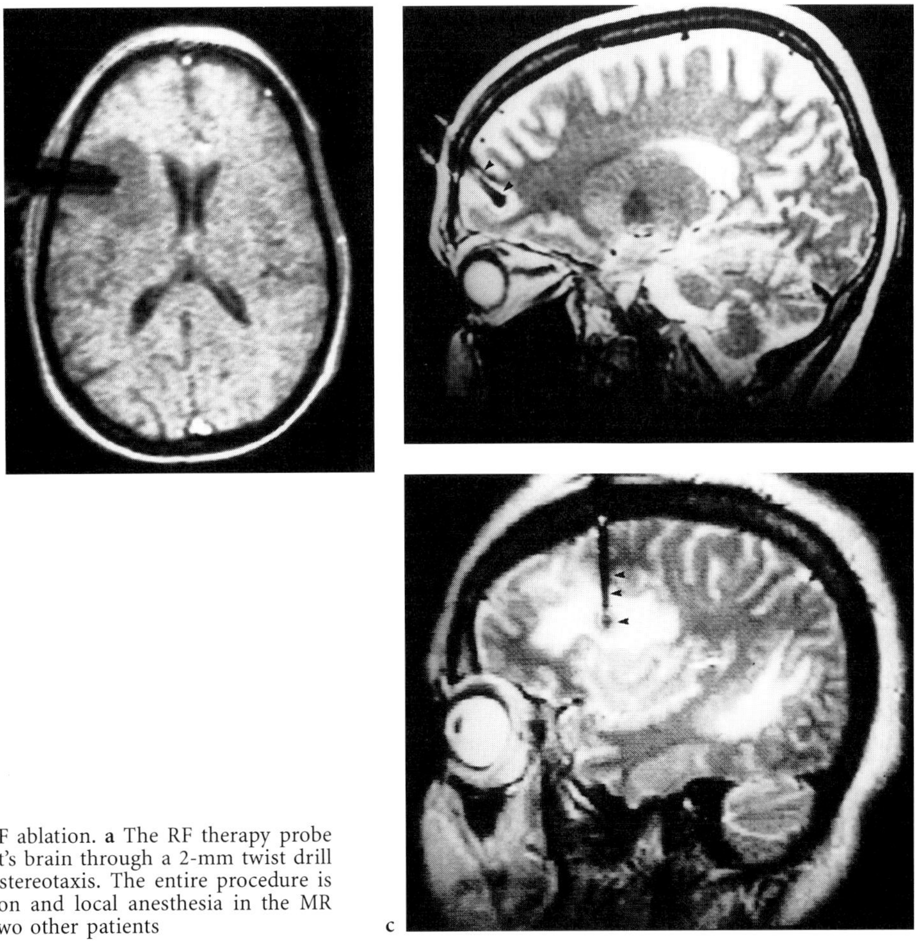

a b c

Fig. 6a–c. MR-guided RF ablation. **a** The RF therapy probe is placed into the patient's brain through a 2-mm twist drill hole using MRI-guided stereotaxis. The entire procedure is done under light sedation and local anesthesia in the MR suite. **b, c** Examples in two other patients

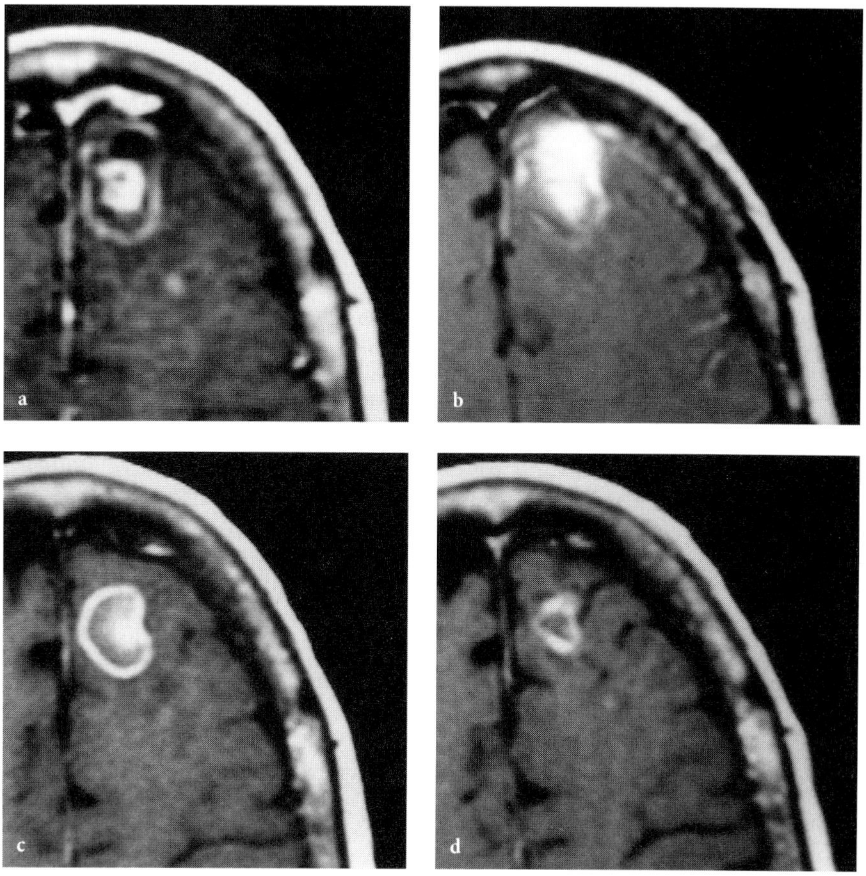

Fig. 7a–e. Contrast-enhanced MR images of a patient who underwent MRI-guided RF ablation of a metastatic adenocarcinoma. **a** pretreatment. **b** Immediately after RF ablation. **c** One week posttreatment. **d** One month posttreatment. **e** Five months posttreatment

ful to visualize vascular structures surrounding the planned trajectory of the RF probe. The RF lesion was detected in posttreatment MRI as a low signal region on T1-weighted images and as a high signal region on T2-weighted images within 20–30 min of the RF ablation. Gadolinium-enhanced T1-weighted images demonstrate a rim of enhancement which outlines the zone of tissue necrosis. A total of 15 tumors were treated in 11 patients. During the 2-year follow-up period seven tumors were controlled by treatment while eight tumors recurred. Five tumors had a durable response to treatment (11.9–23.8 months follow-up, median 15.1 months; Fig. 7). Neurological complications were few and transient except for one patient who still has mild expressive speech difficulty at 10 weeks after treatment.

MRI-guided RF thermal ablation promises to be a safe, minimally invasive treatment of brain tumors. This technique may become an effective palliative measure and may serve as an adjuvant to radiation therapy. However, unlike radiation therapy, which is contraindicated by accumulative toxicity, RF ablation can be repeated as many times as necessary to treat recurrences. Greater efficacy is anticipated as improved MR-compatible RF generator and therapy probes are developed to allow real-time artifact-free MRI of the ablation procedure. As with interstitial laser therapy, the heating effects of the RF ablation can be monitored by temperature-mapping MRI sequences during the application of RF power to confirm the destruction of target tissue before physiological changes become apparent.

■ High-Intensity Focused Ultrasound Ablation

High-intensity focused ultrasound (HIFU) is a new technique of thermal ablation by remote heating. An extracorporeal ultrasound transducer focuses vibrational energy to a point inside the patient's body so that only the tissue within a small focal zone is heated to lethal temperatures

(60 °C or above for thermal coagulation and protein denaturation) while the surrounding tissue experiences only a slight temperature increase. HIFU ablation under ultrasound imaging guidance has been used in clinical trials to treat glaucoma, benign prostatic hyperplasia, tumors of the brain, breast, liver, kidney, and bladder [55–59]. The greatest advantage of HIFU over other thermal ablation techniques is that no surgical invasion is required to access the target provided there is a sonic path clear of bone and air. However, noninvasive methods to measure the temperature of the focal heating zone must be developed to provide adequate control.

By combining the high soft-tissue contrast and the temperature sensitivity of MRI with HIFU ablation a powerful minimally invasive therapy technique can be developed. Several researchers have demonstrated the feasibility of using MRI to guide and monitor HIFU ablation procedures [34, 36, 60, 61]. Fast T1-weighted gradient echo sequences can be used to track in real-time the high-temperature focal zone which appears as a hypointense region to guide the positioning of the ultrasound transducer. Tissue changes secondary to HIFU heating can be detected easily on T2-weighted images as with interstitial laser therapy. Although practical application of HIFU to the intracranial region necessitates the removal of a skull bone flap to expose the dura, surgical invasion of the brain parenchyma can be avoided and the potential for infection and other complications greatly reduced. Clinical application of HIFU in neurosurgery awaits the further development of MRI-compatible HIFU therapy systems and MRI temperature-mapping techniques.

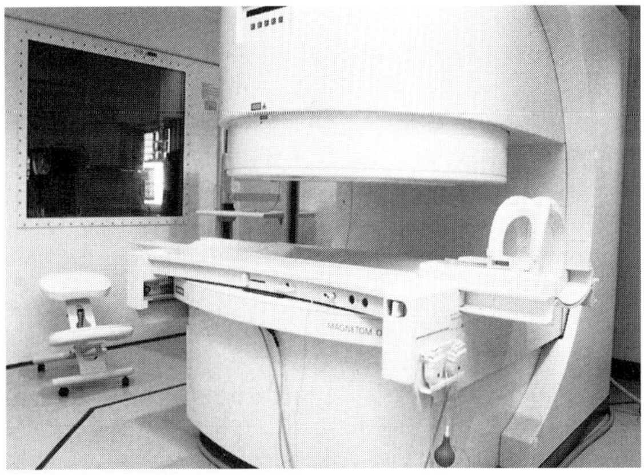

Fig. 8. View of the Heidelberg intraoperative 0.2 T MR scanner (Siemens Open, Erlangen)

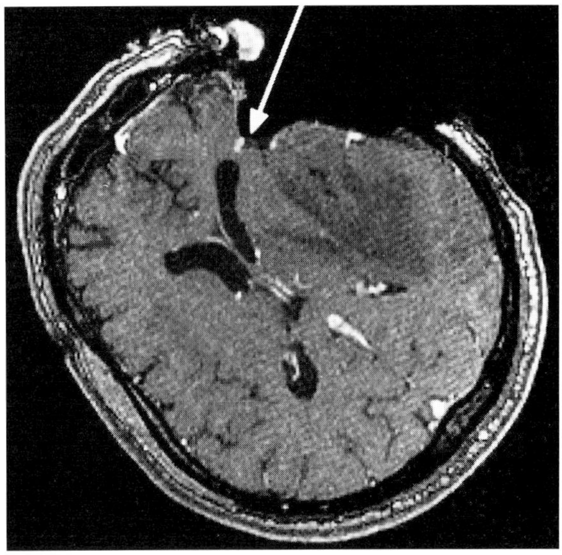

Fig. 9. Axial intraoperative T1-weighted image of a patient during open craniotomy for resection of glioma. In this postcontrast study gadolinium enhancement is present at the margin of the resection (*arrow*)

■ MR-Guided Open Surgical Procedures of the Brain

One of the most fascinating concepts is the use of an open-field MRI in open neurosurgical procedures for intraoperative resection control and protection of neighboring structures. There are currently two concepts of the intraoperative use of MRI for surgical procedures. The "Boston concept" [62] makes the operating room (OR) an MR suite and vice versa using an high-field magnet with an 0.5 T surgical field in between two separated magnets in a double-doughnut fashion (Signa SP, General Electric, USA). This intraoperative MR system allows the surgeon to stand between the magnets during the whole procedure and carry out different types of brain surgery as well as spinal cases. The system is coupled with an MR-compatible microscope and optical navigational device with a LED tracking device mounted to different instruments. The constantly updated images guide the surgeon through the procedure eliminating the errors of brainshift, which usually arise with preoperative images for conventional frame based or frameless procedures. Further advantages are the reduced operating time and the possibility of intraoperative tumor resection control. Disadvantages are the difficult sterile draping of the whole system, the limited space for the surgeon and the exposition of the OR staff to a high magnetic field, and the exclusive dedication of an OR to this type of procedure.

A different concept has been proposed by the Heidelberg group [63]. A low-field (0.2 T) scanner (Siemens OPEN, Erlangen) is placed in the sterile environment of the OR adjacent to an OR in an shielded RF cabin and connected to the OR via an RF-sliding door (Fig. 8). The advantages of this system are the separate use of OR and MR if necessary, the surgeon's comfort during the procedure using his standard instruments, drills, navigational systems, and OR microscope. No interference occurs using electronic devices or delicate intraoperative monitoring as microelectrode recording. The low-field scanner does not need helium tanks for cooling supply, but can be cooled via the hospital water lines. Therefore reduced space is required. Brain shift can be corrected with intraoperative reregistration using fiducial markers placed around the craniotomy site.

After scanning the patient the data are fed into the navigational workstation, and tumor remnants can be resected, if necessary, under navigational control. This has been accomplished in 16 patients with histological confirmation of tumor in twelve (Fig. 9). Disadvantages are the necessity of a patient transport system, which is accomplished in Heidelberg with an carrier system on an air cushion to carry the patient safely to the scanner and back, a special docking mechanism and a modified OR table which slides into the scanner had to be constructed. Due to the limited gap between the two magnets patients must be positioned in supine or prone position. Patients in a lateral position or spinal cases can not be scanned intraoperatively. The patients transport adds 60–90 min to the operating time

The advantages of both systems compared to intraoperative CT are the excellent contrast resolution in soft tissue differentiating a pathological lesion from surrounding brain tissue and the ability of using nonreformatted three dimensional images for surgical planning and excision. Another advantage is the avoidance of ionizing radiation.

Problems which must to be solved are the supply of the full range of MR-compatible instruments and the recognition and correction of local distortion artifacts created by these instruments. Another important point which must be stressed is the creation of surgically induced blood-brain barrier disruptions, which can lead to contrast enhancement and false positive tumor presentation. Especially critical are the use of hydrogen peroxide and the different CUSA systems. Finally, cost-benefit analyses must be carried out including the installation costs, maintenance costs, duration of surgery, additional personnel, length of hospital stay, and life tables relating not only to the length of patients survival but relating to quality of life.

Conclusion

MRI has traditionally been criticized as an expensive diagnostic technology. However, when compared with more costly open surgical procedures and the associated higher patient morbidity, hospitalization costs, and lost time from work, MRI-guided minimally invasive interventions can potentially lower the final cost of medical care in selected patients. More work is clearly warranted in this exciting field to determine its ultimate areas of application in neurosurgery.

References

1. Mueller P, Stark D, Simeone J et al (1986) MR-guided aspiration biopsy: needle design and clinical trials. Radiology 161:605–607
2. Lufkin R, Teresi L, Hanafee W (1987) New needle for MR-guided aspiration cytology of the head and neck. AJR Am J Roentgenol 149 (2):380–382
3. Lufkin R, Layfield L (1989) Coaxial needle system for MR and CT guided aspiration cytology. J Comput Assist Tomogr 13 (6):1105–1107
4. To S, Lufkin R, Chiu L (1989) MR compatible winged infusion set. Comput Med Imaging Graph 13 (6):469–472
5. Anzai Y, Black K, DeSalles A et al A new technique for MR guided thermal ablation of brain tumors. AJNR Am J Neuroradiol (in press)
6. Kratimenos G, Thomas D (1993) The role of image-directed biopsy in the diagnosis and management of brainstem lesions. Br J Neurosurg 7 (2):155–164
7. Wen D, Hall W, Miller D et al (1993) Targeted brain biopsy: a comparison of freehand computed tomography-guided and stereotactic techniques. Neurosurgery 32 (3):407–412
8. Kelly P (1990) Stereotactic imaging, surgical planning and computer-assisted resection of intracranial lesions: methods and results. Adv Tech Stand Neurosurg 17:77–118
9. Lufkin R, Jordan S, Lylyck P et al (1988) Magnetic resonance imaging with topographic EEG electrodes in place. AJNR Am J Neuroradiol 9:953–954
10. Lunsford L (1988) Magnetic resonance imaging stereotactic thalamotomy: report of a case with comparison to computed tomography. Neurosurgery 23:363–367
11. Kelly P, Sharbrough F, Kall B et al (1987) Magnetic resonance imaging-based computer-assisted stereotactic resection of the hippocampus and amygdala in patients with temporal lobe epilepsy. Mayo Clin Proc 62:103–108
12. Uematsu S, Rosenbaum A, Delong M et al (1987) Magnetic resonance planned thalamotomy followed by X-ray/CT-guided thalamotomy. Acta Neurochir Suppl (Wien) 39:21–24
13. Lunsford L, Martinez A, Latchaw R (1986) Stereotaxic surgery with a magnetic resonance- and computerized tomography-compatible system. J Neurosurg 64:872–878
14. Leksell L, Leksell D, Schwebel J (1985) Stereotaxis and nuclear magnetic resonance. J Neurol Neurosurg Psychiatry 48:14–18
15. Burchiel K (1992) Image-based functional neurosurgery. Clin Neurosurg 39:314–330
16. Kondziolka D, Dempsey P, Lunsford L et al (1992) A comparison between magnetic resonance imaging and computed tomography for stereotactic coordinate determination. Neurosurgery 30 (3):402–406

17. Derosier C, Delegue G, Munier T et al (1991) MRI geometric distortion of the image and stereotaxy. J Radiol 72:349–353
18. Villemure J, Marchand E, Peters T et al (1987) Magnetic resonance imaging stereotaxy: recognition and utilization of the commissures. Appl Neurophysiol 50:57–62
19. Bakker C, Moerland M, Bhagwandien R et al (1992) Analysis of machine-dependent and object-induced geometric distortion in 2DFT MR imaging. Magn Reson Imaging 10 (4):597–608
20. Fitzpatrick J, Chang H, Willcott M et al (1990) A technique for improving accuracy in position and intensity within images acquired in the presence of field inhomogeneity. Book of abstracts: 9th annual meeting of the Society of Magnetic Resonance in Medicine. SMRM, New York, p 426
21. Takizawa T (1993) Isocentric stereotactic three-dimensional digitizer for neurosurgery. Stereotact Funct Neurosurg 60 (4):175–193
22. Maciunas R, Galloway RJ, Fitzpatrick J et al (1992) A universal system for interactive image-directed neurosurgery. Stereotact Funct Neurosurg 58 (1–4):108–113
23. Kato A, Yoshimine T, Hayakawa T et al (1991) A frameless armless navigation system for computer-assisted neurosurgery. J Neurosurg 74:845–849
24. Vining E, Duckwiler G, Udkoff R et al (1991) MRI of the thalamus following cryothalamotomy for parkinsons disease and dystonia. J Neuroimaging 1 (3):146–147
25. Gatenby RA, Hartz WH, Engstrom PF et al (1987) CT-guided laser therapy in resistant human tumors: phase I clinical trials. Radiology 163:172–175
26. Higuchi N, Bleier A, Jolesz F et al (1992) Magnetic resonance imaging of the acute effects of interstitial neodymium:YAG laser irradiation on tissues. Invest Radiol 27:814–821
27. Robinson J, Lufkin R, Castro D et al (1992) Magnetic resonance imaging of laser phototherapy: initial experience. Eur Radiol 2:24–28
28. Anzai Y, Lufkin R, Castro D et al (1991) MR imaging-guided interstitial Nd:YAG laser phototherapy: dosimetry study of acute tissue damage in an in vivo model. J Magn Reson Imaging 1 (5):553–559
29. Castro DJ, Saxton RE, Layfield LJ et al (1990) Interstitial laser phototherapy assisted by magnetic resonance imaging: a new technique for monitoring laser-tissue interaction. Laryngoscope 100 (5):541–547
30. Jolesz FA, Bleier AR, Jokab P et al (1988) MR imaging of laser tissue interactions. Radiology 168:249–253
31. Anzai Y, Lufkin R, Hirschowitz S et al (1992) MRI and histopathological correlation of thermal injuries induced by interstitial Nd:YAG laser phototherapy in the chronic model. J Magn Reson Imaging 1 (3):671–678
32. Jolesz F, Moore G, Mulkern R et al (1989) Response to and control of destructive energy by magnetic resonance. Invest Radiol 24:1024–1027
33. Matthewson K, Coleridge-Smith P, O'Sullivan JP et al (1987) Biological effects of intrahepatic neodymium:yttrium-aluminum-Garnet laser photocoagulation in rats. Gastroenterology 93:550–557
34. Matsumoto R, Mulkern R, Hushek S et al (1994) Tissue temperature monitoring for thermal interventional therapy: comparison of T1-weighted MR sequences. J Magn Reson Imaging 4 (1):65–70
35. Stollberger R, Fan M, Ebner E et al (1993) Mapping of temperature changes in heterogeneous tissues for the monitoring of hyperthermia. Book of abstracts: 12th annual meeting of the Society of Magnetic Resonance in Medicine. SMRM, New York, p 156
36. Cline H, Schenck J, Hynynen K et al (1992) MR-guided focused ultrasound surgery. J Comput Assist Tomogr 16 (6):956–965
37. LeBihan D, Delannoy J, Levin RL (1989) Temperature mapping with MR imaging of molecular diffusion: application to hyperthermia. Radiology 161:401–407
38. Dickinson R, Hall A, Hind A et al (1986) Measurement of changes in tissue temperature using MR imaging. J Comput Assist Tomogr 10 (3):468–472
39. Parker D (1984) Applications of NMR imaging in hyperthermia: an evaluation of the potential for localized tissue heating and noninvasive temperature monitoring. IEEE Trans Biomed Eng 31 (1):161–167
40. Ascher P, Justich E, Schrottner O (1991) A new surgical but less invasive treatment of central brain tumours preliminary report. Acta Neurochir (Wien) 52:78–80
41. Blond S, Caparros-Lefebvre D, Parker F et al (1992) Control of tremor and involuntary movement disorders by chronic stereotactic stimulation of the ventral intermediate thalamic nucleus. J Neurosurg 77:62–68
42. Laitinen L, Harriz M, Bergenheim T (1992) Leksell's posteroventral pallidotomy in the treatment of Parkinson's disease. J Neurosurg 76 (1):53–61
43. Tomlinson F, Jack C, Kelly P (1991) Sequential magnetic resonance imaging following stereotactic radiofrequency ventralis lateralis thalamotomy. J Neurosurg 74:579–584
44. Hassenbusch S, Pillary P, GH B (1990) Radiofrequency cingulotomy for intractable cancer pain using stereotactic guided by magnetic resonance imaging. Neurosurgery 27:220–223
45. Matsumoto K, Shichijo F, Fukami T (1984) Long term follow-up review of cases of Parkinson's disease after unilateral or bilateral thalamotomy. J Neurosurg 60 (5):1033–1044
46. Kelly P, Gillingham F (1980) The long term results of stereotaxic surgery and L-dopa therapy in patients with Parkinson's disease. J Neurosurg 53 (3):322–337
47. Siegfried J (1977) 500 percutaneous thermocoagulation of the gasserian ganglion for trigeminal pain. Surg Neurol 8 (2):126–131
48. Organ L (1976) Electrophysiologic principles of radiofrequency lesion making. Appl Neurophysiol 39:69–76
49. Rosomoff H, Brown C, Sheptak P (1965) Percutaneous radiofrequency cervical cordotomy: technique. J Neurosurg 23 (5):639–644
50. Aronow S (1960) The use of radiofrequency power in making lesions in the brain. J Neurosurg 17:431–438
51. Sweet W, Mark V, Hamlin H (1960) Radiofrequency lesions in the central nervous system of man and cat. J Neurosurg 17:213–225
52. Anzai Y, Desalles A, Black K et al. (1993) Interventional MR imaging. Radiographics 13 (4):897–904
53. Matsumoto S, Shima F, Hasuo K et al (1992) MR imaging of stereotactic thalamotomy using radiofrequency methods. Nippon Igaku Hoshasen Gakkai Zasshi 52:1559–1564
54. Black K, DeSalles A, Anzai Y et al MRI-guided thermal ablation of metastatic and primary brain tumors-initial experience of 12 cases. J Clin Oncol (in press)
55. Foster R, Bihrle R, Sanghvi N et al (1993) High-intensity focused ultrasound in the treatment of prostatic disease. Eur Urol 23 [Suppl 1]:29–33
56. Vallancien G, Harouni M, Veillon B et al (1992) Focused extracorporeal pyrotherapy: feasibility study in man. J Endourol 6:173–181
57. Silverman R, Vogelsang B, Rondeau M et al (1991) Therapeutic ultrasound for the treatment of glaucoma. Am J Ophthalmol 111 (3):327–337
58. Fry F, Johnson L (1978) Tumor irradiation with intense ultrasound. Ultrasound Med Biol 4 (4):337–341
59. Burov A (1956) High intensity ultrasonic oscillation for the treatment of malignant tumors in animals and man. Dokl Akad Nauk SSSR 106:239–241
60. Cline H, Hynynen K, Hardy C et al (1994) MR temperature mapping of focused ultrasound surgery. Magn Reson Med 31:628–636
61. Hynyen K, Darkazanli A, Unger E et al (1993) MRI-guided noninvasive ultrasound surgery. Med Phys 20 (1):107–115

62. Schenck JF, Jolesz FA, Roemer PB et al (1995) Superconducting open-configuration MR imaging system for imag-guided therapy. Radiology 195:805–814
63. Tronnier VM, Wirtz CR, Knauth M et al. Intraoperative diagnostic and interventional MRI in neurosurgery. Neurosurgery

Microtherapeutic MR and Endoscopy for Low Back Pain Therapy

2

D. H. W. Grönemeyer, R. Seibel, A. Melzer, M. Deli

Introduction

Acute and chronic back pain, either with or without disc herniation, is one of the major medical problems in health care worldwide. Patients often suffer from radicular pain caused by herniations, pseudoradicular pain caused by facet joints, or local pain caused by the iliosacral joints. In the case of disk herniations both joints must be treated if they are painful. Routine treatments at many centers include such microinvasive techniques as computed tomography (CT) guided techniques for microinvasive periradicular therapy (micro-PRT) [1], mechanical percutaneous nucleotomy (PNT) [2–4], percutaneous laser nucleotomy (PLNT) [1], and CT-guided facet joint and iliosacral joint therapy. Microinvasive interventional magnetic resonance imaging (MRI) is a new tool in guidance technology [5, 6].

Percutaneous techniques for the treatment of lumbar disk herniation are becoming increasingly important. The main interest of all PNT techniques is to reduce the volume and the pressure of the affected disk by leaving all other structures unaffected. The first percutaneous lumbar diskectomy was described in 1975 by Hijikata et al. [7]. Friedman [8] and Schreiber et al. [9] added discoscopy by using a dorsolateral access. In 1986 Ascher et al. [10] and Yonezawa et al. [11] introduced neodymium-yttrium-aluminum-garnet (Nd-YAG) laser techniques for percutaneous disk surgery. CT-guided PLNT for treating disk herniation was developed by our group in 1989 [12]. The indications for PNT techniques are limited to disk herniation without dislocated free fragments. In 1990 we began employing microendoscopy under combined fluoroscopic and CT guidance for treatment of disk herniation with small free fragments in the foramen and the spinal canal and for lysis of epidural scar tissue.

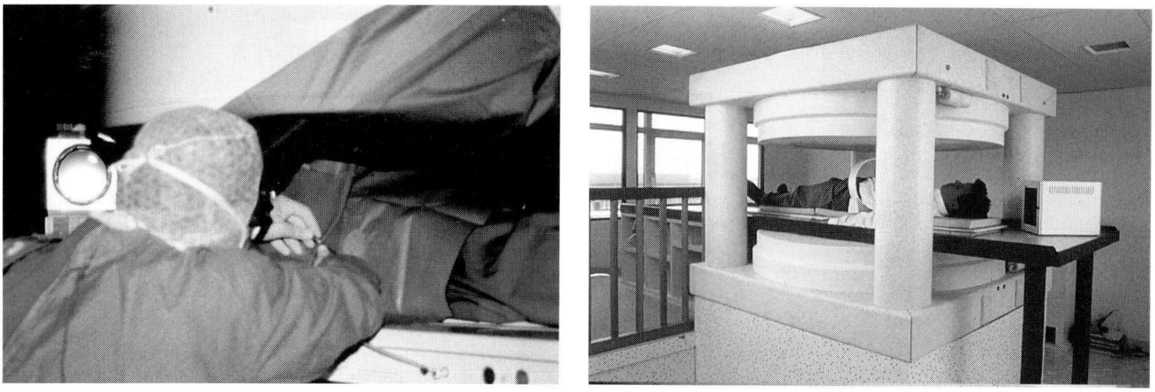

a b

Fig. 1. Open MRI systems for performing microinvasive interventional procedures. **a** Magnetom Open (Siemens). **b** Access (Toshiba)

■ Material and Methods

Scanners

For microtherapeutic interventional MRI procedures we use a low-field 0.064-T open-design MRI scanner (Toshiba Access; Fig. 1.) and 0.2-T system (Magnetom Open, Siemens, Erlangen, Germany). The treatments were carried out with 18- to 21-G cannulae of nitinol (Cook, Denmark), titanium, stainless steel, and flexible microendoscopes of a portable MRI compatible endoscopy systems. For PLNT a we use double-head Nd-YAG or holmium laser (all instruments from Micromed, Bochum, Germany; 0.4 mm fiber, 10 W, 1 s impulse, 1 s gap; over all: up to 180 impulses).

Below we describe the sequences used in the open MRI system:

- Fluoroscopic mode (implemented by Radiologic Imaging Laboratory, San Francisco, CA; USA; developed by Riederer et al. [13]): GE, TE 9 ms, TR 80 ms, FA 70°, matrix 128×180, field of view 18×26×1.5 cm
- Modified keyhole sequences (developed by Busch, Friebe et al. in Mülheim and Bochum): three-dimensional (3D) RUKSE; 3D rotational k-space updating keyhole sequence [14]: GE, TE 20 ms, TR 80 ms, FA 55°, matrix 256×256×8, 30×30×0.45 cm, 256×32×2 keyhole, 256×32×2 update, TA_{ref} 163 s, TA_{key+up} 10 s

We compared two interventional CT scanners: Siemens Somatom Plus S and Philips Tomoscan M. The acquisition time for a single scan was 1–4 s, matrix 512×512, helical mode or workstation for 3D reconstruction.

Instrumentation

Special introducer sets with diameter a of 1.2–4 mm were developed for the procedure (Micromed). The smallest fiberscope, with a diameter of 0.29 mm, fits into a 22-G coaxial interventional needle set. Good view is obtained with endoscopes having a diameter greater than 0.6 mm; the best view is provided by endoscopes with flexible tip and a diameter of 1.8 mm (Micromed; Table 1). Two endoscope systems with chip camera (CCD) were used: the Masy system (Krauth, Hamburg, Germany) and the Integrated Endoscopy System Piccolo (Micromed). We developed and manufactured microinstruments with 0.9-mm diameter which can be used in the spinal canal (EFMT, Bochum, Germany). Microforceps, scissors and other instruments can be introduced

Table 1. Microendoscopes for spinal use

Type	Outer deflectable diameter tip (mm)	Introduced length (cm)	Angle of view	Minimal radius (mm)	Image fibers	Observation depth (mm)
ME 002/0.29	0.29	150	52°	6	1600	1–10
ME 003/0.6	0.6	150	70°	10	6000	2–20
ME 004/0.8	0.8	150	70°	10	6000	2–20
ME 005/1.0	1.0	90	70°	20	12000	3–∞
ME 201/0.8	0.8	65	70°		3000	2–20 (90°: 25)
ME 211/1.5[a]	1.8	65	70°		6000	2–50 (90°: 25)

[a] This endoscope has a working channel with 0.5-mm diameter.

through a 18-G needle or catheter. We use two laser systems. A Nd-YAG laser (MBB, Munich, Germany) and a double-head laser with Nd-YAG and Ho-YAG (Micromed). This system allows both laser pulses to be applied through the same laser fiber. An interventional Somatom plus S (Siemens) is used for tomography. This CT allows two or three surgeons to perform the procedure. For fluoroscopy we use digital C arch (Siemens).

■ Guidance Technique

CT/MRI guidance is used as a stereoguide and a macroscope. The benefit of CT/MRI is the visibility of all structures in the surgeon's field. In prone position the spine, joints, or disks are scanned in axial plane. Access to free fragments or scar tissue must be determined through the foramen or interlaminar. The region of interest is determined, and the angle of approach is marked on the monitor. The entry is marked on the skin of the patient. After local anesthesia a needle or a catheter can be placed. CT is used only for intraspinal approach. Step-by-step tomographic control is used to reduce the risk of injuries of nerve roots or thecal sac. Loss of pressure indicates penetration of the ligament. It is necessary to push away the thecal sac by injection of saline after puncture of the ligamentum flavum. This is possible with a very thin needle (22-G). Local anesthesia of the nerve roots or epidural injection of local anesthetics should be avoided to control sensitivity.

A larger introducer set (1.2–2.8 mm) can be inserted. Microendoscopes with diameters of 0.29–1.8 mm are introduced through this needle. Structures in the spinal canal can be seen after infusion of saline solution. A second access for microtherapy can be placed in the same way if necessary. Under endoscopic guidance the epidural fat and the thecal sac are carefully removed by further injection of saline and manipulation with instruments. After this procedure the spinal nerve roots can be seen. Fibrous tissue or herniated material can be extracted or vaporized. We use a Nd-YAG or holmium laser or microinstruments to perform the dissection. Step-by-step scar tissue must be removed under endoscopic view. Even hard fibrotic tissue can be carefully dissected with instruments without risk of injury of the thecal sac or nerve root. In contrast to Nd-YAG lasers, holmium lasers have only small thermal reactions, which makes them laser suitable for use close to nerve structures in the spinal foramina and the spinal canal.

In addition, PLNT is performed with an Nd-YAG laser (wavelength 1.064 nm) to reduce intradiscal pressure. This procedure should be performed with transforaminal access under CT and fluoroscopic guidance. At the level of L5/S1 the puncture must sometimes be oblique, traversing several CT scans, for example, to avoid nerve injury. The combination of fluoroscopy and CT enables the guidance of the needle in the third dimension.

The technical procedure for treatments in open MRI is carried out with the patient in prone or lateral position. After using a 3D localizer, which shows one image in three planes (Toshiba) or three images in one plane (Siemens) within 15 s, the target region is defined. After marking the distances for the treatment on the monitor and on the skin, fluoroscopic or modified keyhole sequences are acquired. After ensuring a sterile operation field, the entry point on the skin is marked by finger pressure and the instruments inserted in local anesthesia. All treatments are performed with a belt coil and inside the magnet.

For documentation high-resolution T1- and T2-weighted spin echo and 3D sequences were acquired after the treatments.

Patients and Indications

This study compared CT and MRI in examinations of 340 patients (mean age 51 years, range 26–75): PLNT in 80, facet joint therapy in 100, PRT in 100, and iliosacral joint infiltrations in 60. These included 100 endoscopic procedures of the facet joints and herniated disks to achieve a new and safe access. Before microtherapy 81% of the patients (n=144) with acute and chronic disk herniations had neurological deficits such as weakening of the patellar reflex as an expression of disk pathology at L2–L4, weakness of the tibialis anterior, weakness of the extensor hallucis brevis, or decreased ankle jerk. Before treatment the patients had pain scores of 70–100 on the visual analogue scale. Each patient was treated four times, at intervals of 14 days. In 50 cases in which the cortisone treatment was not sufficient for facet joint therapy the patient received 0.7 cc 96% ethanol for neurolysis. Follow-up time was 6 months.

Facet Joints. Facet anesthesia is generally used for acute radicular pain caused by functional disorders and for diagnosis before ethanol injection. Percutaneous ethanol instillation for lysis is important for chronic pain caused by spondyloarthrosis or chronic prolapse. Pain caused by post-

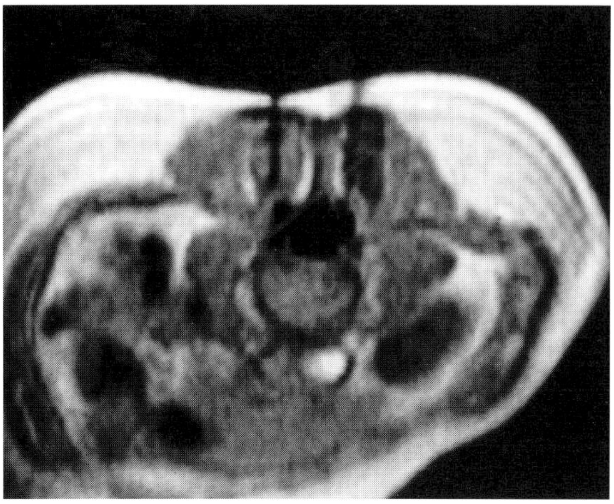

Fig. 2. Microinvasive MRI-guided facet joint therapy with anesthetic agents and 50% ethanol (*left*) and PRT (*right*). The cannula was guided beside the facet joint to the segmental nerve

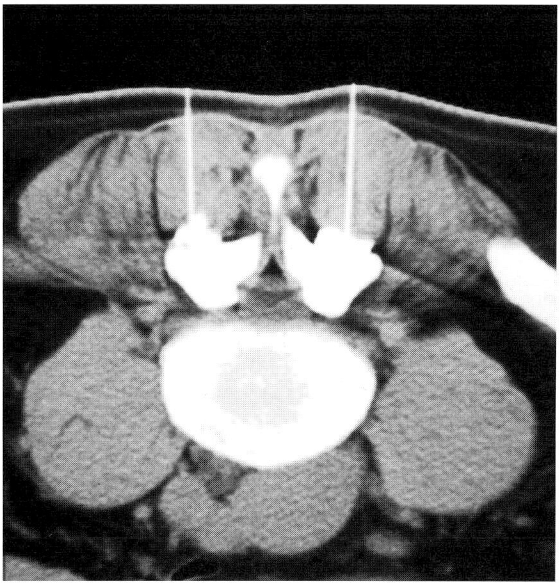

Fig. 3. Microinvasive CT-guided facet joint therapy with contrast medium

diskectomy syndrome can also be treated very easily with facet anesthesia and/or iliosacral joint therapy. A total of 100 patients with facet joint problems were treated (Figs. 2, 3). Endoscopy was carried out in 20 cases.

Iliosacral Joints. Acute and chronic pain caused by sterile inflammation (sacroiliitis) can be treated as acute and chronic pain if the iliosacral joints are locally dolent. This kind of local pain therapy is available for patients with Bekhterev's disease, Boeck's disease, Reiter's disease, brucellosis, and tuberculosis. This therapy technique is very helpful in combination with facet joint therapy, PRT, epidural treatments, and nucleotomy/diskectomy. In this study 80 patients received iliosacral joint treatments (Fig. 4). For both joints the local treatment consists of 1 cc of short-acting and 1 cc long-acting anesthesia (mepivacaine 1%, bupivacaine 0.5%) before 10 mg triamcinolone (Volon A). With both CT and MRI 1 cc of diluted contrast media is given before ethanol injection to demonstrate the spreading of the solution and thus avoid the risk of damaging the segmental nerve or the spinal canal. With MRI no contrast media must be given in local cortisone administration because there is a contrast change in signal intensity after injecting local anesthesia. The signal decreases after the instillation of anesthetic agents in muscle and fat in the T1-weighted sequences. The T2-weighted signal intensity in-

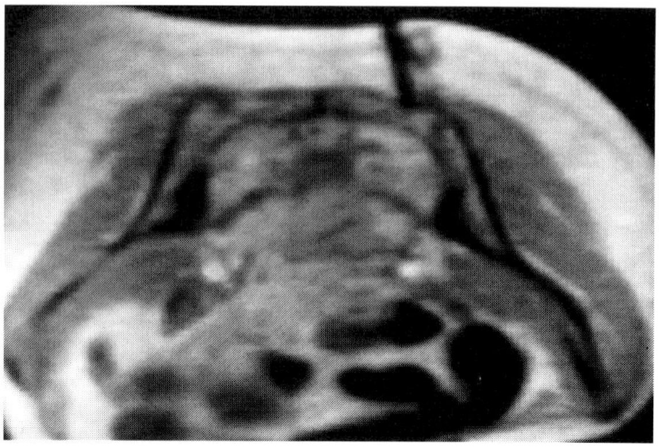

Fig. 4. Micro-invasive MRI-guided iliosacral joint therapy with anesthetic agents and cortisone

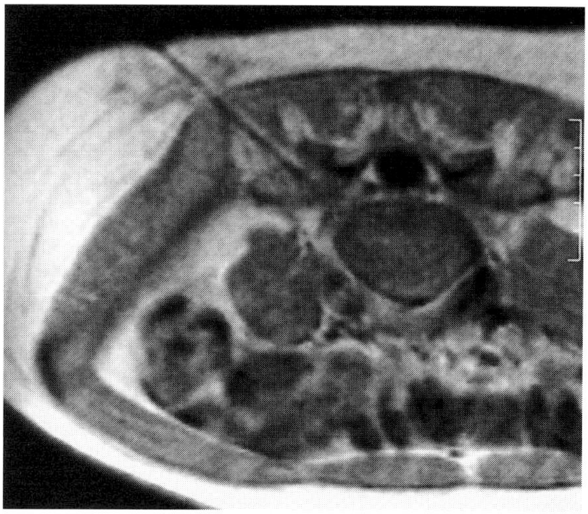

Fig. 5. Micro-invasive MR-guided PRT with anesthetic agents and cortisone

creases after ethanol instillation (virtually isointense to muscle in T1-weighted imaging).

PRT. Chronic disk protrusion or lateral scar tissue after operation are important indications for this kind of microtherapeutic procedure. A total of 100 patients were treated (Fig. 5). Each patient was treated eight times with 40 mg triamcinolone (Volon A) at intervals of 21 days. Before injection of cortisone 0.2 ml contrast media is instillated onto the nerve root. Anesthetic agent is given for local hypesthesia.

PLNT. Endoscopy and lasers can be used to treat acute or chronic disk herniation with lateral lesions after 6 weeks of conservative therapy without success and also mediolateral scar tissue with. Twenty patients underwent endoscopic treatment intraspinally and 60 treatment through the foramen intervertebrale (Figs. 6–8).

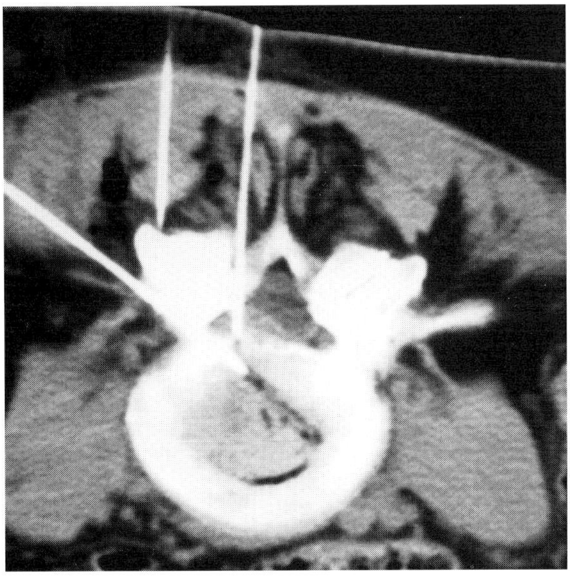

Fig. 6. CT-guided PLNT; two cannulae for the laser inside the herniation (epidural and intraforaminal) and one cannula for facet joint blocking with long-acting local anesthesia

Contraindications

Mass herniation and sequesters are contraindications for PLNT. For PRT, facet and iliosacral joint therapy are among the contraindications to cortisone in the field of nonsterile inflammations, diabetes mellitus, and ulcers. All techniques must be performed under normal hemostatic conditions.

Radiological Diagnosis

Before each treatment it is important for diagnosis to carry out X-ray and MRI study of the affected region, if necessary also functional radiography. These studies can rule out inflammations, degenerative disorders, tumors, osteoporosis, and spondylolisthesis. CT must be performed to obtain information about bones, such as the facet and iliosacral joints. MRI must be performed after 6 weeks of unsuccessful conservative treatment for back pain or in the presence of neurological deficits. Our ex-

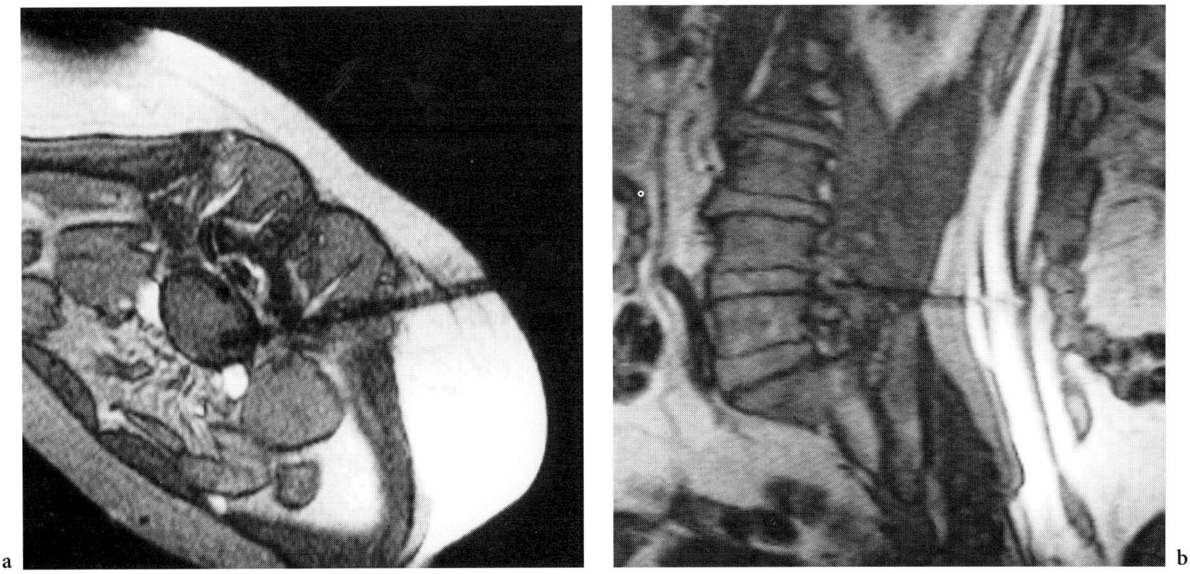

Fig. 7. a MRI-guided PLNT; one cannula for the laser in the center of the disk (axial plane,). **b** MRI guidance of the cannula to the foramen intervertebrale of a patient, sagittal view

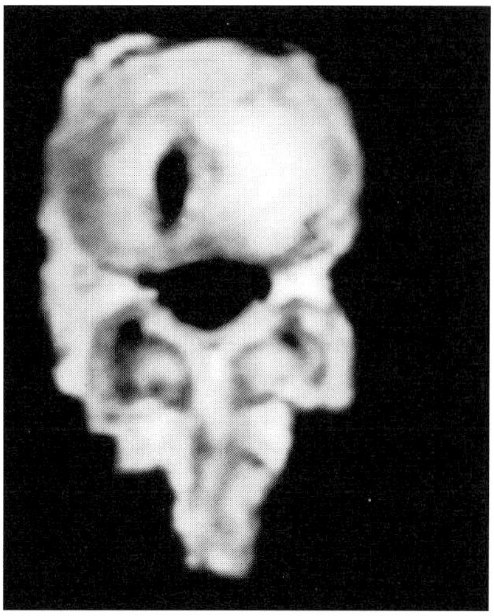

Fig. 8. After laser treatment (Nd-YAG 1064 μm) with 10-W, 3-min continuous pulses, a defined local necrosis is seen (cadaver study)

perience demonstrates that neither MRI nor CT are used as frequently as they should be.

Results

Clinical

The average pain score before therapy was 86%, after treatment it decreased to 7%. Improvement was reported by 87% of patients in reflexes or weakness immediately after the endoscopic microtherapy with the Nd-YAG laser (73% at follow-up). In 92% of cases Lasegue's sign decreased more than 50° or was negative. A greater than 50% overall improvement in pain symptoms was reported by all patients immediately after microendoscopy. Some 90% of patients in the intraspinal group (n=18) reported pain relief greater than 50% on the visual analogue scale at follow-up. Ethanol was given in 40 cases of facet joint therapy. In the iliosacral joint group 37 patients received microinvasive treatment on the right side and 23 on the left.

In 89% of patients in the PRT group (n=55) there was pain reduction of more than 75% (visual analog scale) directly after the treatment. Neurological symptoms such as paresthesia, hypesthesia, and hypofunction of the reflexes improved in 74%. Good results were obtained by PRT in 85% (pain reduction of more than 50% and/or decrease in neurological deficits at a mean follow-up of 1.7 years). The most effective cycle phase was the third and fourth treatments (more than 50% improvement).

Complications and Side Effects

There were no complications of CT- or MRI-guided spinal endoscopy. Nine patients complained of slight nerve root irritation at the treated level. This occurred during the night or the day after endoscopy and lasted several days, sometimes up to 2 weeks. Conservative treatment and PRT with CT-guided injection of cortisone around the nerve root and epidurally was necessary in five patients. This symptoms were related to mechanical irritation by pressure to the nerve root during PLNT. In these cases the routine MR control excluded spondylodiscitis and hematoma as the cause of pain. Three of these five patients suffered from pseudoradicular pain. This was treated by CT-guided blockade of both facet joints (three times over 8 days) by injecting a local anesthetic agent. Two patients reported cramps in the leg.

Technical Aspects

In all, 30 microendoscopies were performed inside the foramen intervertebrale and 30 inside the disk after PLNT. The segmental nerve can be differentiated from the disk inside the foramen intervertebrale, and small vessels are also visible. Inside the disk the laser-induced cavity and the laser treatment can be documented. In CT the gas spreading inside the disk can be very well documented at once. In MRI the heating effect of the laser changes the tissue contrast of the disk and the end plates if the energy is high or the tip near.

The best view is obtained using endoscopes with a diameter of 1.8 mm diameter and an angle of 70°. The deflectable tip is very useful for examining the posterior ligament in front of the dural sac and inspecting the region behind the lamina. It is easy to examine the field of interest in the spinal canal after injection of saline or inflation of air. In this way the dural sac can be pushed away to spread the epidural space. Under endoscopic guidance and CT control the sequestrectomy can be performed safely through a second puncture. It is difficult to see the nerve root in the spinal foramen because of the surrounding fat. In addition to sequestrectomy, PLNT was performed in all patients to reduce the volume and pressure of the affected disk.

A very good overview is obtained of the surface of the facet joints with a 0.6-mm flexible microendoscope, but only a noisy impression with the 0.29 mm system. Twenty procedures were carried out; saline and gas must be inserted to visualize the joints. The instillation of ethanol can be controlled, thus avoiding damage to the capsule.

The tip tracking of the instruments is easy in CT but not in MRI, because the visualization of the instruments is different. In CT the tip and the edges of the instruments are defined with high precision within 0.2 mm and in MRI within 3.5 mm due to artifacts. Vital structures such as nerves cannot be discriminated in MRI within this region of 0–3.5 mm.

In comparing the acquisition time of the two systems, the Somatom Plus S requires 10 s for menu time, 1 s for scan-time, and 10 s for reconstruction time. One movement into the gantry together with the localizer scan requires 8 s, the positioning time for defining the treatment position and bringing the patient into the treatment area outside the gantry is 10 s, and the automatic couch time for moving the table for the next scan into the gantry is 5 s. Overall the total acquisition time is 44 s for one movement and the first scan in the therapy procedure, 36 s for the next scan – a total of 80 s for two scans. The average of the movements and scans are 5 and 188 s machine time (four to seven scans).

The acquisition time for the open MRI is as follows: menu time 5 s, scan time 2 s, reconstruction time 16 s, localizer time 18 s, positioning time 5 s, and couch time 0 s. Overall there are 45 s for the first movement and 23 s for the next scan – a total of 68 s for two scans. The average time for five scans is 137 s. After the first movement the patient does not have to be moved out of the gantry, and the treatment can be carried out by fluoroscopic or keyhole technique inside the magnet.

Treatment time can therefore be shortened by these fast imaging sequences and therapy in an open MRI system. However, the spin echo and 3D sequences before and after the fluoroscopy mode for documentation are time consuming. No radiation is produced by MRI.

■ Discussion

Various types of percutaneous procedures are available for treating diseases of the vertebral column and intervertebral structures. The method described here may be helpful in a large number of patients with disc herniation and pseudoradicular pain, thus allowing conventional surgery to be avoided.

A number of endoscopic techniques are today known in the field of neurointervention. The principal indications are biopsy of brain tumors, evacuation of hematomas and cysts, endoscopic treatment of hydrocephalus and the spine, for example, drainage of syringomyelia and spinal cysts. The first endoscopic techniques were introduced by L'Espinasse in 1910 [15], and Dandy followed in 1922 [16]. The first endoscopic techniques in the spinal canal were reported in cadavers by Burman in 1931 [17]. Spinal endoscopy began to be used for clinical diagnosis in 1967 [18]. At that time equipment for microendoscopy was not available, and the endoscopic techniques offered no advantages over other techniques. A few years later CT became the noninvasive diagnostic tool for spinal column. After development of flexible microendoscopes in the late 1980s the indications for minimally invasive techniques in the brain and spine expanded.

Percutaneous procedures offer various types of treatment for diseases of the vertebral column and intervertebral structures. In the past it was not possible to treat free fragments by PNT. CT-guided video-microendoscopy of the spinal canal offers a new possibility for treatment of dislocated herniations. CT allows a safe and easy access by injection of saline solution epidurally as well as control of the structures around the field of interest. In addition, microendoscopy gives a good view of the surgeon's field. The combination of these two techniques provides the greatest safety for microtherapy in the spinal canal and the foramen.

Low back pain caused by the facet or iliosacral joints can be treated by anesthesia, ethanol (facet joints), or corticosteroids in the case of chronic pain. In 1971 Rees [19] introduced multiple bilateral percutaneous lumbar facet denervation with the scalpel. This method was modified by Shealy [20] who separated the nerves with an electrocoagulation probe. Since then this method has been termed facet denervation. Further developments of the procedure involved it being performed with fluoroscopically guided injections of local anesthetic agents, corticosteroids, or ethanol. The administration of local anesthetic helps in treating acute pain and both joints at all levels of the spine.

Ethanol can be used as an agent for neurolysis of the small sensory facet nerves in cases of chronic pseudoradicular pain [21]. The toxic effect of ethanol in human tissues is known: local dehydration with denaturation of proteins and necrosis [22] and denervation (e.g., lumbar sympathicolysis) [23]. Complications after intravascular ethanol injection have also been described. Cox et al. [24] and Rabe et al. [25] described colon/renal infarctions and abscesses in 1982, Löhr et al. [26] and Lammer et al. [27] skin necrosis in 1985, and the same group a spinalis anterior syndrome [27]. In our department we have experienced no complications after injecting ethanol. Our experience includes approx. 1000 cases of fa-

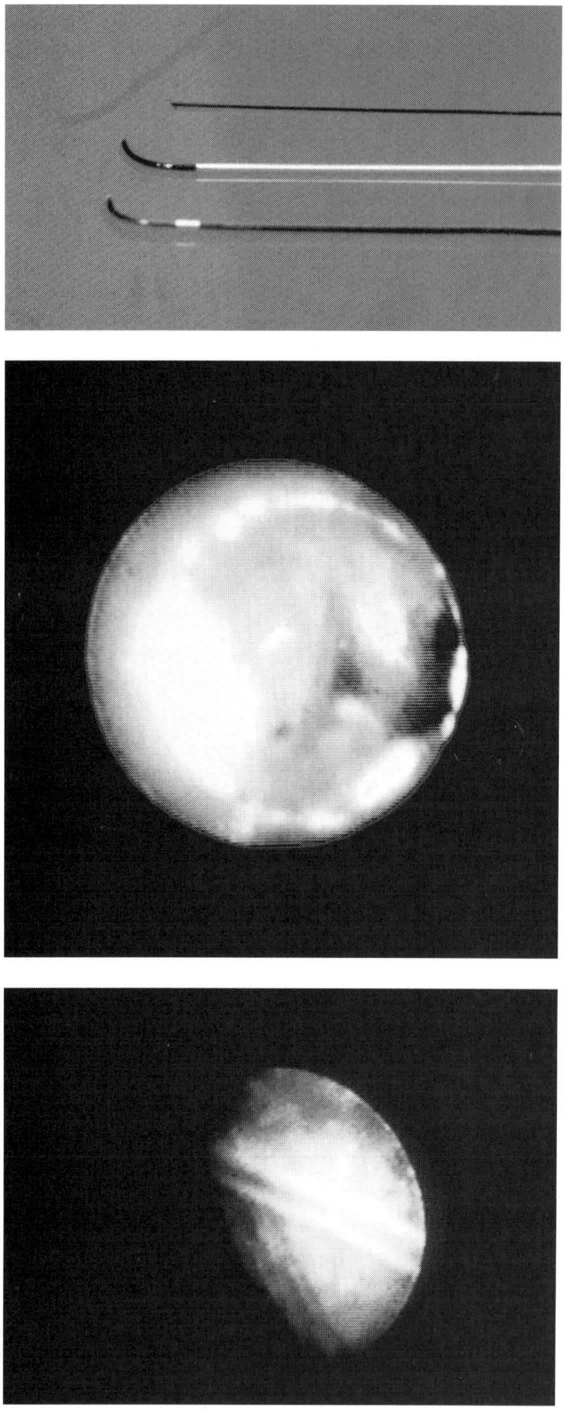

a

b

c

Fig. 9. a Microendoscopes with various diameters. **b** Microendoscopic view inside the foramen intervertebrale of a patient (L4/L5). View onto the segmental nerve and disk

cet joint denervation, percutaneous ethanol instillation for local cancer therapy [28], and sympathicolysis per year. It is important that the ethanol not be injected inside the facet capsule because there is a risk of inflammation, and also the ethanol can flow inside the spinal canal. Therefore MRI-guided endoscopy of the facet joints (Fig. 9) can avoid damaging the capsule and lead to the field of interventional selective laser or radiofrequency ablation of the sensory nerves.

The ethanol is injected very slowly and carefully, without pain to the patient. For safety we used 50% ethanol for the first treatments in an MRI system (96% in CT). The use of 50% ethanol cannot damage the segmental nerves. This dilution is always important when the ethanol treatments are close to the segmental nerve and the epidural space. With ethanol the patient may feel local pain in the following few days. If this back pain is too severe, long-acting anesthesia mixed with 10 mg triamcinolone can be injected twice every 2 days. In this study group the patients had good pain reduction without side effects.

Good 6-month follow-up results were also obtained in the treatment of iliosacral joints. Treatment of these joints was difficult in the past. Tilscher and Eder [29] reported that the injection of dye solution into the joint without image guidance was reached in only 14.5%. The X-ray fluoroscopic mode is not helpful because bony and soft tissue structures are not differentiated. The joint is very hard to reach because there is a complex interindividual anatomic variation of the os ilium, os sacrum, and lumbar spine. There is also a risk if the instruments are introduced without CT or MRI guidance. They can reach into the abdomen and damage vital structures such as arteries. The long-acting local anesthesia bupivacaine causes an allergic reaction in some patients; in this case antihistaminic agents and cortisone must be injected immediately.

Chronic spinal disease caused by intervertebral herniation of the disk is difficult to treat. In many cases microinvasive PRT can significantly reduce or even cure pain syndromes and chronic functional disorders of the spinal column and/or neurological changes. In our study most patients had a continual improvement in state of health of greater than 50%. Most patients suffered from a chronic intervertebral disk which had been treated unsuccessfully. Spontaneous healing was improbable. Infiltration of the pathological structures is routinely determined by CT, but precision is greater using MRI. This is carried out by the very precise positioning of the needle tip in CT and documentation of the drug distribution around the segmental nerve and epidurally by using contrast media for documentation.

The success rate of the PLNT method described here is also high. The immediate improvement of

87% in this study and 92% in a previous study of ours [12] surpasses our previous results with CT-guided diskectomy using an Onik nucleotome [1–3].

The reason for our good results is the atraumatic puncture technique under optimized image control by CT and fluoroscopic guidance, which was developed by our group in 1988 for new access in interventional surgery [1], small diameter (<1 mm), flexibility of the guidance needle, and accurate placement of the tip of the instruments precisely into the region of herniation. A further factor is the laser technique. The Nd-YAG laser which is used for nucleotomy allows heating and vaporization [12]. The vaporization enables efficient and precise excision of parts of the nucleus pulposus, while the heating simultaneously shrinks the disc.

We prefer an energy level between 3 and 10 W to reduce gas development inside the disc, which can damage the anulus and enter the spinal canal. The development of gas is well seen immediately by CT. We have encountered this much more frequently in elderly patients and in old disc herniations. In our opinion, the amount of gas development depends on the water content of the disc. For the use of lasers – especially in estimating the amount of laser energy at the beginning of the PLNT – it would be helpful to determine the age of the disc by MRI and/or spectroscopy. To avoid the development of excessive gas inside the disc we combine our laser technique with the Onik nucleotome workstation for forced suction, shorten the time of laser exposure (0.1–1 s), and reduce the laser energy used in the treatment. To avoid nerve damages and heating pain in the treatment of foraminal and extraforaminal herniation we decreases laser exposure time to 0.1 s and laser energy to 3 W. With this technique we are able to treat lesions with lasers and microinstruments 2 mm from the segmental nerve by CT guidance (see Fig. 6). An advantage of MRI over CT in PLNT is that high temperature alters tissue contrast.

The advantages of an open system in MRI guidance are that there is no radiation, and the patient can be treated inside the magnet. For both the patient and, especially, the therapist the avoidance of radiation is an important advance in guidance technology in microinvasive therapy. The time required to perform the treatment is virtually the same in interventional CT and interventional MRI. There is the possibility of controlling the guidance of the instruments almost in real-time in open MRI fields, but documentation sequences take much more time than CT today.

Both ethanol and local anesthesia installation in muscle and fat tissue alters the contrast in MRI (see Fig. 5) without contrast agents [30]. Fast keyhole sequence facilitates on-line instrument guidance and 3D detection of instruments. Generally the control of the instrument tip is better documented in CT. MRI guidance is helpful if the treatment is not close to vital structures such as in low-risk areas of facet or iliosacral joints. Image quality in the fluoroscopic mode is poorer than in the normal acquisition mode. For good image quality more sequences in one to three planes must be acquired before and after treatment. Thus diagnostic imaging increases interventional MRI time much more than interventional CT.

The benefit of both CT and MRI techniques is the visibility of all structures in the surgical field. Both offer a safe access. This is why we define both tomographic systems as "macroscopes" in the field of minimally invasive therapy – in analogy to "microscopes." With vital structures such as nerves and vessels in so-called high-risk areas CT is the gold standard of guidance technology as in nucleotomies and treatments inside the foramen intervertebrale or spinal canal.

In the near future, heating and cooling of the facet joints using lasers, radiofrequency or cryotherapeutic techniques will be realized. In MRI systems tissue contrast changes caused by temperature change or laser/cryotherapy ablation are visible. Also, tissue temperature measure-

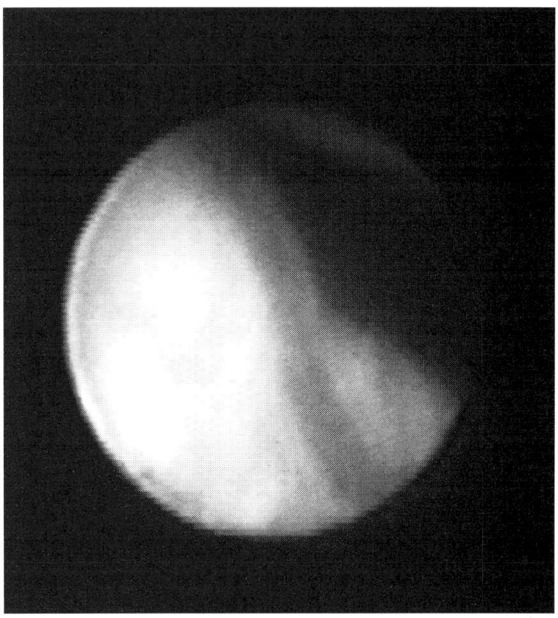

Fig. 10. Microendoscopic view of the surface of a facet joint (L4/L5)

ments for defined applications may become possible in MRI on a "touch-free" basis without using measurement probes [31–34]. This would also be helpful in the field of lasers [31], for example, for PNT [12] (see Figs. 7–9). The combination of interventional MRI or interventional CT guidance with endoscopy techniques improves safety in both nucleotomy and facet joint denervation techniques [35] (Fig. 10), which will also open the field also for laser, radiofrequency, and cryotherapy ablation techniques. If necessary, inspections of the joints with microendoscopes can be used for the specific guidance of ablation instruments.

References

1. Grönemeyer DHW, Seibel RMM, Melzer A, Schmidt A (1998) Microtherapy of disc herniation by MR guidance. In: Jolesz FA, Youws IR (eds) Interventional MR. Dunitz, London, pp 375–388
2. Onik G, Helms CA, Ginsberg L, Hoaglund FT, Morris J (1985) Percutaneous lumbar diskectomy using a new aspiration probe: porcine and cadaver model. Radiology 155:251–252
3. Onik G (1988) Percutaneous automated diskectomy technique. In: Onik G, Helms CA (eds) Automated percutaneous lumbar diskectomy. Rad Res Educ Found Univ Cal Print Dep, pp 77–110
4. Seibel RMM, Grönemeyer DHW, Sörensen R (1992) Percutaneous nucleotomy with CT and fluoroscopic guidance. J Vasc Interv Radiol 3:571–576
5. Lufkin R (1990) MRI asserts potential in interventional care. Diagn Imag 119
6. Grönemeyer DHW, Seibel RMM, Kaufman L, Schmidt A, Rothschild P (1991) Low-field design eases MRI-guided biopsies. Diagn Imaging 47:139–143
7. Hijikata S, Yamiagishi M, Nakayama T, Oomori K (1975) Percutaneous diskectomy: a new treatment method for lumbar disc herniation. J Toden Hosp 5:5–13
8. Friedman WA (1983) Percutaneous discectomy an alternative to chemonucleolysis? Neurosurgery 13:542–547
9. Schreiber A, Suezawa Y, Leu HJ (1989) Does percutaneous nucleotomy with discoscopy replace conventional discectomy? Clin Orthop 238:35–42
10. Ascher PW, Holzer P, Sutter P, Tritthart H (1991) Nucleus pulposus – Denaturierung bei Bandscheibenprotrusionen. In: Siebert WE, Wirth CJ (eds) Laser in der Orthopädie. Thieme, Stuttgart, pp 169–172
11. Yonezawa T, Tanaka S, Watanabe H, Onomura T, Atsumi K (1989) Percutaneous intradiscal laser discectomy. In: Mayer HM, Brock M (eds) Percutaneous lumbar discectomy. Springer, Berlin Heidelberg New York, pp 197–204
12. Grönemeyer D, Seibel R, Schmidt A, Kremer G, van Leeuwen P (1993) Atraumatic CT controlled percutaneous laser nucleotomy. Minim Invasive Ther 2:247–255
13. Riederer SJ, Tasciyan T, Farzaneh F, Lee JN, Wright RC, Herfkens RJ (1988) MR fluoroscopy: technical feasibility. Magn Reson Med 8:1–15
14. Friebe M, Busch M, Hellwig S, Grönemeyer D, Seibel R (1993) Keyhole sequence with rotational K-space updating as a means of fast, high quality low-field interventional MR imaging. Presented at the Annual Meeting of the Society for Magnetic Resonance in Medicine. Abstract 161
15. L'Espinasse VL (1943) Cited in: Davis Neurological surgery, 2nd edn. Lea & Febiger, Philadelphia, pp 442
16. Dandy WE (1922) An operative procedure for hydrocephalus. Bull Johns Hopkins Hosp 33:189–190
17. Burman MS (1931) Myeloscopy for the direct visualisation of spinal cord. J Bone Joint Surg 13:695
18. Ooi Y, Satoh Y, Sugaware S, Mikanagi K, Morisaki N (1977) Myeloscopy. Int Orthop 1:107
19. Rees WS (1971) Multiple, bilateral subcutaneous rhizolysis of segmental nerves in the. treatment of the intervertebral disc syndrome. Ann Gen Pract 26:126–127
20. Shealy CN (1975) Percutaneous radiofrequency denervation of spinal facets Treatment for chronic back pain and sciatica. J Neurosurg 43:448–451
21. Swetlow GI (1926) Alcoholic injections into nerve tissue for the relief of pain. Am J Med Sci 171:397–407
22. Kaufmann G, Richter G (1988) Embolisationsmaterialien. In: Günther RW, Thelen M (eds) Interventionelle Radiologie. Thieme, Stuttgart
23. Seibel RMM, Grönemeyer DHW, Balzer K, Carstensen G, Sehnert C (1990) The CT-guided lumbar sympathetic trunk neurolysis for the treatment of the occlusive arterial disease. In: Seibel RMM, Grönemeyer DHW (eds) Interventional computed tomography. Blackwell, Oxford, pp 211–225
24. Cox GG, Lee KR, Price HI, Gunter K, Noble MJ, Mebust WK (1982) Colonic infarction following ethanol embolization of renal carcinoma. Radiology 145:343–345
25. Rabe FE, Yun HY, Richmond BD, Klatte EC (1982) Renal tumor infarction with absolute ethanol. Am J Roentgenol 139:1139–1144
26. Löhr E, Schmidt-Neuerburg P, Heckemann R (1985) Embolisationstherapie von primären Weichteiltumoren und metastatischen Raumforderungen im Beckenbereich. Indikationen, Ergebnisse und Risiken. Radiologe 25:359–363
27. Lammer J, Justich E, Schreyer H, Pettek R (1985) Complications of renal tumor embolization. Cardiovasc Intervent Radiol 8:31–35
28. Grönemeyer DHW, Seibel RMM (1993) Microinvasive CT-guided cancer therapy of soft tissue and bone metastases. Wien Med Wochenschr 12:313–321
29. Tilscher H, Eder M (1989) Reflextherapie. Hippokrates, Stuttgart, p 75
30. Anzai Y, Desalles AAF, Black KL, Sinha S, Farahani K, Behnke EA, Castro DJ, Lufkin RB (1993) Interventional MR imaging. Radiographics 13:897–904
31. Jolesz FA, Bleier AR, Jakob P et al (1988) MR imaging of laser tissue interactions. Radiology 168:249–253
32. Knuettel B, Juretschke HP (1986) Temperature measurements by nuclear magnetic resonance. Recent Results Cancer Res 101:109–118
33. Le Bihan D, Delannoy J, Levin R (1989) Non-invasive temperature mapping using magnetic resonance imaging of molecular diffusion application to hyperthermia. Radiology 171:853–857
34. Busch M, Friebe M, Schaldach M, Koch M, Grönemeyer D, Seibel R (1993) High-field noninvasive thermometry sequence with SE keyhole technique. RSNA book of abstracts, 963
35. Grönemeyer DHW, Melzer A, Seibel RMM (1998) Interventional CT and MR combined with microendoscopy for low back pain therapy. Minim Juras Ther Allied Technol 7:223–232

Interventional Magnetic Resonance Imaging in the Head and Neck

3

A. Borges · P. Villablanca · D. Castro · E. Abemayor
J. Sercarz · Y. Anzai · T. Vogl · M. Mack · R.B. Lufkin

Introduction

In addition to the impact that magnetic resonance imaging (MRI) has made in the *diagnosis* of head and neck pathology, one of the more exciting novel areas of investigation is its use to guide interventional procedures directly.

Newer surgical techniques have been developed to increase exposure or visualization of a surgical field to perform definitive treatment. A prime example is in surgery of skull base lesions. The actual therapeutic part of surgery is often a small fraction of the procedure. However, the exposure (e.g., infratemporal fossa surgery) itself can cause significant morbidity. This has prompted investigation of newer techniques which use minimally invasive treatments to decrease overall morbidity and patient costs. By providing physicians with visualization alternatives, MRI, when combined with a therapeutic procedure, can achieve these goals.

The head and neck consists of small, closely spaced anatomical structures which require an intimate knowledge of normal spatial relationships and anatomic variations. Lesions often lie near vital structures, complicating intervention. Improved visualization during a procedure can therefore provide the physician with critical information, allowing innovative procedures and enhanced outcomes. MRI has the potential to evolve from a purely diagnostic tool into a guide for more invasive procedures.

While computed tomography (CT) remains ideal for imaging cortical bone, the superior soft tissue contrast in MRI makes it well suited not only for spatial localization but for early and sensitive detection of tissue changes during therapeutic interventions. Unlike in CT, the high flow sensitivity of MRI permits delineation of blood vessels without the use of contrast agents. Furthermore, the characteristics of MRI which make it such a powerful clinical diagnostic imaging tool also make it appealing for use in guiding interventional procedures in the head and neck. Oblique and multiplanar imaging capabilities and the lack of ionizing radiation are particularly valuable. The sensitivity of the lenses to ionizing radiation, a problem in CT studies, also makes MRI especially valuable. The absence of beam-hardening artifacts from bones allows more comprehensive visualization to guide approaches which may be difficult or impossible with other modalities such as conventional CT. In addition, many experts now consider MRI to be the best imaging technique for guiding interventional procedures of an *interstitial*, rather than endovascular or endoluminal, nature.

Despite these advantages MRI has a number of shortcomings which have thus far frustrated researchers' attempts to combine it with invasive procedures in a clinical setting. These problems are steadily being solved with advanced MRI technology. These include slow image acquisition and high cost. However, with faster imaging techniques, the costs decline. Early scanner designs limited access to the patient; a new generation of MRI instruments feature open magnets which greatly improve patient access. Furthermore, despite its value as a diagnostic tool, MRI has been criticized as being a high-cost technology that in some cases may increase the expense of medical care. However, if MRI is considered as part of a direct therapy system, the economic factors change.

Interventional MRI procedures have the potential to cost less than many other treatment options, especially those involving operating room time. Open surgical procedures are associated with known patient morbidity, elevated hospitalization costs, and lost time from work. When these factors are compared with closed MRI-guided interventions, the potential savings are great. Interventional MRI may prove to be the most significant cost saving clinical application of MRI technology since its introduction as a diagnostic device over a decade ago.

■ Aspiration Cytology

Fine-needle aspiration (FNA) cytology is a diagnostic tool with high sensitivity and specificity. In one large series the accuracy rates for FNA in the head and neck ranged from 85% to 98% [1]. Even lymphoma patients can now be evaluated using flow cytometry on aspirates. The ability to obtain tissue specimens from deep regions using FNA without surgical intervention has had a dramatic impact in the management of a variety of head and neck lesions [10, 11]. Although some lesions may be aspirated under direct palpation, there are many cases in which a lesion is deep-seated and recognized only through tomographic imaging. Imaging-guided aspiration cytology is particularly useful for such nonpalpable deep lesions.

CT-guided aspiration cytology was previously used [1], but MRI is rapidly replacing CT in this area because MRI permits precise needle placement in often relatively inaccessible areas. As stated above, there are a number of locations, such as the skull base and submandibular region, where beam-hardening artifacts limit the effectiveness of CT. In addition, other advantages of MRI over CT include the lack of need for carrier needle tip localization by the ability of MRI to obtain an image along the course of the needle without repositioning the patient [9–11, 15, 17, 18] and finally, the newer, open MRI systems with MRI "fluoroscopy" which greatly simplify these approaches (Fig. 1).

Procedure

MR-guided FNA begins with the same patient preparation and draping and the same local anesthetic that are used for aspiration cytology procedures guided by other imaging techniques. A stereotaxic device may improve needle placement [16], but positioning by hand suffices in many situations in the head and neck. A V-shaped surface marker helps determine surface relationships, depth and necessary angle of needle insertion [24]. Various images are used to localize the lesion and determine the best approach.

During the procedure we routinely use commercially available high nickel content needles with a *coaxial* needle system which allows multiple samples to be obtained from a single skin entry site (Fig. 1) [14]. The system uses a 26-gauge needle, of variable length and curvature, which fits through the lumen of a 22-gauge needle. The larger needle is placed in to the lesion, and multiple samples are obtained with the smaller needle. This system is especially useful in the head and neck where even a small amount of tissue trauma to surrounding neural and vascular structures may be deleterious.

Approaches

The following general approaches have proven useful for aspiration cytology of head and neck lesions.

Subzygomatic/Infratemporal. This approach is valuable for parapharyngeal and infratemporal fossa lesions. The patient's mouth is held open, using a bite block if necessary, and the temporomandibular joint is palpated along the inferior border of the zygoma. The coronoid process can be felt anteriorly. The window between the zygoma, coronoid process, and mandibular condyle forms a triangular space through which the needle can be inserted (Fig. 2).

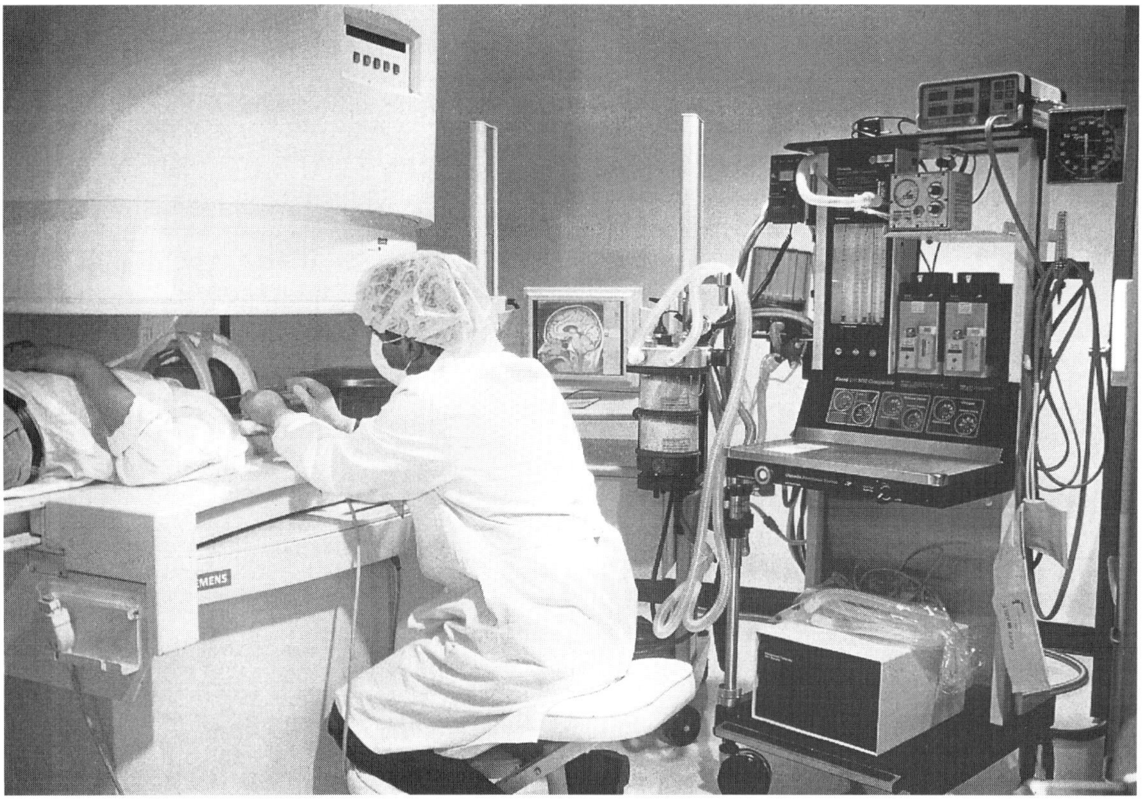

a

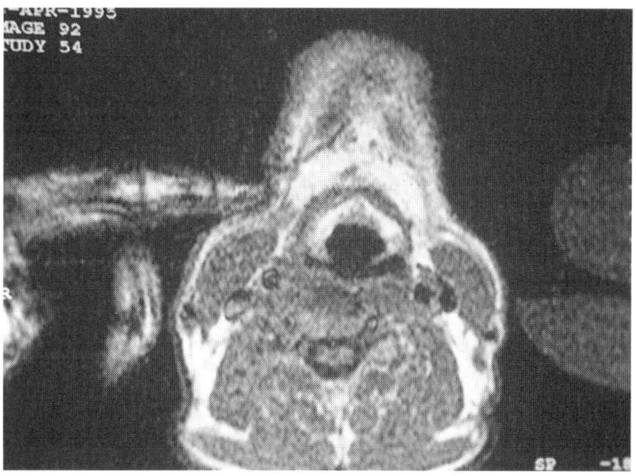

b

Fig. 1 a, b. Open-design MRI systems for use with head and neck procedures. **a** A 0.2-T open-design system with in-room monitor. Note MRI-compatible anesthesia equipment (Siemens Open, Erlangen, Germany). **b** High-speed "fluoro" type MRI sequences improve "free-hand" head and neck biopsy approaches. The physician's finger is shown to aid in biopsy positioning

Retromandibular. This approach is used for parapharyngeal, carotid, parotid, retropharyngeal, and masticator space lesions. The angle of the mandible is palpated and the needle placed posterior to the angle. In order to avoid the major proximal branches of the facial nerve beyond the stylomastoid foramen, the needle should not be placed higher than 1 cm below the bottom of the tragus. The carotid artery should be palpated below the angle of the mandible and controlled during needle placement (Fig. 3).

Submastoid. This approach is useful for lesions of the skull base. The needle should be placed approximately 1 cm below the mastoid tip, along the anterior aspect of the sternocleidomastoid muscle. Again, the carotid artery should be palpated below the angle of the mandible and controlled during needle placement.

Direct. This is used for superficial lesions, such as those in the thyroid or parotid glands. It is important to avoid the airway and major vascular and neural structures when approaching these lesions.

Fig. 2 a–c. Subzygomatic approach. **a** The needle is placed inferior to the zygoma between the coronoid and condyle of the mandible in the open mouth position as shown. **b** Image during biopsy using this approach (*arrowhead*, needle position). Patient had a history of treated juvenile angiofibroma. Biopsy was performed to rule out recurrence. Cytology sample was negative. **c** High infratemporal fossa MRI-guided biopsy of recurrent squamous cell carcinoma. The needle is visible (*arrowheads*) between the coronoid and the condyle

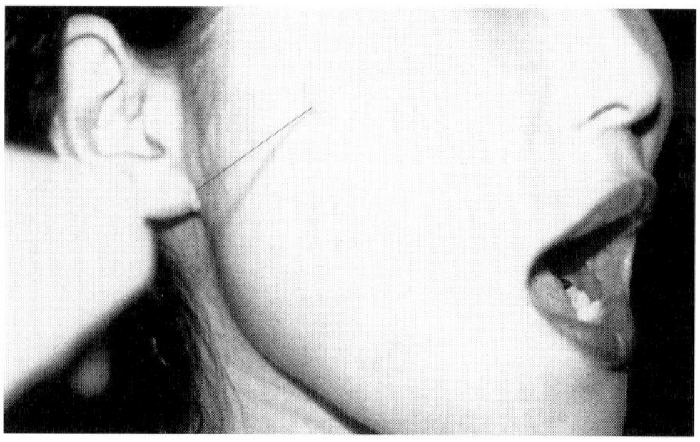

a

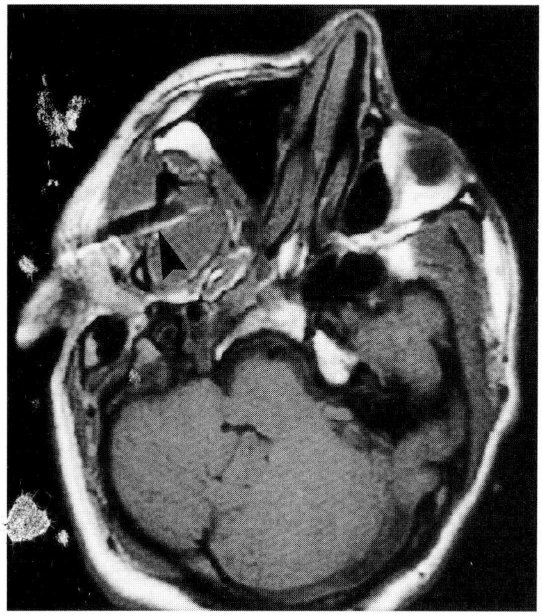

b

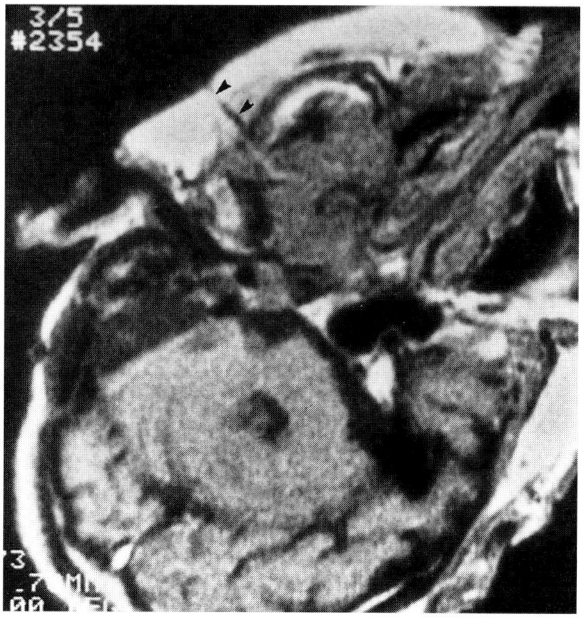

c

Other less common paths include the infraorbital canal to reach the infraorbital nerve, the anterior subzygomatic approach to reach Meckel's cave, and the transnasal approach for deep nasal cavity lesions (Fig. 4).

■ Treatment

While facilitated visualization for biopsy is clinically valuable, MRI is particularly appealing for therapy guidance. The possibility of a probe being placed within a target tissue and therapy (either chemical or thermal) administered is being actively investigated. MRI can demonstrate thermal changes as well as immediate tissue characteristics secondary to treatment with greater sensitivity than CT. Sequential MRI acquisition, coupled with image subtraction and display in the examination room, provides an environment in which the therapy session becomes an iterative process. Projects are underway to develop accurate and reproducible methods of thermal dosimetry using MRI, providing the physician with feedback on therapeutic effects during the procedure [2, 3, 12, 13, 19]. Monitoring these interventions intraoperatively with MRI has become possible with the installation of equipment that allows access to patients.

The development of these therapies are especially relevant in the head and neck. Current surgical treatment often requires extensive dissection for exposure and produces residual functional and cosmetic deformities, particularly in cancer therapy [5]. Also, MRI-guided therapies are ideal for patients who are elderly and/or have multisystem disease that may preclude a lengthy general anesthesia and major surgical exploration. A number of therapeutic applications of interventional MRI are currently under investigation.

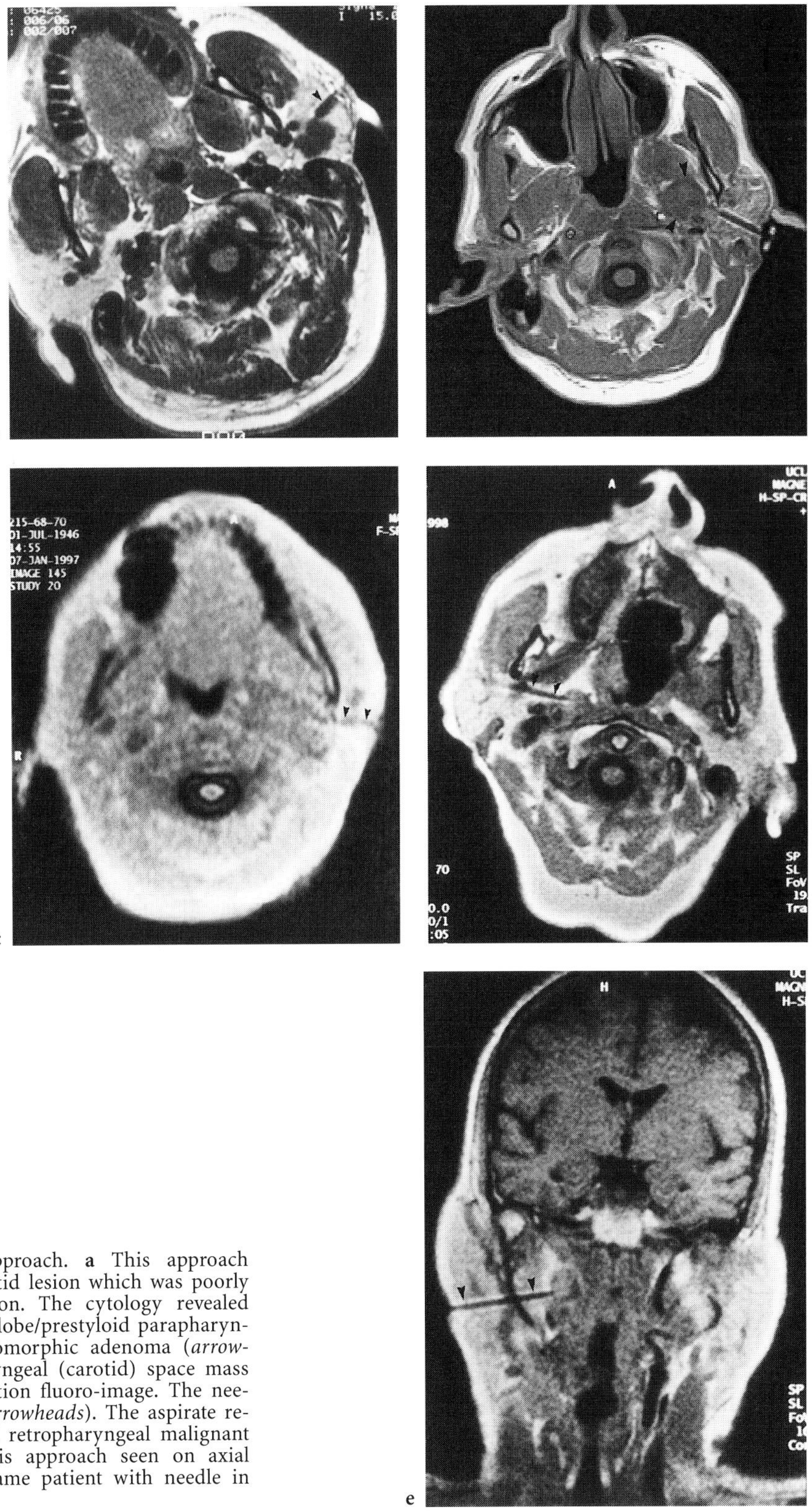

Fig. 3a–e. Retromandibular approach. **a** This approach used on a superficial lobe parotid lesion which was poorly palpable on clinical examination. The cytology revealed pleomorphic adenoma. **b** Deep lobe/prestyloid parapharyngeal space aspiration of a pleomorphic adenoma (*arrowheads*). **c** Poststyloid parapharyngeal (carotid) space mass seen on high speed, low-resolution fluoro-image. The needle is a thin low signal area (*arrowheads*). The aspirate revealed glomus tumor. **d** Lateral retropharyngeal malignant adenopathy aspirated using this approach seen on axial view. **e** Coronal view of the same patient with needle in place (*arrowheads*)

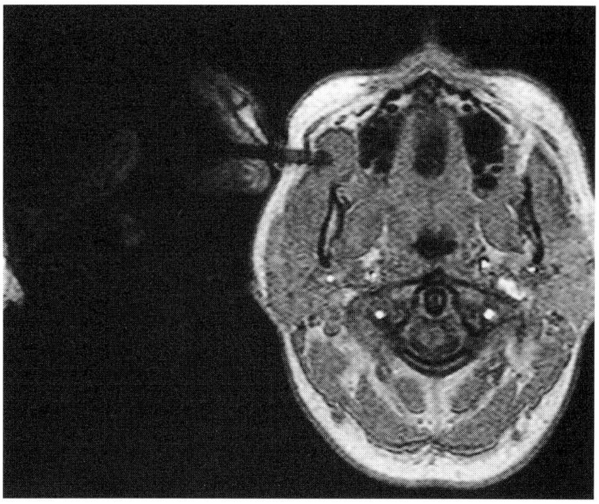

Fig. 4. Anterior direct approach in a patient with a small hemangioma

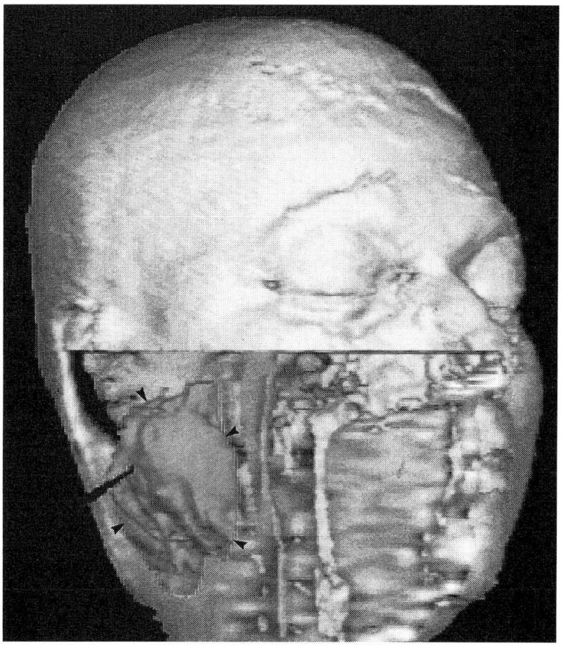

Fig. 5. Three-dimensional MRI of patient with recurrent metastatic breast cancer (*arrowheads*) to the parotid who received palliative treatment with MRI-guided laser

peutic interventions in such cases may provide physicians with tools to palliate advanced, recurrent, or unresectable tumors (Fig. 5). Studies have already shown the effectiveness of laser palliation of tumors in the head and neck using a variety of image guidance systems [6, 7, 8, 22]. The detail provided by MRI is especially important in these patients because their anatomies are often deformed by multiple surgeries and radiation.

In a prospective study, 12 patients underwent laser induced thermotherapy (LITT) of the head and neck under MRI guidance using an interventional subzygomatic approach for recurrent tumors of the nasopharynx and parapharyngeal space (Fig. 6). Lesions of the floor of the mouth and the larynx were directly punctured. Pretherapeutic MRI revealed tumor recurrence in all patients. All patients had already had surgery and/or chemotherapy before LITT intervention. [22, 23] Of the 12 patients 11 tolerated the procedure well. One patient with a recurrent squamous cell carcinoma and infiltration of the sublingual gland developed pain 5 min after starting the laser. No long-term side effects related to treatment were observed. The 2-year MRI control study of the patients with the pleomorphic adenoma showed no recurrent tumor.

MRI thermometry enabled on-line display of the hyperthermic effects, seen as progressively decreased signal from spaces surrounding tumor. Criteria for evaluating success of treatment included clinical data such as pain or other local symptoms as well as pre- and posttherapeutic changes in signal and tumor morphology. It was possible to induce coagulative necrosis (Figs. 7, 8) in all patients (volume range: 3–25 cm^3) and to reduce clinical symptoms in seven patients.

■ Possible Clinical Applications

Palliation in Tumor Treatment Failures

About one-half of patients with head and neck cancer experience persistent or recurrent disease [4]. Current treatment regimens include radiation therapy, which has finite dose limitations, and chemotherapy, which can produce undesirable systemic toxicity and dose limitations. Benign tumors such as pleomorphic adenoma also have high recurrence rates. Use of MRI-guided thera-

Minimally Invasive Primary Treatment

A new study currently underway is testing the viability of using laser heating for primary treatment of head and neck metastatic lymph nodes. A single nodal metastasis approximately halves a patient's prognosis, and surgical removal can produce some loss of function, often making these patients reluctant to undergo such therapy. Using MRI-guided laser to ablate these cancers followed by radiation therapy may potentially provide as effective a treatment as neck dissection but with reduced morbidity. This may serve as a model for treatments of other head and neck tumors.

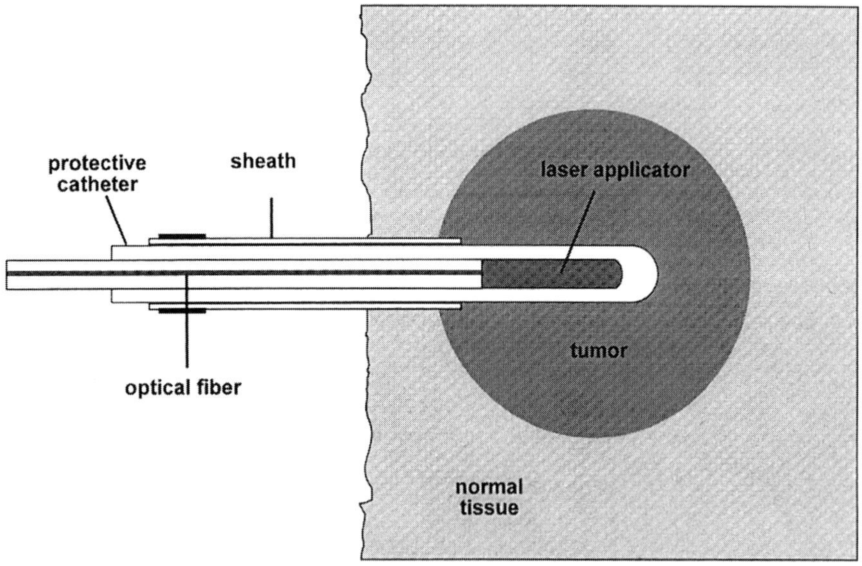

a

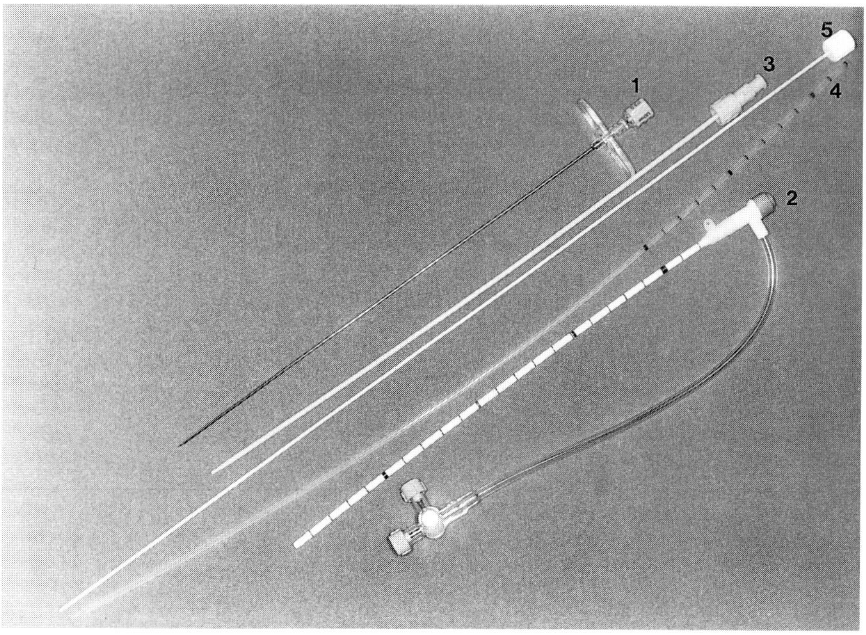

b

Fig. 6. a LITT setup. **b** Laser application kit, consisting of a cannulation needle (*1*) with a tetragonally sharpened tip, a sheath with an additional side port (*2*), and the corresponding stylet (*3*). The protective catheter (*4*), which prevents the direct contact of the laser applicator with the patient, is closed at the distal end and is also provided with a stylet (*5*)

■ Conclusion

Interventional MRI of the head and neck is in its early stages of development. While the value of MRI-guided aspiration cytology in this area has already been confirmed with human clinical studies, the ultimate role of MRI-guided therapy remains to be established. With the new dedicated interventional MRI units now available the future of interventional MRI as a viable therapeutic tool appears promising.

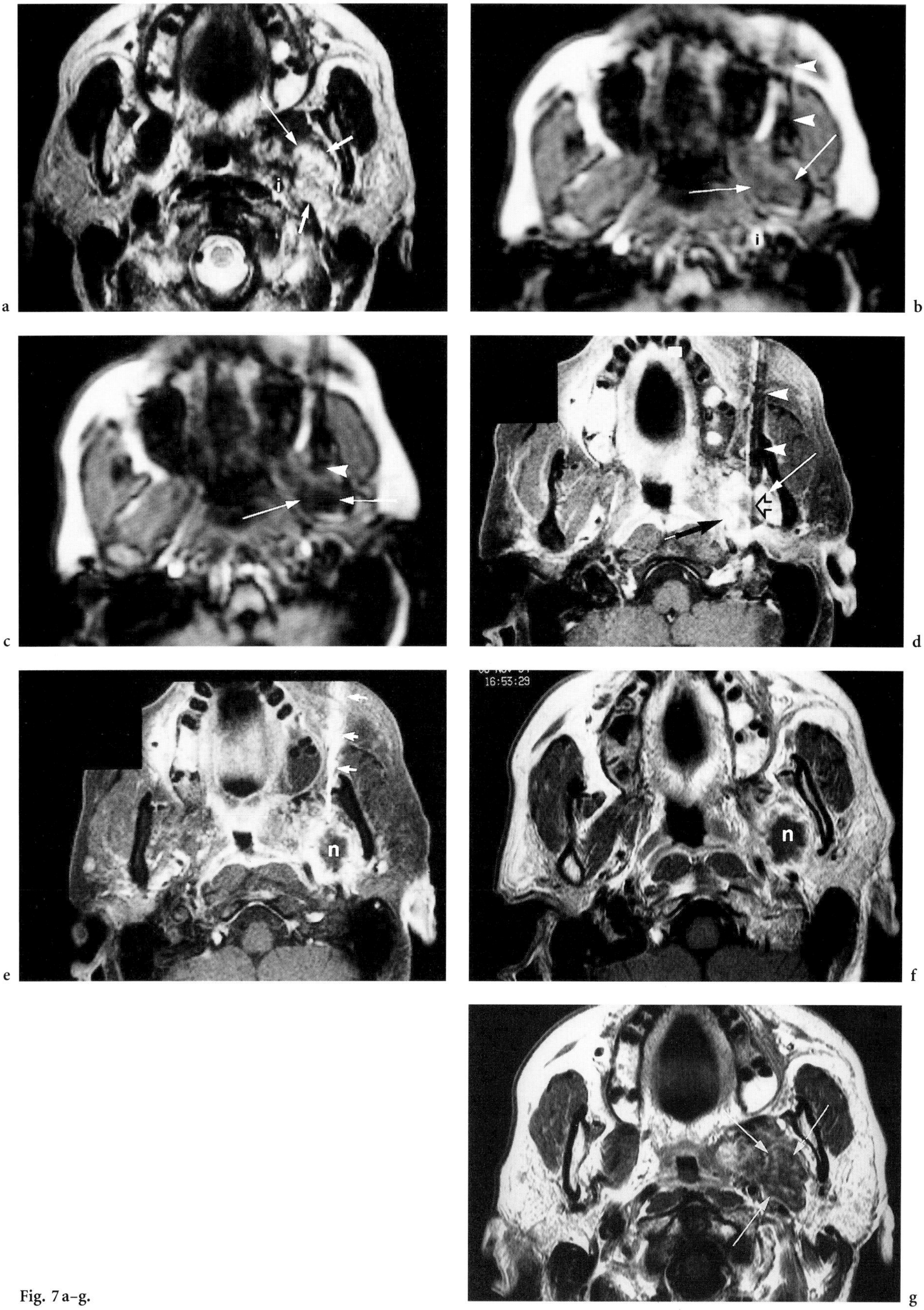

Fig. 7 a–g.

◀
Fig. 7 a–g. Demonstration of MRI thermometry and LITT results in a patient with a recurrent pleomorphic adenoma. **a** The T2-weighted image (TR/TE=3000/90) in transverse slice orientation demonstrates before LITT the recurrent pleomorphic adenoma in the left parapharyngeal space with inhomogeneous signal intensity pattern (*arrows*). Note the close relationship to the internal carotid artery (*i*). **b** Thermo-turbo-FLASH image (TR/TE/TI=7/3/400) demonstrates the lesion (*arrows*) isointense to muscle structures before the beginning of LITT. Note the high signal intensity within the internal carotid arteries (*i*) due to flow phenomena and the end of the magnitude marker (arrowhead). **c** Thermo-turbo-FLASH image (TR/TE/flip angle=400/8/15°) 13 min after starting the laser at 5 W/min. Note the significant signal loss with a diameter of 20 mm in the surrounding of the laser tip (*arrows*) and the end of the magnitude marker (*arrowhead*). **d** The fat-saturated, contrast-enhanced, T1-weighted image (TR/TE=500/15) immediately after LITT in transverse slice orientation demonstrates the adenoma with a hypervascularized border (*arrows*) the introduced laser applicator with the active zone of the laser (*open arrow*) and the magnitude marker (arrowheads). **e** The fat-saturated, contrast-enhanced, T1-weighted image (TR/TE=500/15) 2 days after LITT shows a central non-enhancing area of low signal intensity due to coagulative necrosis (*n*). Note the thin rim of high signal intensity surrounding the area of low signal intensity, which most likely represents reactive changes and the reactive changes in the puncturing canal (*arrows*). **f** The contrast-enhanced, T1-weighted image (TR/TE=700/15) 6 weeks after LITT again shows the laser-induced coagulative necrosis (*n*) and still a rim of high signal intensity surrounding the area of low signal intensity, regressive compared to **e**. **g** The contrast-enhanced, T1-weighted image (TR/TE=700/15) 1 year after LITT demonstrates a further regression of the reactive changes. Only scar tissue can be visualized at the 1 year follow-up control within the lesion (*arrows*)

a
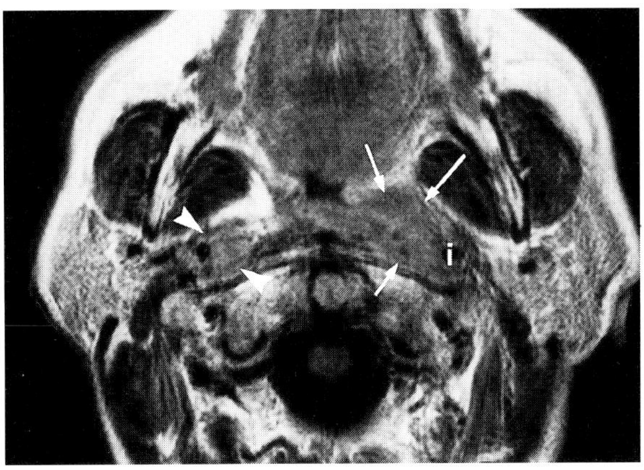

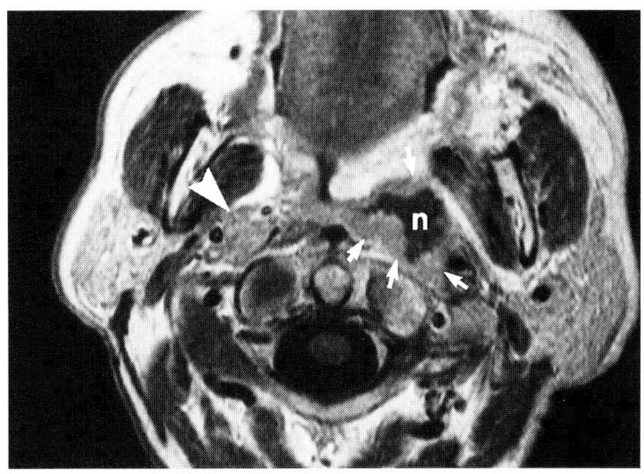

b

Fig. 8 a, b. Recurrence of a squamous cell carcinoma in the left parapharyngeal space. **a** The contrast-enhanced, T1-weighted image (TR/TE=700/15) before LITT reveals the tumor recurrence with homogeneous enhancement on the left side (*arrows*) with circular invasion of the internal carotid artery (*i*) and a lymph node metastasis on the right side (*arrowheads*). **b** The contrast-enhanced, T1-weighted image (TR/TE=500/15) 1 week after LITT allows an excellent delineation of the laser-induced necrosis (*n*). Note the remaining tumor tissue (*arrows*) with high contrast enhancement and the lymph node metastasis on the right side (*arrowhead*). After the therapy the patient reported a significant decrease in clinical symptoms

■ References

1. Abemayor E, Ljung B, Larsson S et al (1985) CT-directed aspiration biopsies of masses in the head and neck. Laryngoscope 95
2. Anzai Y, Lufkin RB, Castro DJ et al (1991) MR imaging-guided interstitial Nd:YAG laser phototherapy dosimetry study of acute tissue damage in an in vivo model. J Magn Reson Imaging 1:5
3. Anzai Y, Lufkin RB, Hirschowitz S et al (1992) MR imaging-histopathologic correlation of thermal injuries induced with interstitial Nd:YAG laser irradiation in the chronic model. J Magn Reson Imaging 2:6
4. Blackwell KE, Castro DJ, Saxton RE et al (1993) Real-time intraoperative ultrasonography as a monitoring technique for Nd:YAG-laser palliation of unresectable head and neck tumors initial experience. Laryngoscope 103:5
5. Castro DJ, Lufkin RB, Saxton RE et al (1992) Metastatic head and neck malignancy treated using MRI guided interstitial laser phototherapy an initial case report. Laryngoscope 102:1
6. Castro DJ, Saxton RE, Ward PH et al (1990) Flexible Nd:YAG laser palliation of obstructive tracheal metastatic malignancies. Laryngoscope 100:11
7. DA K, Fisher R, Kreusky B (1987) Prolonged survival and effective palliation in patients with squamous cell carcinoma of the esophagus following endoscopic laser therapy. Cancer 59
8. Dachman RA, McGehee JA, Beam TE et al (1990) US guided percutaneous laser ablation of liver tissue in a chronic pig model. Radiology 176
9. Duckwiler G, Lufkin R, Teresi L et al (1989) Head and neck lesions MR-guided aspiration biopsy. Radiology 170
10. Frable W, Frable M (1974) Thin needle aspiration biopsy in the diagnosis of head and neck tumors. Laryngoscope 85
11. Frable M, Frable W (1982) Fine needle aspiration biopsy revisited. Laryngoscope 92
12. Jolesz FA, Bleier AR, Jokab P et al (1988) MR imaging of laser tissue interactions. Radiology 168
13. LeBihan D, Delannoy J, Levin RL (1989) Temperature mapping with MR imaging of molecular diffusion application to hyperthermia. Radiology 161

14. Lufkin R, Layfield L (1989) Coaxial needle system for MR and CT guided aspiration cytology. J Comput Assist Tomogr 13:6
15. Lufkin R, Teresi L, Hanafee W (1987) New needle for MR-guided aspiration cytology of the head and neck. AJR Am J Roentgenol 149:2
16. Lufkin R, Duckwiler G, Spickler E et al (1988) Technical Note MR body sterotaxis an aid for MR guided biopsies. J Comput Assist Tomogr 12:6
17. Lufkin R, Teresi L, Chiu L et al (1988) A technique for MR guided needle placement in the head and neck. AJR Am J Roentgenol 151
18. Mueller PR, Stark DD, Simeone JF, Saini S, Butch RJ, Edelmann RR, Wittenberg J, Ferrucci JT Jr (1986) MR-guided aspiration biopsy: needle design and clinical trials. Radiology 161
19. Robinson J, Lufkin R, Castro D et al (1992) Magnetic resonance imaging of laser phototherapy initial experience. European Radiology 2
20. Sinha S, Sinha U, Lufkin R et al (1989) Technical note pulse sequence optimization for use with a biopsy needle in MRI. Magn Reson Imaging 7:5
21. Trapp T, Lufkin R, Abemayor E et al (1989) MR guided aspiration cytology of the head and neck. Laryngoscope 99
22 Vogl TJ, Muller PK, Hammerstingl R et al (1995) Malignant liver tumors treated with MR imaging-guided laser-induced thermotherapy Technique and prospective results. Radiology 196:257–265
23 Vogl TJ, Mack MG, Muller P et al (1995) Recurrent nasopharyngeal tumors Preliminary clinical results with interventional MR imaging-controlled laser induced thermotherapy. Radiology 196:725–733
24. Wenokur R, Andrews J, Abemayor E et al (1992) Magnetic resonance imaging-guided fine needle aspiration for the diagnosis of skull base lesions. Skull Base Surg 2:3

Interventional Magnetic Resonance for Biopsy and Drug Instillation in Cancer Therapy

4

D. H. W. Grönemeyer

■ Introduction

Interventional procedures in the abdomen and pelvis are performed mostly for biopsies, but they are also sometimes carried out for sympathectomies, drainages, and increasingly for cancer therapy. Puncture guided by computed tomography (CT), fluoroscopy, and ultrasound (US) have been reported in the literature for nearly 30 years. Nordenstrom reported the first series of percutaneous fluoroscopically guided lymph node biopsies [1]. Various approaches have been described, including transperitoneal, translumbar, and transvascular, using a number of different image modalities [2–11].

Fine-needle biopsies are most often performed for cytological and histological diagnosis in the abdomen, retroperitoneum, pelvis, lymph nodes, bones, and joints. In general the results with percutaneous aspiration techniques are very good. Success rates for obtaining cytological diagnosis of more than 80% have been reported [8, 11, 12].

US- and CT-guided biopsies are established diagnostic techniques [3]. However, US-guided methods have been replaced increasingly by CT guidance. Magnetic resonance imaging (MRI) techniques for clinical treatments are new and have the potential to replace conventional techniques [14–20]. Initially, however, they must be used carefully in so-called low-risk areas (LoRA), where no vital structures are vulnerable [20].

Tomographic scanners today made routinely possible the biopsy of tumor masses, drainage of fluid collections such as cysts or abscesses [7], percutaneous tumor therapy with ethanol ablation

[21–27], radiofrequency (RF) [28], or lasers [29–30], and interventional pain therapy [1].

When real-time diagnosis of histological or cytological pathology is available, tumor treatment may be performed directly after the biopsy through the same guidance cannula. This shortens the therapy time and is emotionally helpful for the patient. In the field of pain therapy, especially if the tumor mass infiltrates bony structures, percutaneous sympathectomy with ethanol reduces this kind of pain at once in more than 75% of patients.

■ Biopsy

There are various concepts of guidance techniques. Normally physicians perform biopsies with frameless devices in US and CT. In all MRI systems this technique can be performed (Fig. 1) in almost the same manner as in CT [31–32]. Another approach long known in neurosurgery uses stereotactic frames for guidance procedures in predefined virtual image environments. Also in use are interactive guidance systems connected with the instruments via robotic arms (e.g., viewing wand, ISG, Toronto, Canada) or directly with the instruments (e.g., Radionics, MA, USA). These units are stand-alone systems and are helpful in all MRI units by installation of a separate workstation. The guidance procedure is possible only with prescanned images in a virtual volume. One interactive concept is that of the dedicated open MRI system of GE. Here the image plane is automatically referred to a hand-held or a fixed probe over the region of therapy. The position of the probe is identified constantly, and the radiologist can define up to three orthogonal image planes that are related to the axis of the probe interactively.

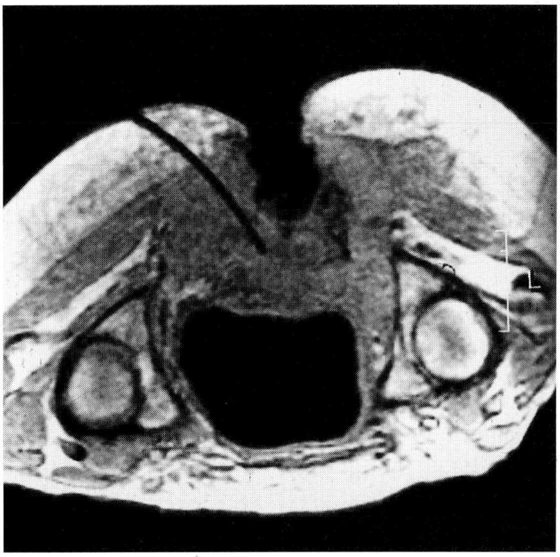

Fig. 1. MR-guided biopsy. The cannula is inserted into a metastasis of a colon carcinoma. On the upper pole of the metastasis tumor tissue was dissected by conventional operation (1989: Openfield MRI (0.06T Diasonics))

Contraindications

Biopsy should not be performed in patients receiving anticoagulant therapy and in those with blood-clotting disorders. Prior to biopsy clotting status and platelet counts must be determined. No other general contraindications are known.

Complications

There are rarely complications when CT-guided techniques are carried out in high-risk areas and MRI-guided techniques carefully in low-risk areas with artifact-free instruments by physicians with substantial experience. No significant complication has occurred since 1988 in our clinic when we initiated clinical interventional procedures in CT, electron beam tomography, and open MRI [20, 32].

Guidance Technique

In MRI a large belt coil (Siemens, Toshiba, Fonar) or flexible coil (GE) is fixed around or onto the patient prior to the biopsy with target volume in the center of the coil (Fig. 2). Using T1-weighted 2D FLASH sequences in "breathhold" the intervention is planned comparable to a CT intervention. The distance from an anatomic landmark within the image plane that can be palpated accurately is determined on the screen (Fig. 3). From the palpated structure the distance is marked on the skin. Subsequent to disinfection and sterile covering, a MRI-compatible cannula is introduced and advanced under "fluoroscopic" FISP or FLASH 2D sequence. An image rate of one per second can be achieved in Toshiba Access or one per 2 seconds in Siemens Open. The biopsy is performed while verifying the needle position with a FLASH 2D sequence in breathhold (Fig. 4).

Before biopsy the patients are positioned comfortably so that the probe can be introduced in the easiest puncture direction avoiding vital structures. By introducing the guidance cannula local anesthesia is injected into the skin and after guidance of biopsy probe into areas where the patient feels pain. The procedure generally takes about 35 min.

a

b

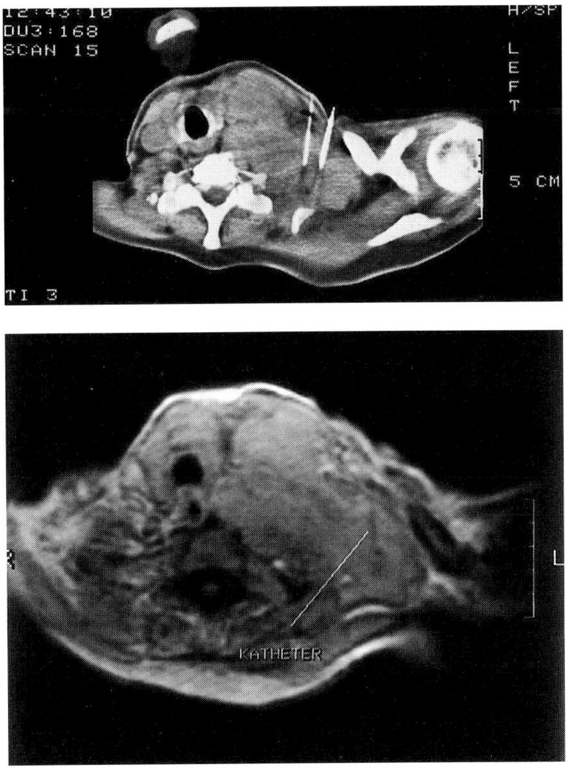

Fig. 2a,b. Imaging of lymphoma patient with biopsy cannulae in place. **a** CT scan. **b** Open field MRI (Diasonics)

■ Liver Biopsy

Indications

The radiological differential diagnosis of focal liver lesions is subject to a considerable uncertainty. This uncertainty is the cause for the increasing interest in CT- and increasingly MRI-guided procedures. The CT-guided technique is safer than US- and MRI-guided biopsies [32], especially in small and deep-seated lesions. Furthermore, the ability to avoid high-risk biopsy routes and to collect material from the nonnecrotic tumor margins is also best in CT. A general advantage of the CT-guided biopsy is the better control of the needle tip and improved documentation of the needle position. Indications for CT-guided liver biopsy are any focal lesions where a suspicion of malignancy cannot be excluded and where obtaining the diagnosis can be followed by therapy.

Contraindications

A significant coagulopathy is a contraindication to this technique. Earlier reports concluded a high risk from hemangioma puncture, but more recent articles have shown a much lower risk of hemorrhage [33–36]. Prior to the puncture of any cystic lesion echinococcosis must be excluded serologically.

Technique

The access route to a liver lesion is determined by the topography. Normally the shortest distance is preferred. However, in cases where a hemangioma is in the differential diagnosis a longer intraparenchymatous puncture tract should be selected. This longer tract can self-tamponade after a hemorrhagic puncture. The longer puncture tract is especially helpful for lesions located close to the liver surface. In cases of subphrenic masses a transpleural access is technically easier to perform than a puncture-directed medial and superior, which avoids the pleural space. When pleurocentesis cannot be circumvented with a maximum inspiration, it is recommended to perform the puncture at maximum expiration or with the patient in the lateral position because under these conditions the pleural recesses contain little or no lung tissue.

We normally use an 18-G set for fine-needle aspiration. Higher success rates in biopsies with large diameter cannulas than in those with needles having a small lumen have also been reported by other authors [35, 36]. Additionally, the specificity with the use of a cutting biopsy is higher than in fine-needle aspiration because histochemical examinations can also be conducted. A large number of aspirates per biopsy is frequently needed; therefore biopsy material should be obtained at least four different times.

The possibilities of incorrect cytological diagnosis are well known. Apart from the quality of the material and its preparations, difficulties can arise from the differentiation of pseudoatypical changes caused by inflammation from genuine atypical cells, which is always difficult and can sometimes be impossible.

The value of a cutting biopsy is often greater than a fine-needle aspiration, especially in cases of benign processes. CT-guided fine needle punctures with needles smaller than 20 G should preferably be performed only in the neighborhood of high-risk structures, such as the vicinity of the porta of the liver or within the subphrenic region. Otherwise, it is recommended to use a 20-G needle (DTMB 20-15 SIN, Cook, Denmark) because even with this small caliber a cutting biopsy is still possible. Another advantage of the 20-G needle is that the needle can be inserted in a fanlike fashion into different tumor areas as with the puncture for aspiration biopsy (Fig. 5).

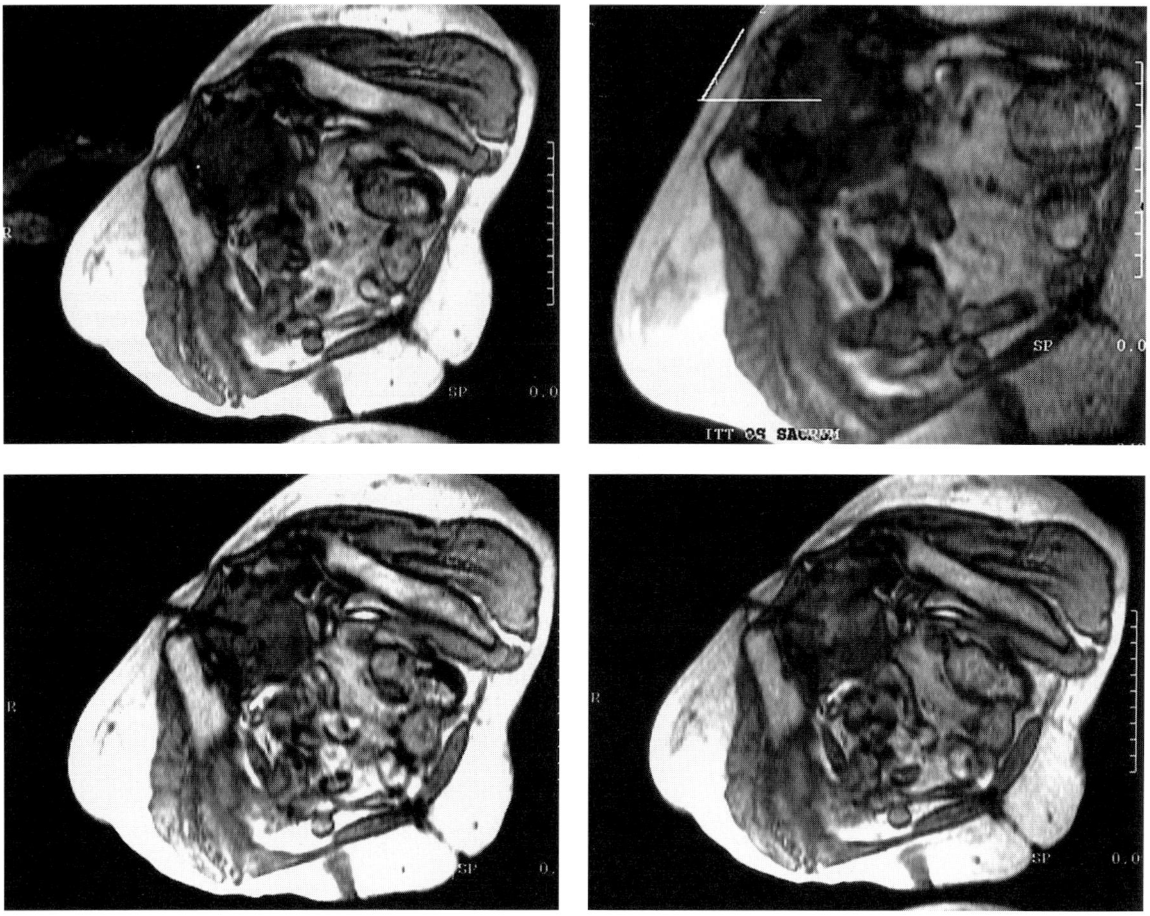

Fig. 3 a–d. MRI guidance for percutaneous ethanol instillation (PEI) into bony metastasis of os sarcum: microinvasive therapy inside a magnet. **a** Fingerprint for localizing. **b** Before contrast medium. **c** After contrast medium. **d** Ethanol instillation

MRI is helpful in lesions more than 1.0 cm in diameter although the tip of the instrument is not exactly detectable; MR fluoroscopy mode is available for nearly real-time guidance and multiplanar imaging. Real-time pathological analysis would help shorten therapy time for the patient. When guidance cannulas are used for biopsy, the tumor can be treated through it, for example, with laser and drugs.

Fig. 4. Biopsy of abdominal mass in Magnetom Open (Siemens) ▶

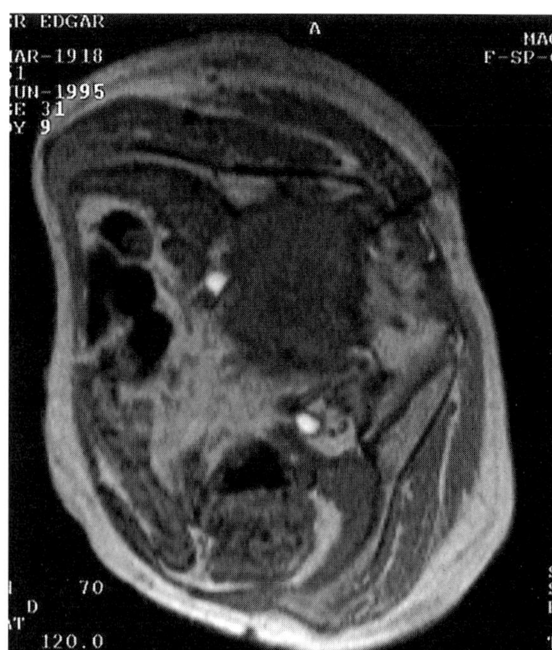

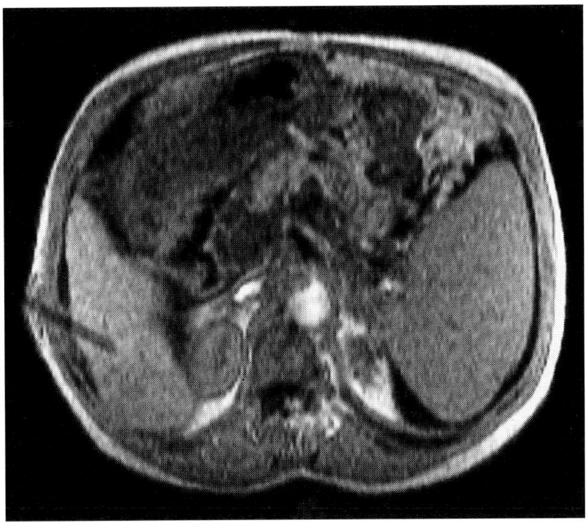

Fig. 5. Liver biopsy in Magnetom Open (Siemens)

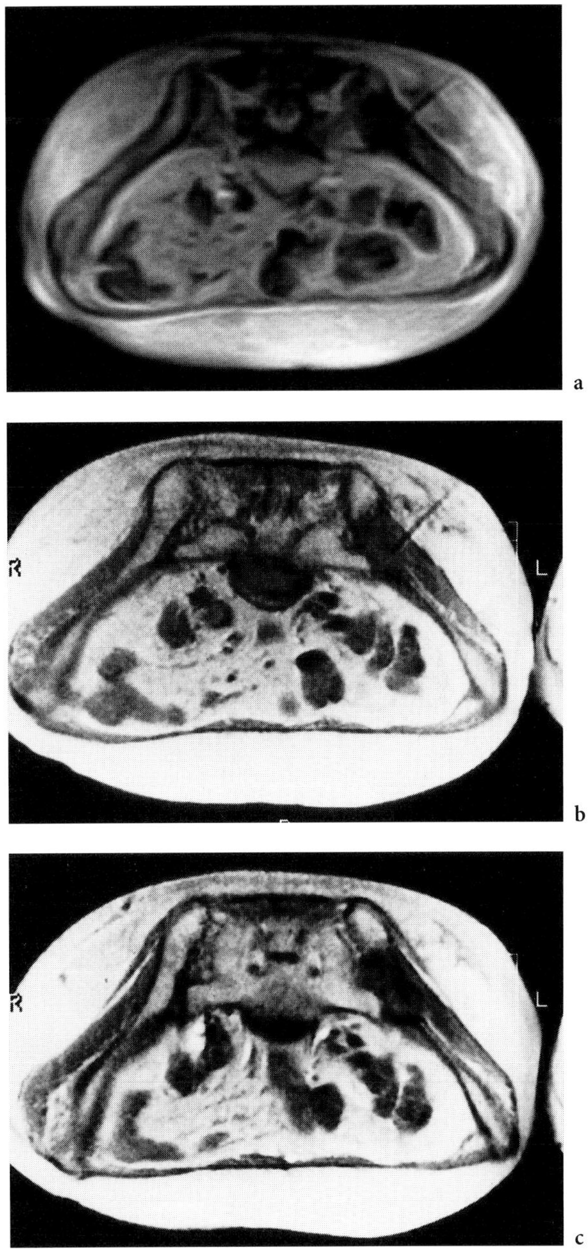

Fig. 6 a, b. PEI for cancer treatment in bony metastasis in os ilium of breast carcinoma with MR guidance. **a** Before contrast medium and ethanol installition. **b** After contrast medium and ethanol instillation. **c** Instillation of 1 cc of ethanol after contrast medium

■ Cancer Therapy

Cancer with metastatic disease worsens the prognosis of patients. Infiltration into abdominal tissues such as the liver and pancreas can be painful, and bone infiltration causes one of the most intense types of pain that exists. Effective tumor therapy must therefore deal with three important parameters: fast pain relief, effective reduction in tumor growth, and stabilization of bone or of the vertebral body to prevent paralysis. New, effective concepts with less traumatic treatments by tomographic guidance for these patients are now available.

Almost all treatment modalities used in the past under CT or US guidance are normally possible in MRI. Today, however, only few instruments and electronic equipment for artifact-free guidance in MRI are available on the market. The easiest method of percutaneous cancer therapy is local administration of highly concentrated ethanol (percutaneous ethanol instillation, PEI) or chemotherapeutic agents (percutaneous drug instillation) [37, 38]. The disadvantage of this technique is that the controlling fluid spreading inside tissue is not exactly assignable; however, ethanol instillation is helpful in providing fast pain relief and in calcifying and stabilizing infiltrated bony structures (Figs. 6, 7).

Other possibilities include intratumoral hyperthermia such as in liver, neck, and brain using Nd:YAG lasers [39–43], RF ablations [44], cryotherapy [45], hyperenergetic US [46–47], and brachytherapy. Imaging of temperature changing in tissues are possible only in MRI, and the therapist can control exactly the depth of the temperature infiltration. New imaging modalities in the open MRI system using temperature sensitive sequences and interactive image subtraction have been developed and are helpful in controlling the predefined treatment area.

Percutaneous sympathectomies [48–50] at all levels of the spine are also helpful as a first step in pain therapy using CT or ultrafast electron

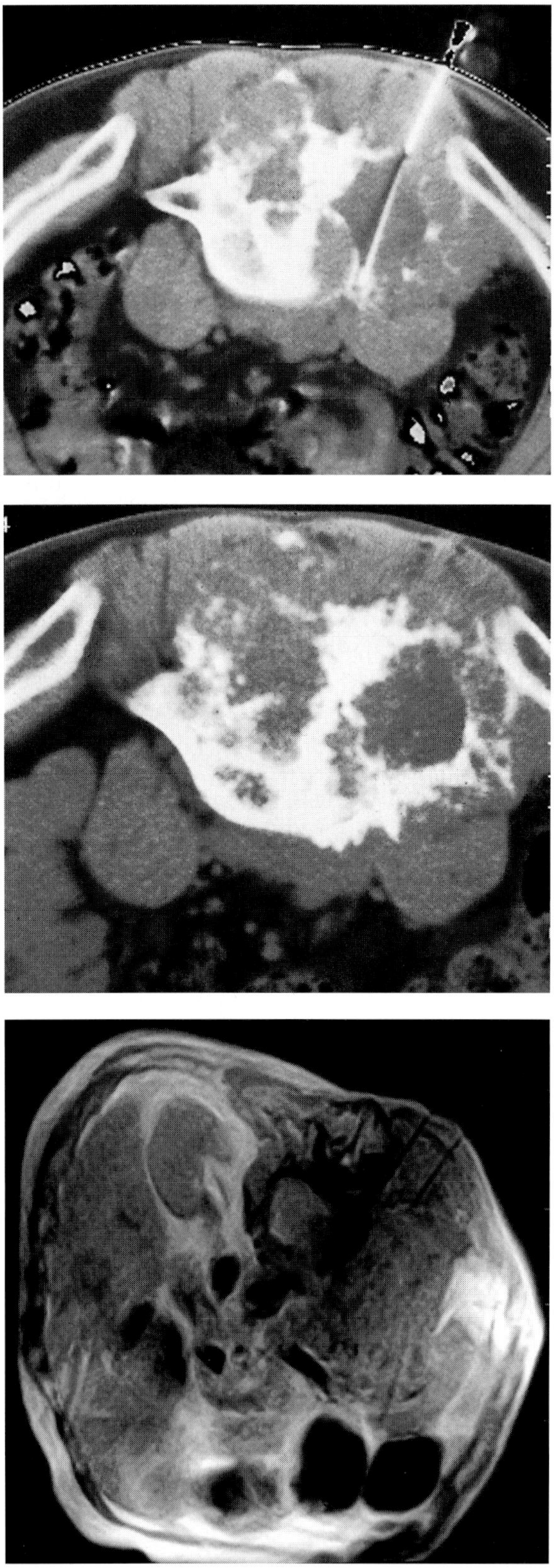

a b c

Fig. 7a–c. PEI of metastasis of renal cell carcinoma in left spine/os ilium area. **a** Before treatment in CT. **b** Three months later with calcification and statilization between left spine and os ilium. **c** MRI guidance (Toshiba Access)

beam tomography with or without combined endoscopy and RF ablation or 96% ethanol instillation.

Psychological and Pain Diagnosis

In addition to radiological and interventional examinations before therapy, psychological diagnosis is most important for the therapeutic concept of cancer patients. The diagnosis of "cancer" incites six types of fear in the patient [51]:

- Fear of death
- Fear of bodily deterioration
- Fear of insufficient therapy
- Fear of intractable pain
- Fear of being helpless
- Fear of being socially isolated

Therefore it is basic to any tumor therapy not to leave the patient alone with his fears but to initiate individual strategies for overcoming these fears and clarify diagnosis and therapy concepts. Additionally, the pain level can be reduced with more physician time and devotion to the tumor patient.

An intensive detailed history and interdisciplinary examinations are necessary prior to any treatment, especially if new symptoms appear in addition to those of the primary diagnosis. A questionnaire is helpful for analyzing the stage of tumor illness as well as the quality and quantity of pain. Characterizing the nature, location, and intensity of tumor pain can be very difficult due to the complexity of pain, psychological situation, and pain perceptibility. Furthermore, predicting whether a tumor will cause pain or what type of pain is due to which type of tumor is not possible. Bone pain and retroperitoneal pain are almost always very intensive types of pain. Nerve infiltrations, compressions, and abdominal obstructions generally also result in severe pain. However, tissue tumors and parenchyma tumors often do not produce pain.

Therefore every physician dealing with oncological patients must have a comprehensive knowledge of the various pain patterns, diagnostic procedures, and treatment strategies of malignant diseases.

Image-Guided Cancer and Tumor Pain Therapy

There are different procedures possible in the field of interventional tumor therapy. Percutaneous drug instillation and laser therapy are most common. Percutaneous ethanol injection for cancer therapy was used first for small liver tumor

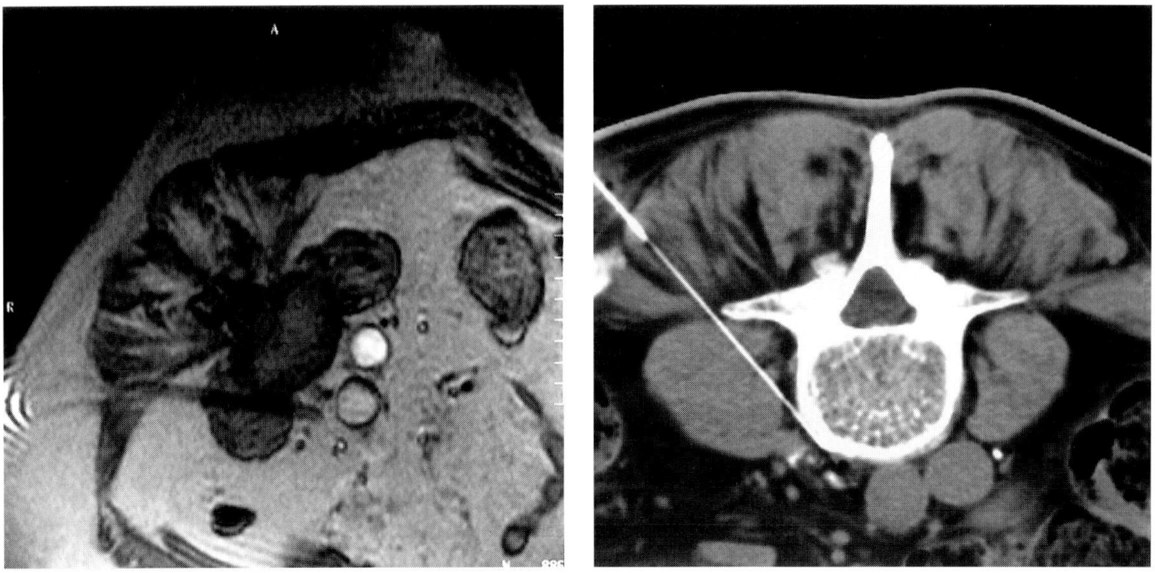

a b

Fig. 8a,b. Percutaneous lumbar sympathectomy. a MR guidance. b CT guidance

by using US guidance [23]. Today hybrid combinations of different imaging systems with CT and increasingly with MRI (Fig. 7) are being used for interventional microtherapy. Both techniques are by far superior to fluoroscopy and US. They provide not only precise, detailed, and reproducible images of the anatomy but also high-resolution and high-contrast information of the pathology.

Even a less well-trained physicians can become familiar with cross-sectional CT/MRI images much more quickly than with the moving real-time images of US. Tomographic images provide an accurate reproducibility of certain slices at any time for cancer therapy and drug instillation in high-risk areas. Tumor pain therapy has proven successful at our institution since 1988. Percutaneous neurolysis of the sympathetic system at multiple levels can be very successful especially in tumor patients who despite pain-relief drug therapy (oral opiates, antiphlogistic drugs, peridural anesthesia, local radiation therapy) continue to have intractable pain (Fig. 8).

Requirements and Indications for Drug Instillation

Requirements for performing this treatment protocol are tumor progression after surgery, radiation therapy, and/or systemic chemotherapy. Patients had contraindications to radiation therapy and chemotherapy for various reasons. These lesions can be treated for a relatively long period of time. Indications include tumor pain and neurological deficits caused by the rapidly growing tumor. Bone metastases and pathological fractures, which have immobilized a patient, are very sensitive to this kind of therapy.

Technique of Intratumoral Drug Instillation

After prescanning the tumor region the entry point of the treatment is defined. Either a transabdominal or a dorsal approach can be used. After local anesthesia of the skin through a guidance cannula the therapy needle is inserted very carefully into the tumor area. This procedure must be performed stepwise by interactive CT/MRI and injection of saline solution for both hydraulic tissue deviation and for anesthetic reasons. To avoid pain during drug administration, a short-acting local anesthetic agent (1% Mepivacaine) is combined with an long-acting agent (0.5% Carbostesin) at a relationship of 1:1 and is injected into the tumor before the specific drug instillation. Also, diluted contrast media is instilled into the tumor before the treatment. This is important for safety in documenting that the needle tip is located outside vessels and in visualizing the drug distribution. Injection with a 15- to 20-cm 22 G cannula is performed with 1.5–5 ml 50%–96% ethanol or with a local acting cytostatic drug of low toxicity: Mitoxantrone 2–20 ml (2–10 mg). We present use low-dose 50%–96% ethanol (1–5 cc and also 50% nearby vital structures). Treatment sessions are necessary every 3–14 days depending on the size of the tumor. The drug is administered every time at another location within the tumor [21].

Complications

Infection and hemorrhage may occur when working with punctures using a fine needle. If a motor nerve is punctured, neurolysis is possible. If the spinal canal is hit, arachnitis, neurolysis, shock, and even death can occur. Therapy of the pancreas includes the possibility of pancreatitis. Vascular complications (false aneurysms) must be considered if arteries are lacerated. We have seen none of these complications any of our own patients [52–54].

■ Conclusion

Summary

Treatment with alcohol can produce severe pain if the dose of local anesthesia or drugs and concentration are not calculated precisely according to the individual clinical situation of the patient. Burning sensation and muscular aches sometimes continue for several days following treatment with ethanol; these can be controlled by antiphlogistic drug therapy. The syndrome of neurolysis after accidental injection of ethanol into a motor nerve can be treated with opiates. The toxic effect of ethanol in human tissues is known: local dehydration with denaturation of proteins and necrosis, and denervation (e.g., lumbar sympathicolysis). Complications after intravascular ethanol injection have also been described. In our department we have never experienced significant complications after injecting ethanol; our experience includes annually about 1000 facet-joint denervations, percutaneous ethanol instillations for local cancer therapy and sympathicolysis.

Only diluted ethanol (50%) and small amounts (<2 ml) should be delivered in the vicinity of vital structures (intestine, skin, spinal canal). Injection of contrast media before the injection of alcohol is absolutely necessary to demonstrate the distribution of the volume. Following each step (change of the angulation of the needle, injection of fluid) a new CT of the region of interest must be performed to ensure the safe site. The distribution of contrast media must be followed in craniocaudal fashion with a slice thickness of 8 mm. Three-dimensional reconstruction images are ideal.

A three-dimensional volume would also facilitate the calculation of the ethanol fractions to be injected. We recommend calculating the entire tumor volume, similarly as in planning prior to radiation therapy, and determining the amount of fractions before starting the treatment. The tumor must be divided in several sections, and the amount and concentration of the ethanol to be instilled can thus be predicted. It should be calculated that for within 1 cm of the spinal canal the ethanol must be diluted by 50%. If the needle tip is near the spinal canal, Mitoxantrone must be used because the latter has no toxic reaction to vital structures such as nerves. It is known that 50% or less of ethanol leads to damage only to the sympathetic nerve fibers, and that it does not significantly affect motor nerve fibers.

The excellent success of ethanol administration in pain therapy is probably due to the fact that it eliminates small sensitive neural branches. The effect of further dilution of ethanol has yet to be confirmed, as well as the combination of ethanol and local cytotoxic agents.

It is still uncertain whether there is a relationship between the amount of injected drugs to the size and the histology of the tumor. Successful intratumoral treatment with ethanol of small hepatic, abdominal, and tracheobronchial tumors has been described by various authors [21, 37, 55–58]. A 100% survival after treatment of a single small hepatocarcinoma with a diameter less than 20 mm has been discussed in the literature [8]. High amounts of ethanol (8–50 cc) for intratumoral therapy are also common. We prefer low-dose ethanol for avoiding complications.

The possibilities and prospects of direct intratumoral administration of cytotoxic agents must be further evaluated. We have already started treating soft tissue metastases in lower abdomen and metastatic disease to the spinal cord with Mitoxantrone. In contrast to radiation treatment, percutaneous ethanol instillations into bone metastasis causes immediate, dramatic relief of pain, and the stabilizing effect of the area of tumor destruction seems to begin earlier. Further controlled studies should evaluate whether intratumoral therapy can be used before radiation therapy or hyperthermia.

Single or repeated neurolysis of the sympathetic nervous system should be added to the therapeutic armamentarium of every physician dealing with patients suffering from metastatic disease.

Future Prospects

More treatments in the abdomen and pelvis will be carried out in near future. Well-organized centers are able today routinely to perform biopsies of tumor masses with a diameter greater than 1.5 cm in low-risk areas and by stereotactic guidance in high-risk areas. RF, cryotherapy, and laser techniques have a great potential for treatments of all tumors if equipment is available. The next steps in developing guidance procedures will include endoscopic minimally invasive therapy procedures and minimized open surgery in open MRI systems in the abdomen and retroperitoneum. Combined MRI and endoscopic therapy especially for obstetrics, gallbladder, urinary tract, and colon will be used routinely if endocoils and/or MRI compatible endoscopic system are developed.

■ References

1. Nordenstrom B (1967) Paraxiphoid approach to the mediastinum for mediastinography and mediastinal needle biopsy: a preliminary report. Invest Radiol 2:141
2. Göthlin JH (1976) Post-lymphographic percutaneous fine needle biopsy of lymph nodes, guided by fluoroscopy. Radiology 120:205
3. Grönemeyer DHW, Seibel RMM, Arnold WH, Kauffmann GW, Kramann B, Richter GM, Starck E: Atlas of CT-guided biopsies, in Seibel RMM, Grönemeyer DHW (eds) (1990) Interventional Computed Tomography. Oxford, Blackwell 3–6
4. Haaga JR, Alfidi RJ, Havrilla TR (1977) CT detection and aspiration of abdominal abscess. Am J Roentgeno 128:465
5. Jaques PF, Staab E, Richey W (1978) CT-assisted pelvic and abdominal aspiration biopsy in gynecological malignancy. Radiology 128:651
6. MacErlean DP (1980) Pancreatic pseudocyst. Management by ultrasonically guided aspiration. Gastrointest Radiol 5:255
7. Pagani J (1983) Biopsy of focal hepatic lesions. Comparison of 18 and 22 gauge needles. Radiology 147:673
8. Macintosh PD, Thomson KR, Barbaric ZL (1979) Percutaneous transperitoneal lymph-node biopsy as a means of improving lymphographic diagnosis. Radiology 131:647
9. Rüttimann A (1968) Ilias lyph node aspiration biopsy through paravascular approach: preliminary report. Radiology 90:150
10. Seibel RMM, Grönemeyer DHW, Weigand H (1990) Thorax - Biopsy: Lunge - Pleura - Mediastinum, in Seibel RMM, Grönemeyer DHW (eds): Interventional Computed Tomography. Oxford, Blackwell 15-26
11. Pereiras PV, Meiers W, Kunhardt B (1978) Fluoroscopically guided thin needle aspiration biopsy of the abdomen and retroperitoneum. Am J Roentgenol 131:197
12. Haaga JR, Alfidi RJ (1976) Precise biopsy localization by computed tomography, Radiolgoy 118:603
13. Dumoulin CL (1993) Real-time position monitoring of invasive devices using magnetic resonance. Magn Resn Med 29:411–415
14. Grönemeyer DHW, Seibel RMM: CT-guided cervical blockades and methods of therapy for lesions of the plexus, in Seibel RMM, Grönemeyer DHW (eds) (1990) Interventional Computed Tomography. Oxford, Blackwell 161–179
15. Grönemeyer DHW, Seibel RMM, Melzer A, Schmidt A (1995) Image-Guided Access Techniques. End Surg 3:69–75
16. Hermann SD, Friedmann LS, Radecki P, Caroline DF (1986) Incidential prostatic carcinoma detected by MRI and diagnosed by MRI/CT-guided biopsy. Am J Roentgenol 146:351–352
17. Lufkin R, Teresi L, Hanafee W (1987) New needle for MR-guided aspiration cytology of the head and neck. Am J Roentgenol 149(2):380–382
18. Mueller PR, Stark D, Simeone J (1986) MR-guided aspiration biopsy: needle design and clinical trials. Radiology 161:605–609
19. Silvermann S, Collick BD, Figueira MR, Khorasani R, Adams DF, Newman R, Topulos GP, Jolesz F (1995) Interactive MR-guided biopsy in an open-configuration MR imaging system. Radiology 197:175–181
20. Grönemeyer DHW, Jolesz F, Lufkin R, Seibel RMM (1996) Image-guided access enhances microtherapy. Diagnostic Imaging Suppl 11:2–5
21. Grönemeyer DHW, Seibel RMM, Schindler O, Schattauer K, Lange S, Schmidt A (1995) Die mikroinvasive, CT-gesteuerte peri-radikuläre Therapie zur Behandlung von chronisch bandscheibenbedingten Funktionsstörungen. Wiener Medizinische Wochenschrift 145:129–139
22. Grönemeyer DHW, Seibel RMM (1990) New forms of interventional tumor therapy in radiology, in Seibel RMM, Grönemeyer DHW (eds): Interventional Computed Tomographie. Oxford, Blackwell 137–152
23. Livraghi T, Festi D, Monti F (1986) US-guided percutaneous alcohol injection of small hepatic and abdominal tumors. Radiology 161:309–310
24. Seki T, Nonaka T, Kubota Y, Mizuno T, Samashima Y (1989) Ultrasonically guided percutaneous ethanol injection therapy for hepatocellular carcinoma. Am J Gastroenterol 84:1400–1407
25. Sheu JC, Huang GT, Chen D (1987) Small hepatocellular carcinoma: intratumor ethanol treatment using new needle and guidance systems. Radiology 163:43-44
26. Silvermann S (1996) Percutaneous abdominal biopsy: recent advances and future directions. Semin Intervent Radio 13:3–15
27. Unger E: MR-guided alcohol ablation of the body, in Black K, Lufkin R (eds) (1994) Interventional MRI. Marina del Rey, pp 154–158
28. Anzai Y (1995) Preliminary experience with a technique for MR-guided thermal ablation of brain tumors. AJNR 16:39–48
29. Jolesz F, Bleier AR, Jakob P (1988) MR imaging of laser tissue interactions. Radiology 168:249–253
30. Grönemeyer DHW, Seibel RMM, Schmidt A, Kremer G, van Leeuwen P (1993) Atraumatic CT-controlled percutaneous laser nucleotomy. Minimally Invasive Therapy & Allied Technology 2:247–255
31. Schmidt AM, Melzer A, Seibel RMM, Grönemeyer DHW (1996) Tomographic guided biopsy and cell aspiration of neoplasms. Minimally Invasive Therapy & Allied Technology 5:249–254
32. Grönemeyer DHW, Seibel RMM, Erbel R, Schmidt A, Melzer A, Plaßmann J, Schmermund A, Baumgart D, Welsch R, Ge J, Görge G (1996) Equipment configuration and procedures: Preferences for interventional microtherapy. Journal of Digital Imaging 9:81–96
33. Kramann B: CT-gesteuerte Leber Biopsie, in Grönemeyer D, Seibel R (eds) (1989) Interventionelle Computertomographie. Berlin, Ueberreutes Wissenschaft, pp 291–295
34. Pagani J (1983) Biopsy of focal hepatic lesions. Comparison of 18 and 22 gauge needles. Radiology 147:673
35. Feuerbach S (1988) Perkutane Biopsie. In Claussen C, Felix R, (eds) Quo vadis CT? Springer, Berlin Heidelberg New York, pp 284–293
36. Lüning M (1989) CT-gestützte Feinnadelbiopsien bei Leberraumforderungen. Ein Vergleich der Ergebnisse einer Arbeitsgruppe von zwei Zeiträumen. Röntgenpraxis 42:1974
37. Grönemeyer DHW, Seibel R, Erbel R, Schmidt A, Melzer A, Plaßmann J, Deli M, Schmermund A, Baumgart

D, Welch R, Ge J, Goerge G (1996) Equipment configuration and procedures: Preferences for interventional microtherapy. Journal of Digital Imaging, 9:81–96
38. Livraghi T, Vettore C, Lazzaroni S (1991) Liver metastases: results of percutaneous ethanol injection in 14 patients. Radiology 179:709–712
39. Gewiese B (1994) Magnetic resonance imaging-controlled laser – induced interstitial thermotherapy. Invest Radiol 29:345–351
40. Higuchi N, Jolesz F, Colucci V, Morris J (1992) MRI of acute effects of interstitial Nd: YAG laser irradiation on tissues. Invest Radiol 27:814–821
41. Kahn T, Bettag M, Ulrich F, Schwarzmeier HJ, Schober R, Furst G, Modder U (1994) MRI-guided laser-induced interstitial thermotherapy of cerebral neoplasms. J Comput Assist Tomogr 18:519–532
42. Vogl T (1996) MR imaging-guided laser-induced thermotherapy. Minimally Invasive Therapy & Allied Technologies 5:243–248
43. Anzai Y (1995) Preliminary experience with a technique for MR-guided thermal ablation of brain tumors. AJNR 16:39–48
44. Organ L (1976) Electrophysiologic principles of radiofrequency lesion making. Appl Neurophysiol 39:69–76
45. Gilbert J (1985) Real time ultrasonic monitoring of hepatic cryosurgery. Cryobiology 22:319–330
46. Cline H (1994) MR temperature mapping of focused ultrasound surgery. Magn Reson Med 31:628–636
47. Yang R (1993) Liver cancer ablation with extracorporal high-intensity focused ultrasound. Eur Urol 23:17–22
48. Seibel RMM, Grönemeyer DHW (1990) CT-guided neurolysis of the presacral and precoccygeal sympathetic trunk, in Seibel RMM, Grönemeyer DHW (eds): Interventional Computed Tomography. Oxford, Blackwell, pp 193–194
49. Schild HH (1989) Perkutane Neurolyse des Plexus Coeliacus, in Grönemeyer D, Seibel R (eds) Interventionelle Computertomographie. Berlin, Ueberreuters Wissenschaft, pp 291–295
50. Bonica JJ (1953) The management of cancer pain, in Zimmermann M, Irings P, Wagner R (eds): Pain in cancer patients. New York, Springer, pp 13–27
51. Seibel RMM, Grönemeyer DHW, Balzer K, Carstensen G, Sehnert C (1990) The CT-guided lumbar sympathetic trunk neurolysis for the treatment of the occlusive arterial disease, in Seibel RMM, Grönemeyer DHW (eds): Interventional Computed Tomography. Oxford, Blackwell, pp 211–225
52. Cox GG, Lee KR, Price HJ, Gunter K, Noble MJ, Mebust WK (1982) Colonic infarction following ethanol embolzation of renal carcinoma. Radiology 145:343–345
53. Rabe F, Yun HY, Richmond B, Klatte EC (1982) Renal tumor infarction with absolute ethanol. Am J Roentgenol 139:1139–1144
54. Lammer J, Justisch F, Schreyer H, Pettek R (1985) Complications of renal tumor embolization. Cardiovasc Intervent Radiol 8:31–35
55. Fujisawa T, Hongo H, Yamaguchi Y (1986) Intratumoral ethanol injection for malignant tracheobronchial lesions: a new bronchofiberscopic. Endoscopic Surgery 18:188–189
56. Burgener F, Steinmetz SD (1987) Treatment of experimental adenocarcinomas by percutaneous intratumoral injection of absolute ethanol. Invest Radiol 22:472-477
57. Sironi S (1991) Small hepatocellular carcinoma treated with percutaneous ethanol injection: MR imaging findings. Radiology 180:333–336
58. Vargas H (1991) Ethanol injection of hepatic tumors. J Invest Surg 4:291–298

Interventional Magnetic Resonance Imaging in the Abdomen

5

S. G. Silverman · D. S. K. Lu

■ Introduction

Interventions guided by magnetic resonance imaging (MRI) represent a natural extension in the continuing growth of interventional radiology. As new imaging techniques are developed and used to detect and diagnose human conditions, the same techniques can be used to guide the interventional diagnosis and treatment of them. This occurred as fluoroscopy, computed tomography (CT) and ultrasound (US) were developed, and it is now occurring with MRI. This has been due in part to the important principle of intervention: that it be guided by the imaging modality which images the lesion best. More importantly, interventional MRI techniques were developed because MRI provides a wealth of image-based information about tissues and tissue function not available with fluoroscopy, CT, or US. When MRI was postulated as potentially guiding therapy, interventional MRI procedures took on greater significance and expanded potential.

The initiation of interventional MRI procedures in the abdomen required work in several areas, such as open configuration MR scanner development, MR-compatible instrumentation, interventional MRI suite design, and safety issues of caring for patients in an MRI environment [41]. These topics are generic to the field of interventional MRI and discussed elsewhere. At this early stage of research and development the specific role of MRI-guided intervention in the abdomen has not been defined for any procedure or any disease. However, preliminary experience is beginning to accumulate. We review here what has been developed and preliminarily researched to date and postulate where, when, and why MRI-guided interventions in the abdomen will prove to be of benefit in the future.

■ MRI-Guided Biopsy in the Abdomen

Although many forms of MRI-guided therapy are being envisioned, all of these procedures are in essence extensions of a diagnostic biopsy procedure, since almost all procedures depend on the ability to position a needle tip under MRI guidance into a predetermined target lesion. Therefore the development of a reliable, easy-to-use, and practical system for MRI-guided biopsy is of paramount importance. Indeed, the ability to perform abdominal biopsies under MRI guidance is now increasingly important, as improving technology is enabling more and more abdominal, and especially hepatic, lesions to be detected which are not otherwise visible by US or CT [8].

MRI-guided biopsies are possible even with standard closed magnets. Mueller first described successful "MRI-guided" biopsies of the liver in 1986 [31] and later in 1989 [32] using prototype nonferromagnetic needles. These early reports used US to guide needle placement, and when the patient was brought to a closed MRI system, MRI confirmed that the needle was placed in the lesion. These landmark studies were the first to demonstrate the use of an MR-compatible needle. Van Sonnenberg et al. also performed MRI-guided biopsy using a wire-sheath system in a closed system [48]. During these early years, conventional spin-echo pulse sequences with relatively long imaging times were used. More recently, much faster gradient echo sequences have been used to guide liver biopsies in closed magnet systems [27].

Despite providing shorter imaging times than were used earlier, these closed systems limit the access of the interventional radiologist, assistants, and nurses to the patient. This limitation is especially important when upper abdominal (e.g., liver) lesions are being considered for biopsy or other intervention. These regions simply can not be easily reached during imaging with closed systems. Therefore patients need to be moved out of the magnet bore to conduct the intervention and thus be intermittently imaged (as is done typically with CT-guided procedures). Since most upper abdominal structures move with respiration, targeting such lesions usually requires multiple needle adjustments, and because each adjustment necessitates movement of the patient out of the magnet bore, these techniques are relatively cumbersome and time consuming [39].

Recently the development of open configuration MRI systems solved the problem of patient access. The first report of MRI-guided biopsies of the abdomen in which MRI was used to target the lesion, and the entire procedure was carried out during MRI with continual patient access by the radiologist was by Silverman et al. [40]. This technique used a 0.5-T vertically open configuration MRI system specifically designed to guide interventions and surgery (Signa SP, GE Medical Systems, Milwaukee, WI) [36]. The design and construction of the scanner included an integrated optical localizer and tracker which allowed interactive control of the biopsy needle such that the biopsy could be guided by MRI alone. Since then MRI-guided abdominal biopsies have been reported using other open configuration systems, including those employing a horizontally open design (Magnetom Open; Siemens Medical Systems, Erlangen, Germany) [9, 25]. Open configuration MRI systems are offered now by virtually all major MR scanner manufacturers [12] and their design and capabilities are described elsewhere. Virtually all of them, whether open horizontally or vertically, offer better patient access for interventional purposes than conventional scanners. Some of these scanners were originally designed to combat claustrophobia and as such do not contain an integrated interventional guidance system. Only the Signa SP provides both access to the patient (because it is open) and frameless stereotactic guidance to direct the needle during performance of a biopsy because it contains an integrated interventional guidance system. Although Signa SP uses an optical tracking system as its interventional guidance method, other methods of localization (e.g., mechanical sensors; radiofrequency, RF, localizers; tip tracking [7, 21]) are also available and can be effective "stereotactic" localizers. Open systems without these integrated localizers can be used alone, or with an adjacent needle localizer, to guide the entire biopsy procedure with MRI. These systems successfully guide biopsy because they allow simultaneous imaging during needle manipulations and near immediate image feedback onto an in-room display monitor so that biopsy needles can be repositioned.

MRI-guided abdominal biopsy can be performed using conventional MRI scanners in which fundamental localization techniques employed in CT are used. Here skin markers are used to locate the skin entry site relative to the target. Images are reviewed intermittently and targeting is based on estimated trajectories. Laser guidance systems can be used to mark the skin entrance site, or a special grid designed for MRI taped to the skin surface can be used [13]. Even the radiologist's finger could be used as a skin marker [26], which at the same time can approximate the needle angulation needed. Once the skin entrance site and needle angulation has been set, the needle is advanced toward the lesion. Unfortunately, unlike the brain or head and neck, because upper abdominal structures move substantially during respiration, the original planned needle trajectory may not match the true needed trajectory, and therefore angulation adjustments are necessary. This is where real-time, or nearly real-time, image updating becomes a powerful tool. On both the 0.2-T vertical field system and the 0.5-T double-ring system, an in-room display monitor showing rapidly updated images using repeated gradient echo sequences are possible. The biopsy techniques that have been optimized and reported for the respective open magnet systems are described below separately.

0.5-T Vertically Open Configuration MRI System

The first vertically open configuration MRI system was installed at Brigham and Women's Hospital in 1994 (Fig. 1). As part of its installation an interventional MRI suite was constructed [41]. In the interventional suite which houses the system, all equipment is MRI compatible and includes an MR-compatible anesthesia delivery system (XL10 MRI Compatible Anesthesia Station, Ohmeda, Madison, Wis.). The equipment includes a patient monitoring system with a pulse oximeter, a non-invasive blood pressure monitor, an airway carbon dioxide monitor, and ECG (MagLife ODAM, Bruker, Wissembourg, France), and two-way audiovisual communication devices. Additional custom-made or modified devices include a laryngoscope containing lithium batteries, aluminum oxygen tank, and MR-compatible stethoscope and intravenous pole. Service connections are provided for vacuum, air and anesthetic gases, as well as for electrocautery, laser and cryotherapy devices. Adjacent to the interventional MR procedure room are rooms for the scanner console and for computer hardware. The rest of the suite contains decontamination and clean rooms for handling and assembling instruments as well as a three-bed holding area for preoperative and post-operative care.

The homogeneous part of the magnet is located in its center (12 pp mover 30 cm) within which images can be generated. Since conventional RF body coils also limit patient access, specially designed flexible surface coils are used that operate as both RF transmitters and receivers. These coils are applied to the surface of the patient overlying the anatomic region of interest. Imaging is achieved in either a standard mode (as in a conventional scanner) or an interactive mode. When imaging in the interactive mode, the radiologist verbally communicates the selected plane to the technologist in the control room via the two way audio system. The plane is referenced to a hand-held probe held over the region of interest. The images are displayed to the radiologist on a video screen mounted above the scan region inside the system.

The interactive mode image planes are determined in the following way. An optical tracking system constantly identifies the position of the probe. A three-dimensional optical digitizer (Pixsys 5000 Flashpoint Position Encoder, Image-guided Technologies, Boulder, Colo.) employs three video sensors (built into the system on a rail above the interventional field), which localize the spatial position of two infrared light-emitting diodes (LEDs) mounted on a hand-held biopsy probe. The spatial information provided by the probe's LEDs is used to generate a normal along the handle of the probe and a position located at a specified offset from the probe. This spatial information is transmitted to a workstation (Sun Sparc 20, Sun Microsystems, Mountain View, CA), which uses menu-driven applications to define the scan plane obtained by the MRI scanner. Thus, the position of the biopsy probe determines the scan plane.

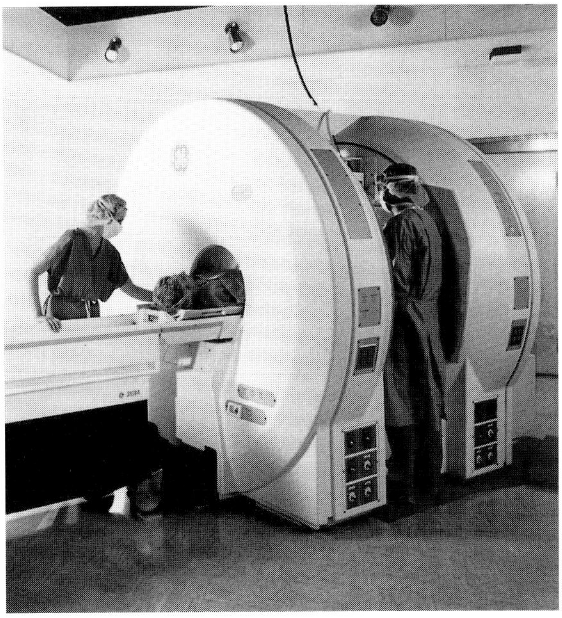

Fig. 1. Interventional MRI system, Signa SP, used at Brigham and Women's Hospital, Boston, Massachusetts. The magnet is constructed using two interconnected cryostats with an opening to permit access to the patient. MRI is possible over a spherical volume about the center of the gap. An optical tracking system with sensors embedded above the interventional field determine the spatial location of a hand-held probe which in turn determines the scan plane which is then displayed on the monitor

The radiologist verbally communicates a desired plane to the technologist in the control room. Any plane may be selected. For example, standard axial, sagittal, and coronal planes can be obtained at the needle tip. Typically three orthogonal image planes relative to the axis of the probe are selected (Fig. 2). When the so-called in-plane mode is selected, the image is in the plane of the long axis of the probe. When a perpendicular plane is selected, the image is in a plane perpendicular to the probe's long axis. Although more planes could be viewed, only these three

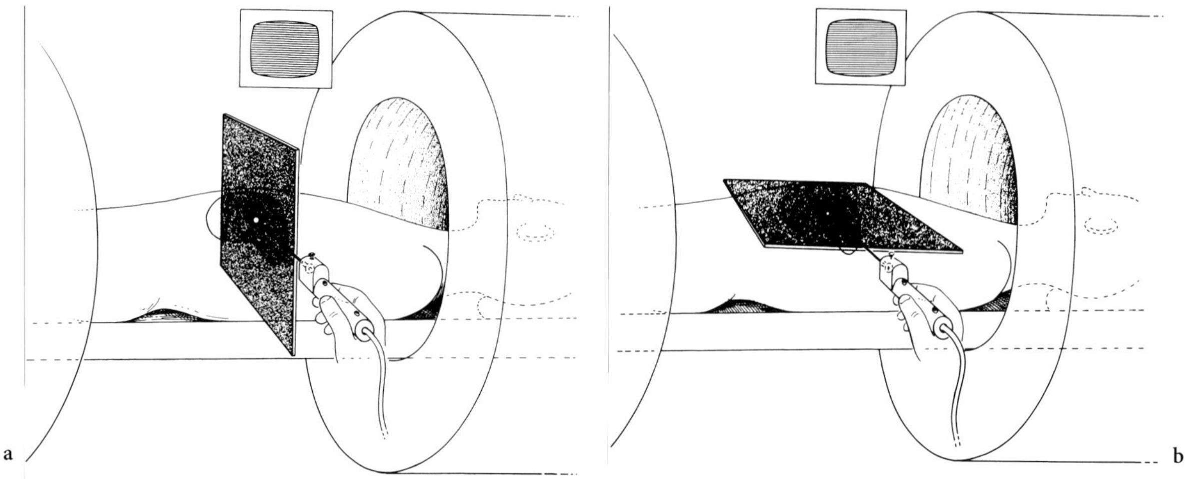

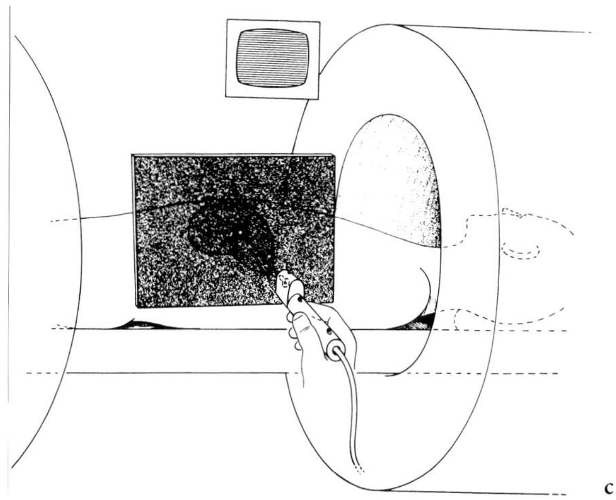

Fig. 2a–c. Diagrammatic representation of the three orthogonal planes shown on the video display inside the MRT system relative to the probe. The "in-plane 90°" plane results in an image that is in the plane of the needle's long axis and is perpendicular to the floor. The "in-plane 0°" plane which results in an image that is both in the plane of the needle's long axis and in a plane that is 90° to the "in plane 90°" view, and the "perpendicular" plane results in an image that is perpendicular to the long axis of the needle at the level of the needle tip

have been used. The nomenclature in-plane 90° results in an image that is in the plane of the needle's long axis and is perpendicular to the floor. The nomenclature in-plane 0° results in an image that is both in the plane of the needle's long axis and in a plane that is 90° or perpendicular to the in-plane 90° image. The perpendicular plane mode results in an image that is perpendicular to the long axis of the needle at the level of the needle tip. The displayed plane is only relevant to the probe position and not to the patient or the magnet. During a side entry with the axis of the probe parallel to the floor, in-plane 90° is axial-like; when the probe is held in a vertical position perpendicular to the floor, however, in-plane 90° is sagittal-like. When the biopsy needle is attached to the end of the probe and an in-plane image is selected, the image is in the long axis of the probe and contain the needle. When there is needle bending, however, the entire shaft (including the tip) may not be on the displayed image. When a perpendicular plane is selected, the image is perpendicular to the needle and shows the needle tip.

Spatial information describing the location of the LEDs can be used to extrapolate the path of the needle and the position of the needle tip if the needle length is known and the needle is straight. When the radiologist holds the probe attached to a biopsy needle and is targeting, the expected trajectory of the needle is displayed as an icon. This predicted trajectory is superimposed on the video-screen image in the magnet bore as a white vertical contiguous line followed by a dashed line. The end of the contiguous line represents the predicted position of the needle tip. The dashed line displays the path the needle would take if it were advanced further. During the procedure, as the needle is advanced, the display constantly updates the radiologist with (a) the actual position of the needle and its tip and the structures that have been transgressed, (b) the predicted path of the needle and the structures in the region of the path should it be advanced, and

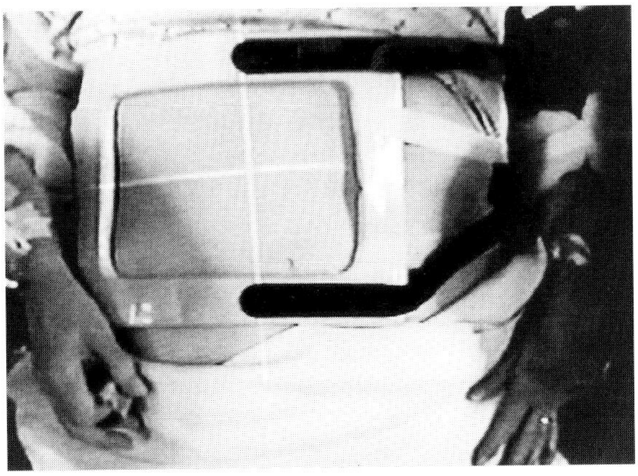

Fig. 3. The transmit/receive flexible surface coil used in the Signa SP system shown in position from an overhead view during an MRI-guided abdominal biopsy. The rectangular region is the surface area in which the cutaneous entry route is chosen

(c) when in-plane, the distance the needle should be advanced for the needle tip to reach the target.

Using a prior MRI or CT scan, the flexible surface coil is positioned such that the entry point and lesion are within the imaging volume, and such that the probe was within the field of view of the videosensors of the optical tracking system (Fig. 3). Then standard, noninteractive scanning using gradient echo and T1-weighted and T2-weighted spin echo pulse sequences is performed to check the surface coil placement. Image parameters are selected to provide optimal tissue characterization for both the lesion and surrounding structures.

Following this initial imaging, the region is scanned in the interactive mode using a nonsterile biopsy probe without an attached needle. To interactive scan we use a fast gradient echo se-

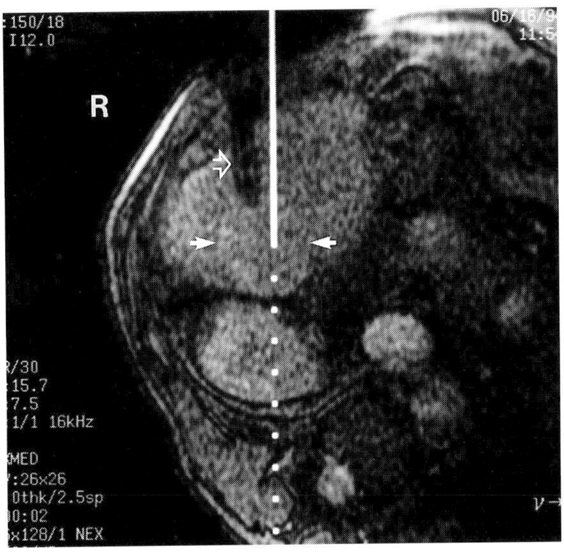

a

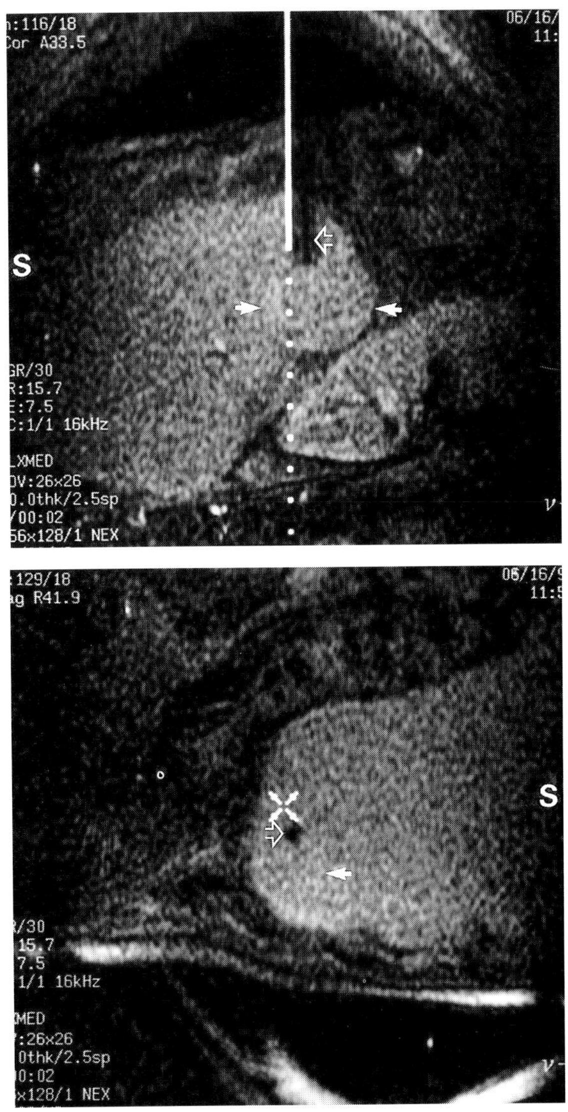

b

c

Fig. 4 a–c. Interactive MRI-guided biopsy of a small hepatocellular carcinoma (*arrows*) using a right anterior epigastric approach shown on "in-plane 90°" (**a**), "in-plane 0°" (**b**), and "perpendicular" plane (**c**) views. The needle icon tip projects in the lesion on each view. The expected path of the needle is displayed as a white line annotation (needle icon) superimposed on the in-plane views. The end of the contiguous line is the predicted position of the needle tip; *dashed line*, the expected path of the needle if it were advanced further. The cross-hairs show the expected position of the needle tip on the perpendicular view. During biopsy, with the needle (*open arrow*) attached, both the needle icon and needle are viewed using the same planes. The lack of an exact match of icon and needle is because of needle bending secondary to liver moving during respiration. *R*, Right; *S*, superior quence (TR=15.7, TE=7.5, flip angle 30°, 10-mm-thick sections) such that images are updated every 1.5 s. The optimal entry point and angle to the lesion are determined by showing the needle icon projecting within the lesion on all three orthogonal planes. The skin site is then marked. A sterile interventional field is prepared along with a specially designed MRI-compatible procedure tray, which includes a ceramic MRI-compatible blade (MicroSurgical Techniques, Fort Collins, Colo.). All biopsy needles are MRI-compatible (EZ-EM, Westbury, N.Y.; Cook, Bloomington, Ind.). A needle of sufficient length to reach the lesion is chosen based on the depth of the lesion in the planned path. The biopsy needle is attached to the probe and the needle advanced (and viewed in the three orthogonal planes) along the planned path. Once the needle tip reaches the target lesion, it can be viewed in the lesion in all three planes (Fig. 4). The depth of needle insertion is determined by the images, not by the depth estimate.

An active clinical trial of percutaneous biopsies using Signa SP at Brigham and Women's Hospital has enrolled 66 patients, of which 61 had their masses biopsied. Biopsies could not be performed because of equipment failure (n=3), lesion invisibility (n=1), and claustrophobia (n=1). Most masses were intra-abdominal (n=50) including liver (n=24), kidney (n=4), adrenal gland (n=5), pancreas (n=6), and lymph node (n=4), among others. Thus far, of 56 verifiable patients there have been 42 with true positive biopsy results, 9 with true negative results, and 5 with false-negative results (sensitivity=0.89, negative predictive value=0.64). There were no complications. Patients with cardiac pacemakers, cerebral aneurysm clips, or other MRI-incompatible devices and implants were not biopsied. Also, patients with a history of active ischemic heart disease (ischemia on ECG or recent symptoms of angina) were not biopsied because ST and T wave ECG changes are distorted, and therefore intraprocedural silent ischemia could occur undetected [14]. These preliminary biopsy data suggest that MRI-guided biopsy using this system is safe and accurate. Test characteristics are similar to those reported with US- and CT-guided techniques. MRI can be used to biopsy lesions visible with MRI alone or seen best with MRI. However, although rare, equipment failure, claustrophobia, and lesion visibility may prevent the use of this system.

0.2-T Horizontally Open Configuration MRI System

This is an iron-core resistive open MRI system (Magnetom Open, Siemens Medical Systems, Erlangen, Germany) which employs a vertical C-shaped magnet design. The two magnet poles are 42 cm apart which allowed for a horizontally oriented open field for patient access (Fig. 5). A specially designed MR-compatible chair situates the clinician next to the patient table. An adjustable optical light bundle is provided to illuminate the interventional field. A mobile console with MR-compatible active matrix liquid crystal display (LCD) monitor (1024 lines and 1280 pixels/line resolution), has been designed for selected scanning operations and viewing of images inside the MR suite. The height and angle of the LCD screen can be adjusted for optimal viewing by the physician. An RF-shielded mouse allows interaction with menu-driven functions of the scanner, including selection of pulse sequences. Therefore scanning can be controlled from within the room if desired, which facilitates the work of the MR technologist who is also assisting with the biopsy procedure.

At University of California at Los Angeles Medical Center, where one of the first of the above scanner systems has been installed, an abdominal biopsy technique has been developed utilizing a free-hand technique with no need for additional stereotactic devices [25]. This technique, reported in biopsying the liver, uses a conventional axial diagnostic sequence (T1 spin-echo, T2 fast spin-echo, or gradient echo sequence) to find the plane containing the target lesion. A T1-weighted gradient echo (FLASH) sequence is preferred because it is faster. Once the lesion is identified, the radiologist chooses either that axial plane for needle advancement or an alternate plane, if needed. The coronal plane is preferred because many hepatic lesions are located in the dome of the liver, and it is often more desirable to choose a lower skin entrance site and angulate the needle cranially in order to avoid the pleural reflection. A 10-s breath-hold, three-section, coronal T1-weighted gradient echo sequence (FLASH) is then performed centered on the lesion, based on the reference axial image, with the radiologist's finger in the imaging plane and marking the skin entrance site. This is repeated until both the radiologist's finger and the lesion are reliably seen in the center slice. At the same time, the radiologist's finger may also be used to give an approximation of the degree of cranial angulation needed to target the lesion.

After the skin entrance site is marked and sterilely prepared, the skin is punctured, and the

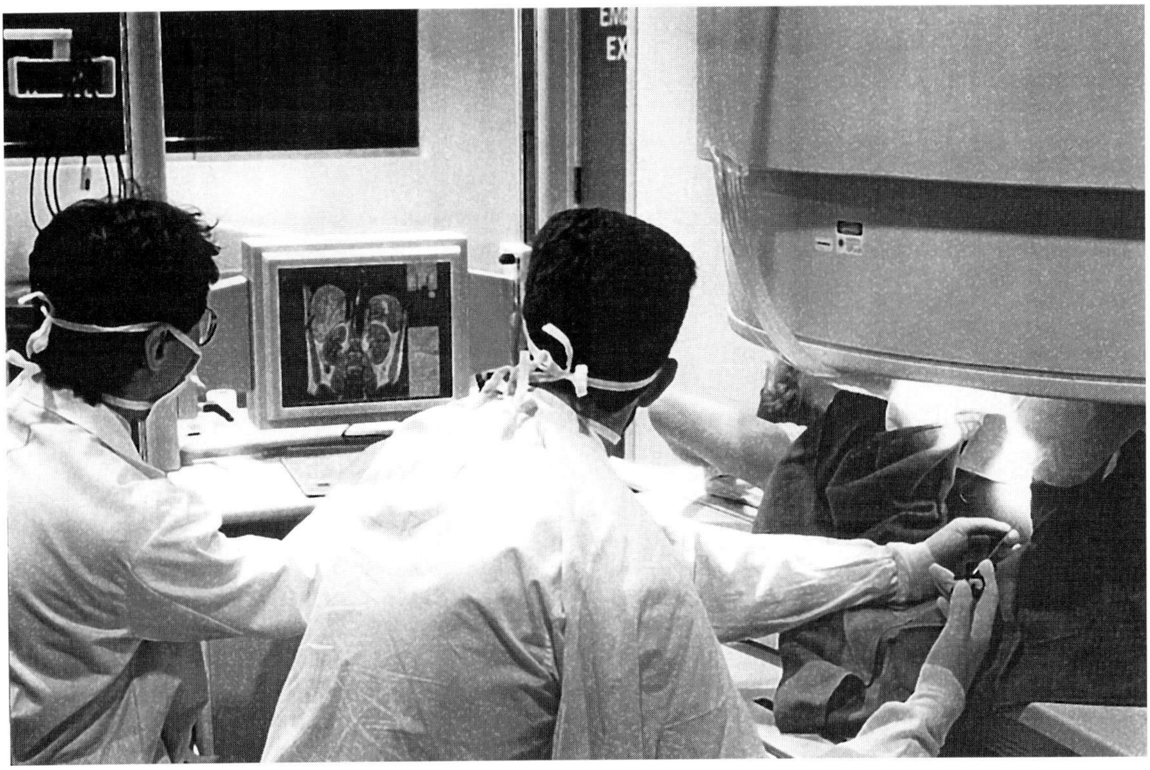

Fig. 5. Photograph of a liver biopsy in the 0.2 T Magnetom Open Scanner system. The patient is lying inside the scanner between vertically oriented magnet poles (*far right*). Note the horizontally open access to the patient by the treating radiologist, who is continually holding the biopsy needle as it is advanced into the liver. At the same time, the radiologist is actively viewing the latest image updates on the LCD monitor (which is showing the needle halfway towards the lesion) so that rapid interactive needle adjustments can be made. The technologist (*far left*) may control the scanner from inside the room next to the radiologist by using menu-driven functions through a mouse attached to the monitor

MR-compatible biopsy needle is advanced toward the lesion. Fine needle angulation adjustments are made stepwise based on repeated image updating using the same coronal 3-section gradient echo sequence. Departures of the actual needle course from the planned needle path can be identified both in-plane and off-plane, the latter by seeing the needle in the adjacent sections. Because it takes only 10 seconds for each image acquisition and another 3 seconds for image display, and usually only several steps are necessary, the time it requires for initial skin puncture to accurately position the needle tip within lesion is approximately 2–3 min (Fig. 6).

The above liver biopsy technique could theoretically be applied in any open configuration MR scanner and in several regions of the abdomen as long as the lesion is visible on an imaging sequence (e.g., FSE or GRE) which is fast enough to allow the needle to be repositioned. In addition to the liver, Frahm et al. have reported successful MRI-guided biopsies of adrenal and pelvic masses using the Magnetom Open scanner [9].

A significant current limitation of the horizontally open magnet design is that some regions of the abdomen (e.g., left lobe of liver, pancreatic body, omentum) cannot be accessed using an anterior approach. It may be possible for small patients to be positioned inside the scanner in the lateral decubitus position so that the anterior abdomen can be accessed. However, few patients are small enough to be so positioned, patients with anterior masses that require an anterior approach are not good candidates for biopsy in this type of scanner. At this stage of development, although experience with MRI-guided abdominal biopsies using the 0.2-T open configuration scanner is early and limited, the initial results are encouraging.

Development of MRI-guided abdominal biopsy has gone beyond the feasibility stage and is now used clinically in our centers. Since US- and CT-guided abdominal biopsies are so efficient and accurate, MRI is preferred rarely (particularly when cost is considered). However, there are patients with lesions which are not seen well with US and

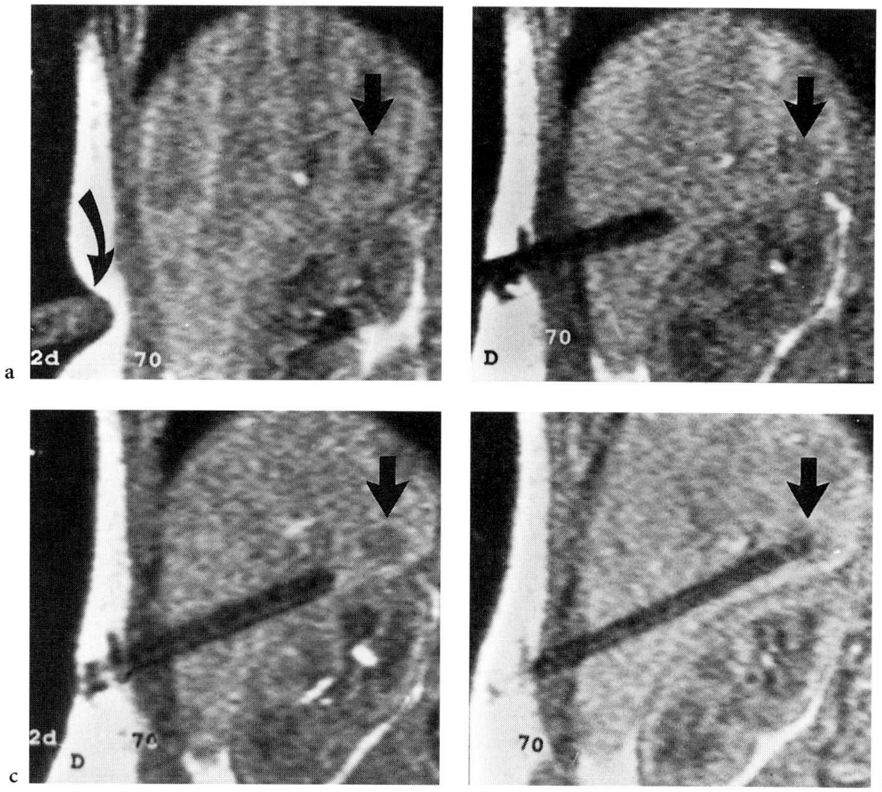

Fig. 6. MR-guided biopsy of hepatocellular carcinoma. Sequential coronal FLASH images (TR/TE 66/9, 70 degree; *from upper left to right, then lower left to right*) demonstrates intermittent image updates during a biopsy. Note the radiologist's finger marking the skin entrance site (*curved arrow*) and approximate angulation towards the lesion (*short straight arrow*), with subsequent advancements of the needle

that are seen equally well with CT and MRI. To choose between CT and MRI guidance one can begin to make an argument for using MRI because (using the above described techniques) it provides continuous patient access and multiplanar imaging which do not exist with current CT-guidance techniques. For example, some hepatic masses located in the dome of the liver and adrenal gland masses are difficult to biopsy using CT guidance because (a) an axial approach would transgress the pleura (and in some cases the lung) and introduce the risk of a pneumothorax, and (b) there may be significant changes in position of the lesion due to respiration which makes targeting with CT difficult.

MRI-guided biopsy techniques provide both a multiplanar approach so that the pleural space and lung can be avoided, and near-real time image feedback that allows targeting a "moving target." Therefore MRI-guided abdominal biopsy is likely to be reserved for the following special circumstances. These include: (a) Lesions seen with CT and MRI and not with US that require an angled or oblique approach to target. (b) Lesions that are viewed best (or only) with MRI. This adheres to the basic principle that the interventional guidance modality should be the modality that visualizes the lesion the best. This makes targeting easier. Lesions not visible with US or unenhanced CT may be biopsied using an enhanced CT, but this is difficult because the lesion may be visible temporarily during a portion of the contrast enhancement. Such lesions are rare but as diagnostic MRI techniques improve, more liver, pancreas, and prostate lesions are being detected only with MRI [8]. (c) Lesions which may also need MRI-guided therapy or have been treated with MRI-guided therapy. If MRI-guided therapy is planned, MRI can be used to biopsy the lesion both before and after treatment.

Despite the promise of MRI-guided biopsy we should caution that there are limitations to MRI-guided biopsy in general that are common to all modalities. As we have learned, some lesions may be well-visualized using a conventional closed (often 1.5 T) MRI system but may not be visualized with an interventional MRI system of lower field strength. Indeed, some lesions may be seen with US and CT and not on any MRI system. Therefore MRI may not be able to be used to guide the biopsy or the treatment of them. Also, as stated above, there are current limitations specific to an MRI environment, such as the inability to detect silent cardiac ischemia, which may prevent the use of MRI to guide any invasive procedure. Nevertheless, the field of interventional MRI is relatively new and some of these limitations are likely to be overcome.

MR-Guided Cancer Therapy (Tumor Ablation)

MRI has been suggested as the principal cross-sectional imaging technique in conceiving an integrated minimal invasive therapy environment [17]. The advantages of multiplanar imaging and excellent soft-tissue contrast make MRI ideal for aiding minimally invasive therapies, including percutaneous tumor ablation. MRI has many of the qualities that would be particularly helpful in guiding interventional and surgical therapies, such as the depiction of pathology and anatomy (including blood vessels) without always needing contrast material, and the ability to characterize tissue function. For example, MRI could aid some percutaneous therapies for cancer by characterizing tissue temperature changes when a thermal-mediated energy such as interstitial laser thermal therapy and cryotherapy is used to ablate the tumor [6, 18]. MRI can provide rapid multidimensional maps of relative temperature changes, show phase changes when tissue coagulates upon heating, and show loss of signal upon freezing when water protons become immobile within ice crystals [10, 18, 19, 29]. Therefore with continuous MRI monitoring treatment potentially can be limited to the pathology and stopped before it affects too much of the surrounding normal tissue. Thus MRI has the potential to monitor and control thermal therapies better than any other image guidance technique.

In the abdomen there are several malignancies which may be suited for percutaneous, image-guided ablation, such as colon cancer metastatic to the liver. There are approximately 160,000 new cases of colon cancer reported in the United States every year. Over 50% of these patients develop hepatic metastasis. Surgical resection of metastatic lesions has shown proven benefit, with 20%–40% 5-year survival rates. Unfortunately, only up to 10% of patients are eligible for liver resection [15]. Other metastatic tumors to liver such as islet cell tumors and some sarcomas may also benefit from resection. Another important common malignancy is primary hepatocellular carcinoma, which is one of the most prevalent malignancies in the world and accounts for approximately 1.25 million death per year [6]. Surgical resection has also shown proven benefit, with up to 30% 5-year survival, and liver transplantation has shown up to 60% 3- to 5-year survival. However, liver transplantation is not widely available, and only up to 30% of patients are candidates for surgical resection due primarily to poor hepatic reserve secondary to cirrhosis.

Several less invasive options have been developed over the past few years for ablation of these liver tumors. Detailed discussion of these techniques is beyond the scope of this chapter and is presented elsewhere in this volume. Rather, these techniques are discussed in relationship to their potential synergy with MR guidance in the following categories.

Laser Ablation

Many investigators are evaluating the use tumor ablation using laser energy deposited through optic fibers, which are small enough to be placed through standard 19-G needles. Much attention has been focused on laser ablation of hepatic tumors, and initial clinical trials have been encouraging with up to 82% of treated lesions achieving greater than 50% tumor necrosis [1]. The most difficult challenge in laser ablation for liver tumors is the small size of the "zone of kill" a single fiber can create, which is up to 1.7 cm, relative to the larger size of most hepatic tumors [47]. Investigators are now looking into ways to maximize laser lesion making by using diffuser tips at the end of the fibers and also by using multiple laser fibers. With simultaneous application of four fibers spaced 1.5 cm apart lesions as large as 4 cm can be created experimentally [2].

Until recently laser ablation has been performed under US and CT guidance. However, after the lesion is targeted, there has not been adequate means by which the ablation process could be monitored [3]. As described above, MRI can also be used for guidance of needle placement, but in addition, MRI can also provide excellent visualization of the reversible and irreversible effects of laser energy deposition, which would be useful for monitoring and control of the ablative process [4]. One of the most important mechanisms for tissue destruction by laser is in fact nonspecific thermal heating, and MRI is ideally suited for temperature monitoring. Vogl et al. recently demonstrated such on-line monitoring

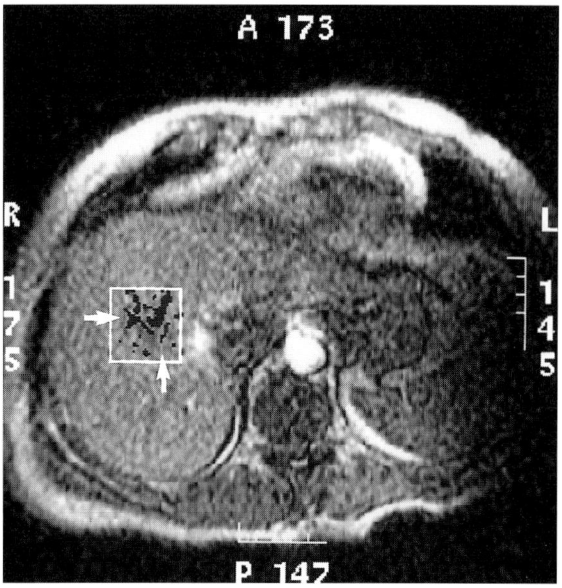

Fig. 7. MRI-guided laser thermal ablation of a solitary focus of metastatic leiomyosarcoma (*arrows*). Nearly real-time thermal monitoring using T1-weighted FSE intraprocedurally demonstrates the effect of the laser therapy (Nd:YAG laser, 2 W, 8 min). *Dark pixels within box*, color-encoded pixel subtraction of a baseline image from one obtained during lasing with the region of interest (*box*)

using thermo sequences in 20 patients with 33 liver lesions, which was accurate in up to 85% of lesions treated [49]. The MRI findings during laser ablation following US-guided laser fiber placement have been shown to be correlated with thermal necrosis on CT at 24 h [34]. Clinical trials using Signa SP are investigating whether using this system, which allows for the complete procedure to be done under MRI guidance and therefore the alteration of fiber position and number based on real-time MRI of thermal effects, will improve the results of laser ablation (Fig. 7).

Radiofrequency Ablation

In this technique an RF probe is introduced percutaneously into the body, and heating is generated at the probe tip by a remote RF generator. While clinical studies have demonstrated effective use of RF lesion making in the head and neck [28], its effectiveness for treating relatively large hepatic tumors is still being investigated. Initial clinical trials have shown encouraging results. Exciting research is also being conducted to maximization RF lesion size by simultaneous saline perfusion of the tumor [45], and by use of a recently developed perfusion probe [11, 24, 43]. If reliable and adequate sized RF lesions could be created, then RF hepatic tumor ablation may become a more practical treatment option.

Where MRI may help in RF tumor ablation is in MR's ability to image heat effects in tissue. Much work is being carried out to develop pulse sequences with maximal sensitivity to temperature changes [10, 18, 19, 30]. This topic is generic to all forms of thermal ablation including interstitial laser ablation, and is covered in more detail elsewhere in the book. The ultimate aim would be the development of a system where a real-time temperature map can be generated, possibly coded in color, which would be superimposed over the tumor, such that the ablation would be terminated only if all of the tumor has reached adequate temperature threshold for cell death. Another limiting factor that needs to be overcome is development of a MR compatible RF generator and MRI methods which can be used during RF heating.

Ethanol Ablation

Percutaneous ethanol injection therapy (PEIT) of hepatocellular carcinoma is now used commonly in parts of the world where hepatocellular carcinoma is endemic. Up to 42%–76% 3-year survival has been achieved in patients with Child's class A cirrhosis [23, 37]. Most investigators are using US or CT guidance for this procedure. However, because most patients with hepatocellular carcinoma have cirrhosis, many lesions may not be visible by US or CT [6]. Therefore lesions that are detectable only with MRI require MRI guidance if PEIT is used. Conventional MRI has been shown to be effective in depicting delayed postethanol effects in tissue [42]. Recently MRI using water-suppressed T2-weighted RARE sequences depicted the deposition of ethanol in liver in vitro [38]. Acute T1 and T2 MR signal changes have also been demonstrated in vivo in porcine liver during ethanol infusion [25] (Fig. 8). Therefore MRI could be used to guide percutaneous ethanol injection therapy of lesions not visible with US or CT. By monitoring the precise intra and peritumoral diffusion of ethanol, MRI may improve the intraprocedural control of PEIT of all lesions.

Cryoablation

Cryosurgery is another experimental method for treatment of a variety of conditions, including metastatic liver tumors [20, 33]. In this technique a cryoprobe is inserted into the lesion under intraoperative US guidance, and liquid nitrogen is

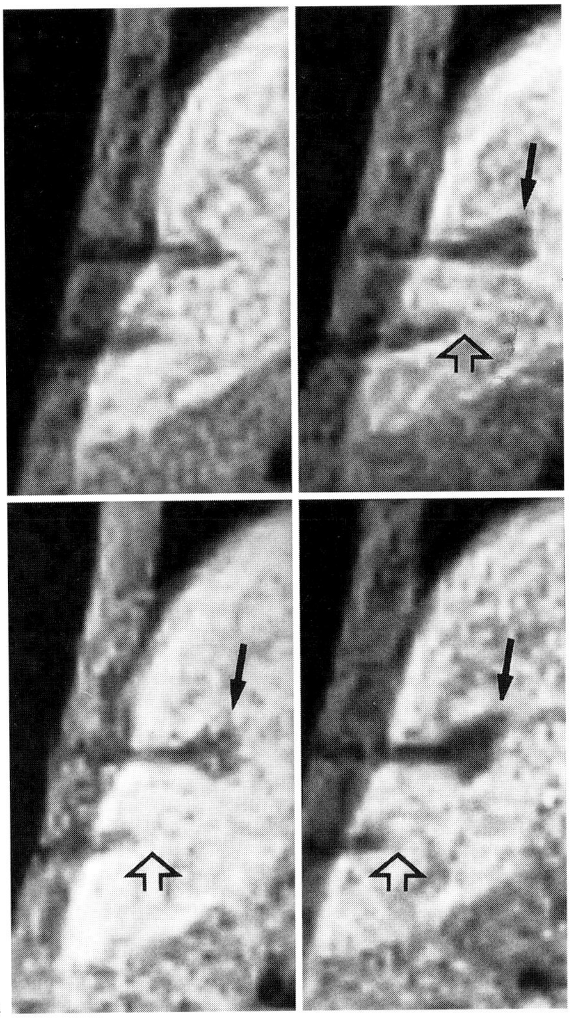

a

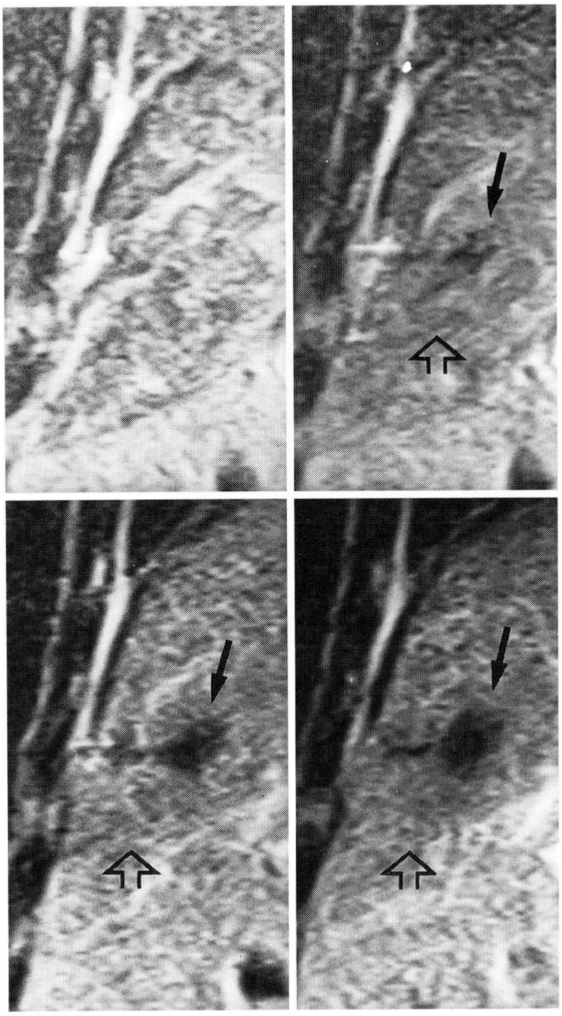

b

Fig. 8a,b. Experimental in-vivo ethanol ablation of porcine liver tissue under MRI guidance: (**a**) sequential coronal T1-weighted FLASH images and (**b**) corresponding T2-weighted TSE images showing enlarging T1 and T2 hypointense ethanol lesion (*black arrow*) at tip of needle. Images were obtained preinjection (*upper left*), after 1 ml (*upper right*), 5 ml (*lower left*), and 10 ml 96% ethanol. Corresponding volumes of saline was injected via second needle (*open arrow*) but no MR signal changes were detectable [26]

circulated through the probe to freeze tumor tissue exposed to the probe tip. MRI can depict tissue changes secondary to freezing [30]. However, hepatic cryosurgery still requires laparotomy, because of the large size of the cryoprobes. Currently, intraoperative US is considered effective in guiding cryotherapy, but the US appearance of the cryolesion is one that shows the front line of the iceball and acoustic shadowing behind [20]. Therefore the control is not as precise as it could be if the entire lesion and the tumor were seen.

Cryosurgery for metastatic liver cancer, despite being used experimentally for more than 10 years, is not used widely. The survival statistics are approximately the same as those using conventional hepatic resection [44–46]. The failures have not been due to inadequate freezing or inadequate "surgical" margins but from the development of new lesions. Therefore, although it is conceivable that MRI will become a primary guidance tool during intraoperative cryotherapy, especially in an integrated open MRI-operating room suite [17], there has been little enthusiasm for employing cryotherapy in patients who are to be operated on anyway. However, if cryotherapy could be administered nonoperatively, MRI may be useful in guiding percutaneous cryotherapy because of its imaging advantages over US. It is possible that smaller probes will be developed in the future such that percutaneous cryotherapy may be performed.

Focused Ultrasound

Focused ultrasound (FUS) is another exciting ablative technique which not only does not require surgery, it does not even require skin puncture [5, 16, 50]. Early work has demonstrated excellent MRI depiction of lesions created in tissue. It may find application within the abdomen and pelvis where there is no intervening bone or air between the US probe and the target lesion. However, current FUS systems are designed for fixed targets. Because of this current constraint, applications in the upper abdomen with targets which move with respiration are not possible now. However, just as US is used today to image the liver, FUS may be used to treat liver tumors in the future [5].

It is evident that MRI has immense potential in guiding multiple forms of nonsurgical cancer therapy in the abdomen, which is an exciting field of active research. Most of the early work has concentrated on liver tumors, but the same techniques may be applied to any organ in the abdomen. Once the technique has been fully developed and tested, other clinical indications may arise. The timing was ripe for the introduction of open configuration MR scanners, and more refined scanners are expected to be developed with time. Combined with inevitable advancement in tumor ablation techniques, MRI-guided therapy may play an important role in the minimal invasive treatment of abdominal diseases in the future.

■ References

1. Amin Z, Brown SG, Lees WR (1993) Liver tumor ablation by interstitial laser photocoagulation review of experimental and clinical studies. Semin Intervent Radiol 10:88–100
2. Amin Z, Bown SG, Lees WR (1993) Local treatment of colorectal liver metastases: a comparison of interstitial laser photocoagulation (ILP) and percutaneous alcohol injection (PAI). Clin Radiol 48:166–171
3. Amin Z, Buonaccorsi G, Mills T et al (1993) Interstitial laser photocoagulation: evaluation of a 1320 nm Nd-Yag and an 805 nm diode laser: the significance of charring the fibre tip. Lasers Med Sci 8:113–120
4. Anzai Y, Lufkin RB, Castro DJ et al (1991) MR imaging-guided interstitial Nd:YAG laser phototherapy: dosimetry study of acute tissue damage in an invivo model. J Magn Reson Imaging 1:553–559
5. Cline HE, Hynynen K, Watkins RP et al (1995) Focused US system for MR imaging-guided tumor ablation. Radiology 194:731
6. D'Agostino HB, Solinas A (1995) Percutaneous ablation therapy for hepatocellular carcinomas. AJR 164:1165–1167
7. Dumoulin CL, Souza SP, Darrow D (1993) Real-time position monitoring of invasive devices using magnetic resonance. MRM 29:411–415
8. Ferrucci JT (1990) Liver tumor imaging: current concepts. AJR 155:473–484
9. Frahm VC, Gehl HB, Robberg WA (1996) Technique or MR-guided core biopsy of abdominal masses using an open low-field scanner: feasibility and first clinical results. Fortschr Rontgenstr 164:1:62–67
10. Gilbert JC, Rubinsky B, Roos MS, Wong STS, Brennan KM (1993) MR-monitored cryosurgery in rabbit brain. Magn Reson Imaging 11:1155–1164
11. Goldberg SN, Gazelle GS, Solbiati L, Livraghi T, Tanabe KK, Mueller PR (1996) Large volume radio-frequency tissue ablation: increased coagulation with cooled-tip electrodes (abstract). Radiology 201 (P):387
12. Gronemeyer DH, Kaufman L, Rothschild P et al (1989) New possibilities and aspects of low-field magnetic resonance tomography. Radiol Diagn (Berlin) 30:519–527
13. Hajek PC, Gylys-Morin VM, Stava J et al (1987) Localization grid for MR-guided biopsy. Radiology 163:825–826
14. Hughes CW, Bell C (1993) Anesthesia equipment in remote hospital locations. In: Rogers MC, Covino BJ, Tinker JH et al (eds) Principles and practice of anesthesiology. Mosby, St Louis
15. Hughes K, Simon R, Adson MA et al (1988) Registry of hepatic metastases: resection of the liver for colorectal carcinoma metastases – a multi-institutional study for indications of resection. Surgery 103:278–287
16. Hynynen K, Freund W, Cline HE, Chung A, Watkins R, Vetro J, Jolesz FA (1996) A clinical noninvasive MRI monitored ultrasound surgery method. Radiographics 16:185
17. Jolesz FA, Shtern F (1992) The operating room of the future: report of the National Cancer Institute Workshop – imaging-guided stereotactic tumor diagnosis and treatment. Invest Radiol 27:326–328
18. Jolesz FA, Silverman SG (1995) Interventional magnetic resonance therapy. Semin Intervent Radiol 12:20–27
19. Jolesz FA, Bleier AR, Jakab P et al (1988) MR imaging of laser tissue interaction. Radiology 168:249–253
20. Kane RA (1993) Ultrasound-guided hepatic cryosurgery for tumor ablation. Semin Intervent Rad 10:132–142
21. Leung DA, Debatin JF, Widermuth S et al (1995) Real-time biplanar needle tracking for interventional MR imaging procedures. Radiology 197:485–488
22. Livraghi T, Bolondi L, Lazzaroni S et al (1991) Percutaneous ethanol injection in the treatment of hepatocellular carcinoma in cirrhosis. A study on 207 patients. Cancer 69:925–929
23. Livraghi T, Lazzaroni S, Pellican S et al (1993) Percutaneous ethanol injection of hepatic tumors: single-session therapy and general anesthesia. AJR 161:1065–1069
24. Lorentzen T (1995) Modified needle technique for large-lesion ablation by using monopolar RF electrosurgery under US control: an in vitro study (abstract). Radiology 197 (P):200
25. Lu DSK, Lee H, Farahani K, Sinha S, Lufkin R (1997) Biopsy of hepatic dome lesions: semi-real-time coronal MR guidance technique. AJR 168:737–739
26. Lu DSK, Sinha S, Lucas J, Farahani K, Lufkin R, Lewin K (1997) MR-guided percutaneus ethanol ablation of liver tissue in a 2-T open MR system: preliminary study in porcine model. J Magn Reson Imaging 7:303–308
27. Mahfouz AE, Rahmouni A, Zylbersztejn C, Mathieu D (1996) MR-guided biopsy using ultrafast T1- and T2-weighted reordered turbo fast low-angle shot sequences: feasibility and preliminary clinical applications. AJR 167:167–169
28. Matsumoto R, Selig AM, Colucci VM et al (1992) Interstitial Nd:YAG laser ablation in normal rabbit liver: trial to maximize the size of laser-induced lesions. Laser Surg Med 12:650–658
29. Matsumoto R, Oshio K, Jolesz FA (1993) Monitoring of laser and freezing-induced ablation in the liver with

T1-weighted MR imaging. J Magn Reson Imaging 3:770–776
30. Matsumoto S, Shima F, Hasuo K et al (1992) MR imaging of stereotactic thalamotomy using radiofrequency methods. Nippon Acta Radiol 52:1559–1564
31. Mueller PR, Stark DD, Simeone JF et al (1986) MR-guided aspiration biopsy: needle design and clinical trials. Radiology 161:605–609
32. Mueller PR, Stark DD, Simeone JF et al (1989) Clinical use of a nonferromagnetic needle for magnetic resonance-guided biopsy. Gastrointest Radiol 14:61–64
33. Ravikumar TS, Kane R, Cady B et al (1991) A 5-year study of cryosurgery in the treatment of liver tumors. Arch Surg 126:1520–1524
34. Roberts HRS, Paley M, Sams VR et al (1997) Magnetic resonance imaging control of laser destruction of hepatic metastases: correlation with post-operative dynamic helical CT. Min Invas Ther Allied Technol 6:53–64
35. Rossi S, Di Stasi M, Buscanni E et al (1996) Percutaneous RF interstitial thermal ablation in the treatment of hepatic cancer. AJR 167:759
36. Schenck JF, Jolesz FA, Roemer PB et al (1995) Superconducting open configuration MRI system for image-guided therapy. Radiology 195:805–814
37. Shiina S, Tagawa K, Niwa Y et al (1993) Percutaneous ethanol injection therapy for hepatocellular carcinoma: results in 146 Patients. AJR 160:1023–1028
38. Shinmoto H, Mulkern RV, Oshio K et al (1997) MR appearance and spectral features of injected ethanol in the liver: implication for fast MR-guided percutaneous ethanol injection therapy. J Comput Assist Tomogr 21:82–88
39. Silverman SG, Bloom DA, Seltzer SE et al (1992) Needle-tip localization during CT-guided abdominal biopsy: comparison of conventional and spiral CT. AJR 159:1095–1097
40. Silverman SG, Collick BD, Figueira MR et al (1995) Interactive biopsy in an open configuration MRI system. Radiology 197:175–181
41. Silverman SG, Jolesz FA, Newman RW et al (1997) Design and implementation of an interventional MR imaging suite. AJR 168(6):1465–1471
42. Sironi S, Livraghi T, Angeli E et al (1993) Small hepatocellular carcinoma: MR follow-up of treatment with percutaneous ethanol injection. Radiology 187:119–123
43. Solbiati L, Tiziana I, Goldberg SN et al (1997) Percutaneous US-guided radio-frequency tissue ablation of liver metastases: treatment and follow-up in 16 patients. Radiology 202:195–203
44. Steele G Jr (1994) Cryoablation in hepatic surgery. Semin Liver Dis 14:120–125
45. Steele G Jr, Ravikumar TS (1989) Resection of hepatic metastases from colorectal cancer: biologic perspectives. Ann Surg 210:127–138
46. Steele G Jr, Bleday R, Mayer RJ et al (1991) A prospective evaluation of hepatic resection for colorectal carcinoma metastases to the liver. Gastrointestinal Tumor Study Group protocol 6584. J Clin Oncol 9:1105–1112
47. Steger AC, Lees WR, Shorvon P et al (1992) Multiple-fibre low-power interstitial laser hyperthermia: studies in the normal liver. Br J Surg 79:139–145
48. van Sonnenberg E, Hajek P, Gylys-Morin V et al (1988) A wire-sheath system for MR-guided biopsy and drainage: laboratory studies and experience in 10 patients. AJR 151:815–817
49. Vogl TJ, Müller, Hamerstingl R, Weinhold N, Mack MG, Philipp C, Deimling M, Beuthan J, Pegios W, Riess H et al (1995) Malignant liver tumors treated with MR imaging-guided laser induced thermotherapy: technique and prospective results. Radiology 196:257–265
50. Yang R, Sanghvi NT, Rescorla FJ et al (1992) Extracorporeal liver ablation using sonography-guided high-intensity focused ultrasound. Invest Radiol 27:796–803

Magnetic Resonance Guided Therapy of Breast Tumors

6

H. MUMTAZ, M. A. HALL-CRAGGS

■ Introduction

Recent trends in the management of early breast cancer have moved towards breast conservation, the safety of which has been validated in several prospective randomized trials which have shown no differences in disease free interval and overall survival in patients who have had breast conservation compared to mastectomy [13]. The aim of breast conserving surgery is to achieve maximal cosmesis and minimal psychological morbidity, without compromising local control and overall survival.

The development of minimally invasive therapeutic procedures has been directed towards reducing surgical trauma by exposing and isolating the smallest segment of the anatomy possible while still allowing access to the target volume with minimal injury. The advantages of such a therapeutic approach are improvement in cosmetic outcome, reduction in length of hospital stay, and potential cost savings. This concept combined with the known safety of breast conservation has prompted research into the application of minimally invasive therapies to breast cancer.

Several forms of minimally invasive local treatment for solid tumors have been described. These include thermal treatment [interstitial laser photocoagulation (ILP), high intensity focused ultrasound (US), and bipolar radiofrequency thermal ablation] and nonthermal techniques (cryotherapy, brachytherapy, and photodynamic therapy). In our unit, interstitial laser photocoagulation of breast tumors has been extensively studied and forms the main focus of discussion in this chapter. The potential application of other techniques in the treatment of breast tumors is briefly discussed.

Interstitial Laser Photocoagulation: Laser Properties

ILP was first reported in 1983 as a minimally invasive technique for localized tumor destruction in solid organs [4]. Tumors are destroyed by direct heating using low power laser light energy delivered via thin optical fibers. However, the size and shape of thermal lesions are difficult to predict due to biological variability [5], fiber tip charring, and changing optical and thermal properties of the tissue during ILP [28]. The application of ILP in primary breast cancer was first described by Stegar et al. [27] in a patient with breast cancer who refused all forms of conventional treatment. Three tumor sites were treated with ILP under local anesthesia and subsequent follow-up by US examination showed reduction in tumor volume. Further preliminary studies evaluating the laser and optical fiber parameters using the semiconductor diode laser showed that precharring the optical fiber bare tip produced significantly larger and more predictable dimensions of tissue necrosis than a clean uncharred fiber tip [11].

To date most experience in the treatment of breast tumors has been with single fibers [11, 18] but this results in a small treated area. Fiber splitters have now been developed whereby a single input fiber is coupled to four fibers via a beam splitter allowing equal delivery of energy down each fiber simultaneously. This has successfully facilitated multiple fiber therapy in the treatment of liver tumors allowing larger volumes to be treated [2]. The volume of tissue necrosis can further be increased by using a "pullback" technique. This involves repositioning the fiber tips immediately after the initial treatment by withdrawing them 0.5–1 cm within the tumor and repeating the ILP. In our unit preliminary experience with two to four fibers in the treatment of malignant breast tumors has resulted in an increase in the volume of necrosis by a factor of approximately 1.5–2 times, although lesion size appears to be related to the distance between the fibers [20].

Another development in laser technology has been the availability of long laser fibers which allow separation of the laser source from the point of treatment allowing therapy within scanners [either computed tomography (CT) or magnetic resonance (MR) scanners]. In the setting of an MR scanner the laser source must be beyond the 5-gauss line, in most cases outside the scanning room. The long fibers are passed through wave guides in the Faraday cage into the scanner itself.

Treatment Technique

The laser used in our studies, the semiconductor diode laser (Diomed-25; Diomed, Cambridge, UK) has the advantages of being small, compact, portable, easy to use, and does not require any special water cooling or three-phase electrical supply. This laser operates at a fixed wavelength of 805 nm, although a newer generation of semiconductor diode lasers are becoming available with variable wavelength [1]. The laser light source is directly coupled to either a single fiber, or via the beam splitter to multiple fibers. The fibers themselves are freshly cleaved and sterilized, although they are precharred prior to treatment. Precharring is carried out by placing a drop of the patient's blood on the fiber tip and briefly firing it at a high power. The optical fibers measure 400 μm in diameter and thus pass easily through 18-gauge needles.

At treatment the skin at the site of percutaneous needle insertion is infiltrated with local anesthetic in all cases. Intravenous analgesia and sedation are usually required when performing multiple fiber therapy. Using aseptic technique and under US guidance, an 18-gauge needle(s) is passed percutaneously and positioned approximately 1 cm apart within the breast mass. An MR imaging compatible needle is selected if the treatment is to be performed within the scanner. The needle length should be optimized to the depth of the tumor to prevent dislodgment. With deeply sited tumors the "shortest route" approach is made with the needle. With more superficial tumors a longer approach is made in order that the needle is anchored and stabilized by the surrounding breast tissue. The laser fiber is introduced into the needle and positioned with 3–5 mm of bare fiber protruding beyond the needle tip. The laser is set to deliver approximately 1000–1500 J of energy per fiber (2–3 W per fiber for 500 s).

Histological and in some cases cytological grading of tumors is necessary for prognostic stratification and guiding treatment, in particular adjuvant chemotherapy. Complete tumor destruction by ILP results in loss of all tumor tissue. Thus it is critically important as part of this technique to obtain all necessary tissue prior to ILP (e.g. core needle biopsy or fine needle aspiration cytology).

Histopathology

Macroscopically a laser burn in breast tissue appears as a three-zone lesion; a central charred hole corresponding to the position of the laser fiber is surrounded by a broad white zone. At the periphery of the white region is a thin haemorrhagic zone.

On microscopic examination the charred cavity corresponds to complete tissue loss. The white zone is known as the zone of "in situ" fixation and is characterized by morphologically normal appearing cells with intact cell membranes The cytoplasm of these cells is hypereosinophilic, consistent with the presence of coagulated proteins. The nucleus of these cells also show featureless, hyperchromatic appearance. Within the haemorrhagic rim, the cells show less severe structural damage, with unstained, slightly hyperchromatic nuclei that retain their chromatin pattern and nucleoli. All three zones have been shown by immunohistochemical analysis to be nonviable [19]. It has been found that laser tissue heals by dense hypocellular fibrosis in a single patient, who following laser therapy refused surgical excision until 9 months after ILP.

■ Imaging

Imaging is critical to achieving successful tumor ablation. It is necessary for locoregional staging of the disease, guiding accurate tumor localization and optical fiber positioning, and monitoring therapy ideally in "real time". Finally, subsequent evaluation should accurately differentiate between the area of laser induced necrosis and residual viable tumor.

Although US can be used for needle and fiber tip placement it has been found to be grossly inaccurate for measuring the volume of laser-induced tumor necrosis and the extent of the remaining viable tumor [11], a finding similar to that observed in the treatment of hepatic metastases [2]. In the liver this is mainly because areas of coagulative necrosis have similar US characteristics to those of viable tumor. This similarity between treated and untreated tumor makes subsequent targeting of residual viable tumor difficult and is a major obstacle to achieving complete tumor ablation.

Of the currently available breast imaging techniques, contrast-enhanced MR imaging appears to be the most sensitive for tumor detection and staging [10, 21, 22]. It is critically important to show the full extent of disease prior to treatment so that additional multifocal disease is not missed. The sensitivity of contrast-enhanced MR imaging in depicting clinically and mammographically occult tumor foci aids selection of patients suitable for ILP treatment. Multifocal or multicentric disease and the presence of an extensive intraductal component is a contraindication for ILP.

MR imaging offers several advantages in monitoring laser-tissue interactions. It is less operator dependent and has better soft tissue contrast resolution than US. MR imaging is very sensitive to tissue water mobility and distribution and the temperature dependence of MR relaxation parameters such as T1 relaxation times and diffusion coefficients [7, 15] make it particularly suitable

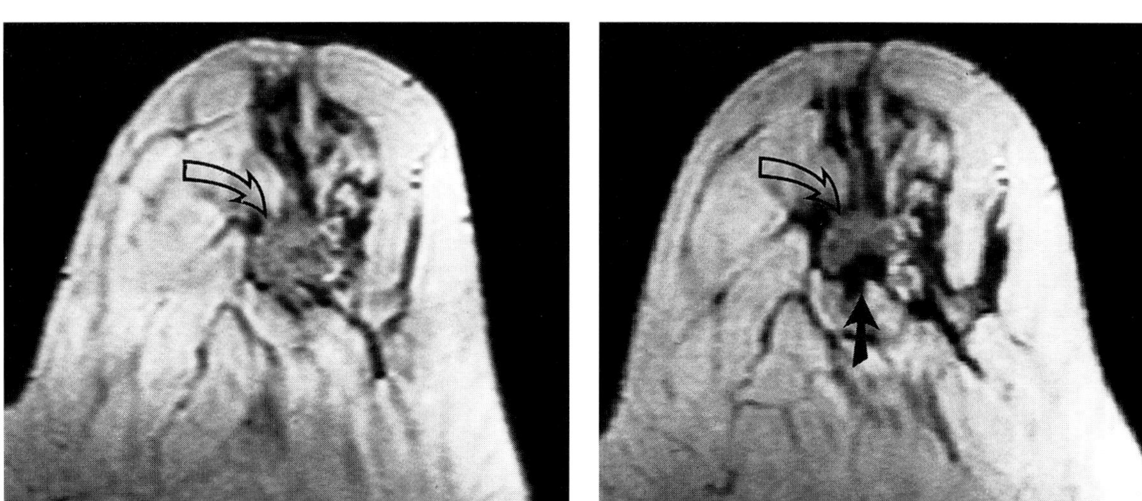

a b

Fig. 1. T1-weighted contrast-enhanced MR images before (**a**) ILP shows a 24 mm irregular homogeneous enhancing mass (*curved arrow*) and 48 h after (**b**) ILP therapy with a single fiber shows a new 9-mm area of nonenhancement (*straight arrow*) consistent with laser induced necrosis. *Curved arrow*, residual tumor

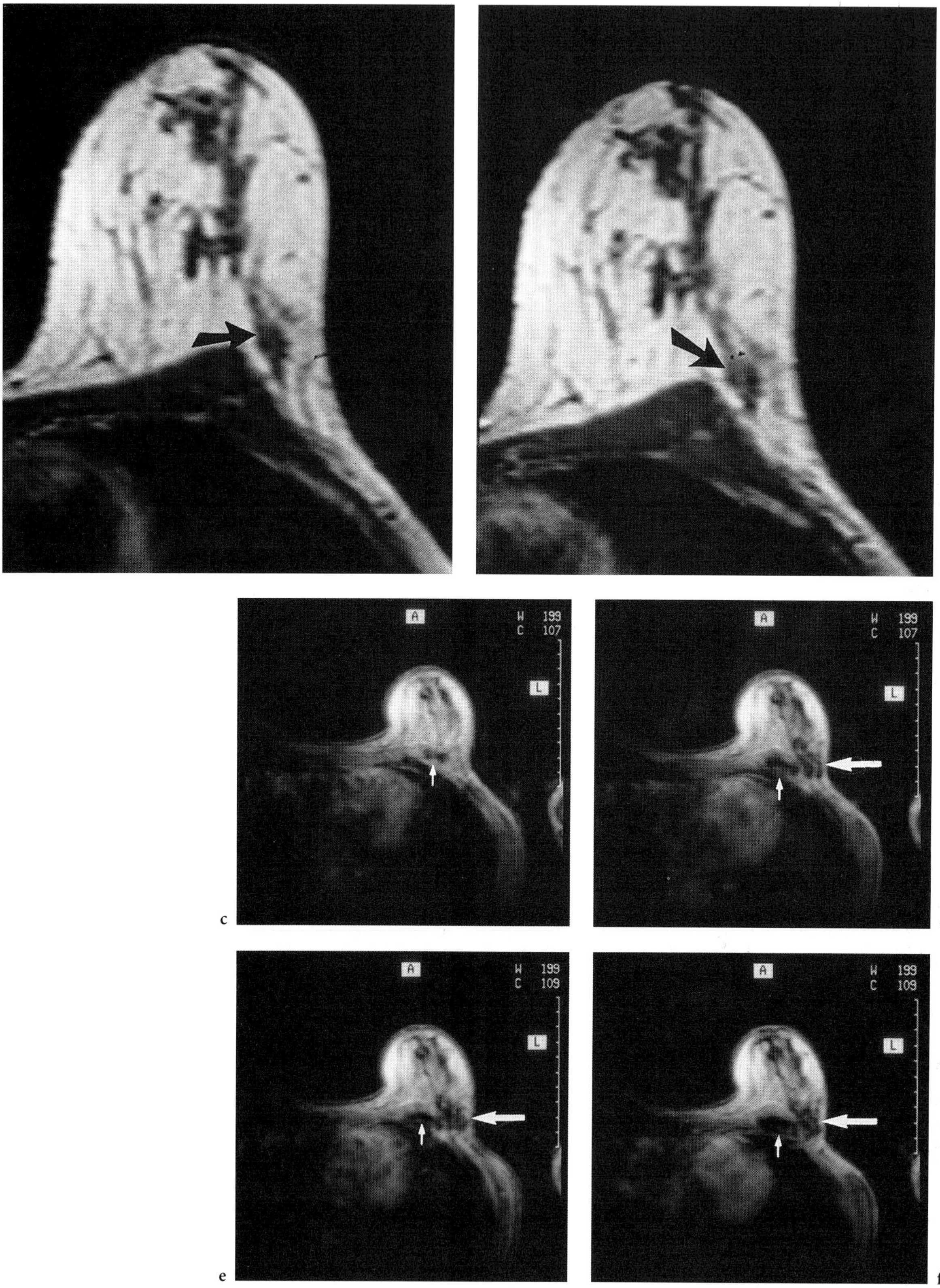

a b c d e f

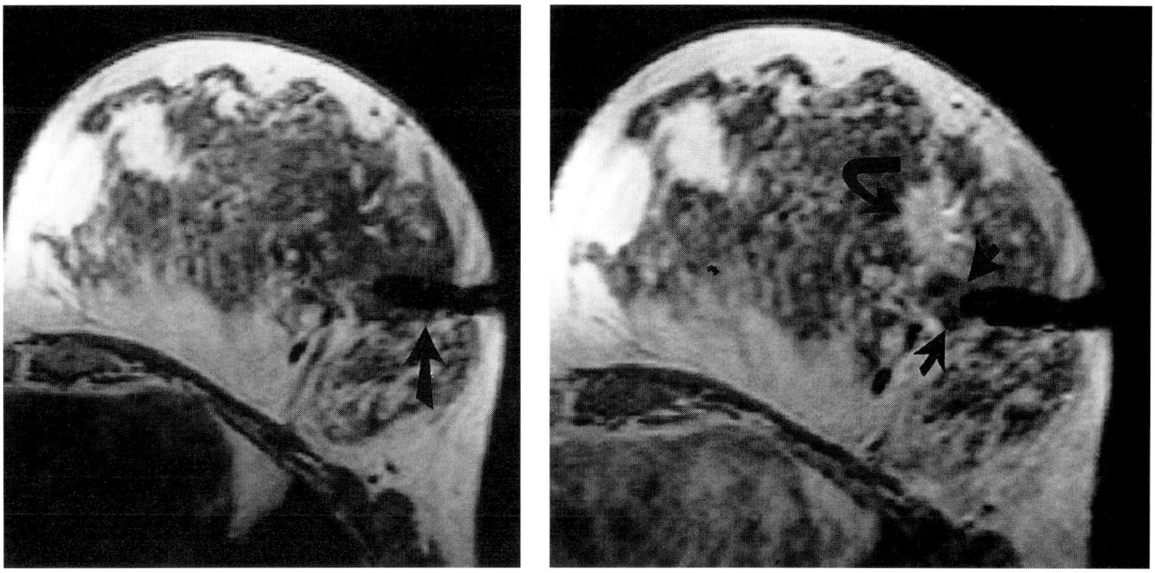

a b

Fig. 3a,b. T1-weighted 3D FLASH MR images in a 41-year-old woman obtained immediately after ILP therapy. Precontrast image with MR needle in place (*straight arrow*; **a**) and contrast-enhanced image (**b**) shows a nonenhancing zone at the needle tip (*arrow*) and residual enhancing tumor superiorly (*curved arrow*). This is the only patient in our series in whom immediately post-ILP contrast-enhanced MR images were correlated with histological findings

for the demonstration and monitoring of thermal energy deposition in tissues. Further advances in the field of MR imaging have delivered fast, temperature-sensitive T1-weighted imaging techniques including diffusion sensitive echo-planar imaging which acquire images on time scales appropriate for essential real-time monitoring of ILP [3]. In addition optical fibers and laser light are not affected by magnetic fields used for MR imaging, nor does the optical fiber disturb the MR signal [14].

We have investigated the accuracy of MR imaging in monitoring the therapeutic effects of ILP in breast cancer and have found that delayed (48 h) contrast-enhanced MR can accurately show the extent of laser induced necrosis and residual tumor after ILP. Early post-treatment images (4 h interval) fail to show the laser effect. Delayed contrast-enhanced MR images showed the laser induced necrosis as a zone of nonenhancement within the residual enhancing tumor (Fig. 1). There is a close correlation between the size of the nonenhancing zone and the histological extent of laser necrosis ($r^2=0.80$) and between residual enhancing tumor on contrast-enhanced MR and histological measurement of residual viable tumor ($r^2=0.86$) [18].

More recently we have evaluated "dynamic" MR imaging of ILP in breast cancer [8] by treating ten patients in a conventional 1-T closed bore magnet but using a side access breast coil (MRI Devices, Milwaukee, USA). During treatment an expanding area of signal loss around each fiber tip can be seen on T1-weighted 2D FLASH images (Fig. 2). The extent of signal loss seen at the end of treatment is closely correlated with the final extent of histological laser-induced necrosis ($r^2=0.80$). Immediate post-treatment contrast-enhanced MR images are not consistently predictive of the extent of laser induced necrosis (Fig. 3).

■ Treatment Outcomes

Single fiber treatment does not produce sufficient large areas of necrosis to treat even the

◄

Fig. 2a,b. Pre-treatment transverse T1-weighted MR images of the right breast in a 58-year-old woman before (**a**) and after (**b**) contrast enhancement shows an ill-defined enhancing mass measuring 9 mm in maximum diameter. Dynamic 2D FLASH images during ILP therapy with four fibers show at 30 s a low signal zone within the pectoralis muscle (*short arrow*; **c**), at 120 s an additional low signal zone within the tumor zone (*long arrow*, **d**). **e** Signal loss at 330 s into treatment. **f** Signal loss immediately after therapy. The signal zone in the tumor area measures 28×15 mm and in the pectoralis muscle 28×8 mm. Operative findings showed a disc of pectoralis muscle necrosis. Histological examination confirmed complete tumor necrosis including a margin of normal tissue smallest tumor. Multiple fiber therapy with "pullback" technique can create laser burns of up to 4 cm. In our studies using the latter technique we have been able successfully to obliterate all viable tumor in a small number of patients. To achieve tumor obliteration consistently it is necessary to select patients with small tumors (<2 cm) and to treat fairly aggressively with larger number of fibers and "pullback" technique.

In the next clinical stage of ILP of breast cancer complete tumor ablation inclusive of a margin of macroscopically normal tissue should consistently be shown to be achieved. Ultimately clinical outcome studies on patients treated with ILP and adjuvant radiotherapy need to be undertaken to assess both the short and long term safety of this approach for treating early breast cancer.

Contrast-enhanced MR imaging accurately show the extent of ILP necrosis, if performed at least 24 h after ILP treatment. Dynamic MR imaging broadly shows the region of necrosis during treatment and could be used to guide therapy.

■ Technical Problems of ILP

Further development of the technique will depend on several technical advances. In order to achieve complete tumor ablation consistently it is necessary to modify treatment during the procedure, to move fibers to areas of untreated tumor and to treat tumor margins. This will be possible only if more rapid "real-time" imaging is developed with image replenishment rates of under 0.5 s. The only significant complication of ILP in our series have been skin and pectoralis burn, and "missed treatments" largely due to misplaced or displaced fibers. "Real-time imaging" would show contrast changes in these tissues during treatment and allow early repositioning of fibers before significant damage to these tissue occurs.

Practical real-time monitoring will need to use the new generation of MR scanners which have easier access to the patient [14]. Development is necessary of artifact-free MR-compatible needles to enable accurate needle positioning and biopsies of the treated margins.

■ Image-Guided ILP of Benign Breast Tumors

In contrast to breast cancer, fibroadenomas present a relatively simple medical problem. The major concern to the patient is usually the presence of a lump in the breast. Consequently treatment does not have to ensure total destruction of the mass and therapeutic success may be regarded as rendering a palpable lump impalpable.

Fibroadenomas can be accurately diagnosed by conventional triple assessment (clinical, cytological and US examination). Conventional treatment includes two options: conservative "watch and see" and surgical excision. Conservative management of fibroadenomas is a safe option in selected patients but is not always acceptable because of variable natural history of these masses. The proportion of fibroadenomas resolving spontaneously over a period of 1–3 years has been reported as no more than 40% [26]. Alternatively, surgical excision may leave scars and deformity particularly in those women with multiple tumors requiring multiple excisions. The development of ILP in the treatment of benign breast fibroadenomas potentially overcomes the pitfalls of conventional conservative and surgical management.

In a small series of 15 women with fibroadenomas treated by one to four fibers ILP in our institution we have observed a mean reduction in tumor size of over 40% at 8-week follow-up. After this the tumor continued to regress slowly. Of these 15 patients 10 refused surgical treatment because of the satisfactory reduction in tumor size. With more aggressive laser therapy to ensure that the entire tumor is necrosed it is likely that the treatment response will improve. In these patients US is useful in follow-up to monitor the reduction in size of the ILP-treated fibroadenomas. MR imaging helps to define the extent of laser-induced necrosis in the tumors that enhance before treatment (Fig. 4) [18].

■ High-Intensity Focused Ultrasound

In this technique US energy of frequency 1–7.5 MHz is generated in an external transducer and brought to a sharp focus at a predetermined depth within the body. With high intensity (greater than 100 W/cm^2) US there is rapid tissue destruction in the focal zone (within 1 s), and the local temperature rises up to 120 °C in vivo. Focal coagulative necrosis is produced by a combination of cavitation and thermal effects, and experimental work in animal liver and tumor models has demonstrated that well-defined zones of coagulative necrosis can be safely and reproducibly induced [12].

The feasibility of MR guidance of focused US therapy has been shown in gel phantoms and in vitro studies [6], and its potential role in the treatment of breast fibroadenomas has been evaluated by Pomeroy et al. [23]. Clinical experience

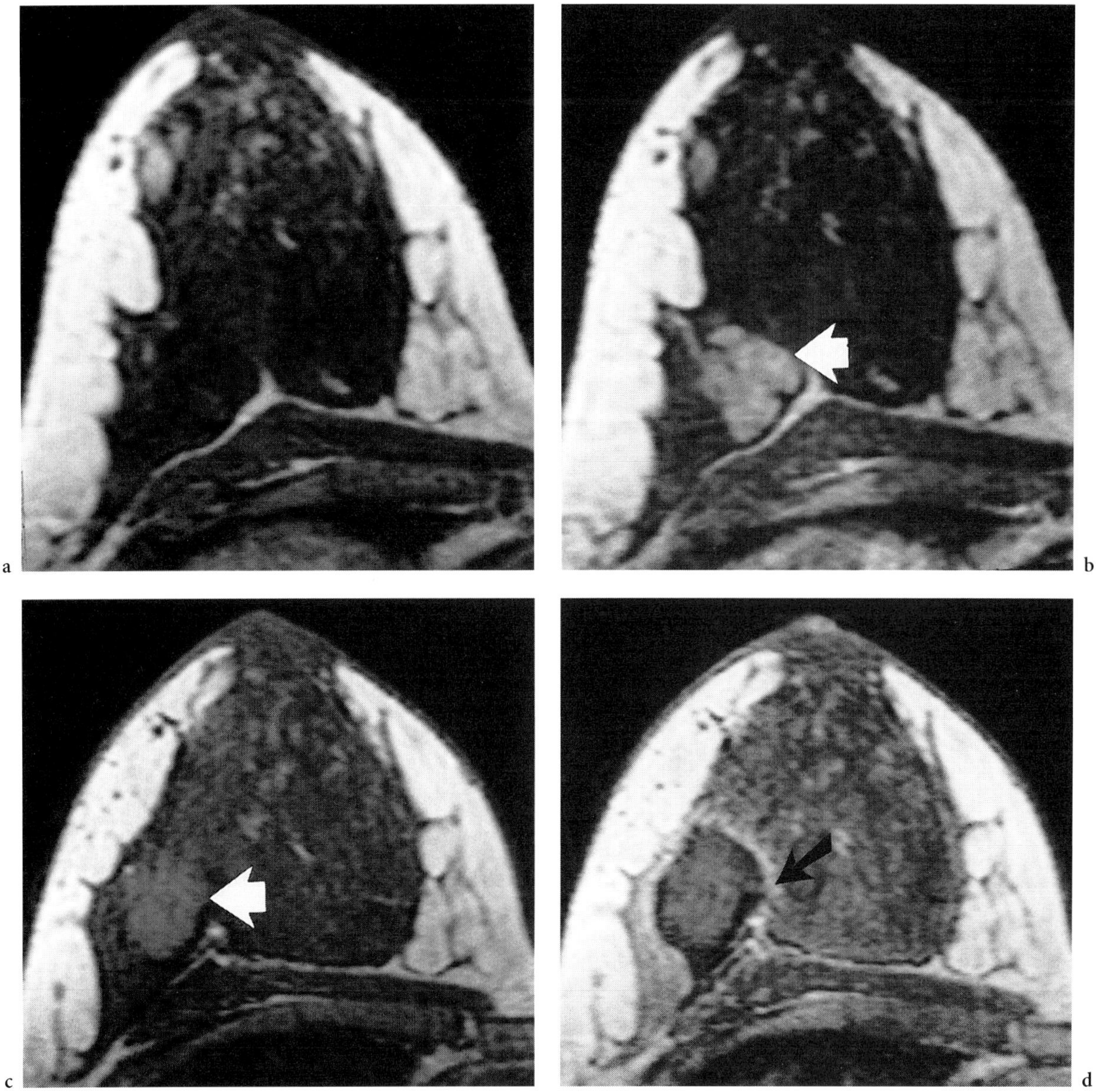

Fig. 4a–d. T1-weighted 3D FLASH images in a 28-year-old woman. Precontrast (**a**) and contrast-enhanced (**b**) images show a 28-mm well-defined lobulated enhancing mass proven on cytology and clinical examination to be a fibroadenoma. Images obtained 2 weeks after ILP therapy with four fibers show an area of increased signal intensity consistent with tissue necrosis (*arrow*; **c**), and contrast-enhanced image (**d**) shows central nonenhancing zone with a thin peripheral enhancing rim. At 6-month follow-up, the lump measured 9 mm on US

is limited, however, and no detailed studies have been published. Hand et al. [9] have described the Sonotherm 6500 scanned focused US system in the hyperthermic treatment of bulky breast tumors, but have not detailed tumor response to treatment.

■ Other Techniques

Radiofrequency electrocautery utilizes a standard electrosurgical generator to deliver radiofrequency energy interstitially via percutaneously introduced fine needle sheathed in nonconductive plastic [17]. The bare needle tip is placed in the desired target, and high-frequency alternating current flows from the uninsulated tip of the electrode into surrounding tissue. Thermal damage occurs by ionic agitation; this results in frictional heating in the tissue around the electrode, rather than the electrode itself being a primary heat source.

Although radiofrequency tumor ablation has been successfully applied in the treatment of hepatic [25] and other tumors, there have been no reports of its role in treating breast tumors. With the development of suitable multi-array electrodes it may, however, prove possible to treat small breast tumors in a manner similar to the experience with ILP.

Cryotherapy involved freezing tumors by cryoprobes is more invasive than ILP due to the bulky probe design. In animal mammary tumor models cryosurgical procedures involving multiple freeze-thaw cycles followed by tumor excision have shown to associated with reduced the local recurrence rate [24]. MR monitoring of cryotherapy to rabbit liver has shown that MR images obtained during the freezing process can accurately depict the area of final necrosis. In addition, the histological changes at each stage of lesion development are correlated with MR signal intensities on follow-up MR images [16]. MR compatible cryoprobes are currently being developed. Clinical experience of cryotherapy is mainly in the treatment of liver metastases and prostate carcinoma, and no clinical studies in breast tumor treatment have been reported.

Photodynamic therapy is a new form of cancer treatment, currently being evaluated in many clinical trials. Although photodynamic therapy has been applied in the treatment of chest wall recurrence after mastectomy, its role in the treatment of primary breast cancer has not been evaluated.

■ Summary

MR imaging offers several advantages in the application of minimally invasive techniques for the treatment of breast tumors. Pre-treatment MR imaging is useful in the loco-regional staging of breast cancer and defining tumor margins. The changes seen during thermal tumor ablation on dynamic MR imaging are closely correlated with the final extent of histological necrosis. Delayed contrast-enhanced MR can accurately define the extent of residual viable tumor. The combination of MR imaging and ILP as an alternative to breast conservation surgery has significant potential in becoming the prototype for using medical technology to improve patient care and health care costs.

■ References

1. Amin Z (1995) Diode lasers: experimental and clinical review. Laser Med Sci 10:157–163
2. Amin Z, Donald JJ, Masters A et al (1993) Hepatic metastases: Interstitial laser photocoagulation with real-time US monitoring and dynamic CT evaluation of treatment. Radiology 187:339–347
3. Bleier et al (1991)
4. Bown SG (1983) Phototherapy of tumours. World J Surg 7:700–709
5. Cheong WF, Prahl S, Welch AJ (1990) A review of the optical properties of biological tissues. IEEE J Quant Elec 26:2166–2185
6. Clive et al (1995)
7. Dickinson RJ, Hall AS, Hind AJ, Young IR (1986) Measurement of changes in tissue temperature using MR imaging. J Com Assist Tomogr 10:468–472
8. Hall-Craggs MA, Mumtaz H, Payley M et al (1996) Dynamic MR guidance of laser therapy to breast cancer. Radiology 201 (P):177
9. Hand et al (1992)
10. Harms SE, Flamig DP, Evans WP et al (1994) MR imaging of the breast: current status and future potentials. AJR 163:1039–1047
11. Harries SA, Amin Z, Smith ME et al (1994) Interstitial laser photocoagulation as a treatment for breast cancer. Br J Surg 81:1617–1619
12. Hill CR, Rivens I, Vaughan MG ter-Haar GR (1995) Lesion development in focused ultrasound surgery: a general model. Ultrasound Med Biol 20:259–269
13. Jacobson JA, Danforth DN, Cowan KH et al (1995) Ten-year results of a comparison of conservation with mastectomy in the treatment of stage I and II breast cancer. N Engl J Med 332:907–911
14. Jolesz FA, Blumenfeld SM (1994) Interventional use of magnetic resonance imaging. Magn Reson Q 10 (2):85–96
15. Le Bihan D, Delannoy D, Levin RL et al (1989) Temperature mapping with MR imaging of molecular diffusion: application to hyperthermia. Radiology 171:853
16. Matsumoto R, Oshio K Jolesz FA (1993) Monitoring of laser and freezing induced ablation in the liver with T1-weighted MR imaging. J Magn Reson Imaging 2:555–562
17. McGahan JP, Browning PD, Brock JM et al (1990) Hepatic ablation using radiofrequency electrocautery. Invest Radiol 25:267–270
18. Mumtaz H, Hall-Craggs MA, Buonnacorssi G et al (1996) Image guided interstitial laser photocoagulation in the treatment of breast fibroadenoma. Radiology 201 (P):176
19. Mumtaz H, Hall-Craggs MA, Wotherspoon A et al (1996) Laser therapy for breast cancer: MR imaging and histopathologic correlation. Radiology 200:651–658
20. Mumtaz H, Hall-Craggs MA, Davidson T et al (1997) Staging symptomatic primary breast cancer with MR imaging. AJR
21. Mumtaz, Hall-Cragg MA, Kissin M et al (1997) Multiple fiber interstitial laser photocoagulation in the treatment of breast cancer. Laser Surg Med
22. Orel SG, Schnall MD, Powell CM et al (1995) Staging of suspected breast cancer: effect of MR Imaging and MR-guided biopsy. Radiology 196:115–122
23. Pomeroy O, Hynynen K, Singer S et al (1996) MR imaging-guided focused US therapy for breast fibroadenomas: a feasibility study. Radiology 197 (P):311
24. Rand RW, Rand RP, Eggerding FA et al (1985) Cryolumpectomy for breast cancer: an experimental study. Cryobiology 22:307–318
25. Rossi S, Di Stasi M, Buscarini E et al (1996) Percutaneous RF interstitial thermal ablation in the treatment of hepatic cancer. AJR 167:759–768

26. Smallwood JA, Roberts A, Guyer DP, Taylor I (1988) The natural history of fibroadenomas. Br J Clin Pract 42:86–87
27. Stegar AC, Lees WR, Walmsley K et al (1989) Interstitial laser hyperthermia: a new approach to local destruction of tumours. BMJ 299:362–365
28. Svaasand LO, Boerslid T, Oeveraason M et al (1985) Thermal and optical properties of living tissue: application to laser-induced hyperthermia. Lasers Surg Med 5:589–602

Interventional Magnetic Resonance of the Thorax

7

J. Goldin

Introduction

Magnetic resonance imaging (MRI) has become an established technique for evaluation of the chest [1–4] and is considered to be superior to other imaging modalities in the evaluation of specific mediastinal [5–7], hilar [8, 9] and chest wall [10–13] abnormalities. MRI should be the perfect modality for imaging the thorax because of the exquisite soft tissue contrast, multiplanar capability, intrinsic flow sensitivity and lack of ionizing radiation. Its utilization in the assessment of the lung has been limited by the signal loss due to magnetic susceptibility artifacts (due to the large number of air and soft tissue interfaces), respiratory and cardiac motion artifacts and poor signal-to-noise ratios. Low-field MR systems offer the advantage of significantly less susceptibility artifact and the potential for better visualization of the lung parenchyma.

Interventional MR (IMR) is receiving great interest as minimally invasive surgical procedures become the preferred method of treatment [14–16]. Developments in computer-assisted tomography and three-dimensional visualization software have given rise to the ability for sophisticated biopsy and surgical procedures to be performed under image guidance. The ability to perform these procedures with a non-ionizing source is of great interest. Currently, interventional magnetic resonance is being developed using open configuration magnets. Early procedures in the thorax have been closely modeled on biopsy and surgical techniques performed under CT or videoscopic guidance. IMR can use previously prepared image data from various different modalities and can also provide cross-section imaging in a near real time frame which is a unique capability of this modality. In addition, the use of high radio frequency (RF) signals specifically targeted by localization offers the potential for the ablation or size reduction of tumors giving rise to a new spectrum of IMR capabilities [14, 16].

The rational use of low-field MR imaging in chest disease requires an understanding of the basic MR physics particular to chest imaging, a familiarity with pulse sequences, techniques of IMR and the clinical conditions in which thoracic MRI has been shown to be of benefit. This chapter reviews these topics and discuss potential uses of IMR in the management of pathology in the mediastinum, lung parenchyma and chest wall.

■ Thoracic MR Physics Principles

Traditional spin-echo sequences remain the most commonly used pulse sequences in imaging the chest. Both 90° and 180° RF pulses are used in spin-echo sequences. These RF pulses rotate the magnetic vector aligned along the z axis into the x-y plane where it produces a detectable signal. By varying the interval between both the RF pulses, images of different characteristics can be obtained determined primarily by the T1 and T2 relaxation times of the tissues encountered.

The T1 relaxation time is a measure of the rate of recovery of the longitudinal or z magnetic vector in a patient and is due to the transfer of energy from the hydrogen proton to the surrounding lattice. T1 varies with magnetic field strength being longer in higher magnetic fields; it tends to be long in water and shorter in fat. Any process that increases tissue water content (e.g., edema) thus lengthens the T1 relaxation time. The interval between successive 90° pulses, known also as the repetition time (TR), determines the ability to differentiate among the relaxation times of different tissues. This is best achieved with short repetition times because tissue relaxation during long repetition times make differentiation impossible. Using a 1.5-T magnet, the usual TR period is about 600 ms for T1-weighted sequences which corresponds to one R-R interval in cardiac gated scans.

The T2 relaxation time is a measure of the time protons take to go out of phase following the end of a RF pulse. It is due largely to two causes: inhomogeneities of the external magnetic field and inhomogeneities of local magnetic fields, from neighboring nuclei, within the tissues. In general, T2 is longer in homogeneous environments (e.g., water where there are no big differences in magnetic field strength) and shorter in inhomogeneous environments (e.g., soft tissue where there are larger variations in the local magnetic fields and the molecules cannot move around so fast resulting in protons getting out of phase faster). An increase in tissue water, (e.g., edema) tends therefore to prolong the T2 relaxation time. A echo time (TE) of less than 30 ms) is considered to be short.

The failure to visualize lung on conventional spin-echo sequences even with relatively short TEs of 20–30 ms is due to the innumerable magnetic field gradients caused by the large differences in magnetic susceptibility between air and soft tissue at each alveolar interface [17, 18]. This is related to the degree of lung inflation being 7 ms at full inflation and 80 ms in deflated, gasless lungs [19]. In pathological states where inflammation or tumor replace air these conventional sequences yield abundant signal [20].

A sequence with a long TR and a short TE is also often employed in which the effects of T1 and T2 are minimized and the contrast results from differences in water or proton density. The resultant images have relatively high signal strength and the lowest signal-to-noise ratio. The degree of contrast is however limited due to the elimination of the positive features of T1 and T2 relaxation.

Conventional MR scanners utilize gradient magnetic fields and two-dimensional Fourier transformation (2-DFT) to obtain spatial localization [21]. The 2-DFT is very sensitive to motion. Motion results in phase changes that result in signal misregistration because signals are incorrectly ascribed to the phase-encoding gradient. This artifact is visible on the images as a band of signal along the phase-encoding direction originating from the moving structure. In the chest such phase-encoding motion artifacts most often arise from the major blood vessels or the heart. It is therefore advantageous to choose a phase-encoding direction that avoids obscuring the region of interest by considering the direction of the expected artifact. A more complex technique to minimize the effect of this phase encoding motion artifact can sometimes be used with discretion in thoracic MR imaging. Unfortunately the result of these complex gradient profiles is that the signal-to-noise ratio on T1-weighted and proton density weighted scans is decreased. The signal arising from flowing blood is also increased which results in further reduction in the contrast between blood and the vessel wall.

Respiratory motion results in a series of ghost images that are seen to extend through the image, being most visible in the subcutaneous fat of the anterior chest wall, oriented along the phase-encoding direction. This artifact can be reduced by altering the sequence in which the phase-encoding views or steps are obtained [22, 23]. This technique in which the respiratory cycle is monitored and the level of phase encoding is chosen according to the level of inspiration is known as respiratory compensation. In the reconstruction process, the phase-encoding steps can be reordered to either shorten the apparent respiratory cycle (high-order sort) or make it appear as if only very long inspiration has occurred (low-order sort). Either of these techniques results in minimizing the respiratory motion artifact without lengthening the scan time or decreasing the signal strength. Respiratory compensation should be used in most thoracic imaging sequences.

A flow artifact arises from blood flowing into the plane at imaging during a scan sequence. The region adjacent to the image volume, in convention multisliced imaging, does not receive RF pulses. As a consequence, the spin momentum of the tissues are completely relaxed. When these relaxed spins enter the image plane they are of relatively high signal intensity. Furthermore, the consequence of flow during the pulse sequence is that the molecules acquire a random phase which results in a large amount of phase-encoding motion artifact. This artifact can be decreased by presaturating and dephasing the inflowing spins with 90° pulses [24] reducing the signal produced by the inflowing blood. This, however, results in increased slice acquisition time and increased power deposition. Spatial presaturation should nevertheless be used in all MR thoracic scans.

■ Thoracic MR Intervention Overview

Open configuration MR systems are designed to allow easy access to the patient. Several systems are readily available. All allow the patient table to be placed along the axis of the magnet with easy access to the patient from either side. If necessary, the table can be placed perpendicular to the magnet access with easy access for an operator at the head of the table.

Conventional spin-echo T1, T2, and other image sequences, are easily obtained on the magnet. These are used as baseline images to localize the area of interest and compare with cross-section or other image data acquired in the previous work-up of the patient. Once the area of interest is localized, care is taken to ensure that the region is included within the central 30 cm of the field; this has been shown to have the most homogeneous flux and defines the region in which electronic spatial coordinate guidance is possible [25]. Once localized, RF transmitter receiver (T-R) coils are placed over the region of interest.

In order to achieve precise placement of either a biopsy needle or RF ablation, a hand-held probe allows the operator to select and control image orientation and location. It is important for close communication between the operator and technologist at the MR console to ensure the relationship of the probe access to the imaging acquisition is known. Current systems have the ability to enable image data collection, processing and display to occur sequentially and simultaneously so that new images may be visualized as fast as every two seconds. Images can be displayed on various consoles including those located within the system to allow the operator real-time feedback.

The ability to advance either RF probe or tip of an instrument to the exact region of interest is of great interest in the development of IMR systems. Currently an optical digitizer systems employing three senses giving rise to a three-dimensional localization of a probe is available. This allows localization and spatial relationship of the probe to be known at all times. Similar techniques are being used to assist with tip localization of various instruments. These include both diagnostic bronchoscopy and laryngoscopes as well as interventional biopsy and RF ablation instruments [26].

■ Thoracic MR Diagnostic Applications Relevant to MR Intervention

Lung Parenchyma

MR has been shown to be more sensitive than CT in the detection of lung nodules that are difficult to distinguish from adjacent vessels on CT examinations [27]. MR has been reported to be as least as sensitive as CT for the detection of pulmonary metastatic nodules larger than 5 mm in diameter [27, 28]. The detection rate of small nodules is improved by using short time inversion recovery (STIR) sequences [29], and may also be improved by the use of low magnet field strengths (0.5 T) rather than the usual higher field strength magnets (1.5 T). The low magnetic field strengths result less induced susceptibility gradients in aerated lung than higher magnetic field strengths. MR imaging can also assist in the better characterization of cystic lesions as a result of the higher signal strength [30, 31] or fluid levels [32] seen on T2-weighted sequences. This differentiation can sometimes be difficult on CT because the high protein content results in soft tissue attenuation in some lesions [33].

MR imaging of the lung parenchyma to date has been of little clinical value [1, 4, 32, 34]. Conventional spin-echo sequences yield little signal intensity from inflated lung parenchyma because of low proton density, the presence of innumerable air/soft tissue (alveolar wall) interfaces which result in large susceptibility induced magnetic field gradient due to internal magnetic field inhomogeneities and intravoxel phase dispersion and cardiac and respiratory motion which results in significant signal loss and image degradation [35, 36]. Currently, normal or subtle lung infiltration cannot be adequately assessed with MRI [37]. Additionally, the inability to reliably detect calcification further results in MR being inferior to CT in the detection and characterization of solitary lung nodules [38]. MR can, however, be useful in differentiating a solitary pulmonary nodule from end-on vessels especially in the perihilar region [27, 38].

Ultrashort TE gradient echo sequences [10] and short TE spin-echo sequences [39, 40] have been developed as a potential solution to some of the problems encountered when imaging the lung parenchyma. The use of ultrashort TE gradient echo sequences does not allow sufficient time for the phase-encoding step of the conventional 2DFT reconstruction process. The use of an alternate projection reconstruction algorithm, similar to that used in CT, does allow TEs as short as 50 ms to be achieved producing proton density weighted images. This technique has been shown to improve visualization of aerated lung parenchyma in peripheral vessels but the effect of physiological motion in the chest is accentuated and the images show little tissue contrast. Moreover, the projection reconstruction algorithm is highly susceptible to magnetic field inhomogeneity which leads to further blurring in the reconstructed images [35].

The use of minimum echo delay (TE 7 ms) has been used to compensate for the very short T2 relaxation time present in inflated lung parenchyma when using conventional spin-echo sequences. The advantage of this technique is that it uses a standard 2-DFT reconstruction algorithm and can be easily performed with only minimal modifications on most current commercial scanners. This technique itself leads to a 3.5-fold increase in the signal-to-noise ratio from aerated lung [39].

MR has been used to quantitate lung water content and to differentiate cardiogenic from noncardiogenic causes [3, 41–44]. Several animal models and small ball magnets have shown that MRI techniques can be used to quantitate absolute lung water content [45] and reliably detect and quantify changes in lung water content and demonstrate its distribution in various types of experimental edema [9, 46]. Recent work in normal volunteers suggest that MRI measurements of relative lung water changes in clinical pulmonary edema should be feasible. In normal volunteers, measurements of average lung density, lung density gradient and pleural pressure gradients on MR were similar to those obtained with more invasive techniques [19]. Disease processes decrease the elastic properties of the lung and thus effect lung density suggesting that MR image determination of lung water content and lung density should prove useful in the assessment of parenchymal lung disease. Differences in MRI characteristics of different types of experimental pulmonary edema have been found in some studies [42], but has not been demonstrated in others [47, 48]. Although high-resolution CT (HRCT) remains superior than MRI in assessing parenchymal disease [49, 50], it has been postulated that MRI has a role in assessing the activity of the disease process [20, 48, 51, 52]. The ability of MRI to differentiate relaxation times of different tissues based on their differences in free and bound water fractions is postulated to offer a potential basis of MRI. It may be able to differentiate between acute and chronic alveolar as well as from chronic fibrosis. In well-establish animal models involving radiation pneumonitis in rats [52] and bleomycin-induced toxicity in mice [41], the T2 values measured in the parenchyma lengthened with the development of acute edema and inflammatory cell infiltrate while T1 shortening occurred with the onset of fibrosis. In clinical studies, MRI has been shown to be equivalent to HRCT in its ability to demonstrate abnormalities correlating with active disease, although HRCT was superior overall in assessing these patients [53]. MR signal intensity has been demonstrated to be correlated with clinical severity of disease and potential response to treatment, with a decrease in signal intensity seen in those patients who demonstrate clinical improvement after treatment [52].

MR has been shown to have a potential role in differentiating various causes of alveolar opacification [20, 50, 54], and is comparable to HRCT in the assessment of alveolar opacification [53]. The pathological appearances are comparable to those seen on the simultaneously acquired MRI images [54]. The presence of alveolar opacification, reticulation, nodules and interlobular septal thickening is reflected best by proton density and T1-weighted MR images. T2-weighted images add no further diagnostic information due to marked fall off of signal intensity.

Fibrosis is often a result of treatment in patients with thoracic malignancies. Due to the different relaxation characteristics, MR should allow differentiation of active inflammatory or neoplastic disease from fibrotic disease. Several reports of using T2-weighted MRI [55], or T1-weighted Gd-DTPA enhanced sequences [56] have shown that fibrosis can be differentiated from recurrent tumor. Unfortunately, because of the inflation-dependent T2 shortening caused by susceptibility artifact, this is not generally applicable. Further differentiation of tumor and associated inflammatory disease is difficult due to overlapping in the influence on both T2 and T1 relaxation curves [55, 57].

The ability to guide biopsy procedures to specific locations of abnormal signal using IMR offers the potential for improved diagnostic yield not possible with conventional CT. This may be of particular benefit in the determination of neoplastic disease from inflammatory tissue or surgery fibrosis in the initial staging and follow-up of patients with lymphoma, lung cancer, and metastatic disease.

The Mediastinum and Hila

MRI is the modality of choice for diagnosing mediastinal or hilar lesions in patients who cannot tolerate iodinated contrast agents and for the imaging of posterior mediastinal or prevertebral masses [32, 58]. The accurate delineation of the spinal cord and spinal canal on MR, together with the ability to perform multiplanar reconstructions, affords MR an advantage over CT in the evaluation of lesions adjacent to the spine [32]. MRI may also be used as an additional imaging modality in the evaluation of the mediastinum and hila following conventional CT examinations in cases where further clarification is required. With MRI there is better inherent soft tissue contrast and the streak artifacts that occur from edges of pulsatile vascular structures, especially in contrast-enhanced CT are not seen. Although not superior than CT in the differentiation of benign from malignant lesions and should not be performed for this purpose [37, 59–61], MRI is occasionally able to characterize fluid-filled or necrotic lesions better than CT. The proteinaceous content of these lesions may result in soft tissue attenuation on CT [33] whereas the prolongation of the T1 and T2 values in these lesions is well demonstrated on MRI [61].

MRI has also been shown to be more accurate than CT in diagnosing mediastinal invasion [62] and vascular invasion by lung cancer [7, 56, 63, 64]. MRI is therefore a recommended secondary imaging modality in the evaluation of lung cancer staging particularly when mediastinal, vascular or cardiac invasion is suspected. Despite early optimism MRI has not been shown to be better than CT in its ability to detect and define mediastinal lymph nodes [29, 62, 63, 65–70]. Although some studies have reported that MRI demonstrates nodes in the aortic-pulmonary window and subcarinal regions [37, 46, 64, 71, 72], because of the ability to image in multiaxial planes, this has not been shown to confer any additional overall advantage in accuracy. MRI is more accurate than CT in the diagnosis of the presence or absence of tracheobronchial lymphadenopathy in patients with lung cancer [7–9, 29, 63], but this may not offer any advantage with respect to clinical management and outcome. MRI is no more sensitive than CT in the differentiation of benign hyperplasia from malignant involvement than CT [73]. The MR appearances of normal thymus and thymic abnormalities have now been well described [1, 74, 75], and although MR is excellent for the diagnosis and evaluation of thymic lesions, it has not been found to have a significant advantage over conventional CT [76, 77].

Heavily T2-weighted MR sequences may be helpful in distinguishing nonobstructive passive lobar atelectasis from atelectasis caused by a hilar-obstructing lesion if CT evaluation has been inconclusive [29, 56, 78, 79]. On T2-weighted images the lung consolidation has a higher signal than the hilar mass where as the nonobstructive collapse has a lower signal intensity [79]. It has been reported that using Gd-DTPA enhanced T1-weighted imaging, this differentiation can be improved further [64]. MR is also useful in identifying underlying mass lesions in the completely opacified hemithorax [80].

Radiation-induced fibrosis and recurrent tumor within the mediastinum can sometimes be differentiated. Due to the similar signal from acute inflammatory tissue and tumor, the differentiation between the two is not possible [55, 57]. MRI has been demonstrated to offer a significant role in the follow-up of patients with treated mediastinal Hodgkin's lymphoma [32, 81]. Following radiation treatment, the residual mediastinal masses on T2-weighted images demonstrated significantly decreased intensity in most patients [81]. The detection in a high intensity residual mass is not specific for tumor but has been used as an indication for the need for biopsy or close follow up [82]. The MR appearances of untreated mediastinal masses associated with fibrosis has also been reported in patients with lymphomas [83] and fibrosing mediastinitis [84].

MRI should be the perfect modality for performing image-guided procedures of the mediastinum and hilum due to the exquisite soft tissue contrast, multiplanar capability, intrinsic flow sensitivity and lack of ionizing radiation. However, respiratory and cardiac motion artifacts are of increased problem during real-time continuous imaging than with the conventional breath-hold imaging techniques. The detection of lesion is improved by using STIR sequences [29] and also may be improved by the use of low-field magnets (0.5 T). There is also better characterization of lesions as a result of the higher signal strength of tumor-containing tissue [30, 31] or fluid levels (25 seen on T2-weighted sequences). This differential can sometimes be difficult on CT because of the high protein content results in the same tissue attenuation in some lesions [33]. This makes the use of low-field MR a useful technique for identifying the nature of the lesion so influencing the nature of the therapeutic or interventional diagnostic procedure being planned.

Chest Wall and Pleural Lesions

MR is an excellent modality for the assessment of the chest wall. T1-weighted sequences are best for the evaluation of tumor invasion of intramuscular fat and assessment of the extent of chest wall involvement. T2-weighted sequences are optimal for differentiation of tumor and edema which produce high signal from the surrounding muscle which has low signal intensity. Although the destruction of cortical bone is better seen with CT, marrow involvement by tumor is better identified by signal changes with MR. As a result of the superior contrast and multiple imaging planes, MR allows better presurgical delineation of the extent of chest wall disease than CT. MR has been shown to reliably assess primary chest wall tumors [64] and chest wall extension of bronchogenic carcinoma [8, 78, 82] and lymphoma [63]. This tissue characterization and spatial resolution allows localization for both biopsy procedures and RF ablation therapy on an open low-field system.

MR appearances of lymph nodes and arteriovenous malformation are characteristic and their diagnosis can be made easily on thoracic MR evaluation. In general, however, there is considerable overlap between the MR signal characteristics of benign and malignant lesions and MR offers no benefit over CT in the differentiation between these two pathologies. It has been suggested that a homogeneous signal intensity and smooth margins are more common in benign tumors while malignant lesions are more likely to have heterogeneous signal and irregular margins [64].

Pleural fluid collections can be easily identified as well as the presence of absence of associated pleural thickening or nodularity. Drainage of a pleural fluid with an interactive feedback as to how much fluid is being drained, and the effect of lung reexpansion can easily be achieved using open MR techniques. This has the potential for improving overall outcome in the drainage and installation of sclerosing agents for a recurrent symptomatic effusions in the setting of malignancy. In addition, direct installation of antibiotic therapy using visualization of the site of deposition may improve the outcome for the treatment of infective pleural collections in immunocompromised patients.

Brachial Plexopathy

MRI provides superior delineation of the normal anatomy of the brachial plexus [85, 86] due mainly to its multiplanar capabilities and superior soft tissue contrast [87–89]. The lack of beam attenuation artifacts from bone and the accurate identification of adjacent vasculature are further advantages of thoracic MR over CT [90]. Although published experience is comparatively limited, MR has been shown to be superior to other imaging techniques for evaluating brachial plexus trauma [87, 91], differentiating fibrosis from tumor [91], and documenting or excluding brachial plexus involvement by malignancy [12, 88, 89, 91].

The suggested MR technique for suspected peripheral brachial plexopathy is as follows: the anatomy is first mapped with T1-weighted images in at least two planes and the study is completed with selective use of other pulse sequences in the appropriate anatomic plane as to delineate lesions and associated (e.g., vascular) pathological abnormalities. Limitations in MR evaluations of brachial plexopathy include limited experience with appropriate use of Gd, limited data concerning differentiation between tumor, fibrosis, and radiation injury, specifically in this region and limited experience with subgross trauma [91] and idiopathic neuritis.

■ Conclusion

The potential for open, low-field IMR techniques seems great. A wide range of minimally invasive procedures ranging from biopsies to RF ablation and minimally invasive surgical resections seem possible. With the advent of increasingly aggressive treatment of severe obstructive pulmonary disease in the form of lung reduction surgery, the potential to perform such procedures using a minimally invasive technique is attractive. IMR techniques may allow these complicated procedures in patients who are highly susceptible to cardiac or respiratory instability to be performed without major changes in the thoracic chest wall function so resulting in decreasing morbidity and overall health care costs. RF ablation may well allow tumors to be shrunk down allowing better outcome following resection. It is likely that interventional therapeutic techniques using three-dimensional imaging modalities with good visualization techniques will become an important part of medical practice. Techniques that allow excellent characterization without exposing patients to radiation will certainly be strong candidates to dominate this exciting area.

References

1. Gamsu G, Sostman D (1989) Magnetic resonance imaging of the thorax. Am Rev Respir Dis 139:254–274
2. Webb WR (1989) The role of magnetic resonance imaging in the assessment of patients with lung cancer: a comparison with computed tomography. J Thorac Imaging 4:65–75
3. Webb WR, Sostman HD (1992) MR imaging of thoracic disease: clinical uses. Radiology 182:621–630
4. Fisher MR (1989) Magnetic resonance for the evaluation of the thorax. Chest 95 (1):166–173
5. Webb WR (1988) Mediastinum and hila. In: Partain CL, Price RR, Patton JA et al (eds) Magnetic resonance imaging, 2nd edn. Saunders, Philadelphia, pp 442–454
6. Brown LR, Aughenbaugh GL (1991) Masses of the anterior mediastinum: CT and MR imaging. AJR 157:1171–1180
7. Webb WR (1986) Magnetic resonance imaging of the hila and mediastinum. Cardiovasc Intervent Radiol 8:306–313
8. Glazer GM, Gross BH, Aisen AM et al (1985) Imaging of the pulmonary hilum: a prospective comparative study in patients with lung cancer. AJR 145:245–248
9. Webb WR, Gamsu G, Stark DD, Moore EH (1984) Magnetic resonance imaging of the normal and abnormal pulmonary hila. Radiology 152:89–94
10. Bergin CJ, Healy MV, Zincone GE, Castellino RA (1990) MR evaluation of chest wall involvement in malignant lymphoma. J Comput Assist Tomogr 14:928–932
11. Haggar AM, Pearlberg JL, Froelich JW et al (1987) Chest-wall invasion by carcinoma of the lung: detection by MR imaging. AJR 148:1075–1078
12. Heelan RT, Demas BE, Caravelli JF et al (1989) Superior sulcus tumors: CT and MR imaging. Radiology 170:637–641
13. McLoud TC, Filion RB, Edelman RR et al (1989) MR imaging of superior sulcus carcinoma. J Comput Assist Tomogr 12:233–239
14. Jolesz FA, Shtern F (1992) The operating room of the future: report of the National Cancer Institutes workshop – imaging-guided stereotactic tumor diagnosis and treatment. Invest Radiol 27:326–328
15. Jolesz FA, Blumenfield SM (1994) Interventional use of magnetic resonance imaging. Magn Reson Q 10:85–96
16. Silverman SG, Collick BD, Figueria MR, Khorasani R, Adams DF, Newman RW, Topulos GF, Jolesz FA (1995) Interactive MR-guided biopsy in an open configuration MR imaging system. Radiology 197:175–181
17. Durney CH, Bertolina J, Ailion DC et al (1989) Calculation and interpretation of inhomogeneous line broadening in models of lungs and other heterogeneous structures. J Magn Reson 85:554–570
18. Morris AH, Blatter DD, Case TA et al (1985) A new nuclear magnetic resonance property of lung. J Appl Physiol 58:759–762
19. Mayo JR, McKay A, Müller NL (1990) T2 relaxation time in MR imaging of normal and abnormal lung parenchyma (abstract). Radiology 177:313
20. Moore EH, Webb WR, Müller NL et al (1986) MRI of pulmonary airspace disease: experimental model and preliminary clinical results. AJR 146:1123–1128
21. Edelstein WA, Hutchison JMS, Johnson G et al (1980) Spin warp NMR imaging and applications to human whole-body imaging (letter). Phys Med Biol 25:751–756
22. Bailes DR, Gilderdale DJ, Bydder GM et al (1985) Respiratory ordered phase encoding (ROPE): a method for reducing respiratory motion artifacts in MR imaging. J Comput Assist Tomogr 9:835–838
23. Wood ML, Henkelman RM (1986) Suppression of respiratory motion artifacts in magnetic resonance imaging. Med Phys 13:794–805
24. Felmlee JP, Ehmann RL (1987) Spatial presaturation: a method for suppressing flow artifacts and improving depiction of vascular anatomy in MR imaging. Radiology 164:559–564
25. Sinha S, Sinha U, Lufkin R, Hanafee W (1989) Pulse sequence optimization for use with a biopsy needle in MRI. Magn Reson Imaging 7 (5):575–579
26. van Sonnenberg E, Hajek P, Gylys-Morin V et al (1988) A wire-sheath system for MR-guided biopsy and drainage: laboratory studies and experience in 10 patients. AJR 151:1088–1089
27. Doppman JL, Pass HI, Nieman LK et al (1991) Detection of ACTH-producing bronchial carcinoid tumors: MR imaging vs. CT. AJR 156:39–43
28. Feuerstein IM, Jicha DL, Pass HI et al (1992) Pulmonary metastases: MR imaging with surgical correlation – a prospective study. Radiology 192:123–129
29. Webb WR, Jensen BG, Sollitto R et al (1985) Bronchogenic carcinoma: staging with MR compared with staging with CT and surgery. Radiology 156:117–124
30. Barakos JA, Brown JJ, Brescia RJ et al (1989) High signal intensity lesions of the chest in MR imaging. J Comput Assist Tomogr 13:797–802
31. Naidich DP, Rumanick WM, Ettenger NA et al (1988) Congenital anomalies of the lungs in adults: MR diagnosis. AJR 151:13–19
32. Weinreb JC, Naidich DP (1991) Thoracic magnetic resonance imaging. Clin Chest Med 12:33–54
33. Mendelson DS, Rose JS, Efremidis SC et al (1983) Bronchogenic cysts with high CT numbers. AJR 140:463–465
34. Gefter W (1988) Chest applications of magnetic resonance imaging: an update. Radiol Clin North Am 26:573–588
35. Bergin CJ, Glover GH, Pauly JM (1991) Lung parenchyma: magnetic susceptibility in MR imaging. Radiology 180:845–548
36. Naidich DP, Weinreb JC, Schinella R (1990) MR imaging of pulmonary parenchyma: comparison with CT in evaluating cadaveric lung specimens. J Comput Assist Tomogr 14:595–599
37. de Geer G, Webb WR, Sollitto R, Golden J (1986) MR characteristics of benign lymph node enlargement in sarcoidosis and Castleman's disease. Eur J Radiol 6:145–148
38. Müller NL, Gamsu G, Webb WR (1985) Pulmonary nodules: detection using magnetic resonance and computed tomography. Radiology 155:687–690
39. Mayo JR, McKay A, Müller NL (1992) MR imaging of the lungs: value of short TE spin-echo pulse sequences. AJR 159:951–956
40. Bergin CJ, Pauly JM, Macovski MA (1991) Lung parenchyma: projection reconstruction MR imaging. Radiology 179:777–781
41. Taylor CR, Sostman HD, Gore JC, Smith GW (1987) Proton relaxation times in bleomycin-induced lung injury. Invest Radiol 22:621–626
42. Schmidt HC, Daw-Guey T, Higgins CB (1986) Pulmonary edema: an MR study of permeability and hydrostatic types in animals. Radiology 158:297–302

43. Cutillo AG, Morris AH, Blatter DD et al (1984) Determination of lung water content and distribution by nuclear magnetic resonance. J Appl Physiol 57:583–588
44. Cutillo AG, Morris AH, Ailion DC et al (1986) Determination of lung water content and distribution by nuclear magnetic resonance imaging. J Thorac Imag 1:39–51
45. Levitt RG, Glazer HS, Roper CL et al (1985) Magnetic resonance imaging of mediastinal and hilar masses: comparison with CT. AJR 145:9–14
46. Webb WR, Jensen BG, Gamsu G et al (1985) Sagittal MR imaging of the chest: normal and abnormal. J Comput Assist Tomogr 9:471–479
47. Vinitski S, Steiner RM, Wexler HR, Rifkin M (1988) Assessment of lung water by magnetic resonance in three types of pulmonary edema. Heart Vessels 4:88–93
48. Cutillo AG, Morris AH, Ailion DC, Durney CH (1989) Clinical implications of nuclear magnetic resonance lung research. Chest 96:643–652
49. Kinsella D, Hamilton A, Goddard P et al (1991) The role of magnetic resonance imaging in cystic fibrosis. Clin Radiol 44:23–26
50. Müller NL, Mayo JR, Lentle BC (1991) Imaging of diffuse lung diseases: past, present, and future. Radiol Clin North Am 29:1115–1121
51. Craig DA, Colletti PM, Ratto D et al (1988) MRI findings in pulmonary sarcoidosis. Magnet Reson Imaging 6:567–573
52. McFadden RG, Carr TJ, Wood TE (1987) Proton magnetic resonance imaging to stage activity of interstitial lung disease. Chest 92:31–39
53. Müller NL, Mayo JR, Zwirewich CV (1992) Value of MR imaging in the evaluation of chronic infiltrative lung diseases: comparison with CT. AJR 158:1205–1209
54. Primack SL, Mayo JR, Hartman TE et al (1994) MR imaging of infiltrative lung disease: comparison with pathologic findings in 22 patients. J Comput Assist Tomogr 18:233–238
55. Glazer HS, Lee JK, Levitt RG et al (1985) Radiation fibrosis: differentiation from recurrent tumor by MR imaging. Radiology 156:721–726
56. Kameda K, Adachi S, Kono M (1988) Detection of T-factor in lung cancer using magnetic resonance imaging and computed tomography. J Thorac Imaging 3:73–80
57. Lee JKT, Glazer HS (1990) Controversy in the MR imaging appearance of fibrosis. Radiology 177:21–22
58. Burk DJ, Brunberg JA, Kanal E et al (1987) Spinal and paraspinal neurofibromatosis: surface coils MR imaging at 1.5 T. Radiology 156:721–726
59. Glazer GM, Orringer MB, Chenevert TL et al (1988) Mediastinal lymph nodes: relaxation time/pathologic correlation and implications in staging of lung cancer with MR imaging. Radiology 168:429–431
60. Ross JS, Donovan PB, Novoa R et al (1984) Magnetic resonance of the chest: initial experience with imaging and in vivo T1 and T2 calculations. Radiology 152:95–101
61. Gamsu G, Stark DD, Webb WR et al (1984) Magnetic resonance imaging of benign mediastinal masses. Radiology 151:709–713
62. Laurent F, Drouillard J, Dorcier F et al (1988) Bronchogenic carcinoma staging: CT vs. MR imaging; assessment with surgery. Eur J Cardiothorac Surg 2:31–36
63. Webb WR, Gatsonis C, Zerhouni EA et al (1991) CT and MR imaging in staging non-small cell bronchogenic carcinoma: report of the Radiologic Diagnostic Oncology Group. Radiology 178:705–713
64. Kono M, Sako M, Adachi S et al (1989) MR imaging in the assessment of lung cancer patients: primary lung cancer staging, evaluation of therapeutic effect and diagnosis of recurrent tumor. Nippon Igaku Hoshasen Gakkai Zasshi 49:831–840
65. Musset D, Grenier P, Carette ME et al (1986) Primary lung cancer staging: prospective comparative study of MR imaging with CT. Radiology 160:607–611
66. Batra P, Brown K, Collins JD et al (1988) Evaluation of intrathoracic extent of lung cancer by plain chest radiography, computed tomography, and magnetic resonance imaging. Am Rev Respir Dis 137:1456–1462
67. Poon PY, Bronshill MJ, Henkelman RM et al (1987) Mediastinal lymph node metastases from bronchogenic carcinoma: detection with MNR imaging and CT. Radiology 162:651–656
68. Grenier P, Dubray B, Carette MF et al (1989) Preoperative thoracic staging of lung cancer: CT and MR evaluation. Diagn Intervent Radiol 1:23–28
69. Patterson GA, Ginsberg RJ, Roon PY et al (1987) A prospective evaluation of magnetic resonance imaging, computed tomography, and mediastinoscopy in the preoperative assessment of mediastinal node status in bronchogenic carcinoma. J Thorac Cardiovasc Surg 94:679–684
70. Platt JF, Glazer GM, Orringer MR et al (1988) Radiologic evaluation of the subcarinal lymph nodes: a comparative study. AJR 151:279–282
71. Batra P, Brown K, Steckel RJ et al (1988) MR imaging of the thorax: a comparison of axial, coronal, and sagittal imaging planes. J Comput Assist Tomogr 12:75–81
72. Webb WR, Jensen BG, Gamsu G et al (1984) Coronal magnetic resonance imaging of the chest: normal and abnormal. Radiology 153:729–735
73. Glazer HS, Gutierrez FR, Levitt RG et al (1985) The thoracic aorta studies by MR imaging. Radiology 157:149–155
73. Panicek DM (1992) MR imaging for pulmonary metastases? Radiology 182:10–11
74. de Geer G, Webb WR, Gamsu G (1986) Normal thymus: assessment with MR and CT. Radiology 158:313–317
75. Molina PL, Siegel MJ, Glazer HS (1990) Thymic masses on MR imaging. AJR 155:495–500
76. Batra P, Herrmann C, Mulder D (1987) Mediastinal imaging in myasthenia gravis: correlation of chest radiography, CT, MR, and surgical findings. AJR 148:515–519
77. Emskotter T, Trampe H, Lachenmayer L (1988) Magnetic resonance imaging in myasthenia gravis: an alternative to mediastinal computerised tomography? Dtsch Med Wochenschr 113:1508–1510
78. Tobler J, Levitt RG, Glazer HS et al (1987) Differentiation of proximal bronchogenic carcinoma from postobstructive lobar collapse by magnetic resonance imaging: comparison with computed tomography. Invest Radiol 22:538–543
79. Herold CJ, Kuhlman JE, Zerhouni EA (1991) Pulmonary atelectasis: signal patterns with MR imaging. Radiology 178:715–720
80. Laissey JP, Rebibo G, Trotot PM et al (1989) Post-pneumonectomy evaluation of the chest: a prospective comparative study of MRI with CT. Magn Reson Imaging 7:55–60
81. Nyman RS, Rehn SM, Glimelius BLG et al (1989) Residual mediastinal masses in Hodgkin disease: prediction of size with MR imaging. Radiology 170:435–440
82. Webb WR (1989) MR imaging of treated mediastinal Hodgkin disease (editorial). Radiology 170:315–316
83. Negendank WG, Al-Katib AM, Karanes C, Smith MR (1990) Lymphomas: MR imaging contrast characteristics with clinical-pathologic correlations. Radiology 177:209–216
84. Rholl KS, Levitt RG, Glazer HS (1985) Magnetic resonance imaging of fibrosing mediastinitis. AJR 145:255–259
85. Blair DN, Rapoport S, Sostman HD, Blair OC (1987) Normal brachial plexus: MR imaging. Radiology 165:763–767
86. Kellman GM, Kneeland JB, Middleton WD et al (1987) MR imaging of the supraclavicular region: normal anatomy. AJR 148:77–82

87. Gupta RK, Mehta VA, Banerji AK, Jain RK (1989) MR evaluation of brachial plexus injuries. Neuroradiology 31:377–381
88. Castagno AA, Shuman WP (1987) MR imaging in clinically suspected brachial plexus tumor. AJR 149:1219–1222
89. Kneeland JB, Kellman GM, Middleton WD et al (1987) Diagnosis of diseases of the supraclavicular region by use of MR imaging. AJR 148:1149–1151
90. Armington WG, Harnsberger HR, Osborn AG, Seay AR (1987) Radiographic evaluation of brachial plexopathy. AJNR 8:361–367
91. Rapoport S, Blair DN, McCarthy SM, Desser TS, Hammers LW, Sostman HD (1988) Brachial plexus: correlation of MR imaging with CT and pathologic findings. Radiology 167:161–165

Subject Index